Cancer Chemotherapy by Infusion

Cancer Chemotherapy by Infusion

Jacob J. Lokich, M.D.

Precept Press, Inc.
Chicago

Published in the USA by

Precept Press, Inc.
160 East Illinois Street
Chicago, Illinois 60611

Published in the UK and Europe by

MTP Press Limited
Falcon House
Lancaster, England

British Library Cataloguing in Publication Data

Cancer chemotherapy by infusion.
  1. Cancer—Chemotherapy
  I. Lokich, Jacob J.
  616.99′4061   RC271.C5

  ISBN 0-85200-680-2

© **1987 by Precept Press, Inc.**

All Rights Reserved

Except for appropriate use in critical reviews or works of scholarship, the reproduction or use of this work in any form or by any electronic, mechanical or other means now known or hereafter invented, including photocopying and recording, and in any information storage and retrieval system is forbidden without the written permission of the publisher.

Library of Congress Catalog Card Number:
86-62057

International Standard Book Number:
0-931028-68-X

91 90 89 88 87   5 4 3 2 1

Printed in the United States of America

For my colleagues and collaborators
on the nursing team
who make medicine possible,
and for my children,
who make my life meaningful

CONTENTS

SECTION II — CHEMOTHERAPEUTIC AGENTS

SECTION IV—REGIONAL INFUSION

SECTION V – SPECIAL CATEGORIES OF INFUSION CHEMOTHERAPY

PREFACE

Chemotherapy for cancer is in a state of evolution. Because some cancers can now be cured with chemotherapy as a singular modality, this therapy can no longer be viewed as simply a palliative contribution. Chemotherapy has assumed an important role as an adjuvant to other modalities, including both surgery and radiation therapy. For some tumors, the primary application of chemotherapy in a combined modality approach to curative therapy has resulted in the application of less radical surgery while achieving substantial cure rates. Nonetheless, with the exception of relatively rare tumors such as childhood tumors, hematologic malignancies, and testicular cancer, the effectiveness of chemotherapy in most tumors is severely limited. At the cellular level, greater understanding of the specific mechanism of tumor cell killing and of the phenomenon of drug resistance are elusive, critical ingredients in the improvement of effectiveness in cancer chemotherapy.

Prolonging the exposure time of the tumor cell to drugs is a concept that was addressed in the early phases of the development of chemotherapy. However, technological limitations inhibited the broader application of chemotherapy by infusion until recent years. Also, the convenience of intermittent therapy on an outpatient basis, with the predominant theory of drug effect based on a dose response as well as the proven effectiveness of this schedule in some tumors, has slowed the process of subjecting infusion chemotherapy to the rigors of clinical trials.

This book represents an effort to bring together the literature on infusion chemotherapy and to critically review that literature as well as ongoing trials. The organization of the book into five sections permits an independent analysis of the rationale and techniques as well as technical considerations involved in infusion chemotherapy, with some overlap of the review of clinical trials as they apply to the individual chemotherapeutic agents and to systemic and regional application of drug therapy.

There are some gaps in the data that may be explored in future editions as ongoing clinical trials progress to their conclusions. These specific areas include extremity infusion and perfusion for melanoma as well as other tumors; the entire spectrum of childhood tumors; and the application of infusion therapy in the delivery of analgesia.

The future of infusion therapy is uncertain, awaiting definitive clinical confirmation by prospective clinical trials. Nonetheless, the basic rationale, the experimental studies both *in vivo* and *in vitro*, and uncontrolled clinical trials all suggest that infusion delivery systems may well contribute substantially to palliative — and potentially, in the future — curative cancer treatment in the same manner that new agents, combination chemotherapy, and adjuvant chemotherapy have been the signposts of progress in chemotherapy over the past three decades.

ABOUT THE AUTHOR

Jacob J. Lokich, M.D., received his medical degree from the University of Pennsylvania School of Medicine. He completed his medical residency at the Peter Bent Brigham Hospital, Harvard Medical School, and then followed with a Hematology fellowship. He currently is assistant professor of medicine, Harvard Medical School, and Medical Director of the Cancer Center, Medical Center of Boston.

CONTRIBUTORS

STEPHEN P. ACKLAND, M.B., B.S., F.R.A.C.P., Fellow, Joint Section of Hematology/Oncology, University of Chicago Pritzker School of Medicine and Michael Reese Hospital and Medical Center, Chicago, Illinois

STEPHEN C. ADAMS, Pharm.D., Coordinator of Drug Information Service, Department of Pharmacy, St. Luke's Episcopal Hospital, Texas Children's Hospital, Texas Heart Institute, Houston, Texas

MUHYI AL-SARRAF, M.D., F.R.C.P. (C), F.A.C.P., Professor of Medicine, Chief of Head and Neck Cancer Service, Division of Medical Oncology, Department of Medicine, Wayne State University and Harper-Grace Hospitals, Detroit, Michigan

CARMEN J. ALLEGRA, M.D., Clinical Pharmacology Branch, Division of Cancer Treatment, National Cancer Institute, Bethesda, Maryland

ROGER W. ANDERSON, M.S., Head, Division of Pharmacy, University of Texas, M. D. Anderson Hospital and Tumor Institute, Houston, Texas

SHAN R. BAKER, M.D., Vice Chairman, Department of Otolaryngology, Head and Neck Surgery, University of Michigan Hospital, Ann Arbor, Michigan

CHARLES M. BALCH, M.D., Head, Division of Surgery; Chairman, Department of General Surgery, University of Texas System Cancer Center, M. D. Anderson Hospital and Tumor Institute, Houston, Texas

ROBERT S. BENJAMIN, M.D., Department of Medical Oncology, University of Texas System Cancer Center, M. D. Anderson Hospital and Tumor Institute, Houston, Texas

JOHN A. BENVENUTO, Ph.D., Department of Medical Oncology, University of Texas System Cancer Center, M. D. Anderson Hospital and Tumor Institute, Houston, Texas

MURRAY M. BERN, M.D., New England Baptist Hospital and New England Deaconess Hospital, Boston, Massachusetts, Assistant Professor of Medicine, Harvard Medical School, Boston, Massachusetts

GERALD P. BODEY, M.D., University of Texas System Cancer Center, M. D. Anderson Hospital and Tumor Institute, Houston, Texas

ALBERT BOTHE, JR., Director, Residency Training Program, New England Deaconess Hospital, Boston, Massachusetts

JEAN-LUC BREAU, M.D. Clinique de Cancerologie, Centre Hospitalier Universitaire de Bobigny, Université Paris Nord, Bobigny, France

JOHN E. BYFIELD, M.D., Ph.D., Associate Director and Chief, Radiation Oncology, Kern Regional Cancer Center, Bakersfield, California

ROBERT B. CATALANO, Pharm.D., Associate Professor of Clinical Pharmacy, Department of Pharmacy, Philadelphia College of Pharmacy and Science; Adjunct Professor of Clinical Pharmacy, Temple University School of Pharmacy; Coordinator of Clinical Research, Department of Medical Oncology, American Oncologic Hospital, Fox Chase Cancer Center, Philadelphia, Pennsylvania

ALFRED E. CHANG, M.D., Surgery Branch, National Cancer Institute, National Institutes of Health, Bethesda, Maryland

BRUCE D. CHESON, M.D., Head, Medicine Section, Clinical Investigations Branch, Cancer Therapy Evaluation Program, Division of Cancer Treatment, National Institutes of Health, National Cancer Institute, Bethesda, Maryland

JERRY M. COLLINS, Ph.D., Clinical Pharmacology Branch, Division of Cancer Treatment, National Cancer Institute, National Institutes of Health, Bethesda, Maryland

ROBERT L. COMIS, M.D., Medical Director and Chairman, Department of Medical Oncology, Fox Chase Cancer Center, Philadelphia, Pennsylvania

GREGORY A. CURT, M.D., Clinical Pharmacology Branch, Division of Cancer Treatment, National Cancer Institute, National Institutes of Health, Bethesda, Maryland

JOHN M. DALY, M.D., Jonathan E. Rhoads Professor of Surgery, Chief, Division of Surgical Oncology, University of Pennsylvania School of Medicine, Philadelphia, Pennsylvania

MERRILL J. EGORIN, M.D., F.A.C.P., Associate Professor of Medicine, Pharmacology and Experimental Therapeutics and Oncology, Head, Division of Developmental Therapeutics, University of Maryland Cancer Center, Baltimore, Maryland

STEFAN EKBERG M.Sc., Department of Radiation Physics, University Hospital, Linkoping, Sweden

GEOFFREY FALKSON, M.D., Department of Cancer Chemotherapy, Faculty of Medicine, University of Pretoria, Pretoria, Republic of South Africa

HUGH A. G. FISHER, M.D., Assistant Attending Physician, Albany Medical Hospital; Assistant Professor of Surgery (Urology), Head, Urologic Oncology, Albany Medical College, Albany, New York

A. GERARD, M.D., Professor of Surgery, Head of the Department of Surgery, Institut Jules Bordet, University of Brussels, Brussels, Belgium

LEIF HÅKANSSON, M.D., Ph.D., Department of Oncology, University Hospital, Linkoping, Sweden

DEBORAH O. HEROS, M.D., New England Medical Center; Assistant Professor of Neurology, Tufts University School of Medicine, Boston, Massachusetts

FRED H. HOCHBERG, M.D., Massachusetts General Hospital; Associate Professor of Neurology, Harvard Medical School, Boston, Massachusetts

GABRIEL N. HORTOBAGYI, M.D., Professor of Medicine, Chief, Medical Breast Service, University of Texas System Cancer Center, M. D. Anderson Hospital and Tumor Institute, Houston, Texas

LUCIEN ISRAEL, Professor and Head, Division of Oncology, Clinique de Cancerologie, Centre Hospitalier Universitaire de Bobigny, Université Paris Nord, Bobigny, France

DON V. JACKSON, JR., M.D., Oncology Research Center, Bowman Gray School of Medicine, Wake Forest University, Winston-Salem, North Carolina

BARUCH KLEIN, M.D., Department of Cancer Chemotherapy, Faculty of Medicine, University of Pretoria, Republic of South Africa

RICHARD LACKMAN, M.D., Assistant Professor, Department of Orthopedic Surgery, Chief, Musculo-Skeletal Tumor Services, Thomas Jefferson University Hospital, Philadelphia, Pennsylvania

YEU-TSU MARGARET LEE, M.D., F.A.C.S., LTC Medical Corps, Chief, Surgical Oncology Section, Department of Surgery, Tripler Army Medical Center, Honolulu, Hawaii; Associate Clinical Professor in Surgery, John A. Burns School of Medicine, University of Hawaii, Honolulu, Hawaii; Clinical Associate Professor, Department of Surgery, F. Edward School of Medicine, Uniformed Services University of Health Sciences, Bethesda, Maryland

SEWA S. LEGHA, M.D., Associate Professor of Medicine, Department of Medical Oncology, Division of Medicine, University of Texas System Cancer Center, M. D. Anderson Hospital and Tumor Institute, Houston, Texas

CYNTHIA G. LEICHMAN, M.D., Assistant Clinical Professor of Medicine, University of Southern California, Los Angeles, California

LAWRENCE LEICHMAN, M.D., Associate Professor of Medicine, University of Southern California, Los Angeles, California

CHRISTOPHER J. LOGOTHETIS, M.D., Chief, Genitourinary Oncology, Associate Internist, Associate Professor of Medicine, Department of Medical Oncology, M. D. Anderson Hospital and Tumor Institute, Houston, Texas

MAURIE MARKMAN, M.D., Department of Medicine, Memorial Sloan-Kettering Cancer Center, New York, New York

CHERYL L. MOORE, R.N., Chief Oncology Nurse, Cancer Center, Boston, Massachusetts

OLALLO MORALES, M.D., Department of Diagnostic Radiology, University Hospital, Linkoping, Sweden

JEAN-FRANCOIS MORERE, M.D., Clinique de Cancerologie, Centre Hospitalier Universitaire de Bobigny, Université Paris Nord, Bobigny, France

HYMAN B. MUSS, M.D., Professor of Medicine, Bowman Gray School of Medicine, Wake Forest University, Winston-Salem, North Carolina

MICHAEL J. O'CONNELL, M.D., Professor of Oncology, Vice Chairman Division of Medical Oncology, Mayo Clinic, Rochester, Minnesota

J.C. PECTOR, M.D., Staff Surgeon, Department of Surgery, Institut Jules Bordet, University of Brussels, Belgium

NANCY PHILLIPS, R.Ph., Oncology Pharmacy Consultant, Fox Chase Cancer Center, Philadelphia, Pennsylvania

MARK J. RATAIN, M.D., Instructor in Medicine, Joint Section of Hematology/Oncology, University of Chicago Pritzker School of Medicine and Michael Reese Hospital and Medical Center, Chicago, Illinois

PHILIP D. SCHNEIDER, M.D., Ph.D., Surgery Branch, National Cancer Institute, National Institutes of Health, Bethesda, Maryland

RUNE SJÖDAHL, M.D., Ph.D., Department of Surgery, University Hospital, Linkoping, Sweden

HANS STARKHAMMAR, M.D., Department of Oncology, University Hospital, Linkoping, Sweden

PAUL H. SUGARBAKER, M.D., Director of Surgical Oncology, Emory University, Robert W. Woodruff Health Sciences Center, Atlanta, Georgia

JOHN SVEDBERG, Ph.D., Department of Radiation Physics, University Hospital, Linkoping, Sweden

EFSTATHIOS TAPAZOGLOU, M.D., Assistant Professor of Medicine, Division of Medical Oncology, Department of Medicine, Director of Hyperthermia Program, Wayne State University and Harper-Grace Hospitals, Detroit, Michigan

ELTON M. TUCKER, B.S.M.E., President, Device Labs, Inc., Medway, Massachusetts

MARSHALL M. URIST, M.D., Associate Professor of Surgery, Chief, Section of Surgical Oncology, University of Alabama at Birmingham, Birmingham, Alabama

NICHOLAS J. VOGELZANG, M.D., Assistant Professor of Medicine, Joint Section of Hematology/Oncology, University of Chicago Pritzker School of Medicine and Michael Reese Hospital and Medical Center, Chicago, Illinois

HARISH M. VYAS, Ph.D., Oncology Pharmacist, New England Deaconess Hospital, Boston, Massachusetts

ARTHUR J. WEISS, M.D., Assistant Professor of Medicine, Division of Medical Oncology, Thomas Jefferson University Hospital, Philadelphia, Pennsylvania

RICHARD H. WHEELER, M.D., Comprehensive Cancer Center, Department of Medicine, Division of Hematology/Oncology, University of Alabama at Birmingham, Birmingham, Alabama

SECTION I

Rationale and Technical Aspects

1

INTRODUCTION TO THE CONCEPT

AND PRACTICE

OF INFUSION CHEMOTHERAPY

Jacob J. Lokich, M.D.

THE CHEMOTHERAPY OF CANCER is distinctive in terms of schedule of delivery from almost every other chronic illness treated by medications. Diseases such as hypertension, infections, arthritis, cardiovascular illness, to name but a few, are all managed by achieving optimal therapeutic drug levels and maintaining such levels continuously over time to ensure control of the disease process.

The rationale for the delivery of chemotherapy for cancer on a bolus or pulse schedule is based upon 4 points (table 1), with the primary basis being the critical role of dose. Frei and Canellos[1] have reviewed the importance of dose in determining the effectiveness of chemotherapy, but only 3 clinical studies have directly addressed the role of dose in optimally designed experimental trials.[2,3,4] In each of the studies, questions may be raised as to comparability of the treatment groups and the interpretation of the data. Nonetheless, preclinical drug studies clearly establish the importance of dose in both in vitro and

Table 1. Rationale for Bolus or Pulse Delivery for Chemotherapy

---

1. Established dose response relationship in experimental and in clinical trials*

2. Convenient outpatient administration

3. Traditional system

4. Cost-effective

---

*See text

3

in vivo animal tumor systems. The most compelling clinical data to support the primacy of dose in the delivery of chemotherapy has evolved more recently from the studies involving autologous bone marrow transplantation.[5] These studies involve removal of a portion of the bone marrow, which is generally the dose-limiting organ system, and reinfusion of the marrow after the administration of potentially lethal doses of single or multiple agents. The bone marrow is capable of "rescuing" the patient by repopulating the marrow through the reinfusion of the patient's own stem cells. Reports from a variety of institutions have identified higher than expected response rates in generally resistant tumors, such as malignant melanoma, as well as responses in patients previously resistant to the same agents administered at the lower doses, such as with ovarian and testicular cancer.

Supernormal doses have also been employed without autologous bone marrow transplantation and have similarly achieved responses in patients previously resistant. The 2 specific examples have been the use of high-dose cytosine arabinoside in leukemia and non-Hodgkins lymphoma and cisplatin in ovary and testicular cancer.[6,7]

An essential aspect of bolus chemotherapy is the intermittency of the schedule. This intermittency is a consequence of the effect of delivering a maximally tolerated dose which, in turn, is measured by the nadir of leukopenia or thrombocytopenia and permits additional dosage to be delivered only with host reconstitution. Thus, for example, the standard schedule of delivering treatment on day 1 and day 21 with a drug regimen using cyclophosphamide and adriamycin is based upon the fact that the nadir occurs approximately between day 10 and day 14. The development of an "adequate" nadir is the goal of bolus chemotherapy and, in fact, the nadir determines subsequent doses. The objective of each dose delivered is to achieve a white count nadir between 1,000 and 2,000 cells per cmm and/or a platelet count nadir of between 50,000 and 100,000 platelets per cmm. For patients achieving nadir white blood counts of greater than 2,000 or platelet counts greater than 100,000, a dose increment of 25% is a standard feature of most clinical protocols. A potential disadvantage of intermittency is the possibility of regrowth of tumor during the absence of drug availability. This clinical phenomenon is most likely to occur in the setting of high-growth fraction tumors.

The intervals between bolus administrations are determined not only by adverse host effects but also by practical considerations for logistics. Thus, the popular day 1, day 8 schedule provides a convenient interval for patients traveling a great distance, as well as allowing for decreased toxicity by spreading the dose of drugs over 2 sessions.

Secondary but important reasons for the bolus schedule chemotherapy relate to the capability of delivering such treatment as an outpatient and therefore maximizing patient and physician convenience. In the treatment of patients with advanced malignancy, it has been an important part of the philosophy of their management that hospitalization time be minimized so that patients are not separated from families and are encouraged to live a normal life. It is clear, however, that because dose is important and secondary immunosuppression is a part of delivering the maximum dose, hospitalization for complications of treatment should be expected. Furthermore, for some agents delivered as a bolus, hospitalization to control the acute gastrointestinal effects is common, particularly with cisplatin chemotherapy.

Finally, the bolus cancer chemotherapy schedule is traditional now by virtue of the fact that it has been the standard for 30 years, and it is also cost-effective compared to alternative schedules. The issue of cost-effectiveness is of particular concern in this era of extraordinary medical costs and the development of diagnosis-related groups (DRGs) as a means of cost containment. Suffice it to state at this juncture that cost-effectiveness, as measured in dollars for chemotherapy delivered by bolus versus infusion, may in fact be quite comparable or even balanced in favor of infusion. The fact that infusion can be delivered as an outpatient procedure obviates the over-whelming cost that was involved in infusion chemotherapy in the past because of the need for hospitalization. In addition, the major modification of drug toxicity that occurs as a consequence of the infusion schedule obviously decreases the medical costs associated with those complications.

Categories of Infusion Chemotherapy

The infusion schedule of delivery denotes the administration of a drug over time, generally for periods of 24 hours or more. The types of infusional chemotherapy may be classified as in table 2. The conceptual basis and rationale for each category is distinctive, as is the clinical effectiveness.

Regional Infusion

Regional delivery represents the oldest category of infusion chemotherapy, exemplified by infusion into the liver. This organ system is of particular appeal not only because it is one of the most common sites of metastasis for a whole

Table 2. Categories of Infusion Chemotherapy

Systemic infusion		
	Short-term	72 to 120 hours
	Protracted	28 days or longer
Regional Infusion		
	Closed space administration	
		Bladder
		Intraperitoneal
		Intrapleural
		Intrathecal
	Arterial infusion	
		Hepatic artery
		Carotid artery
		Hypogastric or iliac artery
		Internal mammary artery
		Bronchial artery
	Arterial perfusion	
		Femoral artery

variety of tumors but also because it is apparent that metastases derive their blood supply predominantly from the hepatic arterial system. It has been demonstrated, however, that the portal vein may provide the vascular nutrients for portions or all of some metastatic lesions and, as a consequence, portal vein infusion singularly or in conjunction with hepatic arterial infusion has been undergoing clinical trials. The rationale for chemotherapy delivered to the liver is based upon the concept of maximizing the dose "topically"; also, because of high hepatic extraction of the cytotoxic agents, host exposure to the drug is minimized, allowing a higher dose to be delivered than would be possible if the agent were to be delivered systemically. Although dose has therefore become the presumed advantage of the direct route of delivery to the tumor, regional chemotherapy also employs the concept of infusion over time.

For head and neck cancers, regional infusion via the external carotid system permits "topical" therapy, but a pharmacokinetic advantage in terms of extraction to minimize host toxicity is generally not the case, as in hepatic arterial chemotherapy. Regional delivery for the treatment of extremity lesions, pelvic lesions, chest wall lesions, or primary or metastatic brain lesions administers the chemotherapeutic agent generally as a bolus or possibly an infusion over 1 or 2 hours. For extremity lesions such as sarcoma or melanoma, the procedure of isolated perfusion by virtue of restricting venous return from the extremity may permit an accumulation of higher doses within the tumor.

Space Infusion

Administration of chemotherapy to a closed-space system exposes the tumor cells to the chemotherapeutic agent over time. For intrathecal or intraventricular chemotherapy, the agent may be delivered as a bolus, but because of a slow egress from the central nervous system, the agents have a maximum time exposure emulating a continuous infusion. Peritoneal chemotherapy is directed at affecting a tumor that implants along the serosal surface. In addition to the topical effect of the drug, systemic absorption for most agents is demonstrable; therefore, recirculation of the drug results in systemic as well as topical application. Intravesical chemotherapy for the treatment of low-grade and superficial bladder tumors is again based upon minimizing host exposure in the course of a brief instillation period. Nonetheless, absorption of most agents employed in this type of chemotherapy is demonstrable.

Systemic Infusion

Systemic delivery of chemotherapy is indicated in most patients, inasmuch as isolated regional localization of metastases to a single organ system is clinically uncommon and many sites do not have a single blood supply. Infusional chemotherapy delivered systemically is generally administered via a central venous access, although at least conceptually, intraperitoneal delivery may be considered as a route of systemic delivery. Two types of systemic infusional chemotherapy may be defined on the basis of different conceptual premises. Short-term infusion is defined as an infusion of 4 or 5 days repeated at 3- to 4-week intervals. The rationale is to maximize the dose of the drug administered, at the same time obviating at least the acute gastrointestinal toxicity. Protracted infusional chemotherapy for weeks or, as a basis for discussion, 30 days, conceptually maximizes tumor exposure based upon the speculation that treatment over an entire tumor doubling time may allow for maximal exposure of the sensitive cell population. By definition, the dose rate of delivery for protracted infusion would be one that does not induce toxicity and thus necessitate treatment interruption.

Rationale for Systemic Infusional Chemotherapy

Table 3 summarizes the basis for applying the infusion schedule for delivery of individual agents. For some drugs and for some tumors, one or more of these reasons may apply; in some instances, the rationale may be contradictory. For example, for rapidly growing tumors with a high proportion of cells in cycle, a single exposure in time may permit a substantial tumor cell kill effect that obviates the need for continuous drug exposure. Similarly, for agents with a prolonged plasma half-life following single bolus exposure, continuous delivery over time at lower doses would seem unnecessary. For most tumors, however, the in-cycle cell population is small, and the plasma half-life for most of the chemotherapeutic agents employed is short. The treatment of acute leukemia with cytosine arabinoside represents an example of the interaction of the issues of drug pharmacology and tumor cytokinetics. Leukemia represents an uncommon tumor in which, at least relative to solid tumors, a high proportion of cells are in cycle, making treatment with bolus delivery reasonable. However, the most effective drug for leukemia treatment is cytosine arabinoside, an agent that has an extraordinarily short plasma half-life and is rapidly inactivated in man as a consequence of the ubiquitous presence of the deaminase in most tissues.

Tumor Cell Cytokinetics

In general, antineoplastics affect a variety of cellular functions or nuclear synthesis of DNA; consequently, they affect predominantly the tumor cell population that is in cycle. Even the alkylating agents that affect preformed DNA and the anthracycline drugs that intercalate in preformed DNA predominantly affect cycling cells. For the most part, solid tumors are composed mostly of

Table 3. Rationale for Continuous Infusion Delivery Schedule for Chemotherapy*

---

1. Pharmacokinetics of antineoplastic agents

2. Cytokinetic profile of tumors

3. In vitro and in vivo experimental data for schedule dependency

4. Clinical trials

---

*See text

cells that are in G_o, or the quiescent phase of the cell cycle, precluding the induction of injury by an antineoplastic drug. Clinical studies of tumor cell kinetics have generally involved the relatively crude method of monitoring the size of a lesion over time and determining by mathematical extrapolation the tumor doubling time. Another method is to expose the tumor cell population to a pulse dose of tritiated, labeled thymidine, and with sequential biopsies one may identify the proportion of cells that are in cycle at any one time. It is evident from such studies that the tumor doubling time for common tumors in particular is measured in months, and that the proportion of cells in cycle at any one point for these same tumors is generally less than 5%. Tumors with the shorter tumor doubling time and a higher labeling index demonstrate higher response rates in general. These tumors include Burkitts lymphoma, small cell carcinoma, testicular cancer, and many of the childhood tumors.

The growth of tumors may also involve an intrinsic autoregulating rhythm in which the proportion of cells that are in cycle (the proliferative thrust) may be greater at some points during a 24-hour period or during a 7-day period than at other times. This circadian rhythm may be fixed for some tumors and variable for others. Studies in animal tumor systems have demonstrated a variation in tumor growth depending upon the light or dark exposure,[8] and clinical studies in man have suggested that response rates may vary according to the time of chemotherapy delivery.[9] In the absence of the ability to identify tumor circadian rhythmicity, the delivery of a drug by continuous infusion may be necessary. On the other hand, the addition of pulse drug at a time when the maximal numbers of in-cycle cells is present could increase drug effectiveness.

Drug Pharmacology

The second major basis for infusional chemotherapy relates to drug pharmacology. Studies of the pharmacology of antineoplastic agents have generally been performed in the context of bolus delivery monitoring blood levels, as well as the accumulation of drug in various fluids such as urine and bile or in stool and cerebrospinal fluid. One can then establish the plasma or serum half-life of an agent, as well as the clearance rate, and thereby extrapolate the timed exposure of the tumor to the drug. As a generality, the half-life of most chemotherapeutic agents is measured in minutes to hours, but the critical determinant of effective chemotherapy is not maintenance of a cytotoxic blood level but rather the intracellular concentration. The pharmacology of antineoplastic agents may vary between patients, since it is related to alterations in the function of individual organ systems such as the liver or kidney, as well as to other undetermined factors. Clinical monitoring of blood levels for these agents is made impractical by the complexity of the assay systems employed, and for some drugs assays may not be available. As an alternative, clinical monitoring is performed, adjusting bolus dose on the basis of drug-induced toxicity, particularly bone marrow toxicity.

The pharmacokinetics of agents delivered by regional delivery similarly support that rationale for this system of chemotherapy. Drug extraction, by the liver, for example, allows for a greater dose on delivery and potentially greater tumor cell effects by minimizing host exposure.

Preclinical Experimental Data Base

The identification of effective antineoplastic agents evolves from preclinical studies in animal tumor systems, such as the transplanted leukemia in mice (L1210), as well as a number of other animal tumor systems, including AKR lymphoma, P388 leukemia, etc. Drug schedule dependency is demonstrable for many of the standard chemotherapeutic agents in these preclinical screening systems, although the extrapolation from mouse to man is not readily translated.

The recent development of the human stem cell assay system offers a new approach to drug development. This system has been able to identify drugs that may be more effective with prolonged exposure times and has the capability of categorizing agents on the basis of the optimal schedule of delivery.[10]

CLINICAL TRIALS

Infusion chemotherapy is being increasingly assessed in clinical trials, predominately in phase 2 settings. Comparative trials of bolus versus infusion chemotherapy are sparse in the literature, but ongoing studies should answer the question of the relative efficacy of the two schedule alternative as well as other important questions relating to the therapeutic index and cost-effectiveness.

Technologic Impetus to Infusional Chemotherapy

The negative inertia affecting the development of infusional chemotherapy has been related in large measure to the limitations of establishing safe and reliable chronic vascular access and the availability of accurate and portable infusion devices that permit ambulatory infusional chemotherapy. The technologic development in these two areas has stimulated the expanded capability of delivering antineoplastics by an infusion schedule.

In addition to technical issues, practical issues related to pharmaceutical aspects of the individual agents are of major importance. Because infusion over time necessitates that an agent not undergo degradation in a drug reservoir to potentially inactive metabolites, drug stability is a critical issue. Stability data for most of the agents have generally been generated on the basis of shelf life or refrigeration life upon reconstitution; because agents are delivered as a bolus, stability over a few hours is generally the optimum available from the pharmaceutical industry. Another important pharmaceutical aspect for infusion is drug solubility, and drugs that require a large volume in order to be maintained in solution may not be practical for ambulatory infusion. Finally, drug interaction with the reservoir or with additional agents that may be administered as an admixture necessitates preclinical studies in order to determine whether infusion over time is practical.

Current Clinical Status of Infusional Chemotherapy

Most systemic and regional infusional chemotherapy is being applied for the treatment of advanced malignancy, with proponents lauding the decreased toxicity and therapeutic benefits. But with rare exception, optimally designed experimental clinical trials have not been performed; as a result, infusional chemotherapy remains an unproven entity for many physicians.

The present status of clinical trials for systemic infusional chemotherapy is indicated in table 4. The importance of prospective randomized trials cannot be overemphasized, but the introduction of this approach has been difficult because of the intrinsic bias of advocates on both sides and because the cost and learning involved in new technology are inhibitory. It will be important in the context of such trials to monitor comparative toxicity, therapeutic impact as measured by response rate and survival, and finally, the relative cost-effectiveness of the two schedules of delivery.

The interdigitation of chemotherapy delivered by infusion with the other therapeutic modalities, radiation therapy and surgical therapy, is in its infancy. So-called "adjuvant" chemotherapy delivered by infusion following surgery requires a more definitive answer from the trials at the phase 3 level in patients with advanced disease. However, ongoing trials that have interdigitated infusion chemotherapy with radiation have demonstrated the feasibility of such an approach. Certainly, if chemotherapy is to function as a radiation sensitizer in such combined modality programs, continuous delivery throughout the period of radiation therapy, generally 2 to 6 weeks, is more rational than the intermittent pulse schedule.

Like bolus or pulse chemotherapy, combination chemotherapy — the delivery of multiple agents simultaneously on a 3- 4-drug regimen — has been the standard and traditional form of treatment since its introduction 20 years ago. With the exception of the use of chlorambucil for chronic lymphatic leukemia, busulfan for chronic myelogenous leukemia, and 5-fluorouracil for the homeopathic treatment of gastrointestinal malignancy, single-agent chemotherapy is virtually unknown. Multiagent infusion programs may involve either the delivery of one agent in a 3- or 4-drug regimen by infusion, or alternatively, by establishing drug compatibilities and developing admixture

Table 4. Current Clinical Status of Infusional Chemotherapy

---

1. Prospective randomized trials comparing the standard bolus schedule with short-term or protracted infusion chemotherapy

2. Combined modality applications, particularly in connection with radiation for sensitization

3. Multiagent infusion chemotherapy employing drug admixtures

4. Evaluation of comparative effectiveness of regional versus systemic drug delivery

5. Adjuvant applications of infusion schedules

---

infusion programs. The latter has been addressed primarily in phase 1 trials.[11,12]

A major impetus to regional chemotherapy, particularly for primary and secondary neoplasia in the liver, has been a consequence of the technologic development of an implanted pump infusion system. Although substantial antitumor effects for this delivery system have been established by a number of centers, the cost of such a program both in terms of dollars and the need for an operative placement has led to prospective trials of this method compared to standard schedules and routes of delivery. Three groups have ongoing trials with a prospective randomized design to determine the role of regional delivery. It is anticipated that such trials will definitively establish the optimum drug and route, as well as dose rate of infusion, and that such trials may serve as a stimulus to infusional trials, both systemic and regional, in other tumor systems.

Summary

The infusion schedule of chemotherapy adds another dimension to the treatment of cancer and has highlighted, to some degree, the issue of the dose versus the schedule of delivery in cancer treatment. In fact, both issues are more complementary than conflictual. High-dose chemotherapy, particularly in conjunction with autologous bone marrow transplantation, increases the response rate, indicating that dose may overcome at least some forms of tumor cell resistance to chemotherapeutic agents. Nonetheless, the concept of continuous tumor cell exposure to drugs has a substantial rationale. Clearly, toxicity is decreased in almost all instances with the infusion schedule, and therapeutic effects are observed; it is not at all clear, however, that the antitumor effects observed are superior to those achieved with a bolus schedule.

Dose advocates are exploring the feasibility, practicality, and cost of autologous bone marrow transplantation and have also been applying the principles developed by the Goldie-Coldman hypothesis by introducing alternating noncross-resistant programs with maximal dose application. Infusion advocates are following the route of prospective comparative trials to influence the nonbelievers. Such trials should not only address therapeutic effects of infusion compared with bolus schedules; trials comparing the bolus to the infusions should also address the issue of the optimal duration of infusion, in that prolonged drug delivery is logistically demanding and imposes substantially upon patient life-style. More critical, however, is the issue of the possible induction of tumor cell resistance as a consequence of chronic low-dose exposure to the cytotoxic drug. Thus, short-term infusion intermittently and protracted infusion may represent two areas of future comparative trials, and pulse delivery superimposed intermittently on an infusion system may be yet another future consideration in developing optimal delivery schedules.

2

EXPERIMENTAL RATIONALE FOR CONTINUOUS INFUSION CHEMOTHERAPY

Mark J. Ratain, M.D., and Nicholas J. Vogelzang, M.D.

Introduction

THE OPTIMAL SCHEDULE HAS not been established for the administration of most antineoplastic agents. This chapter reviews the schedule dependency of antineoplastic agents based on in vitro studies that assess both time- and concentration-dependent cytotoxicity and in vivo studies that evaluate the influence of treatment schedule on tumor response or host animal survival. In vivo experiments suggesting that divided frequent doses of a drug are more effective than single bolus doses are considered to favor the use of infusion chemotherapy. On the other hand, in vitro data suggesting that prolonged exposure (in vitro model for continuous infusion) is pharmacologically efficient (increased cytotoxic effect per concentration-time product) cannot necessarily assess changes in the therapeutic index (tumor regression versus toxicity). Other pertinent data regarding drug stability, mechanism of action, and bolus pharmacokinetics are included where appropriate, but clinical studies of continuous infusion are beyond the scope of this review.

Antineoplastic agents were originally grouped into three classes based on in vitro survival curves and phase specificity.[1] Type 1 agents kill cells in all portions of the cell cycle, and the cytotoxic effect is not significantly affected by the proliferative state. Survival curves are exponential, with a small shoulder. Gamma radiation and nitrogen mustard were originally assigned to this class, also known as radiomimetic agents.

Type 2 agents are phase-specific, and thus the survival curve reaches a plateau, as there is no effect on cells that are not in the optimal phase of the cycle. Vinblastine and methotrexate (amethopterin) were originally assigned to this class.[1]

Type 3 agents are highly cycle-specific, but are active in all or most phases of the cell cycle. Survival curves are exponential, without an apparent plateau. Originally assigned to this class were 5-fluorouracil, actinomycin-D, and cyclophosphamide.[1]

This classification scheme has been modified by other investigators.[2,3] Shimoyama[2] found only two types of action — concentration-dependent (cytocidal) and time-dependent (cytostatic). Drewinko et al[3] found 5 different survival curve patterns following a 1-hour exposure: simple exponential, biphasic exponential, threshold exponential, exponential plateau, and ineffectual.

Drugs that are highly time-dependent, or ineffectual with brief exposure, are those drugs predicted to have greater pharmacologic effect via continuous infusion. Based on these classification schemes, Shimoyama[2] classified the vinca alkaloids, antimetabolites, and L-asparaginase as time-dependent.

Although many pharmacologists associate the concentration-time product ($C \times T$) with pharmacodynamic response,[4] changes in drug concentration or exposure time in vitro may have very different results.[5,6] Eicholtz and Trott[5] constructed the following equation, based on their in vitro studies with methotrexate and Chinese hamster cells:

$$\text{Survival fraction } (C,t) = K_1 \cdot e^{-K_2 t} \cdot C^{-K_3 - K_4 t}$$

Doubling the concentration results in a decrease in survival fraction by $2^{K_3 + K_4 t}$, while doubling the exposure time results in a fractional decrease in survival of $e^{K_2 t} \cdot C^{K_4 t}$.

Rupniak et al[6] also suggest that the product of $C \times T$ is an inadequate representation of a complicated system. They compared the effects of 1-hour and continuous exposure to doxorubicin, cisplatin, vinblastine, and hydroxyurea on human ovarian and colon carcinoma lines in vitro. Their results clearly demonstrate that the major effect of increasing the exposure time is to increase the slope of the concentration-survival curve. Similar conclusions can be drawn from in vivo studies with 5-fluorouracil and ftorafur in mice.[7]

Multiple complex mathematical models have been developed for both in vitro[5,8] and in vivo[8-10] systems using phase-specific agents. It is clear that predicting the optimal schedule of an antineoplastic drug is a very difficult task.

The problem becomes even more complicated when one considers the proliferative rate of the tumor as a contributing factor. In general, a better response to chemotherapy with cell cycle-specific agents is obtained in experimental tumor systems with high proliferative fractions.[11] Since the proliferative state decreases with increasing tumor burden,[12] the treatment of advanced cancer is especially difficult. The optimal schedule for a drug versus a given tumor may depend on the tumor burden.[13] Although intermittent bolus therapy (every 4 days) is optimal for early L1210 leukemia, animals with advanced disease were optimally treated with low-dose daily chemotherapy.[13]

This chapter will focus on each of the major classes of antineoplastic drugs: antimetabolites, plant alkaloids, alkylating agents, and antibiotics. An assessment of the rationale for continuous infusion will be made for each drug, on the basis of in vitro cytotoxicity studies, and in vivo studies of either activity or toxicity of various schedules. Other data (i.e., pharmaceutical) are included where appropriate. This chapter will not discuss several important limitations to the use of continuous infusion chemotherapy. A minimum cytotoxic concentration must be obtained for any effect to occur.[14,15] The minimum concentration needed may be different for each tissue type.[14] It also will vary from tumor to tumor, as some tumors are resistant to even high drug concentrations. Another potential limitation to the use of continuous infusion chemotherapy is drug stability. For example, this has limited the use of etoposide[16] and BCNU,[17] requiring stability testing prior to infusion studies of new drugs. Since these limitations are often not present or significant in in vitro or in vivo systems, they will not be further analyzed.

Antimetabolites

General Considerations

The antimetabolites, which were among the first antineoplastic agents, are probably the best-studied class of anticancer drugs. These compounds are either analogs of nucleotides (cytosine arabinoside, 5-azacytidine, 6-mercaptopurine, 6-thioguanine, 5-fluorouracil) or inhibit the synthesis of nucleotides (methotrexate, hydroxyurea) that are required for DNA synthesis. All of these drugs have short elimination half-lives[18] and are phase-specific,[1,2] therefore making them good theoretical candidates for continuous infusion chemotherapy. In fact, most of the drugs have been employed by continuous infusion in clinical trials,[19] and continuous infusion of cytosine arabinoside is part of many standard treatment regimens for acute nonlymphocytic leukemias[20] and preleukemic syndromes.[21]

Cytosine Arabinoside (ara-C)

There is a clear-cut rationale for the use of ara-C by continuous infusion. The many experiments discussed here should serve as a "standard" to assess the schedule dependency for other drugs. Ara-C has a very short half-life in man, with a terminal half-life of approximately 1–3 hours due to plasma deamination by cytidine deaminase.[22] The drug is stable in solution for up to 192 hours at room temperature.

IN VITRO DATA

Studies by Wu et al[23] clearly demonstrate the schedule dependency of ara-C in vitro, using a sensitive cell line (Raji lymphoma). Although a 1-hour exposure to a low concentration of doxorubicin (25 ng/ml) was highly cytotoxic (8% survival), ara-C demonstrated no activity at up to 25 μg/ml for 1 hour. Similar results were obtained by Drewinko et al,[3] placing ara-C into the group of "ineffectual" agents following a 1-hour exposure. However, with prolonged exposure (14 days), low concentrations (0.1 μg/ml) are cytotoxic (25% survival).[23]

Greenburg et al[24] obtained similar results using granulocyte progenitor cells. There is a consistently increased pharmacologic effect with prolonged exposure in vitro, and both the cytotoxicity and host toxicity would be predicted to be increased by continuous infusion. However, no conclusion can be drawn regarding changes in the therapeutic index based on in vitro studies alone.

IN VIVO DATA

There has been a great deal of interest in determining the optimal scheduling of ara-C during the past 20 years. Kline et al[25] first compared the effects of various schedules of administration of ara-C on L1210 leukemia in mice. A single dose of 1.4 g/kg had little effect, whereas divided doses were quite effective. There was no single best schedule, although there was clearly an increased pharmacologic effect with divided doses, as only a 3 mg/kg/dose was required on a 4 times daily schedule, whereas a 500 mg/kg dose was necessary when the mice were treated every 4 days.

Multiple subsequent reports[9,26-28] have concluded that ara-C is optimally administered in very frequent divided doses. Skipper et al[26] found that the only curative schedule was every 3 hours (8 hours), administered every fourth day. Using a 512 mg/kg/dose, they obtained a cure rate of over 80%, while there were no cures on any of the other schedules using equitoxic doses. Similar results have been obtained by other investigators.[9,27]

Skipper et al[28] also investigated the use of short ara-C infusions (6–24 hours). Their experiments did not show any advantage to short infusion therapy over frequent divided doses. There have not been any reported in vivo experiments using long-term infusions, similar to those used clinically.[20]

5-aza-2'-deoxycytidine

5-aza-2'-deoxycytidine is a derivative of 5-azacytidine, an effective anti-leukemic agent.[29] There are both in vitro[30] and in vivo[31] data to support the use of 5-aza-2'-deoxycytidine by continuous infusion, although similar data are not available for 5-azacytidine.

IN VITRO DATA

Covey and Zaharko[30] performed a series of experiments effectively demonstrating the schedule dependency of 5-aza-2'-deoxycytidine. A 1-hour exposure at 1 μg/ml had only moderate cytotoxicity (35% survival), but prolonged (24 hours) exposure at 0.01 μg/ml achieved a 1-log kill. Using even higher concentrations (1 μg/ml) for 24 hours, a 4-log kill is achievable. These results are even more impressive in light of the observation that 5-aza-2'-deoxycytidine spontaneously decomposes, with a half-life of 15–17 hours.[30]

IN VIVO DATA

Momparier and Gonzalez[31] treated L1210-bearing mice with 1- to 8-hour infusions of 5-aza-2'-deoxycytidine. An 8-hour infusion of 25.6 mg/kg was optimal, with 9/10 "cures." However, equitoxic bolus or short infusion treatments were not tested. They noted that the plasma elimination half-life of 5-aza-2'-deoxycytidine in mice (measured by bioassay) was only 40 minutes, giving additional support to the use of continuous infusion for this drug.

6-mercaptopurine and 6-thioguanine

These two drugs are older agents, usually administered in single oral daily doses. There is a renewed interest in these drugs because of their variable bioavailability when administered orally, which would suggest that intravenous infusion may be preferred.[32] Unfortunately, there are only sparse experimental data on the schedule dependency of these drugs, despite the strong theoretical rationale.

IN VITRO DATA

Greenberg et al[24] assessed the importance of exposure time of 6-thioguanine on granulocytic progenitor cells in vitro. There was no difference in colony-forming cell survival between 1- and 4-hour exposures at drug concentrations ranging from 0.01 to 100 μg/ml.

IN VIVO DATA

There are no in vivo studies of 6-mercaptopurine infusions, but Venditti et al[33,34] have studied the schedule dependency of 6-mercaptopurine versus L1210 leukemia. It was clearly shown that a weekly schedule was inferior to other schedules, but the survival of the mice was similar for schedules ranging from every other day to 4 times daily. There was an increased pharmacologic effect with divided doses, as only 8.4 mg/kg could be given 4 times daily compared to 108 mg/kg on a once-a-day schedule.

Fluorinated Pyrimidines

Multiple studies support the use of 5-fluorouracil (5-FU) and 5-fluorodeoxyuridine (FUDR) by continuous infusion. The rationale for infusion of these drugs is especially strong because of their very short elimination half-life, 10–20 minutes for 5-FU.[35]

IN VITRO DATA

It has been suggested that the pharmacodynamic effect of a 5-FU exposure in vitro can be best predicted by the product $C \times T$.[36] This hypothesis is supported by the data of Calabro-Jones et al,[37] as a 240-hour exposure at 1 μg/ml was as effective as a 2-hour exposure at 100 μg/ml.

However, Drewinko et al[38] suggest that a prolonged exposure is much more important than high peak concentrations, as 2000 μg/ml for 1 hour produced only 80% cytotoxicity, compared to 500 μg/ml for 16 hours (>99% cytotoxicity). However, the drug concentrations in this study were very high, indicating that the cells that were used (LoVo colon carcinoma) were quite resistant. Matsushima et al[39] also compared 1- and 24-hour exposures in vitro. Either 220

μg/ml for 1 hour or 0.23 μg/ml for 24 hours were required to achieve 50% cytotoxicity. This also suggests that the exposure time is much more important and argues against the routine use of the product $C \times T$.

IN VIVO DATA

There are no conclusive in vivo data on the use of 5-FU and FUDR by infusion. Ferguson[40] treated Wistar-Furth rats—a strain with a high incidence of spontaneous mammary tumors—with low-dose oral daily 5-FU (17 mg/kg/day), which significantly decreased (from 28% to 11%) the incidence of these tumors. Other schedules of treatment did not appear to be active. Lin[41] compared the effects of single injection and divided doses of both 5-FU and FUDR on hemolytic plaque-forming cells. Although divided doses of FUDR were significantly more toxic that single injections, there was no significant difference between the two schedules of 5-FU. Henry et al[42] administered FUDR by continuous infusion to beagle dogs without a marked increase in toxicity as compared to single bolus injections. However, it is difficult to make any strong conclusions based on in vivo studies, as the pharmacokinetics of 5-FU infusions are quite species-dependent.[43]

Methotrexate (MTX)

Methotrexate (MTX) inhibits purine and pyrimidine synthesis by acting as a rapidly reversible competitive inhibitor of dihydrofolate reductase.[44]. Multiple in vitro and in vivo studies conclusively demonstrate that MTX is a highly schedule-dependent antineoplastic agent. Because its elimination half-life is only 8–10 hours in man,[44] MTX appears to be a rational candidate for continuous infusion chemotherapy. However, continuous infusion may not be superior to divided oral daily doses.

IN VITRO DATA

Both Eicholtz and Trott[5] and Keefe et al[45] have provided mathematical models of MTX cytotoxicity suggesting that cell survival is affected to a greater extent by exposure duration than by exposure dose. In addition, the model of Eicholtz and Trott suggests that the relative effect of a change in dose or exposure time is dependent on the other independent variable.

Wu et al[23] found a 1-hour exposure to be inactive at doses up to 10 μg/ml, while a 14-day exposure at 0.1 μg/ml yielded no cell survival. Matsushima et al[39] compared the effects of 1- and 24-hour exposure duration. To obtain 50% cytotoxicity, either 97 μg/ml for 1 hour or 0.32 μg/ml for 24 hours were required. Johnson et al[46] compared the effects of MTX on resting and exponentially growing mouse fibroblasts. The resting cells were completely resistant, even at 1mM for 7 days. Their results with the growing cells also demonstrated the predominant effect of exposure time in determining cytotoxicity.

IN VIVO DATA

It has been repeatedly shown that divided doses or infusion of MTX in vivo are more toxic to normal cells than intermittent bolus treatments.[14,41,47-49]

Chabner and Young[14] first demonstrated that there is a threshold effect for MTX cytotoxicity in vivo at a plasma MTX concentration of approximately 0.01 μM, with almost complete suppression of DNA synthesis. The threshold for MTX toxicity may vary from tissue to tissue (small intestine > marrow > Lewis lung tumor).[48] Pinedo and Chabner[47] conclusively demonstrated that MTX toxicity cannot be related to the product $C \times T$ in vivo, as continuous infusion to plasma concentrations of 0.05 μM for 72 hours (product = 3.6 μM hrs) was equitoxic to 10 μM for 12 hours (product = 120 μM hrs).

There have been no in vivo studies comparing the therapeutic index of MTX by continuous infusion with intermittent bolus therapy. Goldin et al[13] showed that the optimal schedule of MTX may depend on the host tumor burden. Daily treatment was the optimal schedule for advanced disease, and it is possible that multiple times daily (or the extreme — continuous infusion) may have an even greater effect. Venditti et al[34] have assessed the therapeutic index (survival) of a variety of schedules of MTX in murine L1210 leukemia. The schedules used ranged from twice daily to weekly, and once daily appeared to be optimal. Thus, it is not clear that continuous intravenous infusion of MTX would be superior to frequent intermittent low doses, which could easily be administered orally.

Hydroxyurea (HYD)

Hydroxyurea (HYD), an older antineoplastic agent, inhibits DNA synthesis through its effect on ribonucleotide reductase.[50] Because it is rapidly eliminated,[51] it is usually given as multiple daily oral doses. As was stated above for MTX, continuous infusion of HYD may not be superior to divided oral daily doses.

IN VITRO DATA

Sinclair[52] found a threshold for cytotoxicity in vitro (Chinese hamster lung cells) of 0.5mM, with a maximal effect reached by 2 hours. A twofold increase in dose did not result in increased cytoxicity, but higher doses were not tested. Rupniak et al[6] suggest that continuous exposure to HYD is required for cytotoxicity, as 1- to 6-hour exposures were ineffective at a dose of 1 mg/ml (13mM). In contrast, there was less than 10% survival using 50 μg/ml (0.66mM) continuously.

IN VIVO DATA

Plager[53] studied the effects of HYD infusions on normal tissues in mice. An infusion rate of 0.47 mg/hr was required to obtain a reduction in mitotic labeling. At higher doses, the reduction was especially rapid.

Both Skipper et al[26] and Venditti[27] have compared the effectiveness of a range of treatment schedules of HYD against L1210 leukemia in vivo. Both studies demonstrated that administering the drug every 3 hours on every fourth day was optimal. This was the only schedule that was curative, although the effect of continuous multiple (every 3 hours) daily doses was not assessed.

Summary

The antimetabolites are highly schedule-dependent in both in vitro and in vivo studies. Although the efficacy of ara-C by continuous infusion has been established,[20,21] further in vivo studies are required for most of the antimetabolites. Because most of these drugs are available in oral preparations, the use of frequent daily dosing should be considered as an alternative to continuous I.V. infusion. Careful comparative in vivo studies are required to improve the rationale for these clinical trials.

Plant Alkaloids

General Considerations

Plant alkaloids are a diverse group of antineoplastic agents. These drugs originally were all thought to cause mitotic arrest via their interactions with tubulin. However, more recent experimental data suggest that the epipodophyllotoxins (VP-16, VM-26) are cytotoxic due to their ability to inhibit topoisomerase II.[54,55] However, all of these agents appear to be phase-specific, with the maximal cytotoxic effect occurring in the G_2 or M phases of the cell cycle.[56]

In contrast to the antimetabolites, these agents generally have long half-lives in man, ranging from 8 hours for VP-16 to 85 hours for vincristine (VCR).[56,57] This is a point against continuous infusion of these agents. These drugs are usually administered by I.V. bolus injections, although an oral form of VP-16 has undergone preliminary testing.[58]

Abundant in vitro data demonstrate that these agents are highly schedule-dependent. However, supportive in vivo studies are generally lacking. Therefore, it may be difficult to show that these agents should be administered by continuous infusion, as intermittent bolus dosing may provide nearly equivalent activity because of the slow elimination of these drugs.

Vinca Alkaloids

Three vinca alkaloids are currently employed in cancer chemotherapy — VCR, vinblastine (VLB), and vindesine (VDS). Despite their similar structures, these drugs have very different pharmacokinetic and clinical properties. VCR is predominantly neurotoxic, whereas VLB is myelosuppressive, with occasional neurotoxicity. In general, vindesine's properties are intermediate between the other 2 drugs. VCR has the longest half-life (85 hours) and the smallest maximally tolerated dose (2 mg).[57] In addition, the cellular retention of these drugs is different, with VLB being rapidly released from cells and VCR released relatively slowly.[59]

As would be expected from the known phase specificity of these drugs, there are multiple in vitro studies demonstrating exposure time-dependent cytotoxicity. However, no definite conclusions can be obtained because of the paucity of supporting in vivo data.

IN VITRO DATA

The vinca alkaloids are very potent drugs that are generally cytotoxic at extracellular concentrations ≥ 1 ng/ml.[60] Wu et al[23] showed that the cytotoxicity of VCR is highly dependent on exposure time. A 1-hour exposure at 10 ng/ml yielded 60% survival, but a 14-day exposure at 1 ng/ml resulted in 100% cytotoxicity. Cytotoxic effects could be demonstrated at VCR concentrations of only 0.1 ng/ml (7% survival).

Ludwig et al[61] obtained similar results with VLB using a human tumor clonogenic assay. When fresh melanoma tissue (a clinically resistant tumor) was exposed to 10 ng/ml for 1 hour, there was approximately 45% survival. However, a 200-hour exposure at 1 ng/ml was highly cytotoxic, with only 3% survival. They tested a total of 77 tumors for VLB sensitivity. Of the 14 sensitive tumors, 42% showed sensitivity only when continuous (200-hour) exposure was used. Wells et al[62] found that even a 20-hour VLB exposure was relatively ineffective; they suggest that a minimum of 45 hours (at VLB concentrations of 1–10 ng/ml) is required for significant activity. Rupniak et al[6] and Mujagic et al[63] have obtained similar results, but used higher drug concentrations (20 ng/ml). However, some tumors (cell lines) do not demonstrate the same scheduling effects. Matsushima et al[39] found a steeper dose-response curve for a 1-hour exposure of PC-7 cells (human adenocarcinoma of lung) to VLB, compared to a 24-hour exposure. With the same cell line, VDS showed only slight schedule dependency, as the dose-response curves were virtually parallel.

IN VIVO DATA

There is solid evidence that the vinca alkaloids are more potent (increased toxicity and cytotoxicity) when given in divided doses,[64] but it is difficult to conclude definitively that the therapeutic index is changed. Feaux de Lacroix and Klein[65] suggest that the fractionation of a VCR dose into 6 small doses over 14 hours is more effective than a single bolus. They carried out their studies with a murine mammary carcinoma in vivo. However, they did not use simultaneous controls treated with single bolus doses. Further studies[66] demonstrated that these differences were most pronounced in the tumor center, where the growth fraction is decreased. Studies with VLB and VDS are needed, as these drugs have shorter half-lives in man than does vincristine.

Epipodophyllotoxins

These drugs are derivatives of podophyllotoxin, which is extracted from the may apple plant.[56] Two epipodophyllotoxins—etoposide (VP-16) and teniposide (VM-26)—are in clinical use. VP-16 has a relatively short half-life (8–11 hours) in comparison to the vinca alkaloids and VM-26. Fairly strong experimental evidence supports the use of divided doses of these drugs, although the superiority of continuous infusion has not been established. However, these agents are highly insoluble[67] and relatively unstable[16], making continuous infusion a relatively impractical option.

IN VITRO DATA

Drewinko and Barlogie[68] first demonstrated the marked time dependency of VP-16 cytotoxicity. At a VP-16 concentration of 1 μg/ml, doubling the exposure time produced a 1-log increase in cytotoxicity. Ludwig et al[61] found that 75% of human tumor explants that are sensitive to VP-16 are resistant when a 1-hour exposure is used. Using HEC-1A cells (human endometrial carcinoma), a 1-hour exposure at 10 μg/ml was equitoxic to a 20-hour exposure at only 0.001 μg/ml (20% survival). This is especially interesting in light of these same investigators' results regarding the instability (60% decay over 72 hours) of VP-16.[16] Matsushima et al[39] confirm the significant schedule dependency of both VP-16 and VM-26 cytotoxicity versus a human carcinoma in vitro.

IN VIVO DATA

Early studies with L1210-bearing mice did not suggest any significant schedule dependency for VM-26.[27] Vietti et al[69] assessed the in vivo cytotoxicity of VM-26 using both an I.V. bolus and 24-hour infusion. The toxicity of the 2 schedules is comparable, as there was little difference in the maximal doses for each schedule. In contrast, there was greater than a 1-log increase in cytotoxicity (vs. L1210) for the infusion schedule. Broggini et al[70] found that divided doses of VM-26 every 3 days were more effective and less toxic than an equivalent single bolus dose.

Dombernowsky and Nissen[71] compared various schedules of VP-16 administration in L1210-bearing mice. They did not use continuous infusion, but assessed the effect of frequent (every 3 hours) small doses on survival. Cures were achievable with all 16 schedules, but a 100% cure rate was achieved only by using 3.75 mg/kg every 3 hours on days 1 and 5. Further studies of these drugs are needed to compare frequent dosing to continuous infusion.

Other Alkaloids

ELLIPTICINE

Ellipticine is a plant alkaloid with significant antileukemic properties.[72] It appears to act via intercalation into DNA. Traganos et al[72] studied the effects of different exposure times on a variety of mammalian cell lines in vitro. The drug appears to be cytostatic, with G_2-phase specificity. A 2-hour exposure at high (6.0 μg/ml) concentration was equivalent in cytotoxicity to a 24-hour exposure at low (0.3 μg/ml) concentrations.

HARRINGTONINE

Harringtonine is a plant alkaloid isolated from an evergreen tree indigenous to China.[73] The drug has significant activity in both leukemia and lymphoma. It appears to act via inhibition of protein synthesis and secondarily inhibits DNA synthesis. Takemura et al (73) demonstrate that the in vitro activity of harringtonine (versus human leukemia and lymphoma cells) is more dependent on exposure time than concentration. There was only minimal cytotoxic activity with 3 μM harringtonine for 1 hour (80% survival), while 0.3 μM harringtonine for 24 hours resulted in a 1-log cell kill. They also found that increasing the exposure time increased the slope of the dose response curve. Therefore, it is reasonable to administer harringtonine (and the related drug homoharringtonine) by continuous infusion, although in vivo studies of harringtonine infusions are needed.

Alkylating Agents

The alkylating agents are a diverse group of drugs with a final common pathway—the covalent binding of alkyl groups of the drug to DNA.[74] The alkylating agents are not phase-specific, but may have an increased effect on cells in cycle. They are usually classified as type 1 agents,[1] which would not be expected to have increased activity with infusion.

The first alkylating agents included cyclophosphamide (CTX), nitrogen mustard, and melphalan (MEL). Other alkylating agents include the nitrosoureas, mitomycin (MIT) (requires bioreduction to active form), and cisplatin (DDP) (and analogues).

Cyclophosphamide (CTX)

CTX is a widely used antineoplastic agent. It is available in both oral and parenteral forms, although the bioavailability of the oral form may have significant interindividual variation.[75] CTX is eliminated fairly rapidly by metabolism and urinary excretion, with a half-life of approximately 7 hours. The activated metabolites appear to have an even shorter half-life.

CTX is inactive in vitro because of the requirement for activation in vivo. However, the in vivo studies addressing the schedule dependency of CTX conclusively demonstrate that the drug should be given in a single bolus dose rather than in divided doses.

IN VIVO DATA

Early in vivo studies in L1210-bearing mice compared single (or weekly) doses to frequent intermittent dosing.[26,27,34] In all studies, a single or weekly dose was optimal. Skipper et al[26] cured 44/79 animals with a single dose of 300 mg/kg i.p., compared to no cures in 30 mice treated with 26 mg/kg daily for 15 days. The latter schedule had only minimal activity, with a 38% improvement in survival.

Nitrogen Mustard

Like CTX, nitrogen mustard is a type 1 agent[1] and would not be expected to have significant time dependency in vitro. There have been few studies of the pharmacokinetics of nitrogen mustard, but it appears to have a very short half-life of approximately 9 minutes.[76] In vivo studies of nitrogen mustard are therefore needed to determine the optimal scheduling of this drug.

IN VITRO DATA

Shimoyama[2] compared 30-minute and 48-hour exposures of nitrogen mustard in 4 different cell lines. There was only a slight decrease in the drug concentration required for 1-log cytotoxicity when the exposure time was lengthened 100-fold (ranging from 23 to 72%). This is the expected in vitro pattern for an alkylating agent.

IN VIVO DATA

Bruce et al[77] compared the in vivo effects of bolus and divided (every 6 hours × 4) doses of nitrogen mustard in lymphoma-bearing mice. Using bolus dosing (0.1 to 0.4 mg/mouse), there was equal effect of the drug on both normal and malignant cells (using colony-forming assays). However, when the same total dose was administered in 4 installments (every 6 hours), there was a five- to ninefold therapeutic advantage versus the malignant cells. Toxicity to normal cells was slightly less, but significantly increased toxicity to malignant colony-forming units was observed. This result is somewhat surprising, and it is not known whether other alkylating agents have decreased myelosuppression when administered in divided doses.

Melphalan (MEL)

Melphalan is a nitrogen mustard analogue that is usually administered by oral dosing. There have been no in vivo studies of the schedule dependency of MEL, but the in vitro data do not favor the use of infusion for administration.

IN VITRO DATA

Wu et al[23] compared the effects of 1-hour and 14-day exposures of MEL on Raji lymphoma cells in vitro. Prolonged exposure did not increase the cytotoxicity of MEL, possibly because it appears to be unstable at 37°. Matsushima et al[39] were able to demonstrate increased cytotoxicity with prolonged exposure, as 2 μg/ml for 1 hour was equivalent to 0.4 μg/ml for 24 hours. However, the effect of lengthening the exposure was small in comparison to many of the other drugs studied.

The Nitrosoureas

The nitrosoureas are unique among the alkylating agents because of their lipophilicity, ability to cross the blood-brain barrier, and delayed toxicity.[74] The nitrosoureas would not be expected to be good candidates for continuous infusion, as they are type 1 agents like the other alkylators. Drug stability is also a problem, particularly for carmustine (BCNU).[78,79]

IN VITRO DATA

Wheeler et al[79] evaluated the importance of exposure time on carmustine cytotoxicity. A major problem they encountered was the instability (half-life of approximately 1 hour) of the drug. However, they were able to show that the survival fraction is related to the total area under the curve of extracellular BCNU:

$$SF = Ne^{-K \cdot AUC}$$

This would suggest that prolonged infusion might have equivalent activity to a single bolus (if the elimination of BCNU is first-order), but does not suggest any advantage to infusion.

IN VIVO DATA

Venditti et al[34] compared the effects of a variety of schedules of BCNU administration on murine L1210 leukemia. A single dose of 96 mg/kg cured 5 of 8 mice and was the optimal schedule. Low-dose daily administration of BCNU (6 mg/kg × 50 days) was effective, with an increase in survival of 463%, but was not curative.

Schmidt et al[80] used an ingenious delivery system in L1210–bearing mice. They used implanted silicone rubber capsules to administer BCNU dissolved in either ethanol or sesame oil. This allows for the slow release of the drug over a 16-hour period. Capsules were inserted both subcutaneously and intraperitoneally and were compared to standard intraperitoneal injections. The delivery of BCNU by slow diffusion was quite effective, with up to 15 of 20 cures (using sesame oil and subcutaneous placement), compared to no cures with intraperitoneal therapy.

Streptozotocin is another nitrosourea that may be a candidate for continuous infusion. Venditti's early studies[27] with L1210 leukemia showed that the only active schedule appeared to be small daily treatments (for 9 days).

In addition to their other unique properties among the alkylating agents, the nitrosoureas may have increased efficacy when administered by infusion. Further studies are needed, although the instability of these drugs may limit the practical testing of this schedule of administration.

Mitomycin-C (MIT)

Mitomycin-C was originally thought to be an antibiotic, but it acts as an alkylating agent when its quinone group is reduced.[81] The elimination and pharmacokinetics of MIT are not well defined, but the drug appears to have an elimination half-life of only 1 to 2 hours.[82] Thus, MIT would be a candidate for infusion if there is significant time-dependent cytotoxicity.

IN VITRO DATA

The cytotoxicity of MIT appears to be a function of the product $C \times T$,[2,83] a property of most alkylating agents. However, Barlogie and Drewinko[83] suggest that there may be less recovery from potentially lethal damage with a short exposure, compared to a longer exposure at equal $C \times T$.

Wu et al[23] suggest that very low concentrations (0.01 μg/ml) of MIT are effective if maintained for 14 days, although the $C \times T$ is higher than that for an equally effective short exposure. Matsushima et al[39] also showed that prolonged exposure of MIT is less pharmacologically efficient than a shorter exposure.

Cisplatin (DDP)

Although DDP is similar to other alkylating agents in its ability to bind DNA, it has several qualities that make it (and other platinum analogues) unique. Cisplatin blocks LoVo cells in S and G_2 phase, suggesting that the drug may be phase-specific.[84] In addition, the ultrafilterable (free) plasma concentration rapidly decreases following bolus administration, with an elimination half-life of less than 1 hour.[85] It also may cause severe nephrotoxicity, requiring special precautions during and after drug administration. The use of continuous infusion of this unique drug might be expected to be superior to standard therapy, but experimental data to date do not strongly support this hypothesis.

IN VITRO DATA

The pharmacodynamics of DDP in vitro are complex. Rupniak et al[6] demonstrate that the slope of the dose-response curve is increased as the exposure time is increased, for both ovarian and colon carcinoma cell lines. However, the colon cell line was more sensitive (greater increase in slope) to changes in the exposure time. For example, with the colon cell line, a 1-hour exposure at 3 μg/ml resulted in 40% survival and a 6-hour exposure of 0.5 μg/ml resulted in only 10% survival. Thus, for equal $C \times T$, the prolonged exposure was more active. With the ovarian cell line, a 1-hour exposure at 5 μg/ml resulted in 40% survival, while a 6-hour exposure at 1 μg/ml resulted in 50% survival. Therefore, there was little difference in activity per $C \times T$ between the 2 schedules for the ovarian line. Most other in vitro studies which address these questions do not suggest any advantage (in cytotoxicity per $C \times T$) to prolonged exposure,[86-88] and there may be a marked disadvantage to prolonged exposure for some cell lines.[23,61] In summary, one can only state that the optimal schedule of DDP in vitro may depend on the tumor line.

IN VIVO DATA

Although there have been multiple human studies of DDP by continuous infusion (see chapter by Ackland and Vogelzang), there has been only one in vivo study of the schedule dependency of DDP activity, using the L1210 leukemia model.[89] The treatment schedules used ranged from bolus infusion (optimal dose = 12 mg/kg) to a 72-hour infusion (optimal dose = 12 mg/kg/d). There was no significant advantage to any schedule when the optimal dose was used, but a 24-hour infusion was inferior to a bolus injection (increased life span of 32% versus 70%) when equal doses (12 mg/kg) were administered.

Antineoplastic Antibiotics

The group of agents generally classified as antibiotics is a diverse, complex set of agents that vary substantially in their schedule dependency in experimental systems. This group includes (1) classical anthracycline antibiotics; (2) anthracenes, which although not anthracycline antibiotics, share the planar ring structure with the anthracyclines; (3) bleomycin and its analogues; and (4) actinomycin D and other agents, including neocarzinostatin. The benefit of continuous infusion of antibiotic agents must be assessed for each agent independently.

Doxorubicin (ADR)

IN VITRO DATA

The schedule dependency of ADR has been the subject of many reports. Shimoyama[2] categorized ADR as a type 1-b drug, a concentration-dependent cytocidal drug with some time dependence. He concluded that for any given exposure duration, an increase in drug concentration results in increased cytotoxicity. Conversely, for a given concentration of drug, extending the duration of drug exposure increased the cytotoxicity.

Ludwig et al[61] examined schedule dependency in a clonogenic assay system and found that either a 1- or 200-hour exposure of tumor cells to doxorubicin was equally effective in inducing cytotoxicity. Matsushima et al,[39] using a clonogenic assay system, found ADR to be the least time dependent of 19 drugs tested against a human adenocarcinoma cell line. Drewinko et al, using the LoVo human colon adenocarcinoma cell line, found that cytotoxicity was maximal (90%) by 2 hours of ADR exposure.[90] No increase in cytotoxicity was observed with drug exposure duration of up to 50 hours.

Using mouse sarcoma cells, Nguyen-Ngoc et al described a classic dose response curve for ADR; cytotoxicity was an exponential function of drug concentration in the media.[91] Cytotoxicity was not an exponential function of exposure time. However, for a given drug concentration (i.e., 1 μg/ml) the cytotoxicity (as measured by tritiated thymidine incorporation) increased with exposure duration (30% at 1 minute, 55% at 3 minutes but only 71% at a 30-minute exposure). These data support Shimoyama's classification of ADR as a type 1-b drug. Wu et al, using a human Burkitt lymphoma line in soft agar, reached a conclusion that ADR ". . . produced a dose-dependent reduction in colony formation following a 1-hour exposure which was further augmented by a continuous exposure to the drug(s)." For example, a 1-hour exposure at 5 ng/ml killed only 30% of the cells, while a 14-day exposure at 5 ng/ml killed all of the Raji cells.[23] Again, this was consistent with Shimoyama's hypothesis.

Krishan and Frei, using human lymphoblasts, found a linear, not exponential, increase in cytotoxicity as the exposure times increased from 1 hour to 24 hours.[92] Barlogie et al reached a similar conclusion using T_1 cells (a human cell line) in culture.[93] These data add further support to the classification of ADR as a type 1-b drug.

Several reports suggest that exposure duration may be more important in achieving cytotoxicity than the ADR concentration. Eichholtz-Wirth, using both HeLa and Chinese hamster cells, reported that ADR-induced cytotoxicity was an exponential function of exposure time up to 4 hours.[94] They did not report results past 4 hours. They elegantly showed, however, that this time-dependent cytotoxicity was a function of the time it took ADR to achieve cytotoxic intracellular concentrations.

Zirvi et al, using a human colon adenocarcinoma cell line, found that all tested anthracyclines, including ADR, were more cytotoxic with low dose/continuous exposure (14 hours) than with high dose/brief exposure (1 hour).[95] Rupniak et al, using a human ovarian cell suspension, found that cytotoxicity was an exponential function of both ADR dose and exposure duration.[6]

One interesting study by Baily-Wood et al examined the effect of bolus and continuous exposure doxorubicin on normal mouse and human marrow cells.[96] A brief (1-hour) high (1 μM) doxorubicin exposure resulted in a loss of 40% of the cells; exposure to a prolonged (7 days) low (0.1 μM) concentration of ADR levels killed only 20% of the cells. The authors concluded that prolonged exposure at low concentrations was more cytotoxic than a brief exposure at higher concentrations, but these reviewers believe that it is consistent with Shimoyama's categorization of ADR.

IN VIVO DATA

Ensminger el al used an ingenious technique to administer either a 3-day continuous infusion or bolus ADR to rats with acute myelogenous leukemia.[97] In this model system, the infusion was slightly more effective, but also more toxic.

Goldin and Johnson concluded that ADR had no schedule dependency in either L1210 or P388 murine leukemia, B-16 melanoma, or Lewis lung carcinoma.[98] A single bolus on day 1 was as effective as a daily × 9 days drug administration schedule.

Sandberg et al, in the L1210 model, concluded that a single bolus of ADR was therapeutically equivalent to daily q 3-hour injections.[99] However, the data revealed that the most survivors occurred when animals were given injections of a q 3-hour basis for the first day only. Venditti[27] reiterated the data of Sandberg et al.

Paccidrini et al, using a murine mammary carcinoma or a Lewis lung carcinoma, treated animals with either a single bolus dose or the same dose of ADR divided over 4 days.[100] They found both increased survival and slightly decreased toxicity (20% early deaths vs 0% early deaths) with divided dose schedules. The intracardiac ADR concentration levels of drug were lower in the animals treated daily × 4. Jensen et al [101] and Solcia et al[102] both reported that cardiotoxicity was more severe in animals given bolus ADR than in animals receiving either long-term infusion or low-dose daily injections.

In conclusion, it appears that ADR is equally effective either as a bolus or as a continuous infusion. The toxicity in vivo appears to be less with continuous infusion.

Other Anthracyclines

There are many analogues of ADR, including older drugs such as daunorubicin, aclacinomycin A and AD32,[103] as well as the newer analogues 4'-deoxy-doxorubicin, 4'-epidoxorubicin, and 4'-0-methyldoxorubicin.[104] The previous comments regarding doxorubicin generally also apply to daunorubicin.[2,27,39,61,98,99,105]

Aclacinomycin A appears to be similar to ADR,[39] but one report[106] suggests that using mouse L cells, a 24-hour exposure to the drug is substantially (greater than 1 log) more cytotoxic than a 1-hour drug exposure to a similar drug concentration. The schedule dependency of the new anthracyclines has been infrequently tested,[95,107] and they appear to follow the pattern of ADR. As some of these agents appear to be noncross-resistant with doxorubicin,[104] further studies of their schedule dependency are needed.

Mitoxantrone

This is the first anthracene derivative to enter clinical trials, and it appears to have activity in breast cancer, acute leukemia, and malignant lymphoma.[108]

Drewinko et al examined the schedule dependency of mitoxantrone against LoVo colon cancer cells.[90] Mitoxantrone was highly cytotoxic to LoVo cells by either bolus or infusion. In this system, prolonged exposure (50 hours) was able to reduce cell viability to 0.01 percent control. Doxorubicin, for the same period, reduced cell viability to only 10% of control.

Fountzilas et al, using human pancreatic adenocarcinoma cells, found that increasing exposure time did not increase cytotoxicity.[109] They could not rule out the possibility that the drug was inactivated under tissue culture conditions after a five-day exposure.

Neocarzinostatin (Zinostatin)

This polypeptide antibiotic is no longer clinically available because of its association with anaphylaxis and death.[110] Shimoyama[2] classified zinostatin as a nonschedule-dependent (type 1-a) drug. Ensminger et al reported that continuous zinostatin was less effective than bolus drug administration in vivo.[97] Further discussions of the schedule dependency of this drug are beyond the scope of this review.

Bisantrene

Bisantrene is one of the anthracenediones which is still in phase 2 trials.[111,112] It has definite activity in breast carcinoma.[113] It is poorly soluble in plasma, regularly causes phlebitis,[114] and therefore has been withdrawn from clinical trials pending reformulation. The drug has a terminal half-life of approximately 30 hours and is clinically given on a q 3- to 4-week bolus schedule.[114]

IN VITRO DATA

Ludwig et al[61] studied 83 clinical specimens in the clonogenic assay and found that 23 tumors (28%) were sensitive to 1-hour exposures to bisantrene. No specimens were sensitive to a 200-hour exposure if they were resistant to a 1-hour exposure. The investigators concluded that bisantrene was not schedule dependent and "should be most active clinically when used in a high dose with an intermittent schedule." Drewinko et al[99] exposed human LoVo colon cancer cells to bisantrene (10 μg/ml) for 1 to 50 hours and found a steady decline in cell survival as duration of exposure was increased. Large increases in bisantrene concentration failed to increase cell kill.

IN VIVO DATA

Citarella et al[111] examined multiple bisantrene schedules in a variety of murine tumors (P388 leukemia, B16 melanoma, Lewis lung carcinoma, etc.). They found equal efficacy with virtually all drug schedules used to treat P388 leukemia, whereas the optimal schedule in B16 melanoma and Ridgeway osteosarcoma was a single bolus dose of the drug.

Bleomycin (BLM)

Bleomycin is a unique antineoplastic agent isolated from a soil streptomyces by Umezawa in the 1960s.[115] It is not a single chemical, but is rather a complex mixture of glycopeptides that can be separated chromatographically into 2 large fractions, A and B, and into 13 different subfractions.[116,117] BLM acts as a mininuclease, causing DNA single strand scissions and release of thymine from the DNA strand.[118,119]

BLM pharmacokinetics were initially performed using bioassays and indium[111] radio-labeled drugs. These assays predicted a very short drug half-life of 16–45 minutes.[120] Development of a radioimmunoassay allowed more precise definition of the initial (1.3 $\pm$ 0.1 hours) and the terminal (3.2–8.9 hours) half-lives.[121,122] In some patients with renal failure, the terminal half-life is considerably prolonged (up to 33 hours).[121]

IN VITRO DATA

Clinical data suggested that continuous infusion or I.M. injections had a therapeutic advantage over bolus I.V. delivery of BLM.[123,124] Six studies[23,39,61,125,126] have reported that BLM cytotoxicity is significantly enhanced with prolonged drug exposure.

There are problems with the studies; for example, the concentrations of BLM used for the in vitro studies usually were not clinically achievable. Broughton et al[121] reported a steady state level of BLM of 0.08–0.3 μg/ml in patients receiving 30 units/day as an infusion, whereas Yee et al reported steady state levels of 0.188–0.32 μg/ml in children receiving similar doses.[122] The most valuable studies in examining the concentration of bleomycin from a clinical point of view were those by Ludwig et al[61] and Matsushima et al.[39]

Ludwig et al[61] found that of 25 clinical tumor specimens tested against BLM, only 6 were sensitive to the drug. However, 4 of those 6 were sensitive only at the 200-hour exposure. The drug concentration for a 1-hour exposure needed to reduce cell growth to 50% of control was 900 times higher than the drug concentration for 200 hours needed to reduce cell growth to 50% of control. The report recommended continuous exposure BLM in clinical human trials. Matsushima et al[39] drew a similar conclusion using the same methodology.

Finally, these studies suggest that at high in vitro BLM doses, an increased duration of exposure increases the fractional cell kill.[125,126] It is unclear, however, whether there is an increased cell kill with increased duration of exposure at low BLM doses. This point has not been clearly defined by the authors of these studies. A classical dose response curve for BLM, that is, a logarithmic increase in cell kill with an increase in drug dose while holding duration of drug exposure constant, seems to exist only for certain cell types[39,126] and not for others.[125]

IN VIVO DATA

There have been few in vivo studies on BLM scheduling, and the data generated have been somewhat contradictory. The study by Takabe et al[127] studied only a 6-hour infusion, but reported an increased tumoricidal effect. Sikic et al[128] and Peng et al[129] directly compared studies of I.V. bolus and infusion schedules in animal models (Lewis lung and P388 leukemia, respectively). Although both studies concluded that infusion was superior to bolus, Peng et al showed only a 0.5-log greater cell kill with infusion than with bolus. Sikic et al likewise showed improvement of less than 1-log cell kill.

The strong opinions of Sikic et al, namely that the infusion of bleomycin caused increased tumor cell kill and decreased pulmonary toxicity, have provided much of the rationale for clinical continuous infusion BLM studies. However, no similar studies have been performed to confirm the findings of Sikic et al.

In conclusion, the in vitro data support the continuous infusion of BLM, whereas in vivo model systems provide equivocal support. These data, combined with the mechanism of action of BLM, namely its cell cycle—specific action, all strongly suggest that continuous infusion of BLM is a superior method for administration of the drug.

Actinomycin D

Actinomycins were first isolated from a soil *Streptomyces* species in 1940.[130] Numerous actinomycins exist, but only actinomycin D is used clinically. Actinomycin D binds to DNA between complementary pairs of deoxyguanosine residues.[131] This intercalation into the DNA helix probably blocks the progression of RNA polymerases along the DNA. The tight binding to DNA may explain why early studies found that actinomycin D is cytotoxic at any phase of the cell cycle.[132] It is usually given on a daily I.V. bolus × 5 days schedule, but recent pharmacokinetic analysis has suggested that single I.V. bolus dosing at 3-week intervals may be equally effective.[131]

IN VITRO DATA

Four in vitro studies have examined the schedule dependency of actinomycin D. Wu et al[23] found that a dose of 0.05 μg/ml for 1 hour allowed 81% survival of Raji-Burkitts lymphoma cells in the clonogenic assay, while a similar exposure for 14 days allowed 0% survival. A dose of 0.5 μg/ml for 1 hour was required to produce 0% survival. Ludwig et al[61] used the clonogenic assay to study sensitivity of 35 human tumors to either 1- or 200-hour exposure to actinomycin D. Only 4 tumors were sensitive, and continuous exposure did not increase the number of "sensitive" specimens. Matsushima et al[39] could not show any schedule dependency of actinomycin D against PC-7 human lung adenocarcinoma cells. Finally, Shimoyama[2] reported that cytotoxicity in mouse and human cells from actinomycin D was concentration-dependent and only slightly time-dependent, and classified it as a type 1-b agent.

IN VIVO DATA

Valeriote et al,[133] using AKR murine leukemia, found that cytotoxicity to leukemia cells and normal cells was concentration-dependent, but paradoxically recommended frequent small doses of the drug. Galbraith and Mellett[134] found that a single nonlethal dose of actinomycin D cured Ridgeway osteogenic sarcoma, and that all animals receiving daily doses (continuous schedule) died. This was attributed to higher drug levels within the tumor. Valeriote et al also found that the single bolus dose was more toxic than daily × 5 bolus schedule.

Miscellaneous Agents

Asparaginase

Asparaginase is a naturally occurring enzyme that hydrolyzes intravascular asparagine, thereby inhibiting protein synthesis. Normal cells are not affected, as they usually can synthesize their own asparagine.[135] There are few experimental data regarding the optimal scheduling of asparaginase, although it is commonly administered in divided doses or by continuous infusion.[136]

Fountzilas et al[109] compared the effects of 1- and 120-hour exposures on a human pancreatic carcinoma cell line in vitro. Asparaginase was virtually ineffective after a 1-hour exposure, but a 10 mM concentration for 120 hours inhibited cell growth by 94%. There are no in vivo studies of the schedule dependency of asparaginase.

Methyl-GAG

Methyl-GAG indirectly inhibits DNA synthesis via its effects on polyamine synthesis,[137] although it may also inhibit the activation of transfer RNA.[138] There are no in vitro studies of the schedule dependency of this investigational agent, but Venditti et al[33,34] have evaluated the schedule dependency of methyl-GAG in the murine L1210 leukemia model. The use of divided doses (2 to 4 times daily) was slightly more effective than single daily doses, with an increase in survival of approximately 25%. A single injection was virtually ineffective, but other schedules were not tested. Weekly administration of the drug appears to be an optimal clinical schedule.[139]

Acivicin

Acivicin, a glutamine antimetabolite, has recently entered clinical trials. Fountzilas et al[109] have shown that a continuous exposure (120 hours) of acivicin is active at extracellular concentrations ≥ 0.1 μM, with $< 10\%$ survival at 10 μM. Ethridge and Von Hoff[140] recently confirmed these results using a variety of human tumors. Using a 1 μg/ml drug concentration, a 1-hour exposure was effective ($< 50\%$ survival) in 9/47 tumors (19%), compared to an efficacy rate of 17/137 (46%) with continuous exposure. There are no in vivo studies of the schedule dependency of this new drug. Infusions of the drug for 72 hours have entered clinical trials; preliminary data suggest an improved therapeutic index.[141]

Pentamethylmelamine

The mechanism of action of pentamethylmelamine is unknown, although it is structurally similar to triethylmelamine, an alkylating agent. Unlike the alkylating agents, it appears to be cytotoxic only with continuous exposure. Wu et al[23] assessed the cytotoxic activity of pentamethylmelamine and other drugs against a human lymphoma cell line. A 1-hour exposure was ineffective at concentrations ≤ 50 μg/ml, but continuous exposure (for 14 days) was effective at concentrations ≥ 1 μg/ml. There are no other studies of the schedule dependency of pentamethylmelamine or its related drug, hexamethylmelamine.

Summary

It should be clear to the reader that the optimal scheduling of antineoplastic drugs is a complex subject. Based on in vitro data, 16 drugs appear to have significant schedule dependency favoring infusion therapy (table 1). Only 2 drugs, nitrogen mustard and neocarzinostatin, have significant schedule dependency against continuous infusion.

However, in vivo studies of divided doses or infusion have been confirmatory in only a subset of the 16 drugs cited above (table 2). There is strong experimental support for infusing the antimetabolites, with the exception of 6-mercaptopuine and 6-thioguanine. Further in vivo studies are required in support of the in vitro results using 5-FU and related drugs.

Table 1. Summary of In Vitro Data Favoring Infusion or Bolus Therapy

Favoring infusion therapy			Favoring bolus therapy
+++	++	+	
Ara-C	5-aza-2'-deoxycytidene	Mitoxantrone	Nitrogen mustard
Methotrexate	5-fluorouracil		Neocarzinostatin
Vincristine	Hydroxyurea		
Vinblastine	Harringtonine		
Vindesine	Acivicin		
VP-16	L-asparaginase		
VM-26	Pentamethylmelamine		
Bleomycin			

There is also a strong rationale for administering the plant alkaloids by continuous infusion. Based on in vitro studies, harringtonine, a new alkaloid, is very promising, and in vivo studies of the infusion of harringtonine should be encouraged.

With the important exception of the nitrosoureas, the alkylating agents appear, in general, to have a decreased therapeutic index by continuous infusion. The apparent efficacy of BCNU by infusion is especially surprising, as the in vitro studies were equivocal. Cisplatin activity appears to be relatively inde-

Table 2. Summary of Experimental Data Supporting Infusion Therapy by Class of Agent

Agent	In vitro	In vivo
Antimetabolites		
Ara-C	+ + +	+ + +
5-aza-2′-deoxycytidine	+ +	+
6-MP/6-TG[a]	N.D.[b]	±
5-FU/5-FUdR	+ +	N.D.
Methotrexate	+ + +	+ +[c]
Hydroxyurea	+ +	+
Alkaloids		
Vinca alkaloids	+ + +	+
Epipodophyllotoxins	+ +	+ +
Ellipticine	±	N.D.
Harringtonine	+ +	N.D.
Alkylating agents		
Cyclophosphamide	N.D.[d]	Inf.
Nitrogen mustard	Inf.	±
Melphalan	±	N.D.
Nitrosoureas	±	+ +
Mitomycin C	±	N.D.
Cisplatin	±	±
Antibiotics		
Anthracyclines	±	±
Mitoxantrone	+	N.D.
Neocarzinostatin	Inf.	Inf.
Bisantrene	±	Inf.
Bleomycin	+ + +	+ +
Actinomycin D	±	+
Miscellaneous agents		
L-asparaginase	+ +	N.D.
Methyl-GAG	N.D.	+
Acivicin	+ +	N.D.
Pentamethylmelamine	+ +	N.D.

[a]Abbreviations of drugs: 6-MP = 6-mercaptopurine, 6-TG = 6-thioguanine, 5-FU = 5-fluorouracil, 5-FUdR = 5-fluorodeoxyuridine
[b]N.D. = Not done, Inf. = Infusion (or continuous exposure) *inferior* to bolus treatment
[c]Optimal schedule may depend on tumor burden
[d]Inactive in vitro, as it requires activation

pendent of schedule, although infusion therapy may potentially ameliorate the severe gastrointestinal and renal toxicity of this important agent.

The antibiotics are a diverse group of drugs. Experimental data strongly support bleomycin infusion, but the data for the anthracyclines and actinomycin are equivocal. In vivo studies are needed for mitoxantrone, in light of the in vitro data.

Finally, several miscellaneous agents appear to be promising candidates for infusion. Acivicin is particularly interesting because of its probable antimetabolic activity, although in vivo studies are needed.

Many of the drugs discussed here have been employed in clinical trials. However, we hope that this chapter will help focus further trials of infusion chemotherapy.

3

THE CLINICAL PHARMACOLOGY OF INFUSIONAL CHEMOTHERAPY

Gregory A. Curt, M.D., and Jerry M. Collins, Ph.D.

INCREASING INTEREST IN ADMINISTERING anticancer chemotherapy via prolonged systemic infusion is predicated on a number of observations. The first is that both acute and chronic normal tissue toxicities may be ameliorated when some agents are delivered as a continuous infusion. It has been reported that the cardiac toxicity of Adriamycin (ADR),[1-4] the pulmonary toxicity of bleomycin (BLM),[5-7] the nephrotoxicity and neurotoxicity of cisplatin (DDP),[8,9] streptozotocin and gallium nitrate,[10] and the bone marrow toxicity of 5-fluorouracil (5-FU)[12-15] are significantly reduced when these drugs are infused over a period of 1 to 180 days rather than as a bolus I.V. injection. Presumably, normal tissue toxicities are related in some way to peak drug concentrations. Importantly, antitumor activity may be preserved through use of these regimens, suggesting improved therapeutic index. Indeed, in some instances, patients may respond to infusional therapy after failing to respond to the same agent administered conventionally.[16]

Infusional therapy is empirically logical, especially for cycle-specific agents. Antimetabolites such as methotrexate (MTX), cytosine arabinoside (ara-C), and azacytidine are selectively cytotoxic in S phase, while BLM is most toxic between M and G_2 of the cell cycle. Although such particularly aggressive human tumors as Burkitt's lymphoma, testicular cancer, Ewing's sarcoma, and diffuse lymphomas may have doubling times of less than 30 days, more common malignancies such as small-cell and squamous-cell carcinoma of the lung and adenocarcinoma of lung, colon, and breast have clinical doubling times in excess of 2 months.[17] Because most cancer chemotherapeutic agents have relatively short half-lives (table 1), the likelihood of "capturing" cells in a sensitive portion of the cell cycle is improved when drugs are administered over a more prolonged schedule.

However, there are also empiric disadvantages to administering drugs via infusion. Chief among these is the potential for selection of drug-resistant clones. Certainly, this concept has a strong in vitro foundation; stepwise selection of resistant cells in sublethal but increasing drug concentrations has been accomplished with a variety of agents.[32] This limitation may be overcome by regional infusion of the involved organ[33] to allow higher local drug concentrations.

Clinical studies should be guided by the principles of pharmacokinetic modeling, which may be important in predicting the relative advantage in giving a specific drug via infusion or a specific intra-arterial or intracavitary route. For some drugs, specialized routes or schedules of administration are scientifically rational; for others, they are not. Irrespective of these guiding principles, the clinical utility of those approaches for most agents await confirmation by well-designed and well-implemented clinical studies. In this chapter, we will review the pharmacokinetic principles of both systemic and regional infusional therapy.

The eventual importance of this approach is predicated on a better understanding not only of the pharmacokinetics but also the pharmacodynamics of anticancer drugs. Through the use of preclinical in vitro screens, it will become increasingly possible to assess the importance of peak drug effects and drug threshold versus "concentration × time" effects. These principles have been successfully translated to the clinic in cardiology and infectious diseases and are likely to become increasingly applicable to cancer medicine as well. Indeed, as the therapeutic index for anticancer drugs is particularly narrow, pharmacokinetic modeling is uniquely important in medical oncology.

Table 1. Half-Lives of Common Chemotherapeutic Agents

Drug	Half-Life (hrs)	Reference
Methotrexate	2 – 8	(18 – 21)
Adriamycin	30	(22,23)
Cyclophosphamide	3 – 10	(24,25)
Vincristine	85	(26)
Cis-platinum	0.2	(27,28)
Cytosine Arabinoside	0.5	(29,30)
5-Fluorouracil	0.5	(31)

Pharmacokinetics of Infusional Therapy

The pharmacokinetic modeling of drugs given by continuous infusion is simplified by the fact that the differential equations that define the transfer processes between compartments can be expressed in simple algebraic terms. For example, the differential equation for a one-compartment model is:

$$V_c \frac{dC_P}{dt} = G - CL_{TB}C_P$$

where V_c is the volume of distribution, C_P is plasma concentration, G is the rate of drug input, and CL_{TB} is the total body clearance. At steady-state, $dC_P/dt = 0$. Thus,

$$C_{ss} = G/CL_{TB}$$

where C_{ss} is steady-state concentration.

For a multicompartmental model,

$$V_c \frac{dC_P}{dt} = G - CL_{TB} C_P + \sum_i [k_{ic} (C_i/R_i - C_P)]$$

where k_{ic} is the exchange rate between the ith compartment and the central compartment. During steady-state conditions, the change in plasma concentration over time (dC_P/dt) is 0, as are the net exchanges between compartments. Thus, the concentration of drug within any compartment, C_i, can be directly expressed as a function (or partition coefficient, R_i) between that compartment and the central compartment:

$$C_i = R_i C_P.$$

As with the one-compartment model, the concentration of drug in the central compartment is directly proportional to the infusion rate and inversely proportional to the clearance of the drug:

$$C_{ss} = G/CL_{TB}.$$

As mentioned previously, one of the basic considerations for infusional therapy is a desire to sustain drug concentrations for a sufficient period to expose cycling cells to effective drug levels. In the past, intermittent bolus doses have been given to partially achieve this goal. The current availability of a variety of delivery devices makes continuous delivery practical in many cases.

The half-life of a drug is the principal pharmacokinetic parameter for deciding between intermittent versus continuous schedules. Figure 1 illustrates the effect of half-life in schedule selection. In the left panel, the drug half-life is very long (48 hours) and the difference is negligible between plasma levels of drug for 5 daily bolus doses versus 120-hour continuous infusion. The panel on the right illustrates the more dramatic differences that are produced for a drug that has a half-life of 2 hours, which is more common (see table 1). The ratio of peak to trough concentrations is greater than 100. Not all drugs have a rationale for continuous infusion, but half-life can be very useful in choosing appropriate cases.

Regional Therapy

Regional chemotherapy can be either intra-arterial (I.A.) or intracavitary (i.e., intrathecal, intraperitoneal, or intravesicular). In each case, the relative advantages of the regional route are dependent not only on the dose-response curve for the individual drug and tumor but also on specific pharmacokinetic principles. For regional drug delivery, the selection of bolus versus continuous infusion schedules is determined by the same principles as for systemic delivery. However, the levels that are delivered to the local area can be amplified substantially.

Figure 2 is a generalized model for regional drug delivery. It is easiest to describe first in terms of I.A. delivery and then to generalize for intracavitary routes. In terms of drug delivery, the relative advantage of the I.A. over the intravenous route of administration for a given drug is defined as: $R_d = C_{arterial}/C_{iv}$ where R_d is the relative delivery advantage, $C_{arterial}$ is the steady-state concentration of drug achieved during arterial infusion therapy, and C_{iv} is the concentration of drug achievable via I.V. infusion. For bolus or intermittent therapy, the same concepts apply if $[C \times T]$ is substituted for concentration.

This relative advantage is determined by both the total body clearance of the drug and the arterial infusion rate:[33] $R_d = 1 + CL_{TB}/Q$ where CL_{TB} is total body clearance of the drug and Q is the flow rate of the artery that is infused. When the organ being infused eliminates or clears the drug itself, there is an additional advantage:

$$R_d = 1 + CL_{TB}/[Q(1-E)]$$

where E is the first-pass extraction ratio from the organ being perfused. The most important concept from these equations is that the simple ratio of clearance to blood flow is the determinant of the relative advantage of the intraarterial route. Furthermore, this information is easily obtained before clinical trials and should guide the design of protocols and drug selection. Specifically, I.A. infusion will provide the most favorable relative advantage in organ sys-

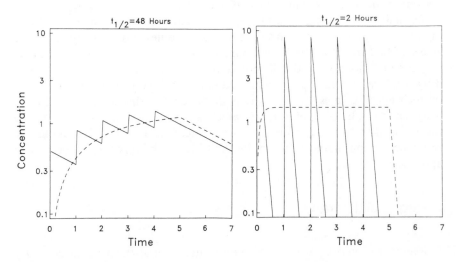

Figure 1. Comparison of 5 daily doses with doses by continuous infusion.

tems with low arterial flow rates. Once a particular artery has been selected, the choice of drug(s) to be infused depends upon both activity against the tumor and clearance from the body.

The same questions are applicable to intracavitary infusions if Q is defined as the exchange rate for the drug between the cavity and the rest of the body. Drugs delivered by the intracavitary route have lower exchange rates than drugs administered intra-arterially, and so have greater drug delivery advantages.

Table 2 ranks some common anticancer drugs in order of total body clearance and predicts the relative advantage in terms of concentration at the target tumor site for flow rates of 10, 100, and 1,000 ml/min. Drugs with high

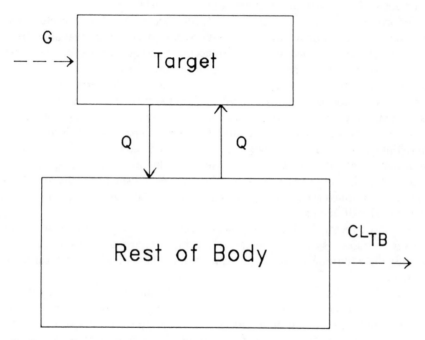

Figure 2. Generalized model for regional drug delivery.

Table 2. Relative Advantage of Regional Infusion for Antitumor Drugs

CL_{TB}	Drug	Q = 10 (ml/min)	Q = 100 (ml/min)	Q = 1000 (ml/min)
25000	FUDR	2500	250	26
4000	5-FU	400	40	5
3000	Ara-C	300	30	4
1000	BCNU	100	10	2
900	Doxorubicin	90	10	2
400	Cisplatin	40	4	1.4
200	Methotrexate	20	3	1.2
40	Etoposide	5	1.4	1.0

Adapted from Collins.[33]

systemic clearance rates (FUDR, 5-FU, ara-C) can be given with significant therapeutic advantage even in organs with high flow rates, but there is little to be gained from administering drugs with low total body clearance (such as etoposide) at such sites. An important corollary of this principle is that drugs requiring activation at a site other than the organ being infused cannot be given I.A. with any therapeutic advantage.

It is here that consideration must be given to the difference between the relatively straightforward measurement of drug concentrations (pharmacokinetics) and the study of drug effects at a given site (pharmacodynamics). While pharmacokinetics study the distribution and elimination of drugs, pharmacodynamics measure therapeutic and toxic effects at the tumor and end organ levels. Our current understanding of the pharmacodynamics of antitumor agents is fragmentary and woefully incomplete.

Improved treatment options for cancer therapy can be expected from approaches that improve the therapeutic index of currently available drugs. Recent technical advances in catheter placement and delivery devices offer new options for both route and schedule of drug administration.

Infusional therapy offers theoretical advantages in terms of reduced toxicity — at a cost of increased effort — over intermittent drug delivery. There is no guarantee that the maximally tolerated infused dose may not be too low to be effective when balanced against tumor cell repair mechanisms and the development of drug resistance. Indeed, a recent comprehensive review of continuous infusion chemotherapy using 40 chemotherapeutic agents concluded that clinical utility had been reasonably established for only ara-C and BLM and cautioned the need for exploratory phase 2 or randomized studies for the majority of agents.[34]

Similarly, regional therapy promises higher drug concentrations at the target site with lower systemic drug levels. Again, this approach must be balanced against the additional effort required as well as the limitations of local organ toxicities.

This chapter has reviewed the theoretical advantages and modeling principles that form the basis for a rational approach in trial design with specific agents and routes of administration. However, the eventual role of these potentially superior treatment options can be answered only by well-designed, randomized and controlled clinical trials.

4

DRUG ADMINISTRATION SYSTEMS FOR INFUSION CHEMOTHERAPY

Elton M. Tucker, B.S.M.E.

Introduction

IT HAS LONG BEEN a goal of physicians to have the ability to deliver drugs to patients by targeted routes and on schedules that optimize the therapeutic benefit and minimize the undesirable side effects of drug therapy.[1] Achievement of this important objective has often been limited by such factors as the delivery system design, stability of the drug, compliance of the patient, the treatment costs, and pharmacokinetics of the drug.

Many delivery methods have been studied to achieve continuous availability of a drug with a short half-life. These methods include the use of frequent bolus injections, timed release of subcutaneous or intracavitary drug deposits and continuous infusion of drugs through implanted or percutaneous catheters.[2]

Progress made over the past two decades in the development of new drugs, and improvements in the effectiveness of existing drugs have created the need for new methods of drug delivery and have encouraged research to optimize the drug, the delivery equipment, and the treatment protocol as a total therapeutic system. With the advancements made in materials technology and the capability to miniaturize complex mechanical and electronic components, major improvements have been made possible in the accuracy, size, and safety of drug delivery systems. Multidiscipline teams of researchers from the clinical, engineering, and pharmaceutical specialities have created alternatives to the use of frequent hypodermic or needle injections for continuous drug availability. Some of these techniques include complex, multifunction electromechanical systems capable of responding to sensor feedback information of the patient's condition for optimizing drug delivery.[3,4]

A variety of systems may be considered when continuous infusion therapy is desired. Each system has certain advantages and limitations that must be clearly understood in relationship to the patient's need. For convenience, continuous or chronic intermittent infusion systems may be organized into such general categories as gravity feed systems, electrically powered bedside systems, patient-worn systems and totally implantable systems.

Two of these systems (patient-worn and totally implantable pumps) offer the obvious advantage of continuous infusion therapy for the ambulatory patient, whereas gravity-fed and electrically powered bedside systems impose serious limitations on the patient's mobility.

When an otherwise active, mobile patient requires infusion therapy, it is desirable to interfere as little as possible with the patient's routine and life-style while providing the necessary treatment. The use of a self-contained, patient-worn or implanted infusion system offers many new possibilities for improving the quality of life when treating infusion therapy patients as ambulatory hospital patients, ambulatory outpatients, or as home care patients.[5]

Patient-worn ambulatory or implanted pumps are generally self-contained systems consisting of a small disposable or refillable drug reservoir, a mechanical pumping and flow-metering system, an electronic control circuit, a malfunction alarm system, and a disposable or rechargeable power system. The components are densely packaged in a small, durable container to be carried in a pouch worn by the patient or, in the case of the implantable system, surgically implanted in the subcutaneous tissue. A drug delivery tube set is used to conduct the infusion fluid from the pumping system to the patient.

Ambulatory systems have been developed to a high level of performance capability, reliability, and safety and are being increasingly accepted by patients and health care staffs. They offer the option of continuous or long-term intermittent infusion therapy for the active, mobile patient while maintaining many of the performance advantages of accuracy, flexibility, and safety of large electrically powered bedside systems.[6] Several alternative pump concepts have been developed for patient-worn and implantable systems for continuous of long-term intermittent chemotherapy. A variety of questions must be considered when selecting a safe, reliable, cost-effective system for the ambulatory patient. The therapy requirements and system demands must be fully defined and understood in relationship to the manufacturer's specifications as they concern:

- drug delivery accuracy
- volume of drug to be delivered per unit of time and per infusion cycle
- flexibility requirements for flow rate adjustments
- frequency of the infusion cycle and duration of the therapy
- compatibility of the drug with the reservoir and drug path
- drug stability under the anticipated environmental conditions
- patient and health-care team training requirements
- capability for close patient follow-up
- infusion site access method
- risks of delivery system damage by patient activities or living environment
- patient safety and protection features.

The above questions require that system selection be considered in very broad terms, including pump performance, system flexibility, drugs to be used, ability of the patient to participate in the therapy, and the availability of an adequately staffed and trained professional team for protocol and patient support.

Patient Worn Extracorporal Systems

In 1963, Elton Watkins Jr., M.D., reported pioneering work from the Lahey Clinic in Boston in the development of a miniaturized mechanical pumping system that could be worn by ambulatory chemotherapy infusion patients.[7] The system provided targeted drug infusion to the liver through a surgically implanted percutaneous catheter. By using a percutaneous catheter placed in the venous or arterial blood supply, it became possible to target the cytostatic delivery to the tumor site, at the same time offering the physician considerable latitude, flexibility, and control of the drug delivery profile. The patient could be treated with long-term continuous infusion, chronic intermittent infusion cycles, or with multiple bolus injections without frequent acute catheterization or repeated venipuncture.

The delivery system (developed in collaboration with United Stated Catheter and Instrument Corporation) first used and reported by Watkins et al was called the Chronometric Infusor and later the Chronofusor. Although production was stopped on the Chronofusor in the mid-1970s, systems were found still in use in some centers in Europe as recently as 1983.

The Chronofusor was a small, self-contained, peristaltic pumping mechanism powered by a precision clock spring motor. A drug reservoir was contained within the housing of the motor and pumping mechanism. Figure 1 shows the fluid schematic of the system and illustrates the component layout of this early ambulatory patient infusion pump. Table 1 lists the published design and performance characteristics.

The disposable plastic reservoir contained 25 ml of a concentrated drug solution that was replaced with a new reservoir every 4 days by the physician or, in some cases, by the patient. After flow rate calibration, sterilization of the drug path was accomplished by exposure to an ethylene oxide gas environment. A special winding key was used by the patient or nurse for rewinding the clock spring motor after each 8 hours of use.[7]

The pumping rate of the system was established by the constant and accurate rotation of the peristaltic pump rollers against a silicone pump tubing. Variations in pump tubing diameters due to manufacturing tolerance required that each tubing set be calibrated in the pump before sterilization and use. Once calibrated, a flow variability of less than $\pm 5\%$ of the established (24-hour) flow rate was achieved.

In operation, the device was positioned on the patient's chest and supported by a strap around the neck. A foam-insulated carrying pouch was used to protect the patient's skin from abrasion and pressure points and to reduce the ticking noise of the clock spring motor. In early studies reviewed by Watkins in

1970,[8,9] ambulatory patients were treated with continuous infusion chemotherapy for as long as 14 months. Interrupted infusion courses were conducted in patients in that study for as long as 3 years.[8,9]

With the successful demonstration of the advantages of chronic percutaneous infusion catheters and miniaturized infusion pumps for ambulatory patients, interest focused on expanding and improving the application of the technique.[10,11] Advancements in ambulatory system designs through use of new materials technology, miniaturized mechanical components, and small, power-

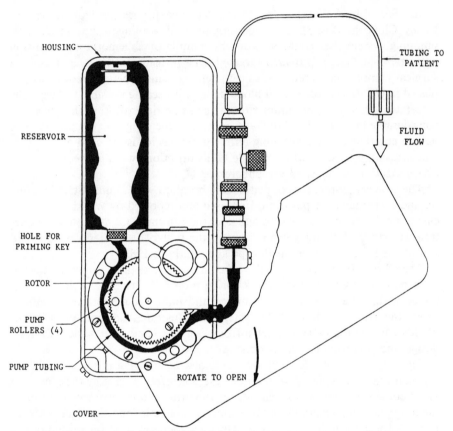

Figure 1. Chronofusor "chronometric" infusion pump.

Table 1. Chronofusor Chronomatic Infusion Pump Features

Delivery Rate	5.0 ml/24 hours ± 0.05 ml standard deviation
Weight:	426 grams
Dimensions:	13 cm × 6 cm × 3 cm
Reservoir volume:	25 ml
Motor drive time:	12 hours per winding

Source: United States Catheter and Instrument Corp., Model 5 – 24 Manual of Instructions (Rev. 5 – 6 – 71).

ful electronic computer circuitry resulted in recognition that continuous or chronic intermittent infusion therapy could be safely and reliably given.

Today, the medical device industry offers a wide variety of ambulatory infusion systems employing many different design concepts. Some of the more common pumping principles in clinical use for extracorporal systems include peristaltic pumps, syringe pumps, pinch tube pumps, and passive elastromeric balloon pumps. Figure 2 shows a typical schematic for a patient-worn pumping system.

Peristaltic Pump

Peristaltic pumps achieve pumping action by progressively squeezing a flexible tube to force the fluid along the tube lumen from the reservoir toward the infusion site. Various mechanisms have been used to achieve the peristaltic pumping action. The most common designs for peristaltic ambulatory pumps are shown in figures 3, 4, and 5.

In the system shown in figure 3-A, the peristaltic action is achieved by the motion of 2 or more rollers located on the periphery of a rotating shaft driven by an electric motor. The rollers are positioned on the shaft in such a way that one roller is always in position to squeeze the tube closed, preventing direct communication between the inlet and outlet ports. This arrangement prevents backflow of fluid from the patient toward the inlet during the rotation cycle.

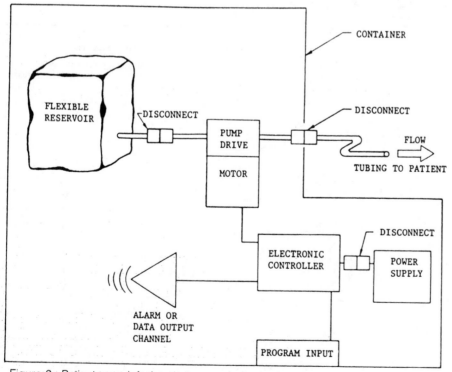

Figure 2. Patient-worn infusion system equipment schematic.

Backflow of fluid in the tube would allow blood to enter the catheter tip and could result in occlusion of the catheter and system failure. In a properly operating system, each roller pushes a column of fluid from the reservoir toward the outlet port as the shaft rotates and never allows fluid backflow. This motion provides continuous fluid flow during the pumping portion of the cycle and is reduced or stopped as the roller passes the outlet port and the pumping action of the next roller begins (figure 3-B).

Figure 4-A shows a variation of the peristaltic pumping action in which a single offset roller moves over the pump tubing and the pump tubing extends for 360° around the housing. In this concept, the tubing is continuously squeezed by the roller, and at the tubing overlap it is squeezed closed at 2 points (inlet and outlet) to prevent backflow of fluid when the roller passes the outlet. Figure 4-B illustrates the resulting flow profile. In a properly designed system, there is one position in the cycle where the roller passes the overlap between the outlet tube and the inlet tube. At this point, the flow of fluid abruptly stops, then immediately resumes at the selected value. There

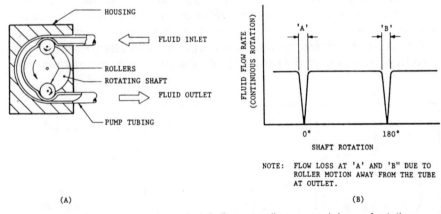

Figure 3. Peristaltic pump schematic—2 or more rollers on periphery of rotating shaft.

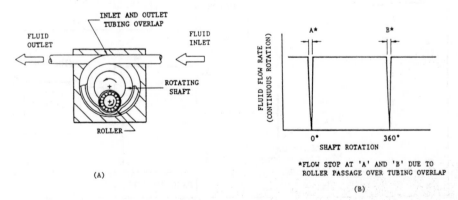

Figure 4. Peristaltic pump schematic—single offset roller.

should be no retrograde flow at this point. To change the flow rate of a continuously rotating system, the motor speed is increased or decreased to the required value. To achieve large changes in the flow rate, a pump tubing of a different diameter may be used. The shape of the flow profile is essentially unchanged by changes in speed or tubing diameter.

A further design variation of the peristaltic pump uses a series of adjacent pressure points or "wave fingers" to progressively squeeze the tube along its length. At least one pressure point along the path is always completely closed to prevent retrograde flow. This concept (shown in figure 5) permits the pump tubing to remain flat, avoiding the need to install the tube around a circular track as required with the rotating designs. Progressive squeezing of the tube along the track moves the fluid down the tube lumen.

Pulse frequency and changes in the internal diameter of the pump tubing can be used in most peristaltic pumps to make flow-rate changes. To achieve large changes in flow rate, or to provide very small flow rates, an intermittent or pulsed power cycle can be used instead of a continuously powered system. Systems using intermittent or pulsed power cycles modify the flow rate by changing the "on time" and/or the "off time" of the motor. Typical flow profiles of continuous and pulsed systems are shown in figure 6. In many applications, the "off time" may be of little or no importance to the pharmacology of the drug, but in cases where the half-life of the drug in plasma is

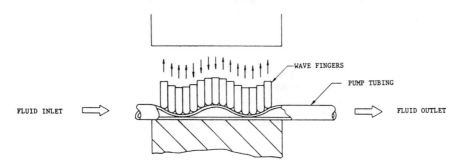

Figure 5. Peristaltic pump schematic—"wave fingers."

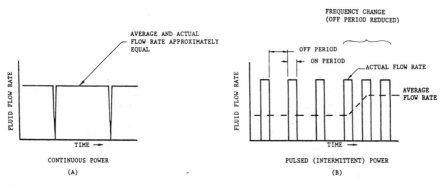

Figure 6. Typical flow profiles of continuous and pulsed systems.

short, drug activity may be undesirably decreased during the no-flow period. With pulsed power systems, it is essential that possibilities for retrograde blood flow into the catheter tip during the off cycle be eliminated. Advantages of peristaltic pumping mechanisms for use in drug delivery systems are shown in table 2.

Piston Pump

Piston pumps using a reciprocating piston in a cylinder (or a diaphragm in a fluid cavity) with mechanical inlet and outlet valves have long been used for fluid and gas pumping. In miniaturized form, these same mechanical concepts are useful for drug delivery. The fluid schematic for a piston or diaphragm pump is shown in figure 7.

An electromagnetic coil or a rotating cam can be used to create the reciprocating motion. When the piston is pulled down, the inlet valve is opened to permit fluid flow from the reservoir into the cylinder (figure 7-A). The outlet valve is closed during this portion of the cycle to prevent retrograde fluid flow from the body. Once the piston reaches the bottom of its travel and the cylinder is filled, the piston direction is reversed to expel the fluid. During this compressive portion of the cycle (figure 7-B), the outlet valve is opened to

Table 2. Advantages of Peristaltic Pumping System Designs

- The drug is always contained within the tubing and does not contact the pumping mechanism.
- The system is self-priming when the rotor is turned.
- There are no rotating fluid seals.
- The system does not require mechanical inlet or outlet valves.
- Flow rate changes are easily accomplished by changing the rotating speed of a continuously rotating system, or changing the pulse duration or pulse frequency in an intermittent pulsed system.

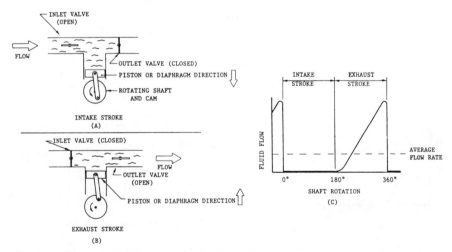

Figure 7. Piston or diaphragm pump schematic.

permit fluid exit, and the inlet valve is closed to prevent fluid flow into the reservoir. Variations in flow rate are achieved by changing the reciprocating frequency for the piston.

Syringe Pump

Syringe pumps achieve fluid delivery in an action comparable to the single cycle of a piston pump, in which the syringe plunger (piston) is progressively forced into the syringe barrel (cylinder) containing the infusion fluid. A schematic illustration of the syringe pump is shown in figure 8-A. Unlike the piston pump, which is usually a multiple stroke or cyclic system requiring inlet and outlet valves as well as a fluid reservoir, the syringe pump uses the syringe cylinder as the reservoir and the syringe plunger as the piston, traveling down the cylinder only one time. This design eliminates the need for inlet and outlet valves. After each cycle, the syringe and plunger set is replaced with a new, prefilled set. A motor-driven screw is used to force the plunger into the cylinder in accordance with a preset linear travel speed. For a fixed motor speed, flow rate (figure 8-B) is maintained constant over the entire reservoir volume, whereas a pulsed or intermittently activated system provides a flow profile as shown in figure 6-B. Because the flow rate of a syringe pump is directly related to the diameter of the syringe barrel and the drive speed of the plunger, large variations in flow rates can be accommodated by using syringes of different diameters and/or varying the plunger travel speed. The flow-rate accuracy of the syringe pump is directly related to the accuracy of the dimension of the syringe barrel internal diameter. To achieve predicted flow accuracy, manufacturer's recommendations relative to syringe selection must be carefully followed.

Pinch Tube Pump

The pinch tube pump uses some features of the peristaltic pump system by incorporating a flexible pump tubing for fluid transfer and some features of a

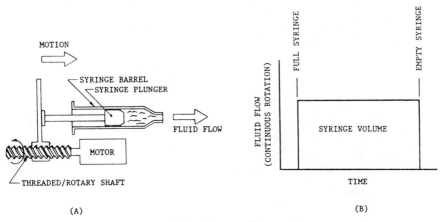

Figure 8. Syringe pump schematic and flow profile.

piston pump by incorporating inlet and outlet pinch valves into the pump tubing. Rather than moving the fluid by peristaltic action, the fluid is cyclically compressed (pinched) in the tube (in sequence with the pinch valves) to force the fluid along the flow path. The pinch tube design is shown in figure 9. As the system operates, it opens the inlet pinch valve and the pump plunger (figure 9-A) while maintaining the outlet valve in the closed position. When the tube lumen has been filled with fluid from the reservoir, the inlet valve is closed. The outlet valve is then opened and the pump plunger pinches the tube walls together to force the fluid from the tube (figure 9-B). The frequency with which the cycle is repeated, the diameter of the pumping tube, and the length of the pinched area determine the fluid flow rate. The system flow profile, shown in figure 9-C, is a pulsatile wave form similar to that of a piston pump. Adjustments in the flow rate can be made by changing the frequency of the cycle or the diameter of the pump tubing.

Elastomeric Balloon Pump

To provide a simple, lightweight ambulatory infusion system, pump designs have been introduced in which the fluid reservoir serves also as the pumping mechanism and power source.[12,13,14,15] In a balloon pump, pumping pressure is created by loading the drug into the balloon reservoir. This stretches the balloon wall, creating a stored compressive force, which then squeezes the drug out of the system during the infusion cycle. By expelling the fluid through a restrictive orifice, a preselected and constant flow rate can be maintained over most of the infusion cycle. This disposable system consists of only a few parts and is intended to be replaced with a new prefilled one at the end of each infusion cycle. A schematic for the elastomeric balloon pump is shown in figure 10-A and the flow profile in figure 10-B.

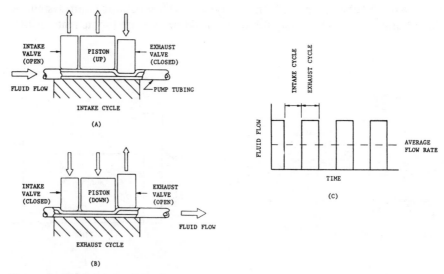

Figure 9. Pinch tube schematic.

Implantable Infusion Systems

For the long-term ambulatory infusion therapy patient, it is desirable to interfere as little as possible with the normal routine of living. For these patients, an implantable pump may be a desirable alternative. These systems, totally implanted in the patient, generally consist of a refillable reservoir, a fluid pumping system, a flow control system, and a delivery catheter.

Although they require surgical implantation, may restrict protocol flexibility, and limit the use of a pump to only one patient, totally implantable pumps offer the patient maximum freedom from external components, percutaneous access problems, and the routine tasks related to care and maintenance of the infusion system.

In the early 1970s, it was recognized that patient quality of life could be significantly improved and some of the risks associated with continuous infusion therapy could be reduced if the infusion system and drug reservoir were totally implanted in the patient rather than carried externally. One of the earliest commercial systems available for total implantation in patients was the one developed by the Infusaid Corp., Norwood, Mass., in collaboration with engineering and medical teams from the University of Minnesota.[16] The system was first used for anticoagulation[17] and later for cancer chemotherapy.[18] After successful and reliable application of the system in these fields, its use was extended into insulin delivery and chronic analgesia.[19]

As shown in figure 11, the Infusaid pump consists of a hollow metal disk separated into 2 chambers by a flexible metal bellows. The inner chamber contains the drug and flow control mechanism, and the outer sealed chamber contains a 2-phase charging fluid of a liquid in equilibrium with its vapor. At body temperature, the vapor pressure exerted by the charging fluid provides the pumping power by exerting pressure on the bellows and forcing the drug from the reservoir. The drug exits the reservoir through a filter and a flow-regulating capillary tube for delivery to the patient. When the drug stored in the reservoir has been consumed, it is refilled for the next infusion cycle by percutaneous injection with a hypodermic needle. Reservoir filling is accomplished by needle penetration through the skin and a self-sealing septum in the reservoir container. Filling of the reservoir expands the volume of the drug

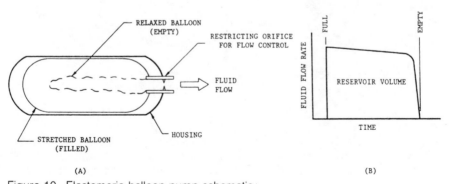

Figure 10. Elastomeric balloon pump schematic.

chamber and simultaneously reduces the volume of the vapor chamber, compressing the charging fluid vapor back into its liquid state in preparation for the next infusion cycle. Each time the reservoir is refilled, the power source is automatically reset for the next infusion cycle.

In its present commercial configuration, the Infusaid pump is a fixed flow-rate system. The flow rate is adjusted at the factory by modifying the length of the flow restrictor capillary tube located in the pump outlet flow path. The flow rate of the pump is defined by Poisseuille equation:

$$Q = \frac{\pi D^4 \Delta P}{128\ \mu L}$$

where Q is the flow rate, D is the inner diameter of the capillary tube, ΔP is pressure differential across the capillary tube, μ is the viscosity of the fluid in the reservoir, and L is the length of the capillary tube. Once the values for D, L, and ΔP are defined during manufacturing, dose rate changes must be made by adjusting the fluid viscosity to change the flow rate or by changing the drug concentration.[19]

To stop the therapy, the drug must be removed from the chamber and replaced with an inactive solution such as heparinized saline to maintain pump flow and system patency.[18]

Design concepts for programmable, implantable infusion pumps are being developed and are reported to be in various stages of clinical testing or commercial introduction.[20,21,22] As presented in the literature, the most common pumping techniques used in programmable systems are similar to the peristaltic or piston pumps described for external systems (figures 3 and 7). Figure 12 presents a component schematic typically used for programmable, implantable systems.

Use of a programmable system rather than a fixed-flow system offers opportunity for easily altering the pump flow rate on a preprogrammed schedule or by direct program intervention. Flow rate programming and alteration

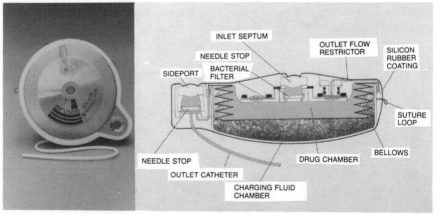

Figure 11. Infusaid implantable pump and catheter (left) and diagrammatic cross-section.

are usually achieved by transcutaneous transmission of programming data to an electronic circuity and memory inside the implanted device. Flow changes can be made on an ad hoc basis or placed into the device memory in such a way that the flow will be automatically altered at some planned future time.

Present programmable systems use batteries for pumping power and/or control circuitry power and therefore have a defined maximum operating life. Most programmable units were developed for drugs of high potency or low-dose requirements and have reservoir capacities limited to 7–20 ml. Use at high dose or with low-concentration drugs requires frequent refills and results in more rapid battery depletion.

Tables 3 and 4 compare various ambulatory patient systems that have been reported in or near clinical use.

Operational Considerations in Pump Selection For Ambulatory Patients

Many issues must be taken into consideration in the selection of an appropriate ambulatory patient infusion system. Some of the important matters to be resolved are not related to the more obvious issues of price, weight, reservoir volume, or aesthetic value, but include such concerns as:

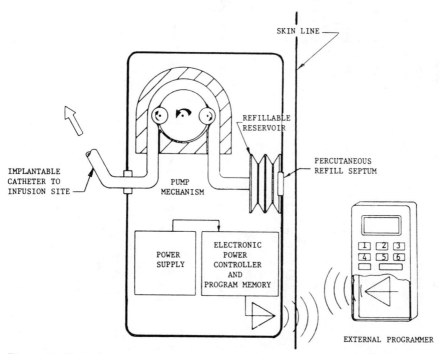

Figure 12. Typical component schematic for programmable, implantable pump systems.

Table 3. Features of Ambulatory Patient Infusion Pumps (External)

Manufacturer*	Model	Power supply	Size cm (L×H×W)	Weight (g)	Pump type	Reservoir Volume (ml)	Alarms/data	Flow rate range (ml / 24 hr.)	Comments
Cormed Inc.	ML 6–4	Rechargeable battery	12.7×8.3×3.8	530	Peristaltic	50	None	4.0 to 20.0	Use separate plug-in flow rate meter for flow adjustment.
	ML 6–6	Same	Same	Same	Same	Same	Same	10 to 50	Same
	ML 6–10	Same	Same	Same	Same	External bag	Same	1,000 to 5,000	Same
	Cormed II	Same	12.2×10.7×3.8	482	Same	60	Low battery, low flow, high flow, electrical malfunction	4.0 to 50	Self-contained flow adjustment and display.
Travenol Laboratories, Inc.	MVP	Rechargeable battery	15.2×8.3×3.8	550	Peristaltic	50	Low battery test	12,24,36,48	Flow rates selected from 1 of 4 rates available.
	Infusor	Stretched elastomeric balloon	3.1 dia.×16 long	33	Fixed pressure through flow control orifice	60	Visual scale for reservoir volume	48 (fixed)	Disposable unit. Flow consistency optimized by use of 5% dextrose and when pump is worn close to patient's body.
	Auto Syringe AS-2F	Rechargeable battery or AC power	18.3×7.3×6.4	482	Syringe	1.0 to 60 (syringe)	Near empty reservoir, pump runaway, occlusion	0.48 to 2,112	Flow rate determined by pump speed and syringe size. Syringes from 1.0 to 60 ml may be used.
Pharmacia Nu Tech, Inc.	Act-A-Pump 1000	Rechargeable battery	10.5×9.5×3.8	425	Peristaltic	75	Low battery, stalled motor	2.0 to 110	Uses separate plug-in flow rate meter for flow adjustment.
Deltec Systems, Inc.	CADD-1	Disposable battery	16.0×8.9×2.8	425	Pinch tube	50	Low battery, pump stopped, wrong delivery, low reservoir	0.0 to 299	Self-contained memory for flow programing. Provides data output concerning program, drug consumed, etc.
Pancretec, Inc.	Provider 2000	Rechargeable battery	15.2×8.6×3.8	660	Peristaltic	External—standard solution bag	Low battery, low reservoir, program error, memory loss, prime overuse, system defective	5 to 1,992	Continuous and intermittent flow profiles. External reservoir allows use of various sizes of standard solution bags.
Parker Hannifin Corp.	Micropump 2000	Disposable battery	7.6×5.1×1.9	75	Diaphragm	External—standard solution bag	—	2.4 to 50	Disposable diaphragm pump cartridge. Self-contained memory for flow programing.
Sharp Co., Ltd. (Japan)	MP-22	Disposable battery	15×7.5×5.2	500	—	40	System defective, low battery	2.5, 5.0, 10.0	Flow adjusted in 3 steps.
Nikkiso Co., Ltd. (Japan)	Myfuser PSW - 11A	Disposable battery	15.2×6.7×2.7	230	Syringe	5 ml syringe	Empty syringe, occlusion, low battery	0.6 to 24	Flow adjusted in 10 steps at 2 speed levels.

*U.S. companies, unless otherwise noted
Note: Product data from sources believed to be reliable, but should be verified by manufacturer.

Table 4. Features of Ambulatory Patient Infusion Pumps (External, continued from Table 3, and Implantable)

Manufacturer*	Model	Power supply	Size cm (L×H×W)	Weight (g)	Pump type	Reservoir Volume (ml)	Alarms/data	Flow rate range (ml / 24 hr.)	Comments
External									
Med Fusions Systems, Inc.	Infumed 200	Disposable or rechargeable battery	10.4×7.6×4.1	364	Peristaltic	75	Over delivery, low battery, depleted battery, under delivery	2.4 to 238	Flow setting in increments 2.4 ml/24 hr.
Graseby Dynamics, Ltd. (England)	MS-16	Disposable battery	16.5×5.3×2.3	175	Syringe	1 to 20 syringe	Flashing light indicates "on"; power shut-off for occlusion or end of syringe	0.48 to 816	Flow adjusted by digital selection over range.
Implantable Pumps									
Intermedics/ Infusaid Inc.	400	2-phase charging fluid	8.7 dia. ×2.8 thick	208	Fixed flow rate, pressurized drug chamber	47	None	1 to 6	Fixed flow rate is factory adjusted to desired level. Dose changes are made by concentration changes with the drug. Contains auxiliary injection port for bolus injection. Models 100 (47 ml), 200 (32 ml), and 500 (22 ml) are available without the auxiliary injection port. Refilled by percutaneous injection.
Medtronics Inc.	8600	Battery	7 dia. ×2.7 thick	175	Peristaltic	20	Not available		Noninvasively programmed to desired profile delivery and rate changes.
Seimans A.G. Frg. (W. Germany)	DFA-1-S	Battery	8.5×6×2.2	170	Peristaltic	10	Catheter overpressure, transmitter control, verify program, motor central	0 to 3.6	Battery life approximately 1 year.

*U.S. companies, unless otherwise noted
Note: Product data from sources believed to be reliable, but should be verified by manufacturer.

- compatibility of the drug path materials with the drugs to be used
- availability of important alarms, status information, and other safety features
- flow rate accuracy
- overhaul and repair services available
- availability of customer training programs and educational materials.

Compatibility of Drug Path Materials

Most pumping systems use various combinations of plastics, elastomers, and/or metals in the construction of the drug flow path. It is essential that materials used in the drug path be identified and assessed relative to the interactions of the materials with the drugs.[23]

As a matter of practice, pharmaceutical firms develop extensive data relative to the stability and bioavailability of drugs for clinical use. For practical reasons, these drugs are usually tested under conditions perceived by the manufacturer to be consistent with anticipated field use, and the data therefore should be reevaluated when considering a new delivery system or technique.[24]

An understanding of the compatibility among the drug path materials, the storage environment, and the drug itself is essential in order to ensure that the patient will be infused with fluids of the predicted dose level, purity, and chemical structure.

Interaction between the drug and the materials of the drug path may result from such physical and chemical characteristics as leaching, sorption, permeation and chemical reactivity.[25] Leaching may occur when plasticizers, material fillers, antioxydants, or antistatic or coloring agents are added to the drug path material. On contact with the drug, these contaminates may be released from the drug path material and migrate into the solution delivered to the patient. If precise knowledge is required concerning leaching characteristics, it should be developed with the proposed drug in contact with the drug path materials under actual-use environmental conditions.

Some materials, such as "medical" grades of elastomers and plastics, have been specifically formulated for medical applications and are readily qualified to meet low-leachability requirements. But because there are numerous formulations of these materials available from suppliers, care must be taken to ensure that the proper medical grade is used in order to avoid leaching problems.

The absorption or adsorption of compounds from the drug into or on the drug path material may also result in an adverse effect on either the drug or the drug path material. The absorption of material from the drug into the drug path material is a physicochemical activity related to the chemistry of the drug and the properties of the drug path material. Chemical interaction may weaken, harden, or otherwise degrade the drug path materials. Adsorption of the drug on the surface of the drug path may alter the concentration, form, or chemistry of the infusion solution. Analyses of drugs in contact with plastics have been conducted over the years and are updated frequently.

Drug permeation of the walls of the drug path occurs when the compound passes through the drug path material into the surrounding environment.

Also, in a reverse situation, materials from the environment (usually air) may pass through the drug path wall into the drug. In applications where water or water vapor is transported through the drug path, possibilities for changes in drug concentrations due to water loss should be considered. Materials commonly used in pump drug-path construction are known to be affected by a variety of compounds and should be evaluated for specific drug interaction.

Alarms and Performance Status Information

Safe use of an infusion system in a hospital setting or with an ambulatory patient requires the availability of accurate pump performance information on a timely basis and in a format that assures proper response to a detected malfunction. Review of pumping systems in use today illustrates that one can choose almost any desired level of sophistication in automation, performance, or information systems. In choosing features required for a specific application, care should be taken to select systems that improve safety and patient therapy management rather than to select systems that have impressive gadgets or unnecessary features creating new possibilities for failure and malfunction. Care should also be taken to ensure that an alarm- or data-output failure does not promote responses that might be more harmful than not having the information in the first place. Useful alarms might include those for low battery power, no flow, occlusion in the output tubing, gas (bubble) detection, fluid spills, and unplanned flow-rate changes.

Flow Rate Accuracy and Precision

Robinson[26] defined pump flow accuracy as "delivering the volume one expects to deliver," and precision as the "flow characteristic as a function of time." In a precise pumping system, one would expect to obtain highly accurate and predictable flow rates at each point of the flow cycle. A pump may be considered "precise" only if the flow profile is accurately repeated cycle after cycle. Because the patient's drug dosage is directly related to the fluid flow rate, the dose inaccuracy is the combined inaccuracy of the drug concentration and the inaccuracy of the pump flow rate. If the drug concentration (or bioavailability) is predictable within 10% and the pump flow rate accuracy is 10%, the patient's delivered dose could be as much as 20% above or below the anticipated value. When these variations are critical in the planned protocol, additional efforts must be made to provide more accurate drug concentrations and/or a more accurate pumping system. Further, when using interrupted flow profiles such as those provided by pulsed pumping systems, peak delivery rate and the "no flow time" must be considered.[27] For highly concentrated drugs in pulsed pumping systems, it may be possible to deliver an acceptable average dose rate by a large flow burst and then stop the flow for some extended period, but an undesirable pattern of cyclic drug plasma levels may be established. This condition is of greater significance if the drug half-life in plasma is short. In some applications, the average dose rate might be satisfactory but the incremental rate could be both excessive and inadequate within the cycle, as shown in figure 13-A. For the condition where large unacceptable variations in drug plasma levels result with pulsed system, the stable flow of a continuously operating system as shown in figure 13-B may be more useful.

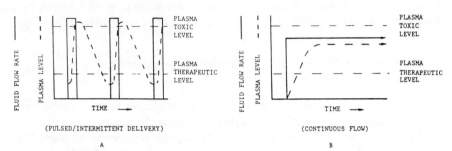

Figure 13. Comparison of plasma levels maintained by pulsed/intermittent delivery pump and continuous flow pump.

As suggested by Robinson,[26] pump volume accuracy is of greater importance when considering drugs of long half-life or when half-life is unimportant in the therapy. Pump precision is of significance when delivering drugs of short half-life or when the drugs must be given in high concentrations and small variation in plasma levels could produce toxicity or become nontherapeutic.

5

TECHNICAL ASPECTS OF VASCULAR ACCESS FOR INFUSIONAL CHEMOTHERAPY

A. Bothe, Jr., M.D. and J. Daly, M.D.

Introduction—Venous Access

THE MAJORITY OF SIGNIFICANT chemotherapeutic agents are administered intravenously.[1] The development of techniques to facilitate vascular access for these medications has minimized logistic barriers to the exploration of various drug combinations and treatment schedules. In the past, difficulty with venous access may have led clinicians to avoid certain vesicant drugs or infusion schedules. Long-term, secure venous access has now allowed continuous and prolonged chemotherapy infusions, more recently on an outpatient basis.[2,3] As described in other chapters, the theoretical advantage of continuous infusion is being studied for its clinical utility. This chapter will consider the techniques for providing vascular access (table 1).

Most I.V. drugs have been given on an intermittent schedule in the hospital through an established I.V. line. Alternatively, direct I.V. bolus injection could be performed on an outpatient basis. Local tissue damage from extravasation of vesicant drugs was always a concern. Short-term continuous infusion for 3–5 days was accomplished by admission of the patient to the hospital. Over the past 5 years, however, there has been a gradual transfer of access technology from other specialties that has given the chemotherapist more latitude in choosing the optimal drug and treatment schedule.

The first major application of chronic outpatient venous access occurred in the nutrition support field. Shortly after the introduction of hyperalimentation itself, equipment and techniques were developed to allow the administration of nutrient solutions at home.[4] By the end of the 1970s, thousands of patients who had otherwise required hospitalization were able to receive their hyperalimentation solutions through "permanent" Silastic catheters.[5] The internal end of the catheter was positioned in the superior vena cava, with the tubing leaving the subclavian vein in the subcutaneous tissue of the chest wall and traveling through a short tunnel to an exit site. The external end of the catheter could then be attached to infusion equipment for solution delivery. Despite long-term problems with infection and thrombosis, this technique remains the standard for permanent delivery of hyperalimentation. Prompted by the demonstrated ability to maintain chronic venous access, a number of similar techniques have been adapted for use in oncologic patients.

Choice of Access Technique

A number of factors should be considered in determining the optimal method of vascular access. No single method of drug delivery is applicable in the oncologic setting to the needs of all patients (see table 2).

The availability of peripheral veins is usually not a problem for the newly diagnosed oncology patient. Peripheral veins may allow the intermittent delivery of nonsclerosing medication if consistent with the treatment plan. Sclerosing medications may also be given initially. However, later during the treatment course the irritative effects of the medication may make access of peripheral veins problematic for even the simplest of infusions. As implied, the property of the infusion can be a critical factor. The tonicity or vesicant nature of certain medications may restrict delivery to a central vein, where

Table 1. Vascular Access Options for Chemotherapy

Method	Advantage	Disadvantage
Peripheral vein cannula	Simplicity	Limited use
Arteriovenous fistula/graft	High flow	Limited patency
Central venous catheter		
(a) peripheral insertion	Ease of insertion	Limited duration
(b) standard central line	Standard procedure	In-hospital use
(c) tunneled central line	Subcutaneous barrier	
Hickman-type catheter	Durable	External enclosure
Venous access disk	Totally implanted	
Arterial disk	Relative ease	External interface
Implanted pump	Self-contained	Expense

Table 2. Criteria in Selection of Access Technique

Site of tumor
Availability
Properties of infusate
Medication schedule
Duration of planned therapy
Regional anatomy
Coagulation status
Home care resources

high-volume blood flow rapidly dilutes the drug before the endothelial wall of the vein is damaged. This is analogous to the dilution required for typical hyperalimentation solutions in which the osmolality is increased 5-fold over normal plasma.

The medication dosing schedule and duration of planned therapy are also important considerations. The needs for vascular access are quite different for a treatment schedule requiring 1 bolus infusion every 3 weeks and a schedule requiring continuous infusion. Similarly, the choice of access route or infusion device may be different for a treatment program lasting for 1–2 weeks and a program with 10 cycles lasting more than 6 months.

Obviously, the choice of the access route may be affected by tumor-related changes in regional anatomy. Previous local surgery or radiation treatment or the presence of a tumor mass may prevent the use of standard methods of access. Also important is knowledge of resources to care for the access device. Delivery of supplies, assistance for dressing and catheter care, and the patient's ability and willingness to participate are all critical factors.

Venous Access Options

The most commonly used method of chemotherapy delivery is the peripheral vein cannula or needle (see table 3). This method is so frequently used for hospitalized patients that it needs little explanation. It is usually simple and effective. It is ideal for bolus or intermittent use and is relatively safe. The risk of phlebitis increases directly with time. However, phlebitis is usually a local problem, rarely causing ascending septic phlebitis or septicemia.[6] The extravasation of certain drugs at peripheral insertion sites can lead to major local wound problems from tissue necrosis. Peripheral vein access has been less than ideal for continuous infusion in the outpatient setting because of the difficulty in maintaining the access route.

The arteriovenous fistula or graft remains the standard access technique for hemodialysis. Application in other fields such as chemotherapy or hyperali-

Table 3. Vascular Access Route Alternatives

Peripheral vein access
   hand/forearm
   antecubital
   cephalic

Central vein access
   subclavian
   jugular
   cephalic/chest wall
   antecubital
   femoral system
   visceral (e.g., gonadal, iliac)

Arterial access
   proximal to tumor
   examples: hepatic, femoral, carotid

mentation has been less satisfactory. Once the fistula is constructed, it is usually well accepted by the patient. The mature fistula usually has a flow rate high enough to tolerate the infusion of most chemotherapy drugs.[1,7] Except in the uremic patient, however, the patency rate and duration has been disappointingly low. The construction of the fistula can be a demanding technical operative challenge, and even in the most experienced hands, the thrombosis rate is high.

The central venous catheter is widely used in several areas, including surgery, anesthesia, cardiology, critical care, nutritional support, and hemodialysis. The access afforded through the central vein allows the insertion of various catheters and devices related to each of the above specialties. For the chemotherapist, the central venous catheter provides a secure, relatively safe route for delivering a wide range of medications.

Central venous catheters inserted peripherally are usually reserved for short-term use. The antecubital or brachial vein routes have been used. Some groups have been successful using this approach, but most have not found this satisfactory for long-term use. Significant problems with infection and phlebitis are common with the usual polyethylene catheters; Silastic catheters may cause less difficulty. Maintaining dressings and minimizing motion at the catheter/skin junction is another difficulty with the arm location, especially for longer infusion periods.

The standard method of central venous catheter insertion in the nonthrombocytopenic patient is the infraclavicular subclavian vein approach. Once such a catheter is successfully placed in the hospitalized patient, it can be maintained for weeks. Careful catheter and exit-site care minimize the risk of infection. The development of occult or clinically significant thrombosis remains a concern. The supraclavicular approach to the subclavian vein is used by some, out of individual preference or training. Likewise, the jugular route may be used in patients with coagulopathy or with problems in the chest wall (e.g., tumor, radiation) precluding the infraclavicular route. With experience, complications related to subclavian vein insertion should be in the 1% range. Important maneuvers to minimize such complications are well described in various texts on bedside procedures.

Several additional steps are routinely employed with chemotherapy patients. The smallest possible dressing is used. Therefore, if a through-the-needle catheter is used, a Seldinger maneuver is performed with a flexible-tipped guidewire.[8] After the standard insertion, the guidewire is placed through the catheter to allow removal of the catheter and needle unit (see figure 1). The needle and needle guard are separated from the catheter and the catheter is trimmed to the appropriate length. The catheter is then reinserted over the guidewire, the guidewire is withdrawn, and a fixation suture is applied to the hub or the junction of the catheter and hub. Nylon suture material is routinely used to fix such catheters. Silk sutures are more commonly associated with "stitch abscess," which may create a significant problem in the immunosuppressed oncology patient.

The tunneled subclavian line technique was initially proposed to move the catheter exit site and I.V. tubing connection away from sources of contamination in patients with tracheostomies.[9] The construction of a short subcutaneous tunnel using a modified Seldinger technique allows the exit site to be moved 2–3 in. away from the usual infraclavicular venipuncture site. Some groups once recommended such a short tunnel for all patients with central lines, but the value of this technique has not been substantiated for routine use. Tunneling of the standard subclavian line does have applicability for outpatient use. The tunnel allows for the catheter exit site to be located in a more convenient location for dressing changes. The tunnel also uses the concept from the Silastic catheter experience of providing an additional bacteriologic barrier by moving the skin opening away from the catheter/vein junction.

The insertion of a tunneled subclavian line for ambulatory continuous infusion requires several additional steps beyond those of the standard infraclavicular subclavian venipuncture. Once the standard venipuncture is performed and the catheter is placed in the subclavian vein, a flexible-tipped guidewire is inserted through the catheter. The catheter and needle unit are then removed. Additional local anesthetic is infiltrated over the proposed course of the tunnel. The same insertion needle used for the initial venipuncture is placed through the skin at the planned exit site. The tip of the needle is then directed through the subcutaneous tissue to the original venipuncture site. When the end of the needle is visualized, the external end of the guidewire is threaded in retrograde fashion through the needle. The needle is removed and the catheter is then threaded over the guidewire from the new insertion site, through the tunnel, and into the subclavian vein. The catheter is fixed at the exit site in the usual fashion and a single suture is used to close the original venipuncture

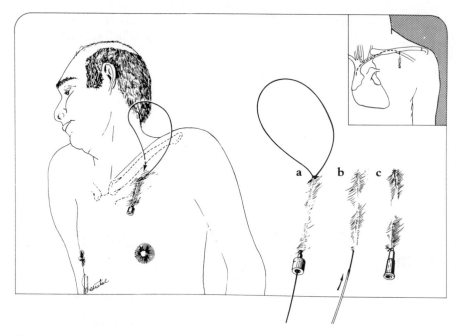

Figure 1.   A Seldinger maneuver is performed with a flexible-tipped guidewire to allow for removal of the needle and tunneling of the catheter.

site. Depending on the catheter material, this catheter can be left in place 3 months. If additional time is required, a new catheter can be exchanged over a guidewire to avoid cracking of the catheter material, which occurs with prolonged use. The more durable Silastic catheters are not affected by such problems.

The development and commercial availability of venous access disks represents an improvement over the tunneled subclavian line for continuous ambulatory chemotherapy.[10,11,12,13] The Silastic septum in a small-volume reservoir allows the entire system to be placed in the subcutaneous position. Access to the system is obtained with a specially designed Huber-point needle placed through the skin into the Silastic septum. The system can be used for either continuous or bolus infusion (see figure 2).

As previously described,[11] the disk system is inserted under local anesthesia. A standard infraclavicular venipuncture is accomplished and a guidewire is placed into the subclavian vein. A subcutaneous pocket is constructed on the anterior chest wall through an incision made approximately over the fourth rib just lateral to the sternal border. The pocket is constructed in the cephalad direction. A tunnel is made for the catheter from the upper end of the pocket to the original venipuncture site and the disk is sutured to the floor of the pocket with nonabsorbable suture. The catheter is trimmed to the appropriate length and then inserted into the subclavian vein through a tear-away sheath introducer that has been threaded over the guidewire (see figure 3).[14] The pocket and infraclavicular venipuncture site are closed, and the system can be used immediately upon confirming satisfactory position of the catheter tip by X ray.

Continuous outpatient infusion chemotherapy is usually delivered by a battery-operated pump containing the desired drug in high concentration. The drug is pumped through a short segment of I.V. tubing, which is attached to a

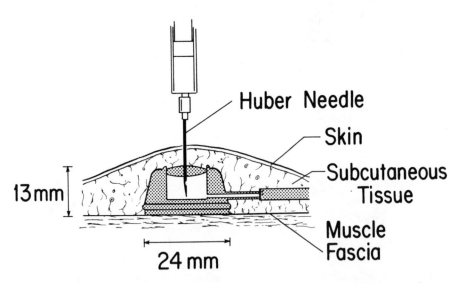

Figure 2.   The disk system is accessed using a specially designed Huber needle.

right-angle Huber-point needle inserted through the skin into the disk. The needle can be left in the same position for 2 weeks. To continue the infusion, a needle is repositioned in the disk through the skin several millimeters away from the former site. When the infusion is completed, the system is simply flushed with a dilute heparinized saline at monthly intervals.

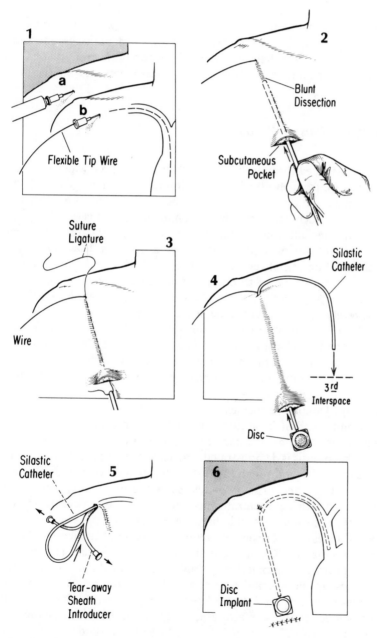

Figure 3.   Step-by-step method of catheter insertion using a disk system.

As with the Hickman or Broviac catheter, the catheter and disk are usually placed in the anterior chest wall and through the subclavian vein. If the subclavian veins are not available because of local changes or previous thrombosis, the catheter may be directed through the jugular vein, with the disk in the usual position, such as the anterior axillary line or lateral suprascapular area, if the chest wall cannot be used for implantation (e.g., radiation fibrosis, tumor, previous local surgery).

Prior to insertion, clotting studies are obtained. Patients who are relatively hypercoaguable are considered for low-dose anticoagulant therapy.[15] Hypocoaguable patients have disk insertion postponed until the abnormality is resolved. Patients who have experienced a thrombotic event related to a previous central line undergo venography to assess patency of the central venous system.

Complications of Venous Access

Catheter-related thrombosis may develop at any time while a catheter is in place, ranging from shortly after insertion to more than a year.[15,16] The most frequent presentation of thrombosis is the development of a dull pain in the ipsilateral shoulder, suprascapular region, or ipsilateral cervical area. Clinical findings may include arm edema, but are usually far less dramatic. There may only be a slight fullness in the supraclavicular fossa or delayed emptying of a jugular vein. Superficial veins in the skin may become prominent in the upper lateral chest. Suspicion of thrombosis should be evaluated by contrast venogram performed from the ipsilateral arm. Contrast injection through the disk itself is rarely of help except to demonstrate tip obstruction. In the case of a fibrin sheath or tip obstruction, contrast may flow retrograde back to the injection site, i.e., "back tracking." The dye runs outside the catheter, but is contained by the mesothelial lining that surrounds the system soon after implantation. Thrombosis most often develops at the site of catheter entry into the vein and rarely propagates far enough to cause an abnormality at the catheter tip. Doppler assessment of a subclavian vein may be useful in complete thrombosis, but its accuracy is limited by operator experience. Partial thrombosis may not be detected at all by ultrasound.

Once thrombosis is demonstrated, I.V. heparin administration is begun. This can be accomplished through the disk or through a peripheral I.V. site. If the patient is to be treated on an outpatient basis, the ambulatory battery-operated pump is filled with a concentrated heparin solution to achieve the same effect. The patient need not be hospitalized unless there is superior vena cava syndrome or unless the discomfort requires parenteral analgesics. Heparin is begun at less than 1,000 units/hour and increased as needed. This usually gives relatively prompt symptomatic relief and more gradual improvement of physical findings. In the hospitalized patient, the heparin dosage can be adjusted upward more quickly until the PTT reaches twice control value. The patient is then converted to oral warfarin at a dosage to give a prothrombin time less than twice control. The dosage is later reduced to just under 1.5 times control for the remaining duration of use. Rarely does the disk system require removal. Coagulation abnormalities can usually be controlled for as long as chronic venous access is required.

Few data exist on the risk of pulmonary embolism related to chronic venous access devices. Older literature in vascular surgery suggested that upper extremity thrombi were rarely the source of hemodynamically significant pulmonary emboli.[17] Given the large number of central vein devices used in numerous specialties and the common incidence of venographically demonstrated thrombi without serious sequelae, the incidence of significant thrombi is likely to be quite low. Nevertheless, investigations are under way to identify those patients at high risk for the formation of catheter-related thrombosis. Also, studies are in progress investigating the various prophylactic regimes to prevent thrombus formation, including less thrombogenic catheter material.[18]

Occlusion of the catheter itself may serve as an harbinger of vein occlusion. If the catheter has a small intraluminal plug, it can usually be cleared.[19,20] On the other hand, the catheter may not flow or allow withdrawal of blood because the tip is involved in thrombosis.

Another area of significant concern is the risk of infection associated with chronic vascular access devices.[21,22,23,24] The earlier hyperalimentation literature reports the incidence of catheter-related sepsis at 2–3%. It is difficult to interpret this figure, given the wide variety of hospitalized patients receiving hyperalimentation and the varying duration of catheterization. More recent reports concerning home hyperalimentation patients suggest an average rate of catheter-related infection as 0.5 episodes per patient year. Clinical experience shows that some patients experience no infectious problems, whereas other patients have numerous infectious complications. This difference may be related to such individual host factors as nutritional state, presence of an abdominal wall ostomy, and adherence to dressing protocols. Also, one would not expect the high incidence of infectious problems in patients with hematologic malignancies to occur in patients with solid tumors.

The two major infectious problems related to permanent access devices are exit-site infections and catheter sepsis. Exit-site infections are the more common phenomenon. For standard Silastic catheters, this may include an abscess or cellulitis at the catheter exit site. These can frequently be managed by local care and culture-specific antibiotics. Any drainage at the exit site is cultured, and small collections are drained and packed. Blood cultures are obtained from the catheter itself and from a peripheral site. If these are positive for the same organism cultured from the exit site, the catheter usually requires removal. If the bloodstream has not been seeded, culture-specific antibiotics are continued, along with local wound care, until the problem is resolved.

Catheter sepsis usually presents as fever or, rarely, a toxic picture. Blood cultures are obtained peripherally and through the access device. If the cultures from the device itself are positive, the catheter usually requires removal after antibiotics are begun. The duration of culture-specific antibiotics depends on whether the patient had experienced a high-grade septicemia. Insertion of a new line at an alternate site is delayed until there is no risk of metastatic infection to the new device. In a fulminant picture, prompt removal of the catheter is required.

Infections at the disk pocket can be managed in the same way as exit-site infections, using traditional Silastic central catheters. Low-grade purulence at the needle insertion site may be treated with antibiotics and local wound care. A small incision for drainage at the site of infection may help resolve the problem. Once the pocket itself becomes significantly infected, it should be opened. This exposes the disk, converting it to an external system. As with the usual Silastic catheters, removal of the access disk is required if it demonstrates a positive culture.

An infrequent problem is the malpositioning of the intravascular portion of the catheter.[11,16] The tip of smaller bore catheters may flip upward into the ipsilateral jugular vein after having been placed in the proper position at the time of insertion. Occasionally, there is a spontaneous reversion to the correct position. This phenomenon is less likely to occur with catheters inserted from the left subclavian route. A catheter tip in the jugular vein should not be used for infusion of any sclerosing agent. Frequently, the catheter can be repositioned by an angiographer, who simply hooks the tip of the catheter with a snare and positions it correctly.

Malpositioning of the disk has been an infrequent occurrence. Rarely, the disk can flip sidewards or upside down in the pocket, thereby preventing needle access. This position, confirmed by a simple radiograph, is due to disconnection of the fixation sutures from the underlying pectoralis fascia. The disk may be remanipulated into the correct position, although refixation in the pocket may be necessary. The angiographer can also be helpful in the rare instances of shearing of the Silastic catheter or disconnection of a catheter from the access disk.[16,26] The distal fragment of the catheter may embolize into the right heart. The high incidence of infectious complications in this situation warrants angiographic retrieval.

The skin overlying the disk can well tolerate multiple punctures. Occasionally, there has been erosion[27] over the puncture site in the setting of a local infection or if the skin becomes taut over the disk. A local infection is treated as above. In both instances, revision of the system will require moving the access disk to another location on the chest wall. If this is not possible, the system can be converted to a catheter with an external end.

Arterial Access

The development of regional systems to deliver chemotherapy is based upon the occasional clinical situation in which a tumor may be confined to a region or organ with a singular arterial inflow to the tumor. Regional delivery affords the opportunity of maximizing the dose of drug to be delivered. In addition, regional extraction of the drug in a "first pass" effect minimizes the systemic host exposure to the agent, thereby limiting the possibility for toxicities, particularly to bone marrow.

A variety of tumor sites lend themselves to regional drug delivery (see table 4). Neoplastic liver disease is the most common application of regional delivery systems, related in part to the frequency of metastases from a variety of primary tumor sites to this organ. Regional delivery to the liver may be provided via the hepatic arterial system or, alternatively, via the portal venous system. Although the portal vein has been a common site of delivery for both adjuvant chemotherapy trials as well as for therapy of metastatic disease alone or combined with hepatic arterial delivery, this route provides a relatively small proportion of the blood supply to hepatic metastases. Regional delivery to the liver fulfills all the criteria for optimal regional delivery in that a continuous infusion schedule is most commonly employed and the liver is a major metabolic organ with a rich vascular supply that allows for drug extraction.

For the other sites of regional delivery, particularly for the extremity, bolus or relatively short-term infusion has been employed, commonly in conjunction with venous occlusion. In most of these clinical circumstances, a radiographically placed catheter is positioned and used for a relatively brief pulse of chemotherapy. For head and neck cancer, however, trials of protracted infusion with arterial catheters in the carotid arterial system have been carried out in a fashion similar to that of trials for hepatic neoplasia.

For most if not all regional systems, the possibility of radiographic placement of the catheter minimizes the need for a direct surgical placement of such a catheter. There are, however, important potential advantages of surgical catheter placement: (1) guaranteed evaluation of the abdomen to ensure that the tumor is confined to the liver; (2) direct confirmation of distribution of the infusion to the entire liver; (3) minimal incidence of hepatic artery occlusion; and (4) the option of using the implanted pump system, obviating the need for an external pump device.

It is not within the purview of this chapter to review the specific features of all types of regional delivery nor to review the technology associated with radiographic catheter placement. Instead, the discussion will focus on hepatic arterial infusion and the use of the implanted pump system, indicating the technical aspects of insertion, complications of regional infusion, and the present status and future direction of implanted pump technology in the management of malignancy.

Operative Placement of the Implanted Pump

With more than 4,000 implantable pumps placed through 1985, the technical aspects of pump placement have been firmly established. A review of the

Table 4. Regional Delivery Sites for Infusional Chemotherapy

Site	Vascular access
Liver	Common hepatic argery
	Gastroduodenal artery
	Portal vein
Extemity	Femoral iliac artery
Pelvis	Hypogastric artery
Chest wall	Internal mammary artery
Lungs	Bronchial artery
Head and neck	Carotid artery

surgical approaches to hepatic neoplasia by Neiderhuber and Enzminger outlines the basic procedure, including an analysis of the various arterial patterns that may be encountered and the management of these complicated vascular configurations.[28]

The operative procedure itself consists of an exploratory celiotomy with visual and manual assessment of the entire abdominal cavity for the presence of extrahepatic metastatic disease. In addition, a meticulous assessment of the disposition of metastases within the liver that may lend themselves to resection is crucial.

The right gastric artery and small branches to the duodenal bulb are ligated and divided, and the area of the porta hepatis and the common bile duct are skeletinized. Catheterization of the gastroduodenal artery is performed after ligation of the right gastric artery and dissection of the common hepatic, proper hepatic, and gastroduodenal arteries. Care is taken to ligate all branches of the gastroduodenal artery, particularly the supraduodenal artery arising within 2 cm of the origin from the common hepatic artery. The gastroduodenal artery is ligated distally and temporarily occluded proximally while the transverse arteriotomy is performed. The beaded Silastic catheter is inserted so that the tip lies just at the junction of the common hepatic and gastroduodenal arteries. In a minority of patients, the gastroduodenal artery is catheterized to allow infusion of the left hepatic artery. A replaced right hepatic artery is cannulated separately and directly using a tapered catheter to allow continual blood flow through the nonoccluded right hepatic artery. Conversely, the gastric duodenal artery may be cannulated to allow infusion of the right lobe of the liver, while a second catheter is placed retrograde into the left gastric artery to infuse the left lobe of the liver. A dual-catheter arterial pump is used to provide bilateral hepatic infusion in the latter 2 circumstances.

After catheterization, 2.0 ml of a fluorescein solution is injected into the side port of the pump and the abdominal contents are exposed to a Woods light to demonstrate a homogeneous uptake in the liver and to ensure absence of infusion to the stomach and duodenum. Following confirmation of optimal catheter placement, the implantable pump is placed in a subcutaneous pocket in either the right or left lower quadrant. Postoperatively, confirmation of the hepatic perfusion is performed using technetium or macroaggregated albumin.

In patients for whom an implanted pump in the abdomen is not possible because of prior radiation to the porta hepatis, or contraindications to operative placement such as comorbid disease, a catheter may be inserted via the brachial artery with radiographic guidance. The catheter tip is placed in the common hepatic artery beyond the origin of the gastroduodenal artery, and the latter artery may be occluded by primary embolization. The catheter may then be connected to an implanted pump, which is placed on the anterior chest wall in the subclavicular area. Such a technique has been employed extensively by Cohen et al[29] with few technical complications.

Special clinical circumstances may arise necessitating unusual adaptations of the basic procedures. For example, the identification of unsuspected hepatic metastases at the time of surgery for a primary tumor of the colon may not permit simultaneous placement of an implanted pump because of the absence of informed consent, knowledge of the vascular supply to the liver, and cost considerations. An alternative to placement of the implantable pump would be the placement of an implantable access disk. The same technique of catheter placement is used employing a beaded arterial catheter, but the disk, rather than the pump, would be inserted in the subcutaneous tissue over the lower ribs in order to ensure easy access. The access device could subsequently be replaced by an implanted pump, or the access device could be infused directly with an external pump.

Another unique clinical situation is one in which hepatic resection is carried out. Regional infusion may be desirable either as an adjuvant to the resection or for the treatment of residual unresectable disease within the liver. Such an approach to hepatic neoplasia is investigational, but studies by Kemeny et al have demonstrated that there are few complications related to regional infusion following partial hepatic resection even for multiple resections.[30]

Complications of Implanted Pump Hepatic Arterial Infusion

The virtues of the implanted pump system are related to the relative lack of complications compared to regional infusion using percutaneously placed catheters to the hepatic arterial tree. Complications that do occur may be separated into those related to the pump and catheter and those related to the actual drug infusion. Pump and catheter complications from collected series are summarized in table 5. Operative mortality is less than 1%. Arterial thrombosis, which occurs in up to 40% of patients with a percutaneous placement of a catheter, develops in less than 3% of patients with implanted pumps. Thrombosis is usually asymptomatic, but may occur in the setting of mild nausea, gastric ileus, and an elevation of liver function tests. More often, however, it is an unsuspected finding noted on the follow-up macroaggregated albumin scan. It may also be suspected with pump flow rate changes during treatment or if gastritis or gastroduodenal ulceration occurs. The development of arterial occlusion generally is irreversible and necessitates discontinuence of regional infusion.

Catheter occlusion is rare and can be treated initially with injection of urokinase in an attempt to dissolve a distal clot. Proper flushing of the

Table 5. Implanted Pump Complications in Hepatic Infusion Studies

Complication	No. patients	Frequency (%)
Tissue erosion	94	0
Wound infection	106	2 (1.9)
Sepsis	103	1 (1)
Pocket seroma	106	2 (1.9)
Catheter replacement	93	1 (1.1)
Catheter occlusion	93	1 (1.1)
Arterial thrombosis	106	3 (2.8)
Drug leakage	94	0
Drug extravasation	84	0
Component migration	94	0
Device failure	106	3 (2.8)

catheter component and prevention of pump overrun should avert such an occurrence. Small seroma that may develop can be managed by simple aspiration or drainage. Pump pocket infection, which may occur in up to 2% of patients, can be minimized by the use of perioperative antibiotics.

Drug-related complications are more common than complications related to the hardware and are only partially related to the implanted pump system (table 6). Agents that are not extracted by the liver can lead to systemic toxicity such as bone marrow suppression. This complication has been observed in conjunction with mitomycin-C and the nitrosoureas. The most common drug employed for regional arterial infusion of the liver is FUDR, which appears to have a unique potential for hepatic toxicity. Depending on the infusion rate, elevation of the hepatic enzymes, especially SGOT, is commonly observed after 2 weeks of infusion. This observation has been correlated with the development of gastric and duodenal ulceration as well. Hohn et al have emphasized that duodenal and gastric ulcerations may be minimized by meticulous elimination of accessory vascular channels to the duodenum.[31] Similarly, cholecystitis may be prevented by routine cholecystectomy at the time of catheter placement. Biliary sclerosis remains a serious and unpredictable complication in a series reporting on the implanted pump device for regional infusion of the liver.[32] Sclerosis of the biliary tract can cause a clinical picture of obstructive jaundice that may be difficult to distinguish from progressive hepatic metastases. The process may continue within the liver and induce hepatic failure over time. The development of biliary sclerosis is an absolute contraindication to continued infusion of FUDR.

The latter complication has not been observed in association with other agents or with the use of other systems of delivery such as percutaneously placed catheters with external pumps.

Regional Delivery, Future Perspectives

The precise role of regional delivery in the treatment of localized malignancy is dependent upon the outcome of prospective clinical trials to confirm early phase 2 trials.[33-35] Such trials are ongoing at least for the regional infusion of hepatic metastases for coloretal cancer. Special applications in hepatocellular carcinoma and in tumors of other sites such as the extremity, head and neck, brain and pelvis continue to be studied in phase 1 and phase 2 trials.

Technological advances in pumps and catheters are continuing. Multiple catheters and multiple pump chambers may permit the simultaneous infusion

Table 6. Drug-Related Complications of Hepatic Arterial Infusion of FUDR Using an Implanted Pump System

Complication	Frequency (%)
Hepatic Enzymopathy	40
Gastric ulcers	40
Acalculous choleceptitis	10
Biliary sclerosis	56

of several sites and the delivery of a variety of agents simultaneously. The spectrum of drugs that can be administered by regional delivery is being expanded as the pump compatibility of other drugs and new investigational agents become available. Finally, the capability of using programmable pumps that permit fluctuations in the rate of drug delivery will increase the flexibility of regional delivery systems.

Summary

Vascular access is a crucial component to infusional chemotherapy delivered either intravenously as systemic therapy or arterially for regional therapy. Technological advances have provided a major impetus to the pragmatic application of the infusion schedule to the treatment of cancer. There are a number of options for venous access, and selection criteria for the use of each option are being identified. The major complications of venous access involve thrombosis of the central veins; various methods of prevention employing anticoagulation are being explored. The use of the venous access portal represents the standard for the infusion of chemotherapy for the present. The precise role of surgically accessed arterial delivery is dependent upon establishing the true clinical effectiveness of such therapy compared to systemic delivery systems.

6

NURSING MANAGEMENT OF INFUSION CATHETERS

Cheryl L. Moore, R.N.

SELECTION OF THE APPROPRIATE type of catheter for the delivery of infusion therapy is influenced by several factors, including the site and stage of disease, anticipated length of therapy, patient educability and compliance, the performance status of the patient, and patient self-image and preference. These issues are addressed carefully by the oncologist with the patient and family during initial discussions concerning treatment options.

In order to provide optimal care of an infusion catheter, regardless of its specific type and location, the number of care-givers must be limited to a minimum of properly trained individuals. These would ideally include the oncology nurse, the I.V. therapist, a designated home care nurse when appropriate, and a significant other person.

Meticulous care of the catheter and its site of exit is vital for maximum protection against complications. Such care requires strict adherence to aseptic techniques during dressing changes, maintenance of occlusive dressings at exit sites, and appropriate flushing techniques and intervals to preserve catheter patency.

Although technical management of the catheters is one of the primary considerations in providing safe infusional therapy, patient and family education parallels this in importance. This chapter will address these issues separately in relation to specific catheter types, including the Hickman and tunneled subclavian catheters, inplanted venous access ports, arterial catheters, and implanted infusion pumps. Complications secondary to indwelling catheters will be discussed in the context of their influence on catheter care and patient education and with respect to their detection and management. The perspective from which this material is presented is largely based on our institutional philosophies and experience.

Hickman Catheters

The Hickman catheter has its primary application in the area of hyperalimentation and the treatment of leukemic patients. The catheter provides chronic venous access, as well as the ability to deliver continuous leukemic maintenance therapy in an ambulatory setting with the use of a portable pump. The Hickman is representative of a number of Silastic catheters used for infusion therapy. Available with a single or double lumen, it has an inner diameter of 1.6 mm, which facilitates the administration of blood products and other high-viscosity solutions.

Operative placement of the Hickman catheter is dictated chiefly by the requirement for the long subcutaneous tunnel that extends from the subclavian or internal jugular insertion site to the sternal area (approximately 20–30 cm). This places the exit site well within reach of the patient, promoting the option for self-care.

The presence of Dacron cuffs in two places along the outside wall of the catheter promotes granulation at the cuff sites, sealing the tunnel against bacterial invasion from the skin surface. Dressing requirements differ greatly between institutions, ranging from a full protective sterile dressing to the complete absence of a dressing once granulation has taken place.[1] Our institutional policies require maintenance of sterile occlusive dressings while the catheter remains in place.

The Hickman catheter is associated with long-term use, and because of its Silastic properties, with proper care it will provide venous access for many months and even years.

Dressing Application

Dressing changes are performed 3 times weekly by the patient or a significant other person who has been properly trained in the procedure. The dressing procedure requires strict sterile technique and the use of sterile gloves and masks. A triple povidone-iodine application is used to prepare the area over which the dressing will be placed. The catheter exit site is covered with a small amount of povidone-iodine ointment, a small gauze square, and finally, an occlusive covering of a sterile Elastoplast dressing. This is secured by a window frame application of paper tape. The catheter is secured to the dressing by a chevron of adherent tape (see figure 1). Finally, a proximal loop of catheter is taped to the dressing surface to avoid excessive strain on the catheter.

The patient is provided with a low-tension smooth clamp for use in preventing blood loss if the catheter is accidentally damaged. However, except under circumstances in which the catheter is disconnected for use, the use of a clamp is not recommended due to the potential for weakening the Silastic material, resulting in an eventual ballooning of the catheter.

When the catheter is not being used for infusion, the open end is protected with a sterile plug adaptor through which heparinization is performed. Patency is maintained by daily heparin flushes in a concentration of 1,000 u/ml of solution with a total volume of 2 ml. This exceeds the amount of maintenance heparin required by many other institutions.[1]

The Hickman catheter is maintained in this way until the patient has completed therapy, at which time the catheter may be removed. Catheter removal does not require an operative procedure and is generally accomplished in the outpatient clinic. After an intravenous injection of diazepam, the surgeon removes the catheter by maintaining a firm, continuous pull on its distal end until the tip emerges from the subcutaneous tunnel. As a rule, the Hickman's Dacron cuffs have granulated into the tissue within the tunnel and remain in the patient without complication.

Patient and Family Teaching

Patient and family education with respect to Hickman catheter maintenance and care varies according to the proposed use for the catheter. Leukemic patients and their significant others are instructed in the dressing change procedures, with particular emphasis on the proper application of sterile gloves and the points relative to sterile technique. The importance of maintaining dressing occlusiveness is stressed, and the possibility of the necessity for more frequent dressing changes to achieve this is suggested.

Because the Hickman catheter exits well below the original venotomy site, the dressing is placed within reach of the patient himself, who may wish to be the main caretaker of the catheter. In this case, it is generally the practice to include a significant other in the teaching process as a support for the patient.

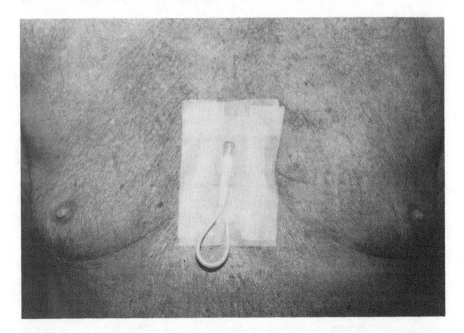

Figure 1.   Hickman and tunneled subclavian catheters are dressed occusively with sterile Elastoplast. Catheters are secured with plastic tape.

Teaching heparinization procedures to maintain catheter patency during dormant periods requires instructions to prepare heparin syringes as well as to inject the catheter with the solution.

All techniques are taught first by verbal instruction and physical demonstration by the oncology nurse. This is followed by a return procedure by the patient (or significant other) until competency is demonstrated.

Additional teaching emphasizes the importance of obtaining prompt attention to any signs of infection noted at the catheter exit site or to generalized symptoms of sepsis. Leakage of infusate near the catheter connector or exit site or blood backflow into the pump tubing may indicate an interruption in the integrity of the catheter itself or the connections between the catheter and tubing. Either could lead to air embolus, infection, or a serious occlusion of the catheter as a consequence of intraluminal clotting.

Subclavian Catheters

Percutaneous subclavian catheters provide venous access for a large number of patients receiving infusional chemotherapy. Continuous infusion of vesicant drugs requires the use of centrally placed catheters to avoid the risk of extravasation. For protocols requiring short-term infusions (e.g., 5–day) during a hospital admission, the catheter is generally inserted for the duration of the drug therapy and removed at the completion of the course before discharge from the hospital. Treatment protocols that promote outpatient status dictate the creation of a subcutaneous tunnel for purposes of catheter stabilization and protection against systemic infection.

The Deseret, representative of a polyvinyl subclavian catheter, has an inner diameter of 1.7 mm and is cut to a length of 20 cm (8 in.) for tunneling and 15 cm (6 in.) for temporary use. This length prevents entry of the catheter tip into the right atrium, where contact with the endocardium may cause obstruction of the tip.

Catheter insertion is accomplished at the bedside, thus allowing completion on an outpatient basis. However, due to the extensive teaching time required to instruct the patient and family in optimal catheter care, a hospital admission for 2–3 days may be offered to facilitate catheter insertion and to provide adequate reinforcement of teaching principles.

Subclavian catheters may be used for leukemic therapy in the initial period of induction. In the leukemic population, the dressing change is performed—as with the Hickman—3 times weekly. However, the major portion of these catheters are used in the solid tumor patient population, in which the frequency of dressing change is twice weekly. The dressing procedure is identical to that required for Hickman dressings but, because of the short subcutaneous tunnel (approximately 5 cm, or 2 in.), the patient is unable to perform his/her own dressing change and the responsibility falls to the significant other.

Heparinization of an uninfused catheter is performed daily with 2 ml heparin, 1,000 u/ml. Because of its tendency to kink or crack near the hub over time, the catheter is routinely exchanged over a guidewire if the catheter duration exceeds 90 days. Catheter removal is accomplished by the oncology nurse after completion of therapy.

Patient and Family Teaching

Instructional issues parallel those of the Hickman catheters. The incidence of clinically detectable venous thrombosis in patients with indwelling polyvinyl catheters has been noted to be substantial (about 30%).[2] Therefore, the patient is apprised of the signs and symptoms of thrombosis and cautioned to alert the primary physician promptly upon presentation of symptoms (see section on complications, below).

Implantable Venous Access Portals

The third type of subclavian catheter is the implanted venous access portal (VAP). This catheter has several advantages over the external catheter systems in terms of aesthetics, decreased patient responsibility, fewer teaching requirements, and decreased risk of venous thrombosis and infection[3] (see table 1 for comparisons in care).

Three implantable portal systems are currently available. Although somewhat variable in configuration and material, all 3 consist of a disk-shaped portal with a central self-sealing silicone septum through which needle access is gained and an attached Silastic catheter (see table 2 for specific feature comparisons).

Because a minor operative procedure is required for insertion and removal, this catheter is usually selected for the patient requiring infusional therapy for at least 6 months or for the patient with suboptimal peripheral access.

The care of the catheter system has been delegated primarily to the oncology nurse and specifically designated individuals such as the I.V. therapist and home care nurse. Because of lessened patient responsibility and the resultant decrease in required teaching time, the patient may achieve catheter/port insertion and treatment initiation on the same day on an outpatient basis. Incisional sutures remain in place for 10 to 14 days after insertion.

Table 1. Subclavian Catheters: Comparison of Routine Care

Catheter	Dressing change	Heparinization	Teaching requirements
Hickman	3x/week	Daily	Dressing change Heparinization
Tunneled subclavian	2x/week	Daily	Dressing change Heparinization
Implanted VAP	None*	Monthly	None

*Weekly by nurse for infusional therapy

Needle Access

The VAP is accessed by a Huber point needle, which is specially beveled to prevent coring the silicone septum upon entry. The most easily used needle configuration is a 90° needle with 22 gauge, 1 inch in length. For those patients with a greater depth of subcutaneous tissue over the implanted port, a 1 1/2-inch needle may be required for more comfortable needle seating. Needles may remain in place for an average of 2 weeks. Frequency of needle change is governed by the condition of the skin at the needle site. Absence of erythema or inflammation at the exit site may allow the needle to remain in situ for as long as 4 weeks.

The postoperative accumulation of fluid in the VAP pocket of some patients has precluded the use of the portal for at least 2 days after the insertion procedure due to difficulty in palpating the device for needle insertion. In order to avoid this problem and the accompanying risk of improper needle seating, a heparinized needle attached to its extension tubing is inserted by the surgeon at the time of surgery, when the site is still anesthetized and before serous fluid has accumulated. In this way, the patient may begin therapy immediately after the procedure, if desired, or the needle may remain in place until therapy is initiated. It is prudent to emphasize here that no drug therapy is initiated via any subclavian catheter before a single-view chest X ray confirms position of the catheter tip in the superior vena cava and the absence of pneumothorax.

Needle access is gained under strict sterile guidelines, requiring the use of sterile gloves and a triple povidone-iodine prep. Masks need not be worn because the port represents a closed system.

The Huber point needle is first attached to an extension tubing and primed with bacteriostatic saline. To obtain access to the portal, the needle should be

Table 2. Specific Features of Implantable VAP

VAP	Reservoir volume	Portal	Septum dimensions	Catheter lumen
Infuse-A-Port (Infusaid Corp.)	.6 ml	Polyethersulfone plastic weight: 16.3 gm diam: 48 mm height: 16.5 mm	diam: 13 mm depth: 6.2 mm	0.6 mm I.D.*-2.3 mm O.D.* 1.0 mm I.D.-2.5 mm O.D.
Mediport (Cormed, Inc.)	.5 ml	Stainless steel Silicone collar weight: 25 gm diam: 33 mm height: 14 mm	diam: 11 mm depth: 7.7 mm	0.5 mm I.D.-2 mm O.D. 1.0 mm I.D.-2.23 mm O.D. 1.5 mm I.D.-3.0 mm O.D.
Port-A-Cath (Pharmacia-Nutech, Inc.)	.4 ml	Stainless steel weight: 28 gm diam: 25.4 mm height: 13.5 mm	diam: 11.25 mm depth: 5.8 mm	0.5 mm I.D.-2.03 mm O.D. 1.02 mm I.D.-2.8 mm O.D.

*I.D. = inner diameter
O.D. = outer diameter

held with a forefinger supporting the needle angle to prevent the needle shaft from swiveling on its hub, which could result in deflection of the point as it enters the skin (see figure 2). Once the needle has pierced the skin over the center of the portal, firm pressure is required to penetrate the silicone septum until the needle point comes to rest against the floor of the portal. The needle should seat perpendicularly against the needle stop. Occasionally, resistance in flushing or inability to aspirate blood (withdrawal occlusion) is caused by improper needle seating, in which the bevel of the needle is placed at too severe an angle to the needle stop or too close to the septal wall. Needle puncture is well tolerated by most patients, and local anesthesia has not been required for access to the portal.

Dressing Application

An antibiotic ointment (Neosporin) is placed at the prepared needle site and covered with a half-inch square of Telfa to preserve the adhesive properties of the occlusive dressing that follows. The needle is dressed by dual overlapping sterile cellophane dressings, which stabilize the needle and seal the needle site from bacterial entry. Care is taken to pinch the dressing beneath the needle hub to prevent skin decubiti and to form an occlusive seal (see figure 3). The outer edges of the dressing are secured with paper tape to maintain occlusiveness.

This deviation from the dressing procedure practices for external catheters resulted from the desire to observe the needle position through the dressing. One of the benefits derived from this variation was that the cellophane dress-

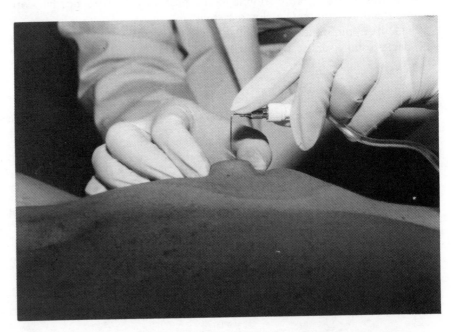

Figure 2.   To prevent deflection of needle upon entry through portal septum, support angle of needle with forefinger. Insert needle perpendicularly to intraportal needle stop.

ing tends to maintain its occlusiveness longer than the Elastoplast dressing; therefore, the frequency of dressing changes has evolved to once weekly by nursing personnel. Except under special circumstances, the significant other is not responsible for the dressing change because of the difficulty in manipulating the transparent dressings and the risk of needle dislodgment during dressing removal. This is the primary reason for the decrease in patient/family responsibility and teaching time required for catheter care. In addition, when the septum is not in use, the access needle is removed, obviating the need for a dressing.

Heparinization of the venous access port is required prior to needle removal or at monthly intervals when the system is in a dormant state. The concentration of heparin required to maintain patency is 100 u/ml, with a total volume of 5 ml to accommodate the capacity of the catheter (1 ml), port (0.2 – 0.4 ml), and the 37 cm (15 in.) extension tubing through which the heparin is injected (3 ml).

Special Considerations

All 3 categories of venous infusion catheters lend themselves to blood sampling and the infusion of I.V. fluids and blood products. The external catheters require routine care after blood sampling, including a flush with 10 ml of

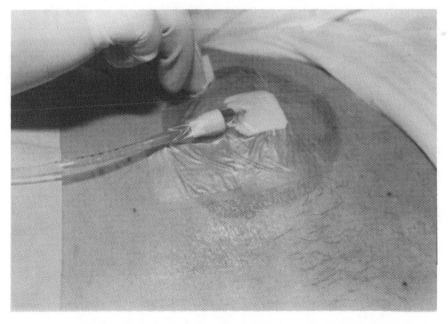

Figure 3.   The VAP needle is secured and covered by 2 overlapping pieces of sterile transparent dressings. The second is pinched under needle hub to form occlusive seal and protect from decubitus.

bacteriostatic saline and a final heparin flush if no infusion is to follow. Fluids and blood products may be administered under gravity flow if desired.

The preservation of the implanted VAP for infusion therapy depends on meticulous care with all infusions and blood samplings due to the presence of the portal, which represents a substantial risk of occlusion if blood is allowed to remain stationary within. Blood sampling from the portal is therefore followed by an immediate flush of 20 ml of bacteriostatic saline, and a final heparin flush if infusion does not immediately follow. Administration of intravenous fluids and blood products is most safely accomplished with a volumetric infusion pump. Constant positive pressure helps to eliminate the possibility of unnoticed interruptions in flow, which could lead to catheter or portal occlusion. Blood product administration should be followed by the flushing procedure recommended for blood sampling.

In addition to blood clotting, occlusion of the VAPs may occur as the result of sedimentation, crystallization, or clumping from the simultaneous infusion of incompatible products such as heparin and Adriamycin. To prevent this from occurring, flushing the septum with a forceful, pulsatile action with 40 ml of bacteriostatic saline to rid the portal and catheter of one product before administering another incompatible product is recommended by one of the portal manufacturers.

Neither external catheters nor VAP needles should be directly connected to the portable pump or intravenous tubing without the benefit of an extension tubing, which may be clamped at any time the pump or infusion tubing is disconnected from the patient. The clamp provides protection against air embolus and blood backflow. It is particularly important with respect to the use of the VAP systems that the clamp be closed prior to needle removal in order to prevent reflux of blood into the catheter tip, which could lead to occlusion. The extension tubing facilitates flushing the system, blood sampling, and other procedures without necessitating dressing removal. The extension is considered an integral part of the catheter system and is changed only when the catheter or VAP needle is changed. (The exception to this is the Hickman catheter, which extends beyond its exit site sufficiently for tubing disconnections.)

Swimming is restricted for any patient with a system in which a dressing is in place. Bathing is allowed with proper waterproof protection, which the patient provides by applying several layers of household plastic wrap over the exit site. The protective covering extends well outside the boundaries of the sterile dressing and is taped occlusively on all four sides. The pump is placed outside the shower stall or bathtub away from contact with moisture.

Management of Local Skin Effects

The presence of an indwelling infusion catheter may result in certain local skin manifestations of varying severity and consequences; these should not be confused with infectious processes.

The most frequently noted local effect is an erythematous area that may occur at the exit site of the external subclavian catheter, often accompanied by slight swelling, but without drainage or extreme tenderness. This condition, which may be noted soon after catheter insertion, has commonly been associated with the use of povidone-iodine ointment. The elimination of the ointment from the dressing application nearly always allows the condition to clear. Neosporin ointment may be substituted with the same result, inasmuch as its use as a bacterial protectant in VAP dressings has not resulted in reactive skin problems.

Less prominent erythematous processes are noted in some patients in a more or less chronic state. These are innocuous in appearance, nontender and noninflammatory, and have required no treatment or corrective measures. The mechanical movement of the external catheter seems to create an irritative focus at the exit site, which may remain in a stable state for the duration of the catheter.

External tunneled subclavian catheters require stabilization with one suture near the exit site. Normal movement of the catheter during patient activity occasionally causes inflammation or erosion in the area of the suture, requiring its relocation.

Skin effects suggesting an allergic component include reactions to tape and adhesives on standard dressing materials. These effects may range from erythema or rash to severe blistering and may motivate the use of an alternative dressing. Paper tape is used exclusively to secure central catheter dressings in our institution because of its hypoallergenic properties. If, however, paper tape does evoke an allergic reaction, the use of tape is eliminated altogether. Allergic reactions to transparent dressings appear rare, as evidenced by our experience with VAP dressings. Therefore, even though they stabilize external catheters less well than standard Elastoplast dressings, they may be used alternatively to eliminate reactions to Elastoplast. Another alternative dressing material is Microfoam, which may be substituted for standard dressings in the face of allergic reactions or chronic excessive perspiration, which destroys the occlusiveness of standard materials.

Escape of infusate through catheter defects or insecure connections sometimes results in exposure of the skin in the area of the catheter dressing to drug. Direct contact of drug with skin creates significant potential for cutaneous damage. Because 5-fluorouracil precipitates to a powdery substance when exposed to the air, it has a greater tendency to adhere to skin than do liquid drugs, becoming a severe topical irritant. Therefore, it is important to remove any traces of drug from the skin as soon as possible. Skin damage may occasionally be severe enough to warrant removal of an external catheter or the access needle in the implanted system to allow air exposure to accelerate the healing process. Generally, however, even in the presence of moderate skin irritation, the infusion may be continued with modification of dressing techniques. Severe excoriative areas should be closely observed for signs of infection and kept scrupulously clean. The patient should be seen by the oncology nurse or physician at least twice weekly for monitoring of the skin condition and dressing changes. Because of its healing properties, a transparent cellophane dressing is usually applied over the catheter or needle exit site, using a minimal amount of skin surface area and eliminating surrounding tape. As much of the damaged skin is exposed to air as possible. Any other interventions, such as topical anti-inflammatory preparations, have not been necessary, and no infectious processes have resulted from this type of complication.

Complications Associated with Subclavian Catheters

Venous Thrombosis

The most problematic complication associated with the use of venous access catheters has been the development of thrombosis in the conduit vein of the indwelling catheter. The incidence of clinically detectable thrombosis in our institution has been lowered from approximately 30% in a patient population in which external polyvinyl subclavian catheters were utilized to 16% in a group of 330 patients in whom implanted venous access ports with Silastic catheters were studied.

Physical symptoms of thrombosis in order of frequency of occurrence include vague discomfort to acute pain in the area of the shoulder, neck or arm; supraclavicular swelling; a pattern of venous distention in the neck, shoulder or chest wall; and evidence of the development of collateral circulation on the chest wall or arm. These symptoms generally occur on the side ipsilateral to the catheter, but occasionally contralaterally. Less frequent signs of thrombotic development have been dysphagia, superior vena cava syndrome, pain in the ear, and headache.

Venous thrombosis is confirmed by arm venography. The major portion of thrombi have been noted to occur in the subclavian or innominate vein around the body of the catheter. A smaller portion formed in the superior vena cava, in some instances near the catheter tip.

Patients who are considered at risk for the development of venous thrombosis are those who have had previous episodes of thrombosis with or without a central line in place, those with intrathoracic disease or other disease processes that might increase coagulability, and those in whom abnormally low antithrombin levels are detected.[3] These patients may be considered for low-dose anticoagulant therapy either by oral administration of Coumadin or by the concomitant infusion of low-dose heparin with compatible drugs such as 5-FU or FUDR in the infusion pump.

Aside from physical symptomatology of venous thrombosis, certain functional catheter complications may occur secondary to clot formation. These problems include withdrawal occlusion, catheter kinking, resistance in catheter flow, and extravasation. These will be discussed in ensuing paragraphs.

Management of Venous Thrombosis

Thrombosis in a patient with an external tunneled catheter is generally managed by removal of the catheter. Once symptoms subside, the catheter may be relatively easily reinserted in the contralateral subclavian at a later date if infusion therapy is to be pursued. In this event, the patient would be placed on prophylactic anticoagulant therapy.

Thrombotic development with an implanted system in place presents a different problem because of the operative nature of removal and reinsertion of the device. In addition, most of these patients have been selected for use of the implanted systems because they require long-term ambulatory infusion. Therefore, an attempt to maintain function of the catheter system is made by placing the patient on anticoagulant therapy until symptoms have abated. The most frequent form of management has been the 24–48° infusion of heparin, which in most cases resulted in the recession of objective and subjective symptoms. The patient is then maintained on Coumadin for the duration of the catheter placement to prevent clot propagation.

Although lytic therapy with streptokinase or urokinase may be instituted, it is generally felt that the risks in this case outweigh benefits. The reason for this is that venous thromboses do not seem to declare themselves symptomatically in the early phases of formation during which lytic drugs would be most effective. Often, early symptomatology includes collateral circulation visible on the chest wall and upon venogram, indicating that the thrombus has been present for a time. In the event that lytic therapy is deemed feasible, a peripheral catheter is imbedded in the clot under fluoroscopic guidance and a 12–24° infusion of the drug is instituted through the catheter.

Explantation of a venous access port in the setting of venous thrombosis may take place because of symptoms refractory to anticoagulation or clot progression at a later date.

Detection and Management of Infection

Local Infections

Although sepsis has been exceptionally rare in our experience, it may occur locally at the exit site of the catheter or Huber needle or in the VAP pocket. It is detected by an erythematous swelling, tenderness, and an exudate that yields a positive culture.

A positive culture results in the removal of the temporary external subclavian catheter; however, the more permanent systems such as the Hickman (provided the infection appears to be confined below the subcutaneous cuff) and the implanted portals are more commonly allowed to remain in place while antibiotic treatment is administered.

When a local infection is suspected, blood cultures are drawn through the external catheters in order to rule out an occult systemic infection. The same applies for the implanted system, but only in the event a Huber needle is in place at the time the infectious process is noted. Otherwise, a potentially infected port pocket should never be accessed with a needle because of the risk of tracking organisms into the catheter and subsequently to the systemic circulation.

Systemic Infections

If bacteremia is suspected in any patient in whom a central line is in place, blood cultures should be drawn both peripherally and through the catheter in an attempt to ascertain whether the catheter is a potential source of infection. The general rule of thumb has been that if the peripheral culture is positive but the central is negative, the assumption that the catheter is not the source of the organism results in the initiation of antibiotic therapy. The catheter remains in place in both the external and implanted systems. However, a positive central culture results in the removal of the external tunneled subclavian catheter; the removal of the Hickman catheter in the leukemic patient is at the discretion of the hematologist. The implanted VAP may remain in place in this situation, with antibiotics being administered until central cultures are negative. If the infection persists after a reasonable trial of antibiotics, explantation of the portal should be considered.

Extravasation

Fortunately, extravasation of infusate into the subcutaneous tissues of the catheter tunnel or port pocket occurs very rarely.

The potential for extravasation during infusion through external catheters is small, and its occurrence would in all likelihood be the result of a crack or defect in the wall of the catheter within the subcutaneous tunnel, allowing drug to escape into the surrounding tissues. This, of course, would be rectified by exchange of the catheter over a guidewire, provided the extravasation occurred with a nonvesicant drug. In the event a vesicant drug was implicated, the catheter ideally should be removed and a surgical consult placed to assess tissue damage and the possible need for intervention. The area should be monitored for a period of weeks for signs of necrosis.

The implantable VAP represents a greater potential for extravasation from the standpoint of continuous Huber needle placement. The great majority of extravasations have been caused by inadvertent needle dislodgment from excessive strain on catheter tubing. Needle dislodgment occurs most rarely in ports that have a greater depth of septum.

A system in which the port and catheter are 2 separate units attached at the time of insertion presents a risk of possible separation, with resultant flow of infusate into the portal pocket (see section on catheter embolus, below). This complication could be confirmed immediately upon single-view chest X ray.

An important phenomenon that has been noted in the VAP system has been extravasation into the infraclavicular space or portal pocket, which on contrast radiographic flow study through the portal is shown to be the probable result of the presence of a thrombus at the tip of the catheter. Flow of the infusate is actually directed by the thrombus in retrograde fashion along the outer wall of the catheter until it deposits into the subcutaneous tissue beyond the venotomy site (see figure 4). This complication can be confirmed only by use of contrast and, if thrombus is seen or suspected as the cause of backflow, arm venography should follow to establish the extent of the clot. This event nearly always results in explantation of the device, since the backflow pre-

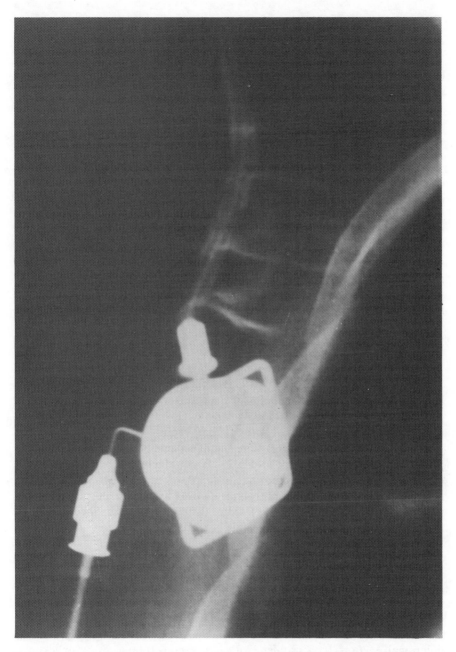

Figure 4.   Contrast flow study through VAP showing retrograde flow of infusate along outer wall of catheter and into subcutaneous tunnel and pocket. This patient had thrombosis in superior vena cava at tip of catheter.

cludes its use and complete clot lysis cannot be expected from anticoagulant therapy.

A defect in the catheter or septum could be suspected in the event of extravasation not otherwise explained. A contrast study through the portal would again be the diagnostic factor.

Catheter Tip Migration

Several patients in whom the Silastic catheter of the implanted system was originally confirmed to terminate in the superior vena cava had incidental chest X rays showing migration of the tip of the catheter to the internal jugular vein. Sequential chest X rays revealed the catheter of one patient with intrathoracic disease as drifting between the superior vena cava and the internal jugular vein. Catheter tip migration is significant in the context of the infusion of sclerosing drugs, for which a larger lumened vessel would be preferred by most practitioners. Malposition of the catheter can be corrected by the radiologist, who may redirect the catheter tip under fluoroscopic guidance by means of a transfemoral snare.

Catheter Embolus

Very rarely, separation of the catheter from the portal in the 2-unit implantable system has resulted in embolus of the catheter to the right atrium, and in one patient, the right ventricle.

The catheters were retrieved without complication under fluoroscopy. The possibility of catheter fracture and resultant separation is small but also worthy of consideration. Careful attention to manufacturer's recommendations for insertion techniques is important to help prevent catheter/portal separation. Additionally, the inability to aspirate blood from the portal, accompanied by extravasation of flushing fluid or infusate, should be investigated by single-view chest X ray to rule out this potentially serious complication.

Catheter Occlusion

Catheter occlusion due to intraluminal clotting may occur in either external or implanted catheter systems. This nearly always occurs in a situation in which the intravenous flow through the catheters is interrupted, either by pump malfunction, by a problem with intravenous tubing, or by unacknowledged completion of the infusion.

Occlusion is most consequential in Hickman catheters because of their relative permanency, and in the implanted venous access port systems due to the difficulty in dislodging or lysing a clot once established within the portal. Tunneled subclavian catheters may be exchanged over a guidewire if a problematic occlusion occurs.

In general, if the occlusion is discovered at an early stage, flushing the septum with a tuberculin syringe of heparin 1:1,000 directly attached to the catheter or Huber needle will dissolve the clot. If heparin fails to restore patency, lysis with streptokinase 10,000 u or urokinase 2000 u diluted in volumes to equal catheter capacity may be attempted. This solution is allowed to remain in place for 10 minutes, after which an attempt to aspirate the clot is made. If aspiration is not achieved, the attempt is repeated at 10″ intervals for 30″, and then again at 24° until aspiration of the clot has been accomplished. An additional 4–5 ml of blood is aspirated and the system is then flushed with 20 ml of sterile saline. Failure to reverse an occlusion would result in removal of the access device.

A second cause for catheter occlusion is drug precipitate. In this case, prevention tends to be curative because once drug crystals become lodged in the catheter lumen or within the portal of the implanted system, they are extremely difficult to dissipate. 5-FU precipitates not only on exposure to air but to cold temperatures as well. Patients should be instructed to protect the ambulatory infusion pumps and tubings from the elements, keeping them well covered by warm clothing when outside in cold weather even for short periods.

5-FU precipitate may be detected in the pump tubing as well as in the medication reservoir of the pump. Although drug precipitate is unlikely to cause occlusion of external catheters, the problem may present itself in relation to VAPs. Because the Huber needle used for continuous infusion is bent at a 90° angle, the precipitate may accumulate at the needle flexure, resulting in cessation of flow through the system. This situation may lead to leakage of drug at connection sites along the pump tubing or expansion of the plastic extension tubing under constant pump pressure. Stoppage of drug flow through the catheter produces the possibility of blood backflow into the catheter tip, with resultant risk of intraluminal clotting.

If it is not possible to introduce flushing fluid through a Huber needle, the used needle should be replaced and another flushing attempt made before portal/catheter occlusion is assumed. In most cases, drug precipitate affects only the needle in place and not the portal or catheter.

One should exercise caution in delivering Mannitol through catheter systems, particularly those of less than 1.0 mm intraluminal size. If Mannitol is insufficiently diluted, it may crystallize, causing a serious catheter occlusion. One such incident was rectified by the application of heat to the chest wall over the catheter tunnel with restoration of catheter patency.

Catheter occlusion may be mimicked by incidental kinking of the catheter. Although a kink may be present from the time of insertion, patient movement or position may create an occlusive bend in the catheter, preventing flushing. Recumbency of the patient may worsen a catheter malformation to the point that a kink can be palpated in the subcutaneous tunnel, particularly at the entry site to the vein. Severe kinking that stops drug flow may result in the development of leakage at catheter connections in the outpatient from constant pump pressure. Catheter kinks are easily detected by X ray because of the radio-opacity of the catheters.

Table 3 provides a guideline for detection of potential complications involving implantable access systems.

Withdrawal Occlusion

The inability to aspirate blood from a catheter or VAP may simply be the function of patient position or variants in intrathoracic pressure. This problem can often be corrected by instructing the patient to change position or alter the depth of respirations.

Needle position in the VAP is extremely important. If the needle is situated at an angle or too close to the sides of the portal, aspiration may not be possible. In the absence of more obvious signs of complications, withdrawal occlusion may be assumed to be temporary or the result of incorrect needle angling.

Thrombosis at the catheter tip or a constrictive clot around the catheter may prevent aspiration of blood. Therefore, withdrawal occlusion in a catheter that

Table 3. Guidelines for Detection of VAP Complications

Problem	Possible causative factors	Action
• Spontaneous blood backflow	• Tubing disconnections	• Tighten all connections
	• Pump battery failure	• Change pump battery
• Leaking connections	• Tubing disconnections	• Tighten all connections
	• Clogged Huber point needle	• If flush with n/s is unsuccessful, change needle
	• Catheter occlusion	• Attempt n/s flush. If unsuccessful, change needle. If occlusion remains, follow guidelines for lysis of intraluminal clots
• Extravasation	• Dislodged needle	• Check needle placement. If no blood backflow, change needle
	• Catheter disconnection from portal	• Attempt to aspirate blood. If unable, x-ray chest
	• Venous thrombosis at catheter tip (backtracking of infusate)	• Radiographic flow study via VAP
	• Defective portal septum or catheter	• Radiographic flow study via VAP
		• Operative exchange of system
• Withdrawal occlusion	• Patient position	• Change patient position
	• Temporary minor catheter occlusion	• 20 ml n/s flush
	• Needle dislodgement	• Check needle placement
	• Improper needle placement in septum	• Reinsert needle ensuring perpendicular angling of needle to needle stop. Avoid placing needle too close to sides of inner reservoir
	• Catheter disconnection from portal	• Chest x-ray
	• Thrombosis	• Venogram
• Resistance in flushing	• Catheter occlusion	• See "leaking connections"
	• Improper needle placement	• See "withdrawal occlusion"
	• Kink in catheter	• Chest x-ray

has previously allowed blood sampling may be predictive of the presence of venous thrombosis, since 50% of those patients with symptomatic thrombus formation had previously developed permanent withdrawal occlusion.

Kinks or curves in the catheter that may occur at the time of insertion are generally found in the catheter tunnel or at the entry to the vein, although as much as a 360° catheter loop has been noted in at least one patient. While a gentle curve may allow infusion, it may prevent blood sampling.

Hepatic Artery Catheters

The fact that tumors derive their blood supply from arterial sources has given rise to the practice of delivering drugs to malignant tumors by infusion through an arterial catheter. Arterial infusion may be administered regionally by various arterial routes, including the external or internal carotid, femoral, and hepatic arteries.

Nursing implications with respect to technical management and patient/family teaching differ little between sites of catheter exits. Thus, for purposes of simplification, hepatic artery catheters, being the vehicle for the most common type of arterial infusion, will be the focus of discussion.

Hepatic artery catheters may be placed either surgically or percutaneously. The less invasive percutaneous method requires a radiographic procedure for insertion. Both methods require hospital admission for catheter placement and a period of postprocedural observation.

Percutaneous approach to the hepatic artery may be achieved via the femoral, axillary, or brachial arteries. Because the transfemoral approach requires the patient to be at bed rest for the duration of the catheter, the primary percutaneous method of hepatic artery cannulation in our institution has been transbrachial. Although the brachial artery is a much smaller conduit and somewhat more difficult to catheterize, it does allow the patient the option for ambulatory infusion and obviates the greater risk of ischemia, bleeding, and brachial plexus damage presented by the transaxillary approach.[4]

The left brachial artery is generally chosen as the site of insertion because of its greater accessibility to the aorta and the increased risk of cerebroembolic events if approached from the right.[4]

Immediate postprocedural nursing responsibilities include checking the catheterized limb at frequent intervals for signs of bleeding, and vital signs. The patient is restricted to bed rest for 24 hours. Catheter patency is maintained by the infusion of normal saline solutions via a volumetric pump.

As soon as the placement of the catheter has been confirmed radiographically, chemotherapy may be initiated via the volumetric infusion pump, with subsequent conversion to a portable pump in preparation for ambulatory infusion at home.

Dressing Application

Sterile and occlusive dressings over the arteriotomy site must be conscientiously maintained to prevent infection and catheter dislodgment. These dressings are changed weekly by the oncology nurse, applying strict aseptic principles. Specific dressing techniques have been suggested previously in the literature.[5]

An important characteristic of a percutaneous hepatic artery catheter is that the catheter is not sutured in place because of the possible need to manipulate or reposition the catheter at some point during the course of treatment. Stabilization of the catheter is accomplished by the use of sterile adhesive strips that firmly anchor the catheter to the skin just below the site of insertion. After a triple skin prep with povidone-iodine, its corresponding ointment is placed at the arteriotomy site and covered with an occlusive sterile dressing.

Another characteristic of the catheter is its tendency to kink or crack, particularly in the area of the stopcock, which is placed on the catheter in radiology. As a preventive, the catheter and stopcock are splinted with a padded tongue blade and taped securely in place over the finished dressing. Special care is taken to create gentle loops in the excess catheter when securing with tape to prevent kinking (see figure 5). The entire dressing, including the secured stopcock and excess catheter, is wrapped in Kling bandage for protection.

Special Considerations

Because of the frequency of catheter displacement in transbrachial catheters (20%),[6] position is routinely checked at weekly intervals by angiography before continuing chemotherapeutic infusion or as dictated by the develop-

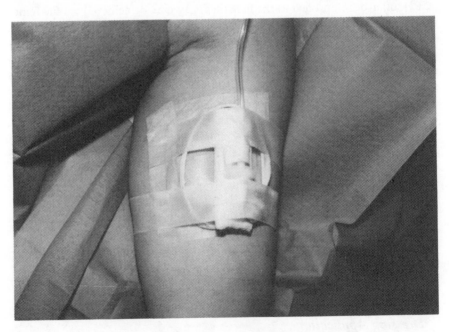

Figure 5. Transbrachial artery catheter dressing illustrating splinted stopcock and gently coiled catheter that prevents cracking and kinking of brittle catheter material.

ment of symptoms that may indicate catheter malposition or other complications. The catheter may be repositioned by simple manipulation unless advancement is required, in which case a new catheter must be inserted because the exposed portion of the one in place is contaminated.

Upon disconnection of the portable pump from the catheter, care should be taken that the stopcock is placed in the "off" position to the catheter to prevent blood backflow, which could result in intraluminal clotting. The catheter is flushed with 10 ml sterile bacteriostatic saline after removal of the pump and again before reconnection to assure patency. (As a general rule, hepatic artery catheters should not be aspirated because of the high risk of occlusion.)

Intraluminal catheter clots may occur at any time during infusion as a result of interrupted flow through the catheter. If resistance is met when flushing the catheter, a persistent effort to override the resistance should *not* be made. Because of the risk of causing an embolic incident or infarction in the event of catheter displacement, the radiologist should diagnose and correct the problem.

Patient and Family Teaching

Patient education, which begins prior to placement of the arterial catheter, encompasses such issues as the anatomical location of the catheter, postinsertion care, and expected scheduling (i.e., weekly outpatient visits and catheter position confirmations with radiology). Possible complications of the arterial catheter and infusional drug are discussed in detail (see table 4).

Postoperatively, the patient is instructed to limit the range of motion of the catheterized limb somewhat because of the risk of displacing the catheter. Because transbrachial artery catheters are generally inserted in the left upper arm, left-handed patients experience more restrictions in relation to hair combing and other such activities.

With respect to patients with surgically placed hepatic artery catheters exiting on the abdominal wall, the significant other must receive instruction as to the principles of sterile technique and the actual procedure for dressing change to be accomplished once weekly at home and once weekly in the outpatient clinic by the oncology nurse.

Patients with transbrachial artery catheters are not instructed in dressing changes because of the fragility and unstable characteristics of the catheters. They may, however, be instructed to change or rewrap the Kling bandage protecting the arteriotomy site dressing. Special emphasis should be placed on avoidance of wrapping the dressing too tightly, thus impeding circulation.

The importance of immediately reporting symptoms of catheter complications is emphasized to facilitate early intervention and prevent serious morbidity. Stress is placed on maintaining a constant flow through the catheter and reporting blood backflow or leakage immediately because of the risk of a resultant catheter occlusion.

The remainder of the instructional process is dedicated to those issues relating to drug side effects and toxicities and pump maintenance.

Catheter Removal

Hepatic artery catheters are removed at the end of the infusion period or in the event of a complication necessitating removal. Surgical catheters may be discontinued in various ways. In our institution, the catheter is allowed to clot by terminating the infusion through it, and then the catheter is cut close to the skin surface. Alternatively, the catheter may be removed by withdrawal at the bedside.

Percutaneous arterial catheters are simply removed by the physician, who simultaneously applies firm pressure on the artery above the area of insertion. The pressure is maintained for at least 10 minutes after removal or until bleeding has ceased.

Implantable Infusion Pump

The totally implanted pump is an appropriate device for the patient who anticipates an extended course of therapy and who prefers freedom from the encumbrance of dressings and external infusion pumps required by other types of arterial or venous access catheters.

The Infusaid pump has been employed to deliver FUDR as well as insulin, morphine, and heparin. The primary oncologic application for this implanted

Table 4. Complications of Transbrachial Hepatic Artery Catheters

Requiring catheter removal	Symptoms
• Visceral artery thrombosis (celiac, splenic, common hepatic)	• Abdominal pain, chest pain • UGI bleeding • Elevated liver enzymes (hepatic artery) • Fever
• Brachial artery thrombosis	• Loss of radial pulse • Cold extremity • Loss of sensation, color of arm
• Bleeding at arteriotomy site	• Bleeding uncontrolled by pressure dressing
• Infection	• Fever, chills • Local exit site redness, tenderness, purulence

Requiring catheter repositioning or replacement	Symptoms
• Catheter displacement*	• Systemic toxicities • Abdominal pain, gastritis, ulcers
• Catheter cracks	• Blood backflow • Leakage of infusate
• Catheter occlusion** (may be 2° to catheter cracks)	• Inability to flush catheter • Leakage of infusate at catheter connections

*May lead to visceral artery thrombosis
**Irrigation of clotted catheter may result in embolic event if catheter is displaced.

pump has been the continuous administration of FUDR, both systemically via the internal jugular or subclavian vein and intrahepatically via the hepatic artery. The pump may be implanted into a subcutaneous pocket on the abdominal wall, with the catheter terminating either in the hepatic artery or, by creating a long subcutaneous tunnel, in the superior vena cava via the subclavian vein. The infraclavicular space, or upper chest wall, also lends itself to implantation with the device, in which case the catheter may be directed into the subclavian vein for systemic infusion or into the left brachial artery for hepatic artery infusion.[7]

Description and Principles of Operation

The Infusaid is a titanium disk that weighs 208 gm without the added weight of infusate and has a diameter of 87 mm. Its substantial "hockey puck" size and shape may preclude its use in some patients who are emaciated or of small stature because of the lack of adequate subcutaneous tissue or body area to comfortably accommodate the pump. The Silastic catheter is provided with an inner diameter of 0.6 mm and an outer diameter of 2.3 mm.

The Infusaid is a hollow pump divided into 2 chambers. The lower chamber, which contains a fluorocarbon or charging fluid, is separated from the upper chamber, or drug reservoir, by a metal diaphragm or bellows. The drug chamber is filled by needle access through a center silicone septum. The instilled fluid compresses the bellows against the fluorocarbon in the chamber below, condensing it to its liquid state. Under the influence of ambient body temperature, the fluorocarbon is converted into vapor which, as it expands, exerts constant pressure on the drug chamber above, expelling drug from the pump and through the catheter.

Pump flow rate will increase correspondingly with increase in body temperature as well as geographic elevation, since atmospheric pressure has a direct relationship to intravascular pressure.

The Infusaid is available in several models that vary slightly in design and capacity. Model 400 is used most commonly for administration of chemotherapeutic drugs because it has a 50-ml capacity and an auxiliary side port that bypasses the drug chamber with direct access to the catheter. The Infusaid is approved for infusion only with the aforementioned drugs via the drug chamber; however, virtually any other drug may be delivered by the side port with proper flushing techniques.

Preparation for Treatment

At the time of implantation, the pump is filled with a plain bacteriostatic solution and heparin. The flow rate of each individual pump is predetermined by the manufacturer. Its performance is based partly on the atmospheric pressure or elevation above sea level of the area in which the patient resides and partly on the addition of 1,000 u/ml of viscosity-controlled heparin to the infusate. Under normal conditions of body temperature and atmospheric pressure, this concentration will result in a relatively constant outflow of drug from the pump. Variations in heparin concentrations will alter the pump flow rates; that is, the less heparin used, the more rapidly the pump will infuse.

Our protocols have required the use of heparin in concentrations of 200 u/ml rather than 1,000 u/ml, and a brand of heparin other than that used in the manufacturer's pump calibrations has been utilized; thus, the preset rates are not assumed for treatment initiation. The actual rate of the pump is always established first by the infusion of heparin 10,000 u/50 ml in a plain bacteriostatic solution (water or saline) for at least a week. The pump chamber is emptied at this point, and the daily flow rate is calculated. The drug concentration to deliver the proper daily dose may then be determined and added to the pump with heparin 10,000 u in a total volume of 50 ml. Because the flow rate is not adjustable, a change in drug dose must be effected by emptying and refilling the pump with an altered concentration of drug.

Catheter position must be confirmed prior to administration of any drug through the pump. Subclavian catheter placement may be confirmed by simple chest X ray, which should show the catheter tip terminating in the superior vena cava. Hepatic artery catheter placement is confirmed by a radioactive nuclide study in which 99^{M}TC-MAA is injected into the auxiliary side port of the Infusaid and followed by a 10–20 ml sterile saline flush.[8] This study should show adequate perfusion of both lobes of the liver and, ideally, the absence of shunting to the lungs or G.I. system. Once proper catheter placement has been determined, the chemotherapy cycle may be initiated. Intrahepatic treatment protocols tend toward 2-week cycles of drug therapy followed by a 2-week infusion of plain solution, repeated to tolerance, treatment failure, or complete remission.

Refilling Procedure

Needle access to the Infusaid drug chamber is gained by the introduction of a straight 1 1/2-in. 22-gauge Huber point needle through a small silicone septum located in the center of the pump. As in all other catheter care procedures, a triple povidone-iodine prep is used and sterile technique is exercised throughout. The refill equipment consists of the Huber needle, a 3-way stopcock, extension tubing with clamp, and an empty 35 to 50-ml syringe, assembled in that order. Needle patency should be tested prior to accessing the pump. The extension tubing need not be clamped.

As soon as the needle pierces the septum and meets the needle stop inside the pump chamber, pressure within the drug reservoir forces the infusate into the empty syringe. Once the flow ceases, the stopcock is turned "off" to the needle to close the system and the extension tubing is clamped and removed from the stopcock, remaining attached to the syringe. The tubing and syringe are set aside so that the contents can be measured for pump rate and dose calculations. The newly prepared syringe containing the refill solution is then attached to the stopcock, which is placed "on" to the needle and syringe. Needle placement is confirmed continually during the ensuing refill procedure by alternately injecting 5 ml and releasing pressure on the syringe plunger to observe back pressure from the pump. To prevent its inadvertent dislodgement, the needle must be held firmly against the pump needle stop during the refill. When the syringe contents have been injected, the stopcock is turned "off" to the needle. The needle is then quickly withdrawn and pressure applied to the injection site.

Failure of fluid to return from the pump upon penetration of the septum may be the result of a defective needle, an empty pump, or pump failure. The pump chamber should never be aspirated in an attempt to obtain flow because of the potential for creating negative pressure within the pump, resulting in backflow of blood into the outlet flow restrictor of the pump and possible permanent occlusion. Differentiation between an empty pump and pump failure may be made by injecting 5 to 10 ml of sterile water into the drug chamber. Failure of the injected fluid to return may indicate operative failure of the pump; its return flow most likely means the pump had become empty at some point prior to this procedure. Since an empty pump may easily lead to catheter occlusion as a result of reflux of blood into the tip, catheter patency should be tested by injection of sterile saline through the side port of the pump.

Auxiliary Side Port Use

The side port is accessed in the same manner as the central septum, except that a 90° Huber needle may be used to facilitate manipulation of the extension tubing and syringes. When a perfusion scan is performed via the side port, the needle's 90° angle and the extension tubing allow the syringe to be handled out of range of the gamma camera.

All bolus injections via the side port should be preceded and followed by at least 10 ml sterile saline. Side port injections should not exceed the rate of 10 ml/min. to avoid subjecting the septum to excessive pressure.

The side port may be used for the continuous infusion of drugs that have not been approved for use in the central chamber or whose doses require flow rates exceeding those offered by the pump (e.g., 5-FU). After access is gained with a 90° Huber point needle, the exit site is dressed and managed in the manner identical to that of the VAP. The exception is that, for the same reasons as with the central chamber, the side port should not be aspirated for blood sampling or needle placement confirmation.

When the side port is used for continuous infusion, a portable infusion pump is used to propel the drug through the catheter. The central chamber should be refilled with plain solution to avoid the possibility of infusing drugs incompatible with heparin.

Caution should be exercised if infusing a vesicant drug continuously because of the possible instability of a needle in a pump located on the abdominal wall and the risk of dislodgment of the needle through patient activity.

Pump Complications

Table 5 refers to complications associated with implanted pump systems. Catheter occlusion and catheter dislodgment may occur with less frequency than with external catheters because many of the causative factors—catheter disconnection, external pump failures (occlusions), excessive patient activity and/or arm movement—have been removed by internalizing the system.

Patient and Family Teaching

Implanted pumps require no technically oriented patient teaching because, except for the above-mentioned use of the side port for continuous infusion, there are no dressings, pump batteries, or medication reservoirs to change.

Although the significant other may be taught the refill procedure, this is more the exception than the rule. Patient/family instruction is more often confined simply to cautions regarding the importance of keeping scheduled appointments for refills to eliminate the possibility of a depleted drug volume and of avoiding certain physical activities that might result in damage to the pump or catheter dislodgement. Patients are apprised of the principles of pump function and the influence of body temperature and atmospheric pressure on flow rate. They are instructed to call the physician if (1) body temperature exceeds 101°F, (2) air travel is anticipated, or (3) a vacation or an extended stay is planned in an area representing a major change in altitude. Long exposure to saunas, hot tubs and steam baths is discouraged. Remaining educational issues relate to drug side effects and toxicities.

Pump removal, accomplished by a minor surgical procedure, may be necessitated by pump malfunction, development of thrombosis in the catheterized vessel or other such complication precluding the use of the pump, or termination of treatment.

Table 5. Implantable Pump Complications

Complication	Probable cause	Action
• Catheter occlusion	• Empty pump • Drug incompatibility • Aspiration of side port or central chamber	• Flush via side port • Use lytic drugs if necessary
• Catheter dislodgement	• Excessive patient activity • Tenuous catheter placement	• Surgical catheter manipulation
• Pump failure	• Mechanical	• Prove failure by 5-10 ml fluid injection into central chamber. Absence of backflow requires pump replacement

• Infection
  • local
  • systemic
	• Postoperative development
	• Access needle contamination
		• Antibiotics
		
		• Possible explantation

Conclusion

Continuous infusion chemotherapy can be safely given in an ambulatory setting with adherence to certain principles of good nursing and medical practice.

Meticulous care of infusion catheters must be employed to provide maximum protection against known complications. Guidelines for aseptic techniques and maintenance of catheter patency must be strictly followed by a limited number of care-givers.

Patient and family teaching must be comprehensive and reinforced at intervals to provide a knowledge base for recognition of reportable signs and symptoms that can lead to serious complications.

Among the goals of safe outpatient care is to provide the patient with the knowledge and ability to manage his/her own care and the assurance that supports are in place when attention is sought.

7

PHARMACEUTICAL ISSUES IN INFUSION CHEMOTHERAPY STABILITY AND COMPATIBILITY

John A. Benvenuto, Ph.D., Stephen C. Adams, Pharm.D., Harish M. Vyas, Ph.D., and Roger W. Anderson, M.S.

Concepts and Definitions

THE INCREASED USE OF small-volume infusions, continuous infusions, and individualized home care infusions in various container materials has necessitated the determination of stability and compatibility of cancer chemotherapy agents under these diverse conditions. The lack of such data can potentially lead to underdosing or administration of toxic degradation products. Because these interactions are a direct result of medication preparation, the establishment of a pharmacy-based infusion service is essential to the delivery of effective infusion therapy. Other rationale for a pharmacy-based infusion service include sterility and accuracy of drug preparation; central location for drug preparation and record-keeping; reduced exposure of other hospital personnel to cytotoxic agents; and expert knowledge of drugs, doses, fluids, and potential hazards.

Increased safety for the patient is obtained by the preparation of all doses in a sterile environment while employing aseptic technique. Accuracy is achieved by precise measurement of both the drug and the fluid in which it is to be administered. The dispensing of all medications and I.V. fluids containing medications in their ready-to-be-administered form is another safety measure. The pharmacist has the expert knowledge to check orders for dosage, stability, or incompatibilities that otherwise might not be detected.

Another benefit of a pharmacy-based infusion service is the reduced exposure to cytotoxic medications among other health care staff members. The pharmacy has in place the specialized equipment and preparation techniques to reduce this potential hazard.

The major pharmaceutical considerations in designing an infusion regimen include stability, compatibility, solubility, in-line filtration, and sterility. Stability may be defined as the amount of time a specific formulation in a specific delivery system retains its identity, strength, quality, and purity. It is a common practice for these infusions to be administered in polyvinylchloride (PVC), polyolefin (PAB), plastic syringes, latex (elastomer), and other materials instead of glass. Indeed, our studies[1] and others[2-4] have shown that glass is not inert and can promote decomposition of some drugs. Unless otherwise stated, 90% of initial concentration is considered the maximum acceptable drug concentration decrease for a drug to be considered stable. Incompatibilities are those factors that adversely affect drug stability; they can be classified as physical, chemical, or therapeutic in nature. Therapeutic incompatibilities are related to undesirable agonist or antagonist activities.

Stability relates to the inherent chemical lability of a compound. Some drugs have very low inherent lability and thus undergo virtually no decomposition under the relatively mild conditions of administration. The many examples of such drugs include antimetabolites such as 5-fluorouracil (5-FU)[5] and cytarabine.[6] Other compounds are so highly labile that they undergo decomposition even under mild administration conditions. Examples of these drugs are carmustine and the nitrosoureas in general.[7] In addition, the interaction of a drug with other drugs in a mixture, with the container, or with the solvent can catalyze the decomposition of the drug. In this case, the reaction rate increases but the reaction products remain the same. This is in contrast to chemical compatibility, in which the reaction of a drug with its environment can lead to drug decrease by conversion to another compound or irreversible interaction such as absorption by the container. Additionally, physical incompatibility can result in precipitation or color changes.

In our studies, 2 predominant pathways for a decrease in drug concentrations: absorption by the container and drug decomposition. Adsorption drug decay curves are biphasic, characterized by a rapid initial phase and either falling to a plateau or declining further because of drug decomposition. This is a saturable process, generally forming a drug monolayer on the inner surface of the container.[8-9] Absorption, on the other hand, is a slow, diffusion-controlled interaction with the container matrix.[9] This is not a saturable process under administration conditions and shows a steady, continuous decline of drug concentration with time. The latter phenomenon gives a similar pattern to drug decomposition, and an analytical technique that can distinguish between the two is recommended.

Physical incompatibility was not observed, but precipitation is suspected in some low temperature studies.[7] Unfortunately, the nature and extent of the present studies do not allow for the exact determination of the mechanisms by which drug decrease occurs. Because of this, and also for convenience, all decrease in drug concentration with time in terms of stability have been defined.

The following procedure is routinely used for stability studies.

Procedures for Study of Stability

Experimental Procedure

SAMPLE PREPARATION

(a) Drug solutions are prepared according to package inserts at concentrations that are clinically relevant. Diluents are 5% dextrose for injection (D_5W) or 0.9% sodium chloride for injection (normal saline, NS).
(b) For each drug, 3 containers are filled with drug solution and 1 with diluent as blank control.
(c) Standard solutions are prepared fresh daily at concentrations bracketing those under study.

QUANTITATIVE AND QUALITATIVE DETERMINATIONS

Qualitative

(a) Color changes in the solution or container are recorded.
(b) Any precipitation or cloudiness of the drug solution is determined.

Quantitative

(a) A stability-indicating assay must be developed. This assay must show no interference from solvent or preservatives and be specific for the drug under study. The stability-indicating ability of the assay can be assessed by spiking the drug solution with appropriate decomposition products or solution additives. Alternately, decomposition of the drug may be achieved by harsh conditions such as pH extremes or oxidation.
(b) A standard curve is run on each day of study to minimize effects of instrument variability. The standard curve is challenged by a sample of known concentration to ensure the validity of the method.
(c) Samples are obtained at 0, 1, 3, 5, 7, and 24 hours. The samples are placed in Teflon coated screw-capped borosilicate glass vials and vials are placed in an ice bath until analyzed.
(d) Samples are analyzed in duplicate.
(e) The pH of the drug solutions is determined at the beginning and the end of the study period using a pH meter. A drug in solution is considered stable if there is less than a 10% decrease in concentration during the course of the study. If a drug does not fulfill this requirement, then the duration of stability or utility time,[10] the time at which a 10% decrease (t_{90}) occurs, is given.

Analytical Procedures

HIGH-PRESSURE LIQUID CHROMATOGRAPHY (HPLC) ASSAYS

HPLC analyses were performed on a Waters Associates instrument equipped with a M6000 pump, a U6K injection, and a 450 variable wavelength UV detector. Peak areas and retention times were determined electronically, using a Waters Data Module. Separations were achieved on a reverse phase ODS column. HPLC conditions for each drug are listed in table 1.

ATOMIC ABSORPTION ANALYSIS

A Perkin-Elmer atomic absorption spectrometer (Model 5000) with HGA Programmer in the flameless mode was used for cisplatin analysis in PAB. Drug samples were diluted 1 to 10 before analysis. A platinum lamp (30 mA) in an argon atmosphere with detection at 265.9 nm was used.

Short-Term Stability

The results of our short-term single-agent stability studies are listed in table 2. As defined previously, a drug is considered stable if there is less than a 10% change in drug concentration for the length of the study. These studies were carried out for 24 hours except for 5-FU and doxorubicin (ADR), which were studied for 48 hours, all at room temperature and not protected from light. For those drugs whose concentrations decreased by greater than 10%, the time at which a 10% change occurred is listed. For those drugs whose concentrations decreased by greater than 10%, the time at which a 10% change occurred is listed. Also listed are the container, diluent, and concentration of the drug solution.

Effect of Container Composition

In most cases, the drugs are stable for a minimum of 24 hours under the conditions indicated, but for some drugs the stability may be much longer. However, variations due to container material and diluent are evident (table 2). It must be remembered that no one container is superior. Depending upon the chemical and physical properties of the drugs and containers, drugs show preferential stability in specific containers. Table 2 shows that some drugs are more stable in PVC (plicamycin), PAB (bleomycin and fluorouracil), or glass (carmustine, fluorouracil, plicamycin). Stability is not the only consideration in the determination of which container to use. Factors such as leaching of plasticizer from PVC and breakage of glass containers are also significant considerations. There is no "best" container; the choice of container must be based upon the drug being administered and the results of stability/compatibility testing.[12]

Because most of the drugs were stable under the conditions studied, only those few that were stable for less than 24 hours will be discussed. The stability of bleomycin was investigated using HPLC. Bleomycin (BLM) was dissolved in D_5W at a concentration of 0.3 u/ml. Samples of drug solutions from PVC, PAB, Travenol glass, and American-McGaw glass were analyzed as indicated in table 1. Nine of the BLM components were separated and detected, but only the major components A_2 and B_2 were quantitated for stability. The identities of A_2 and B_2 were based on their relative percent compositions. The best container for the administration of BLM is PAB, with a utility time of 1.87 hour (T_{90}

of B_2). Because, in this case, 2 components with different stabilities are being considered, the utility time is that of the least stable component, which may or may not be a measure of the antineoplastic activity of BLM. PVC, on the other hand, had a utility time of 0.7 hour. The drug decline in PVC is rapid and saturable, i.e., adsorption; the decline in PAB is a slow, linear decay characteristic of drug decomposition or absorption. In the current situation, we cannot distinguish between the 2 possible mechanisms. The Travenol glass container (utility time 11 hours) is better than the American-McGraw glass (utility time 1.3 hours). The difference in utility times and the inverse component stabilities apparently are due to different container materials. Again, the major decline in this case appears to be from adsorption.

Carmustine (BCNU) is unstable and has limited utility in all containers studied (table 2). In essence, there are equivalent stabilities in PAB and the glass

Table 1. HPLC Conditions for Analysis of Antitumor Agents

Drug	Solvent	Detector wavelength (nm)	Flow rate (ml/min)	Sample volume (μl)	Retention time (min)
Bisantrene	0.05 mM Na H_2PO_4, pH 6/ MeOH/H_2O (23:47:30)	254	1.7	10	4.15
Bleomycin Sulfate	5mM heptane sulfonic acid pH 3.5/MeOH (50:50)	254	1.7	35	A_2 4.65 B_2 5.70
Caracemide	H_2O/MeOH (90:10)	230	1.5	2	7.60
Carmustine	50 mM sodium acetate, pH 4.0/MeOH (50:50)	230	1.0	10	3.70
Cyclophosphamide	H_2O/MeOH (40:60)	210	1.0	25	3.13
Cytarabine	0.01 M $NH_4H_2PO_4$, pH 7	270	2.0	10	3.10
Dacarbazine (PVC)	0.05 M sodium acetate, pH 3.5/MeOH (80:20)	254	2.0	2	5.50
Dacarbazine (PAB)	0.01 M heptane sulfonic acid, pH 4.5/MeOH (50:50)	254	1.2	15	2.25
Dactinomycin	0.01 M NH_4CO_2H, pH 3.5/ MeOH (20:80)	254	2.0	40	2.18
Doxorubicin	5 mM heptane sulfonic acid/ MeOH (30:70)	254	1.3	25	3.10
Etoposide	H_2O/MeOH (50:50)	254	1.0	10	8.40
Fluorouracil	H_2O/MeOH (90:10)	254	1.0		2.43
Leucovorin Calcium	5 mM NH_4CO_2H, pH 3.5/ MeOH (70:30)	280	0.8	5	3.90
Methotrexate	5 mM NH_4CO_2H, pH 3.5/ MeOH (70:30)	254	1.0	20	4.33
Mithramycin	H_2O/MeOH/CH_3CN (19:75:6)	285	1.0	25	2.97
Mitomycin	H_2O/MeOH (50:50)	254	1.0	5	4.13
Pentamethymelamine	0.01 M Ammonium formate, pH 3.5/MeOH (60:40)	254	1.0	25	13.00
Procarbazine	0.01 M sodium acetate, pH 5.15/MeOH (75:25)	254	2.0	10	5.00
Vinblastine Sulfate	0.01 M NH_4CO_2H, pH 3.5/ MeOH (40:60)	265	1.0	20	3.75
Vincristine Sulfate	0.05 M NH_4CO_2H, pH 3.5/ MeOH/CH_3CN (48:41:11)	254	1.0	25	3.45
Vindesine	H_2O/MeOH (80:20)	254	2.0	25	8.00

Table 2. Short-Term Stability

Drug		Container	Diluent	Concentration		Duration of stability (hr.)
Dactinomycin		PVC	D5W	9.8	μg/ml	24.0
		PAB	D5W	7.5	μg/ml	24.0
		Glass T[a]	D5W	9.8	μg/ml	24.0
		Glass A[a]	D5W	7.5	μg/ml	24.0
Bleomycin	A2	PVC	D5W	0.3	unit/ml	0.7
	B2	PVC	D5W	0.3	unit/ml	1.3
	A2	PAB	D5W	0.3	unit/ml	24.0
	B2	PAB	D5W	0.3	unit/ml	18.7
	A2	Glass T	D5W	0.3	unit/ml	24.0
	B2	Glass T	D5W	0.3	unit/ml	11.0
	A2	Glass A	D5W	0.3	unit/ml	1.3
	B2	Glass A	D5W	0.3	unit/ml	24.0
Carmustine		PVC	D5W	1.25	mg/ml	0.6
		PAB	D5W	1.25	mg/ml	7.0
		Glass T	D5W	1.25	mg/ml	7.7
		Glass A	D5W	1.25	mg/ml	8.3
Carecemide		Glass	D5W	20.0	mg/ml	24.0
Cisplatin		PAB	NS	0.1	mg/ml	19.4
		Glass A	NS	0.1	mg/ml	24.0
Cyclophosphamide		PVC	D5W	6.6	mg/ml	24.0
		PAB	D5W	6.7	mg/ml	24.0
		Glass A	D5W	6.7	mg/ml	24.0
Cytarabine		PVC	D5W	1.82	mg/ml	24.0
		Glass T	D5W	1.83	mg/ml	24.0
Dacarbazine		PVC	D5W	1.7	mg/ml	24.0
		PAB	D5W	1.7	mg/ml	24.0
		Glass T	D5W	1.7	mg/ml	24.0
		Glass A	D5W	1.7	mg/ml	24.0
Doxorubicin		PVC	D5W	0.18	mg/ml	48.0
		PAB	D5W	0.18	mg/ml	48.0
		Glass T	D5W	0.18	mg/ml	40.0
		Glass A	D5W	0.18	mg/ml	48.0
Fluorouracil		PVC	D5W	8.3	mg/ml	43.0
		PAB	D5W	8.3	mg/ml	48.0
		Glass T	D5W	8.3	mg/ml	7.0
		Glass A	D5W	8.3	mg/ml	48.0
Leucovorin		PVC	D5W	0.91	mg/ml	24.0
Leucovorin		PAB	D5W	0.91	mg/ml	24.0
Leucovorin		Glass T	D5W	0.91	mg/ml	24.0
Leucovorin		Glass A	D5W	0.91	mg/ml	24.0
Methotrexate		PVC	D5W	0.96	mg/ml	24.0
Methotrexate		Glass T	D5W	0.96	mg/ml	24.0
Plicamycin		PVC	D5W	25.8	μg/ml	24.0
Plicamycin		PAB	D5W	45.5	μg/ml	unstable[c]
Plicamycin		Glass T	D5W	25.8	μg/ml	24.0
Plicamycin		Glass A	D5W	45.5	μg/ml	5.6

Continued

Table 2, Continued

Drug	Container	Diluent	Concentration	Duration of stability (hr.)
Plicamycin	PAB	NS	45.5 µg/ml	24.0
Plicamycin	Glass A	NS	45.5 µg/ml	< 1.0
Mitomycin	PVC	D5W	0.40 mg/ml	2
Mitomycin	Glass T	D5W	0.40 mg/ml	1
Mitomycin	PVC	NS	0.40 mg/ml	24.0
Mitomycin	Glass A	NS	0.40 mg/ml	24.0
Pentamethylmelamine	PVC	D5W		24.0
Pentamethylmelamine	Glass T	D5W		24.0
Vinblastine	PVC	D5W	0.17 mg/ml	24.0
Vinblastine	PAB	D5W	0.17 mg/ml	24.0
Vinblastine	Glass T	D5W	0.17 mg/ml	24.0
Vinblastine	Glass A	D5W	0.17 mg/ml	24.0
Vincristine	PVC	D5W	20.0 µg/ml	24.0
Vincristine	PVC	D5W	20.0 µg/ml	24.0
Vincristine	PAB	D5W	20.0 µg/ml	24.0
Vincristine	Glass T	D5W	20.0 µg/ml	24.0
Vindesine	PVC	D5W	47.6 µg/ml	24.0
Vindesine	Glass T	D5W	47.6 µg/ml	24.0

[a]Glass T - Travenol glass container
[b]Glass A - American-McGaw glass container
[c]Increase of drug concentration with time

containers, with utility times ranging from 7 to 8.3 hours. The decay curves are rapid and linear—most likely indicative of drug decomposition. The utility time of BCNU in PVC is less than 1 hour, with a rapid, biphasic decline in drug content reflecting the highly labile nature of the drug in this container. Glass and polyolefin containers are suitable for the administration of BCNU, but only if the drug solution is kept in these containers for less than approximately 6 hours.

Cisplatin (DDP) was studied in PAB and American-McGaw glass containers. An atomic absorption technique was used that measures total platinum but cannot distinguish between different platinum-containing compounds. However, a decrease in total platinum, which would occur with adsorption or absorption, can be detected. It does appear that DDP is absorbed by the PAB container, inasmuch as a slow, linear decline in platinum occurs. DDP is very reactive and forms aquo compounds in aqueous solutions. These species are probably the active forms of the drug in vivo; however, the actual active compound(s) are still unknown. Thus, the measurement of total platinum is more beneficial than measurement of the individual compounds.

ADR was studied for 48 hours in PVC, PAB, Travenol glass, and American-McGaw glass, using a HPLC assay (see table 1). ADR was stable for 48 hours in PVC, PAB, and American-McGaw glass; however, the utility time in Travenol glass was 40 hours (see table 2). The differences in the utility times of the 2 glass containers probably reflect differences in container compositions.

update of this study revealed no therapeutic advantages to the BLM-containing program.[36]

Holister et al[37] examined the use of continuous infusion VCR and BLM with prednisone as a nonmyelosuppressive combination regimen for refractory non-Hodgkin's lymphoma. The program consisted of continuous infusion of vincristine at 1–2 mg per m²/day for 2 days followed by BLM at 0.25 units/kg given by bolus injection immediately followed by 0.12 units/kg infused daily for 5 consecutive days. Responding patients went on to receive a high-dose methotrexate regimen of 1,500 mg/m² with citrovorum rescue on days 15, 22, 29, and 36. Treatment cycles were repeated every 6 weeks in responding patients. Of 16 patients treated in this fashion, 3 had complete and 5 had partial responses, with a median response duration of 29 weeks. These occurred despite reported "resistance" to the standard bolus method of administration of VCR in all of these patients and to previous bolus BLM in all but 1 of the cases. The study design could not distinguish which agent administered by continuous infusion was responsible for this effect.

The implication of this study is that "resistance" to certain drugs may be schedule-dependent. This intriguing result has yet to be confirmed by other investigators.

Other Tumors

Kolaric et al, in testing BLM infusions combined with radiotherapy in inoperable squamous cell carcinoma of the esophagus, demonstrated a CR and PR rate of 52% in 25 patients.[38] The program consisted of BLM administered at a dose of 15 units/m² over 12 hours twice weekly, with concurrent radiation therapy, to a total dose of 3,600 to 4,000 rads. This trial did not involve a concurrent control group with BLM applied in the form of I.V. bolus injections. However, the same investigator found a response rate of 62% (15/24 patients) with 6 CR and 9 PR in a previous study using I.V. bolus BLM administration. Using this historical control group, one would conclude that BLM infusion combined with concurrent radiation therapy in the treatment of inoperable esophageal cancer presents no advantage over the conventional I.V. bolus method of bleomycin administration. On the other hand, the 12-hour infusion method used is theoretically less than optimal, inasmuch as a BLM infusion not preceded by an I.V. bolus dose would not be expected to reach steady-state levels until approximately 10 hours. One could argue that a 12-hour infusion administered twice weekly does not take full advantage of the potential for long-term BLM infusion. Nathanson[39] has investigated 2 regimens, both of which used continuous infusion BLM in combination with either VLB alone or with VLB plus DDP in the treatment of far advanced metastatic malignant melanoma. The initial regimen consisted of VLB 8 mg/m² given by I.V. bolus injection on days 1 and 2 followed by administration of BLM 20 u/m² by continuous 24-hour infusion for 5 consecutive days. The second regimen employed VLB 6 mg/m² on days 1 and 2, BLM 15 u/m² by continuous 24-hour infusion for 5 consecutive days, and DDP 25 mg/m² administered as a 1-hour of this degradation product is unknown, its presence at any level was considered deleterious. The production of this compound was significantly depressed when the drug solution was protected from light. Using a brown plastic cover, the duration of stability was 24 hours, whereas a black plastic cover increased the utility time to 96 hours.

Procarbazine also was unstable in the PVC container when exposed to room light. When the procarbazine solution was protected from light by storing in a bench drawer, the drug was stable for 24 hours. Etoposide was stable when exposed to room light, as indicated in table 3.

Manufacturers of a number of agents, including ADR, dacarbazine, and methotrexate, recommend that they be protected from light.[14] However, we have found that for at least 24 hours, these drugs are stable when exposed to room light at room temperature in PVC, PAB, and glass containers (table 2). It may be that 24 hours is too short a time to see a significant decrease in drug content.

Effect of Delivery System

In addition to interacting with administration containers, drug solutions also interact with the tubing[9] and filters[15,16] of administration sets. The tubing of these sets is generally PVC, with the attendant problem of leaching. Cellulose filters and plastic filter housings are also likely to cause decreasing drug content. This phenomenon is particularly apparent with ADR, which causes tubing and filters to become bright red. The loss of drug could be exacerbated by the increasing lengths of administration tubing; however, this effect is somewhat lessened by the rapid rate at which the drug solution travels through the set.

Table 4 shows the effects of passage of ADR solution through a manifold filter and tubing. The drug solution was prepared at a concentration of 1 mg/ml in 50 ml D_5W contained in a Travenol Viaflex bag. The bag was attached to a multiple I.V. manifold and filter (Quest Medical, Carrollton, Tex.). The Quest filter uses an acrylic copolymer as its filtering membrane; this membrane type is common in commercial filters. A prefilter sample was obtained after passage through the administration set but before the manifold. Postfilter samples were obtained from the tubing immediately following the filter. Postfilter sample 1 was the initial drug solution passing through the filter; postfilter sample 2 was the final portion of the drug solution to pass through the filter. The third sample was obtained at the end of the manifold tubing. Each sample was analyzed in triplicate by high-pressure liquid chroma-

Table 4. Retention of Doxorubicin by Quest Manifold Filter

Sample	Percent of prefilter sample
Prefilter	100
Postfilter 1	101
Postfilter 2	99
Postfilter and tubing	93

tography using a 5 μm ODS-2 reverse phase column. The eluent was 0.05 M NH$_4$H$_2$PO$_4$, pH 3.5, at a flow rate of 1 ml/min. and detector wavelength of 265 nm.

Although the filter became bright red, there was no decrease in ADR at the clinically relevant concentrations we studied. Apparently, the filter becomes rapidly saturated with only a nominal amount of drug. Greater than 95% of ADR has been reported to be bound to cellulose acetate/nitrate filters;[15,16] however, the ADR concentrations used in these studies were only 1–30 μg/ml. Retention on the filter is a concentration-dependent, saturable process. On the other hand, there is an appreciable loss of drug to the tubing. This phenomenon is likely to be dependent on the length of tubing and the flow rate of the drug solution.

Apparent decreases in toxicity have led to suggestions that filtration of DDP results in a significant loss of drug. To determine the validity and extent of this proposal, we studied the effects of 3 filter types on DDP concentrations. Solutions (100 ml) of 1 mg/ml of DDP prepared in normal saline were filtered through Monoject 20 × 1.5 needles with 5 μm filters, Millipore Millex OR 0.22 μm filters, and Quest 6-port manifold fluid delivery sets equipped with 0.22 μm filters.

DDP was quantitated by high-pressure liquid chromatography after derivatization with sodium diethyldithiocarbamate.[17] We found no significant decrease in DDP content of the solutions passed through the 3 filters. Thus, the apparent decrease in DDP toxicity after filtration cannot be attributed to a chemical or physical loss of drug. The altered biological effect may relate to dose or rate of administration.

As a further test of the observation that filtration does not affect drug concentration, we studied the filtration of plicamycin and vincristine through the Quest manifold filter. These drugs were studied because of their low concentrations in solution and the increased likelihood of observing a decrease in drug concentration. Plicamycin at 0.4 mg/ml was dissolved in D$_5$W contained in a PVC bag. The bag was attached to a Quest manifold filter via a Quest fluid delivery set. Before and after filtration samples were analyzed by high-pressure liquid chromatography. There was no decrease in drug content.

Vincristine at 40 μg/ml was filtered in the same manner as described previously for plicamycin. Again, samples were analyzed before and after filtration by HPLC. No decrease in vincristine concentration was observed. Although this small sampling of drugs cannot predict for all others, it would appear that even at low drug concentrations there is no significant effect of filtration.

Long-Term Stability

To determine whether drug solutions could be prepared long before use and then stored until needed, we studied the stability of 4 specific drugs under a variety of conditions and in a variety of containers. For our initial work, we chose 4 drugs: cytarabine, ADR, 5-FU, and BLM (table 5). These drugs are generally given by continuous infusion and are candidates for home therapy programs using portable infusion pumps. This technique reduces the duration of inhospital time and thus reduces overall cost of treatment.

Cytarabine was reconstituted in bacteriostatic water according to the manufacturer's package insert and then diluted with D_5W to 5 mg/ml for PVC and Travenol Infusor and 12.5 mg/ml for 20 cc plastic syringes. Drug solutions were analyzed by HPLC, using an ODS-2, 5 μm particle size column and 50 mM $NH_4H_2PO_4$, pH 3.5 MeOH (95:15) as eluent. After filling with drug solutions, containers were kept at room temperature, refrigerated (6°C), or frozen (–8°C). On days 0, 1, 5, 10, 20, and 30, samples were removed and analyzed by HPLC. Frozen solutions were allowed to thaw at room temperature. Standards were prepared on days of study and were run periodically during the day. As shown in table 5, cytarabine was stable under all conditions for the 30-day duration of the study.

ADR was diluted with D_5W to achieve concentrations of 3 mg/ml for PVC and Infusor and 7.5 mg/ml for syringes. (The drug solutions were analyzed by HPLC on a Bondapak C_{18} reverse phase column and 5 mM octanesulfonic acid, pH 3.5/MeOH (20:80) as eluent). After being filled with drug solutions, the containers were kept at room temperature, refrigerator temperature (6°C), and freezer temperature (–8°C). On days 0, 1, 5, 10, 20, and 30, aliquots of drug solution were removed and analyzed as described above. Frozen samples were again allowed to thaw at room temperature. Standards were prepared daily and run periodically during the day.

As observed previously (see table 2), ADR is unstable in PVC. The duration of stability at room temperature is 15 days versus the 40 hours observed before. This difference is due to the differences in sampling intervals in the two studies; in the present study, the intervals are days, whereas in the previous study they were hours. The different sampling intervals have varying effects on the estimates for the "best fit" regression analysis equation used to calculate T_{90} valves. ADR was even less stable in PVC at freezer temperatures (table 5). The duration of stability of less than 1 day may reflect the precipitation of drug at this temperature.

For PVC and the Infusor, the 5-FU solution was diluted with D_5W to a concentration of 10 mg/ml. For the syringe, the final drug concentration was

Table 5. 30-Day Stability at Freezer, Refrigerator, and Ambient Temperatures in Infusors,[a] PVC Bags, and Plastic Syringes[b] with D_5W

Drug	Infusor			PVC			Plastic syringe		
	23°	6°	–8°	23°	6°	–8°	23°	6°	–8°
Cytarabine	30[c]	30	30	30	30	30	30	30	30
Doxorubicin	30	30	30	15	30	< 1	30	30	30
Fluorouracil	30	N.D.[d]	N.D.	30	N.D.	N.D.	30	N.D.	N.D.
Bleomycin	30	30	< 1	< 1	30	26	9	< 1	1.6

[a]Travenol Laboratories, Inc.
[b]Monoject 20 cc disposable syringe, Sherwood Medical Industries, Inc.
[c]Values are durations of stability in days.
[d]Not Done. Since fluorouracil is known to precipitate at low temperatures, studies were conducted at room temperature only.

25 mg/ml. Drug solutions were analyzed by HPLC on an ODS-2 (5 μm particle size) reverse-phase column with 50 mM $NH_4H_2PO_4$, pH 3.5, as eluent. After being filled with drug solutions, the containers were stored at room temperature in the dark. On days 1, 5, 10, 20, and 30, aliquots of drug solution were removed and analyzed. Standards were prepared 3 times daily.

Fluorouracil stability was determined only at room temperature because the drug precipitates from solution at refrigerator and freezer temperatures. The drug was stable for the duration of the study (30 days) in the 3 containers. This is in agreement with published reports of fluorouracil long-term stability.[5]

BLM was dissolved in D_5W to a concentration of 0.4 u/ml for PVC and Infusor and a concentration of 1 ml for syringes. Drug solutions were analyzed by HPLC on a Bondapak C_{18} column, using 5 mM heptanesulfonic acid pH 3.5/MeOH (50:50) containing 1% glacial acetic acid as eluent. Separate filled containers were kept at room temperature, refrigerated (6°C), and frozen (–8°C). On days 0, 1, 5, 10, 20, and 30, aliquots of drug solution were removed and analyzed in triplicate by HPLC. Frozen samples were allowed to thaw at room temperature. Standards were prepared on days of study and run periodically during the day.

BLM was the least stable of the 4 drugs studied (table 5). At –8°C in the Infusor there was less than 1-day stability. In PVC at room temperature, there was less than 1-day stability, consistent with our previous results with bleomycin in PVC. This is a saturable process, indicating that adsorption is the main cause of drug decrease. BLM showed poor stability at all temperatures in the plastic syringe (see table 5). Plastic syringes should definitely not be used for the long-term storage and subsequent administration of BLM.

In general, the lowest stabilities were encountered at refrigerator and freezer temperatures for these drugs. Although chemical stability may increase with lower temperatures, physical incompatibilities and precipitation may increase;[7] therefore, the need to determine stabilities of drug solutions at low temperatures is highly important and justified.[18]

Admixtures

Combinations of drugs in solution in the same container present another dimension of complexity to the compatibility of drug solutions. In addition to the effects of container composition, solvent, light exposure, and temperature, the interactions of the drugs must also be taken into account. The possible effects of putting more than 1 drug in solution in the same container are that 1 drug may catalyze the decomposition of the other(s) or may promote precipitation.

We investigated the compatibilities of a number of drug combinations, mainly those containing ADR. The choice of combinations was dictated by current protocols in the use at M.D. Anderson Hospital and the need to know if these combinations could safely be used for home therapy using portable continuous infusion pumps. Table 4 lists the combinations, conditions, and duration of stability of the individual drugs in the combination studied.

The results of the study of ADR and dacarbazine in syringes at freezer temperature again show the phenomenon of decreased stability at low temperature. However, the stability for the duration of the 5-day study of the same combination in syringes at refrigerator temperature and in Infusors at freezer and refrigerator temperatures indicate that the container also affects stability.

The stability of the combination of ADR and vincristine (VCR) under various conditions was investigated for a 7-day period (table 6). Except for VCR in the Infusor at 4°C and ADR in the syringe at 23°C, the two-drug combination is stable. The 4-day stability of VCR and the 5-day stability of ADR are still sufficiently long to allow use of the respective combinations in many situations.

We have investigated the possibility of combining 4 drugs in the same container. Doxorubicin, dacarbazine, and diphenhydramine were stable for

Table 6. Stability of Combinations of Antitumor Agents

Combination	Concentration (mg/ml)	Container	Temperature	Duration of stability (day)
Doxorubicin	0.79	Syringe	−10°	< 1
+Dacarbazine	9.2	Syringe	−10°	< 1
Doxorubicin	0.63	Infusor	−10°	5
+Dacarbazine	7.3	Infusor	−10°	5
Doxorubicin	0.79	Syringe	4°	5
+Dacarbazine	9.2	Syringe	4°	5
Doxorubicin	0.63	Infusor	4°	5
+Dacarbazine	7.3	Infusor	4°	5
Doxorubicin	0.3	Syringe	4°	7
+Vincristine	0.009	Syringe	4°	7
Doxorubicin	0.23	Infusor	4°	7
+Vincristine	0.006	Infusor	4°	4
Doxorubicin	0.28	PVC	4°	7
+Vincristine	0.007	PVC	4°	7
Doxorubicin	0.37	Syringe	23°	5
+Vincristine	0.009	Syringe	23°	7
Doxorubicin	0.23	Infusor	23°	7
+Vincristine	0.006	Infusor	23°	7
Doxorubicin	0.28	PVC	23°	7
+Vincristine	0.007	PVC	23°	7
Doxorubicin	3.0	Infusor	4°	7
+Dacarbazine	33.3	Infusor	4°	5
+Diphenhydramine	1.7	Infusor	4°	5
+Metoclopramide	12.0	Infusor	4°	3
Doxorubicin	3.0	Infusor	23°	5
+Dacarbazine	33.3	Infusor	23°	5
+Diphenhydramine	1.7	Infusor	23°	5
+Metoclopramide	12.0	Infusor	23°	1
Cisplatin	0.86	Glass	23°	4 hr
+Carmustine	1.4	Glass	23°	3 hr

the 5-day duration of the study; however, the fourth drug, metoclopramide was not. The 2.9-day duration of stability at 4°C and 1.3-day at 23°C severely limits the use of this combination in a home therapy program. Again, the decreased stability at lower temperatures suggests that precipitation is the cause of the decrease in drug content rather than decomposition and refutes the belief that increased stability should occur at lower temperature.

Because of the rapid decomposition of BCNU, the stability of the combination of DDP and BCNU was studied for 4 hours in a glass container at room temperature; however, carmustine remained stable for only 3 hours. The administration of BCNU, whether given in combination or as a single agent, should be by rapid infusion.

Conclusion

Container, temperature, exposure to light, concentration, diluent, drug interactions in combinations, filtration, and tubing all can influence drug stability. Even so, the overwhelming majority of antitumor agents are stable under administration conditions. Although these drugs can be very reactive, it is only after metabolic or chemical activation that their cytotoxic activity is manifest. In some cases, e.g., the nitrosoureas, the drugs are inherently labile and have only short stabilities under most circumstances. Unfortunately, it is impossible to predict drug stability under all conditions. It is, therefore, imperative that stability/compatibility testing be conducted on new, untried modes of packing and storing drug solutions. Care must be exercised to ensure that procedures are reliably precise and that analytical procedures are stability-indicating.

SECTION II
Chemotherapeutic Agents

8

ANTIPYRIMIDINES: 5-FLUOROURACIL AND 5-FLUORO-2'-DEOXYURIDINE

Michael J. O'Connell, M.D.

THE FLUORINATED PYRIMIDINES 5-FLUOROURACIL (5-FU) and 5-fluoro-2'-deoxyuridine (FUDR) have been extensively studied as cytotoxic agents for the treatment of human malignant neoplasms since their introduction into clinical trials more than 25 years ago.[1] These compounds were synthesized to produce antimetabolites, closely related to the naturally occurring pyrimidine uracil, which have the ability to block DNA synthesis by inhibiting the enzyme thymidylate synthetase and to further interfere with nucleic acid synthesis by incorporation of the fluorinated pyrimidine directly into RNA.[2,3] FUDR is rapidly cleaved to 5-FU in vivo following administration. FUDR can be converted directly to the active inhibitor of thymidylate synthetase (5-fluoro-2'-deoxyuridine-5'-monophosphate), whereas 5-FU must undergo a series of metabolic conversions to form the active moiety.[4]

5-FU and FUDR are rapidly metabolized in the liver and other tissues to produce biologically inactive metabolites. These are eventually converted to carbon dioxide, which is eliminated via the respiratory tract. Approximately 80% of 5-FU can be accounted for by conversion to respiratory carbon dioxide within 12 hours of administration.[5] Although the fluorinated pyrimidines are excreted into the urine, this route of elimination is not of major importance, accounting for only about 15% of drug excretion. The serum half-life of 5-FU and FUDR is only 10–20 minutes following rapid (bolus) I.V. injection.

Both 5-FU and FUDR are commercially available. The former is supplied in aqueous solution that is stable for 2 years without refrigeration. FUDR is supplied as a sterile powder that must be reconstituted with water. Reconstituted vials should be stored under refrigeration for not more than 2 weeks. FUDR has been demonstrated to undergo less than 5% degradation for periods up to 12 days in a totally implanted drug delivery system.[6]

Clinical Trials of Fluorinated Pyrimidines
Given by Short- and Long-Term Intravenous Infusions

The appeal of the theoretical rationale for administration of fluorinated pyrimidines by infusion technique rather than bolus administration is based on the short serum half-life of these compounds and the large proportion of malignant cells in human solid tumors that are not undergoing active growth and are not, therefore, affected by cycle-active antimetabolites at any one point in time: Longer periods of drug administration might result in a greater percentage of malignant cells exposed to the cytotoxic agent during a sensitive phase of the growth cycle, resulting in an enhanced therapeutic effect. Some pharmacologic studies[4] have also demonstrated more complete metabolism of both 5-FU and FUDR when these drugs are given by continuous infusion as indicated by reduced urinary excretion compared to bolus administration. Presumably, rapid administration of the fluorinated pyrimidines can overload the catabolic enzyme pathways required for metabolic conversion to the active moiety, with more of the inactive parent compounds excreted unchanged into the urine. Other investigators,[7] however, have not observed significant urinary excretion of 5-FU following bolus intravenous administration at a dose of 500 mg/m[2]. Finally, toxicity to the bone marrow should be decreased, because the slow I.V. infusion of 5-FU results in much lower drug concentrations in bone marrow compared to rapid intravenous administration.[7]

A series of controlled clinical trials of 5-FU and FUDR given in 2-hour, 8-hour, and 24-hour infusions in patients with advanced colorectal cancer have been conducted at the Mayo Clinic by Moertel et al,[8-10] as outlined in table 1. These studies indicated essentially no difference in pattern or severity of toxicity when 5-FU was given by 2-hour infusion compared to bolus administration, although a higher dose of 5-FU must be given by 2-hour infusion (25 mg/kg/day for 5 days) contrasted with bolus administration (13.5 mg/kg/day for 5 days) to produce equivalent levels of clinical toxicity.[8] When the duration of 5-FU infusion was increased to 8 hours at a comparable dose

Table 1. Controlled Clinical Trials of 5-FU and FUDR Given by Intravenous Infusion in Patients with Advanced Metastatic Colorectal Carcinoma (Mayo Clinic)

Treatment regimen*	Number of patients	Objective response rate (%) at 8-10 weeks	Reference
1. 5-FU (rapid I.V.)	74	12	7
5-FU (2-hr infusion)	75	12	
2. 5-FU (rapid I.V.)	45	20 ⎫ P = N.S.	8
5-FU (8-hour infusion)	45	11 ⎭	
3. FUDR (rapid I.V.)	63	17 ⎫ P < .05	9
FUDR (24-hour infusion)	65	6 ⎭	

*Treatment given for 5 consecutive days in each study, and up to 4 additional doses every other day in studies 1 and 2 (references 7,8). Courses repeated at 4- 5-week intervals.

level (22.5 mg/kg/day for 5 days), there was a marked decrease in clinical toxicity, particularly myelosuppression.[9] Objective tumor response rates were somewhat lower among patients receiving 8-hour infusions (11%) compared to randomized controls receiving bolus I.V. administration (20%), although these differences were not statistically significant and could have been due to administration of 5-FU at less than its maximally tolerated dose level in patients receiving 8-hour infusions.

In contrast with the pattern observed with 5-FU , the dose level of FUDR must be decreased (2.25 mg/kg/day for 5 days) when administered as a continuous 24-hour infusion; the tolerable dose level of FUDR when given by bolus injection is 40 mg/kg/day for 5 days. A marked difference in toxicity was seen between these two methods of FUDR administration, with significantly more leukopenia following rapid I.V. administration and significantly more stomatitis with continuous I.V. infusion for 5 days (p<.01). The objective response rate associated with 120-hour infusion of FUDR (6%) was significantly lower then the response rate (17%) seen with rapid I.V. administration.[10] Thus, this controlled trial failed to confirm in patients with advanced colorectal cancer the earlier contention of Sullivan et al[11] that administration of FUDR by continuous infusion improves the therapeutic response.

Seifert and associates[12] subsequently conducted a randomized clinical trial of 5-FU given by rapid I.V. administration (12 mg/kg/day for 5 days) compared to 5-FU given by continuous 120-hour infusion in patients with advanced colorectal cancer. In this study, the starting dose of 5-FU given by continuous infusion was 30 mg/kg/day for 5 days, with escalation to 35 to 40 mg/kg/day in patients who did not experience toxicity at the lower dose level. Objective tumor responses were seen in 15 of 34 patients (44%) treated with continuous infusion and 8 of 36 patients (22%) randomized to bolus administration. Patients treated with the bolus schedule had a much higher incidence of severe leukopenia (31% had WBC nadirs <2,000 cells/mm^3), whereas those receiving continuous infusion much more frequently experienced severe ulcerative stomatitis (65% of patients treated). As the authors pointed out, no attempt was made to stratify patients prior to randomization, and substantial differences in clinical parameters (e.g., sex, age, site of indicator lesion, local versus distant metastasis) existed that could account in part for the differences in response rates between the treatment groups.

Early uncontrolled studies of the fluorinated pyrimidines in the treatment of advanced colorectal cancer gave conflicting results with respect to which agent, 5-FU or FUDR , was most active. Curreri and Ansfield[13] reported higher objective tumor response rates with FUDR, whereas Young et al[14] found that both drugs produced essentially the same response rate. To address this issue, a randomized trial of 5-FU versus FUDR was carried out at the Mayo Clinic among 168 patients with advanced colorectal cancer.[15] Treatment with each drug was given by an intensive course technique using rapid I.V. injection with therapy given for 5 consecutive days and then every other day for a maximum of 4 additional doses. Objective tumor responses were seen in 19/84 patients (22.6%) receiving FUDR and 10/84 patients (12.0%) receiving 5-FU. These differences were not statistically significant (P = .08). The average duration of response was 6.5 months for patients treated with 5-FU and 8.3 months for patients receiving FUDR. Therefore, there does not appear to be a substantial difference in therapeutic activity between systemic 5-FU and FUDR when given by bolus administration in intensive courses for the treatment of advanced colorectal cancer.

Summary

In summary, although marked variations in dose levels and patterns of clinical toxicity have been observed with continuous I.V. infusions of 5-FU and FUDR up to 120 hours in duration, there is no convincing evidence of an improvement in therapeutic response from controlled clinical trials among patients with advanced colorectal cancer. Furthermore, there was no apparent improvement in tumor response rates when 5-FU was given by 4-day infusion in combination with either mitomycin-C or methyl CCNU for the treatment of advanced colorectal cancer by the Southwest Oncology Group.[16] In this study, 46 of 269 patients with measurable indicator lesions (17%) had an objective tumor response. The authors concluded that "this burdensome method of 5-FU administration in combination with either mitomycin-C or methyl CCNU appear[s] to offer little advantage over bolus 5 FU alone." Although various uncontrolled studies have reported favorable objective response rates in patients with a variety of other solid tumors treated with continuous infusions of the fluorinated pyrimidines,[11,17] and other studies[18] have demonstrated the feasibility of administering very high doses of 5-FU as a 24-hour infusion (up to 14 grams) to patients with advanced cancer, there are currently no randomized trials comparing this method of drug administration to bolus administration.

Studies of Protracted Venous Infusion of the Fluorinated Pyrimidines

More recently, Lokich et al reported on phase 1 studies of continuous venous infusion of FUDR[19] and 5-FU[20] given for more protracted periods via central venous access using a tunneled subclavian line and ambulatory infusion pumps. A FUDR dose of 0.15 mg/kg/day for 14 days was found to be tolerable, with severe diarrhea dose-limiting at higher drug doses. No toxic effects were seen at FUDR delivery rates ≤0.125 mg/kg/day for periods up to 78 consecutive days. The recommended FUDR dose of 0.15 mg/kg/day for administration by continuous infusion for 14 days represents 1/20th of the maximal tolerated daily dose of 3 mg/kg/day when FUDR is given by continuous infusion for 5 days and 1/266 of the maximal tolerated dose of 40 mg/kg/day when FUDR is given for 5 days by bolus injection. These results confirm previous observations that the tolerated daily dose of FUDR is decreased when the duration of administration is prolonged by continuous infusion.

With 5-FU, stomatitis was dose-limiting at daily doses of 5-FU >300 mg/m²/day for periods of 30 to 68 consecutive days. At 5-FU doses <300 mg/m²/day it was possible to administer continuous intravenous infusions for

as long as 60 days without any hematologic toxicity whatsoever or other significant side effects. Cumulative doses of 5-FU were extended 3 to 4 times beyond
the level that can be administered by bolus or 5-day infusion schedules. The
recommended dosage schedule for phase 3 trials of continuous infusion 5-FU
was 300/mg/m²/day for 30 days. Plasma pharmacokinetics performed in
patients receiving 5-FU by continuous intravenous infusion in another Phase 1
trial[21] demonstrated a mean 5-FU plasma concentration of 0.91 ± 0.4 ng/ml at
a daily 5-FU dose of 300 mg/m².

In a subsequent report,[22] objective tumor responses were seen in 6/22
patients (27%) with a variety of advanced gastrointestinal carcinomas who had
measurable indicator lesions and received continuous venous infusions of 5-FU
at a dose of 300 mg/m²/day for 30 to 180 days. Toxicity was considered
minimal in the overall group of 32 patients treated; it consisted of stomatitis (3
patients), subclavian thrombosis (1 patient), and paresthesias and swelling of
the distal phlanges of the fingers (2 patients). Other investigators[22,23] have also
reported tender swelling of the fingers and toes variably associated with paresthesias and a scaly, erythematous, papular dermatitis. This unique symptom
complex, referred to as the "hand-foot syndrome," seems to be specifically
associated with prolonged continuous intravenous infusion schedules of 5-FU.

The potential for objective tumor regression using protracted venous
administration of 5-FU for patients with advanced colon cancer has been
recently confirmed by investigators from several other institutions with preliminary response rates of 31 to 45%.[24-26] Although most investigators reported
only mild toxicity using this approach, 8/13 patients (60%) in another series[23]
developed dose-limiting toxicity that required discontinuation of therapy. The
toxicity included stomatitis; swelling, redness, and tenderness of the distal
phalanges; and dermatitis. Chemical phlebitis, drug extravasation, diarrhea,
and bacteremia related to the central venous catheter have also been
reported.[23-26]

To place the value of continuous infusion 5-FU into clinical perspective, the
Mid-Atlantic Oncology Group is conducting a prospectively randomized trial
of this method of treatment compared to intermittent bolus administration of
5-FU using a standard intensive course schedule (see figure). The results of this
trial will be awaited with interest. Meanwhile, as summarized in table 2, the

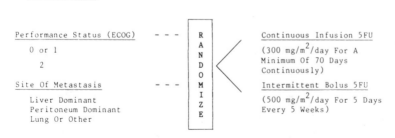

Figure 1.   Schema of Mid-Atlantic Oncology Group protocol for patients with
advanced measurable colorectal cancer.

medical oncologist must weigh the advantages and disadvantages of this more demanding and expensive method of chemotherapy administration that has not as yet been demonstrated to produce an improved therapeutic index by controlled clinical trial.

Table 2. Comparison of Prolonged Intravenous Infusion Versus Bolus
          Administration of Fluorinated Pyrimidines in Cancer Chemotherapy

Prolonged infusion	Bolus injection
Theoretical advantage of exposing greater proportion of cancer cells to cytotoxic agent during sensitive phase of growth cycle	Brief exposure of cancer cells to cytotoxic drug (serum half-life 10-20 min)
Greater cumulative rate of drug delivery	Higher peak serum drug level
Minimal hematologic toxicity	Leukopenia dose-limiting with potential for life-treatening infection
Requires permament central venous access and ambulatory infusion pump	Simple intravenous injection
Stomatitis, bacteremia from central venous line, dermatitis, drug extravasation, diarrhea	Stomatitis, diarrhea
Expensive	Relatively inexpensive
Improved Therapeutic Index (?)	Standard method of administration

9

METHOTREXATE

Carmen J. Allegra, M.D., and Gregory A. Curt, M.D.

Introduction

THE FOLIC ACID ANALOGUE methotrexate (MTX) has gained widespread use in the treatment of malignant disorders since its initial recognition as a potent cytotoxic agent in 1948. This agent was the first to produce impressive remissions in acute leukemia[1] and cures in the treatment of choriocarcinoma in women.[2] Since its introduction, MTX has been given by a variety of regimens. Initially, the drug was administered on a daily oral treatment schedule that was found to be ineffective in the treatment of solid tumors. However, improved response rates were noted with twice-weekly or once-weekly administration of higher doses of drug.[3,4] Djerassi et al were the first to illustrate responses in childhood acute leukemia with higher doses of MTX given by infusion to children refractory to conventional methotrexate treatment.[5]

Over the past two decades, MTX has become an important therapeutic agent in the treatment of choriocarcinoma in women, osteogenic sarcoma, breast cancer, epithelial cancers of the head and neck, acute leukemia, and the lymphomas.[6] In establishing the current "conventional" therapy for each of these diseases, many doses and schedules have been investigated, including high-dose therapy using up to 12 gm/m[2] [8] with leucovorin rescue and therapy with infusions of up to 30 hours duration.[7] These clinical studies have been formulated by the preclinical observation that the cytotoxicity of the antimetabolites, including MTX, is dependent on both the level of drug to which a given cell is exposed and the duration of the exposure time,[8,9] i.e., the concentration $\times$ time ($C \times T$) product. High drug doses given over long infusion periods have attempted to maximize these two variables. In addition, the same principles of dose and schedule have been more recently applied to the complex issue of circumventing cellular drug resistance.

Theoretical Considerations

To appreciate fully the rationale for infusional and/or high-dose therapy with MTX, one must consider the pharmacology of the drug, including its mechanism of action, cellular transport, the mechanisms by which cells become resistant to the drug. Methotrexate is capable of inhibiting certain folate-requiring reactions, most importantly dyhydrofolate reductase (DHFR, $K_i = 10^{-11}M$). Because all folate-requiring 1-carbon transfer reactions use folate in its fully reduced form (tetrahydro), it is the function of DHFR to maintain the intracellular folate pools in the biologically active reduced state. Thymidylate synthase, a critical enzyme in the *de novo* production of thymidylate and DNA synthesis, is the only physiologic enzyme that produces oxidized folate (dihydrofolate) in the process of 1-carbon transfer from 5-10-methylene tetrahydrofolic acid to deoxyuridylate. Inhibition of DHFR by MTX leads to the intracellular accumulation of oxidized folates as a product of ongoing thymidylate synthesis. These oxidized forms of folate inhibit the synthesis of purines, thymidylate, and certain amino acids,[10] ultimately resulting in cell death. Because physiologic folates can displace MTX from binding sites on DHFR, maintenance of intracellular free drug is essential for prolonged enzyme inhibition.

It has been known for at least two decades that the intracellular natural folate cofactors exist in a polyglutamated form, i.e., having up to 6 additional glutamyl residues appended to the terminal portion of the molecule.[11] This property allows for intracellular retention of the folates and concomitantly confers a greater affinity for many of the folate-requiring enzymes, including thymidylate synthase, AICAR transformylase, and methylene tetrahydrofolate reductase.[12-14] More recently, it has been shown by many investigators that MTX also undergoes the process of polyglutamation in a variety of normal and malignant cells both in vitro and in vivo.[15-18] Like the physiologic folates, this metabolism to polyglutamates allows for retention and intracellular accumulation of the drug[18] even in the absence of extracellular MTX. The MTX polyglutamate forms retain a high affinity for DHFR and also acquire potent inhibitory activity against several other critical folate-requiring enzymes.[11-13] The role of inhibition of folate-requiring enzymes other than DHFR by the MTX polyglutamates, unclear at present, is a subject of active preclinical investigation.

The process of MTX polyglutamation has been shown to be a dose- and time-dependent phenomenon, and sensitivity to MTX can be correlated with the ability of a cell to convert MTX to its polyglutamate forms. This correlation has been studied in vitro using 3 breast cancer cell lines. Jolivet and co-workers were able to correlate the sensitivity of these breast cancer cell lines to their ability to polyglutamate and retain MTX.[18] Specifically, polyglutamate species with 3 or more glutamate moieties were selectively retained intracellularly in the absence of extracellular drug and were responsible for maintenance of free drug levels and prolonged target enzyme inhibition.

Cowan and co-workers cloned a human breast cancer cell line that is 1,000-fold resistant to the cytotoxic effects of MTX.[19] The only abnormality that was found to account for drug resistance in these cells was a lack of MTX polyglutamation. Similarly, in small-cell lung carcinoma cell lines whose sensitivity/resistance was developed in vivo, a similar correlation was demonstrated.[20] As in the human breast cancer cell lines, it is the formation of polyglutamate species with 3 or more glutamyl moieties that are selectively retained in the absence of extracellular drug and responsible for prolonged DHFR inhibition.

In all in vitro systems studied to date, polyglutamate formation is time- and concentration-dependent. Drug treatment schedules capable of achieving prolonged elevated drug levels have a theoretic advantage over brief exposures in that prolonged exposures may result in a greater intracellular accumulation of drug through the formation of polyglutamates. As stated above, these forms may contribute to cytotoxicity by the inhibition of enzymes other than DHFR and may be critical in overcoming drug resistance. Another empiric advantage of prolonged drug exposure and intracellular polyglutamate formation is their selective retention and capacity for prolonged target enzyme inhibition.[21]

The intracellular transport of MTX should also be considered in the design of clinical drug schedules, as sensitivity of cells to MTX has been directly correlated with a cell's ability to transport the drug.[23] At concentrations of less than 10 μM, MTX enters the cell by energy-dependent mediated carrier transport.[22] There is an alternate low-affinity mechanism that is poorly understood but appears to participate in drug transport at concentrations greater than 20 μM.[24] This low-affinity system may represent passive diffusion of drug across the cell membrane, as the system does not appear to be saturable.

Infusional therapy capable of sustaining high extracellular drug concentrations has theoretical advantages for inducing cytotoxicity in untreated cells as well as cells that have become resistant to "standard" doses of MTX. The mechanisms by which cells become resistant to MTX include amplification of the target enzyme DHFR, altered affinity of the target enzyme for MTX, defective membrane transport, and altered polyglutamation of methotrexate.[10] Each of these mechanisms has been investigated and correlated with drug sensitivity in vitro;[18-20] most recently, clinical specimens from patients resistant to MTX in vivo have closely paralleled the resistance mechanisms documented in vitro.[25] In particular, amplification of DHFR in clinical specimens has been confirmed in human small-cell lung cancer,[25] acute leukemia,[26,27] and adenocarcinoma of the ovary.[28] As alluded to above, infusional therapy may be advantageous in overcoming several of the resistance mechanisms found in mammalian cells:

1. Enhanced accumulation and retention of drug through polyglutamate formation resulting from more prolonged drug exposures may overcome resistance due to either DHFR amplification or altered affinity for drug.

2. Defective transport mechanisms may be overcome with prolonged high drug concentrations because intracellular drug entry is also dose-dependent and independent of active transport mechanisms at drug concentrations above 20 μM.

3. The presence of extracellular drug for a prolonged period would allow similarly prolonged DHFR inhibition, even in the absence of polyglutamation.

Clinical Investigations

Infusional therapy with MTX appears to have an additional clinical advantage in the treatment of "sanctuary" sites, including CSF and testes. Early investigations by Chabner et al[29] defined a minimum inhibitory concentration of MTX for murine bone marrow cells as 10^{-8} M. Uniform high drug levels in sanctuary sites are critical in achieving adequate therapeutic responses, and multiple investigators have illustrated the usefulness of infusional MTX therapy for achieving high and uniform drug levels in the CSF.[30-32] Bleyer and co-workers found a 1-log difference in CSF drug concentrations in ventricular versus lumbar levels following intrathecal administration.[33] CSF drug levels were studied in 13 children with acute lymphocytic leukemia given infusional therapy with either 500 mg/m^2 or 1,500 mg/m^2 as an I.V. push (1/3 dose) followed by a 24-hour infusion of drug.[30] In the 1,500 mg/m^2 group, CSF levels of 3.5×10^{-7}M were achieved and maintained over the 24-hour infusion. Simultaneous steady-state plasma levels were 30 μM. Shapiro and co-workers[31] achieved CSF levels of 6.4×10^{-6}M in children treated with high-dose 4-hour infusions of 200, 300, and 400 mg/kg. These investigators also found CSF levels of 6×10^{-7}M with 24-hour infusions of 500 mg/m^2. Clinical studies such as these suggest that adequate and uniform drug levels can be achieved in sanctuary sites such as the CSF with infusional therapy.

In vitro investigations by Eichholtz et al[9] performed on 3 cell lines (human adult kidney [HAK], HeLa S-3, and Chinese hamster cells [lung fibroblasts]) have clearly shown that drug concentration and exposure time are critical determinants of cytotoxicity. This type of information was quantitated by Pinedo and co-workers, who studied the rate of depletion of nucleated marrow cells in mice treated with MTX infusions. Marrow toxicity was both time- and drug-concentration dependent; 70% depletion of nucleated cells occurred at 12 hours for a constant drug level of 10^{-5}M, and only after 48 hours for a constant drug level of 2×10^{-7} M.[8]

Given this time and dose dependency, Liguori and co-workers investigated whether the achievement and maintenance of drug levels in human tissues were best accomplished by infusional rather than bolus delivery.[34] These investigators performed serial skin biopsies on patients with solid tumors receiving MTX and compared the tissue drug levels achieved following a 50 mg I.V. bolus to tissue drug levels in patients who received the same dose given as a 12-hour I.V. or intra-arterial infusion. Their results suggest that tissue levels are sustained 2–3 times longer in the infusion groups, but the number of experiments was small and the data too incomplete to draw definitive conclusions.

Many clinical trials have attempted to consolidate the theoretical advantages of infusional therapy into clinical responses. Encouraging preliminary results were reported in the treatment of 10 children with acute leukemia who were refractory to standard therapy with daily oral or twice-weekly I.M. methotrexate.[5] All of these patients achieved a remission with MTX given as an 18-hour infusion of 36 mg/m^2 following an initial loading dose of 12 mg/m^2. These positive results are in contrast to those of Janka and co-workers, who treated 8 children with acute leukemia in relapse with single-agent MTX given as a 24-hour infusion of 500 mg/m^2 followed by leucovorin rescue.[32] Despite achieving steady-state serum concentrations of 2.4×10^{-5} M and CSF concentrations of 4.2×10^{-7}M, no responses were obtained. Similarly, Cohen et al treated 6 patients with advanced acute leukemia who had failed standard therapy that included conventional-dose MTX. These patients with refractory disease were treated with a high-dose (4–12 gm/m^2) MTX infusion over 24 hours.[35] Again, no responses were observed despite maintenance of 2.4×10^{-4}M serum levels of drug for the 24-hour infusion period.

Although the role of infusional therapy with MTX in the treatment of acute lymphocytic leukemia remains controversial, it is clear that high blood levels and uniform CSF exposure can be achieved and maintained throughout the infusion. This capacity may be important in the treatment and/or prophylaxis of this patient population, where the testes or CNS is a frequent site of initial disease and/or relapse.

High-dose infusional therapy with MTX has been shown to play a beneficial role in the treatment of osteogenic sarcoma. The responsiveness of this tumor to MTX appears to follow a steep dose-response relationship so that higher drug levels would be expected to confer greater cytotoxicity.[36] Because most trials using high-dose therapy have given the drug over 4–6 hours, the precise role of more prolonged infusional therapy remains unclear. No randomized trials have defined the effectiveness of various infusion schedules versus bolus injection using high-dose therapy.

Early work by several investigators found that osteogenic sarcoma was poorly responsive to low doses (30–50 mg/m^2) of MTX,[37] and the trials of Rosen and Jaffe have clearly illustrated the benefit of high-dose therapy.[36,37] In the initial treatment of 10 patients with metastatic osteogenic sarcoma with 50–500 mg/kg given as a 6-hour infusion, Jaffe reported 2 partial responses and 2 complete remissions.[37] Interestingly, 3 patients refractory to the 6-hour infusions were treated with identical doses given as a 24-hour infusion. One of three achieved a partial response to the lengthened duration of drug exposure. A recent summary of more than 200 patients given 5,000 doses of high-dose MTX reports a steep dose-response with optimal responses achieved with 4-hour infusions of 12 g/m^2 for younger children and 8 g/m^2 in adolescents.[36] Although few responses were seen with lower doses, these higher doses yielded a 40% complete remission rate and a 68% response rate overall. In an attempt to increase disease response with prolonged drug exposure, Cohen and co-workers treated 6 refractory patients with osteogenic sarcoma with a 24-hour infusion of MTX at a dose identical to one that was ineffective (4 to 12 g/m^2) when given as a 6-hour infusion. No responses were reported.[35]

Squamous cell carcinoma of the head and neck has also been intensively studied in a variety of dose schedules in an attempt to optimize the delivery of MTX, the single most active agent in the treatment of this disease. Two promising studies used 24- and 30-hour infusions of 737 mg/m^2 and 2 mg/kg in the treatment of 44 patients with head and neck cancer.[38,39] These regimens induced a 50–60% response rate compared to a 12–53% response rate for historical controls using bolus therapy.

A randomized study attempting to clarify whether increased dose and/or duration of exposure are important to response in squamous cell carcinoma of the head and neck was undertaken by Taylor and co-workers.[40] This study randomized 47 patients to receive either 1,500 mg/m^2 via 24-hour infusion with leucovorin rescue or 40 mg/m^2 I.M. Both regimens were repeated weekly and both were escalated to toxicity. The response rate in the high-dose group was 32% versus 22% with standard dose. This difference was not statistically significant; however, the mean time to progression was 11 weeks versus 5 weeks in the high and standard regimens, respectively, and this was significant at the p = 0.04 level. Despite an improved disease-free interval, the overall survival for each group was identical at 4.2 months. Because toxicity was significantly greater in the high-dose group, the authors concluded that high-dose MTX in this setting conferred no therapeutic advantage.

These conclusions are supported by those of Woods et al, who randomized 72 patients to receive 50, 500, or 5,000 mg/m^2 of MTX intravenously every week and found no differences in response ($\sim$30%) or survival among the three groups. Interestingly, this study did report 5 patients who progressed at one dose level and who subsequently responded at the next highest escalation. Reinforcing the parallel relation between toxicity and response, DeConti randomized patients with squamous cell carcinoma of the head and neck to receive either 40 mg/m^2/week or 240 mg/m^2/every 2 weeks by I.V. bolus.[42] Although no difference in response rate ($\sim$25%) or survival was noted, both the response duration (105 days versus 42 days) and toxicity were enhanced in the low-dose but more frequent weekly schedule.

Finally, a study by Volger failed to document a correlation between the dose intensity or duration of MTX exposure and response rate.[43] In this study, 281 patients with epithelial carcinoma of the head and neck or with colon or breast cancer were randomized to receive 125 mg/m^2 of MTX orally every 6 hours for 4 doses, 15 mg/m^2 orally every 6 hours for 4 doses, or 60 mg/m^2 by I.V. bolus. All doses were given on a weekly schedule. The authors reported no significant differences in response rates, survival, or duration of response with any of the 3 regimens.

Several other studies have examined the effect of infusional therapy with MTX in a variety of other solid tumors. Notable is a nonrandomized study by Sullivan, who treated 161 solid tumor patients with 5 mg I.V. over 24 hours or in 4 divided doses orally over 24 hours until toxicity developed ($\sim$10–14 days).[44] There was no significant therapeutic advantage to either regimen. In a separate study, 30 patients with a variety of solid tumors were randomized to receive either 25 mg/m^2 of MTX twice weekly or 100–200 mg/kg by I.V. infusion over 6 hours. Again, no difference in response rate or survival was noted between the two groups.[45] Thus, studies on the treatment of tumors other than osteogenic sarcoma so far have failed to show convincing evidence for a dependency of response on either dose or schedule. It is possible that more prolonged schedules of even higher doses may be beneficial in the ultimate treatment of these or other diseases.

In an effort to continue the search for an optimal dose schedule of MTX, a recent phase 1 study has defined a maximally tolerated dose of MTX given by prolonged I.V. infusion at 0.75 mg/m^2/day for 28 days and 1.5 mg/m^2/day for 14 days.[46] The toxicity of these exquisitely low doses demonstrates the importance of dose scheduling and confirms that continuous exposure to 10^{-8}M drug will inhibit DNA synthesis. Stomatitis and mild thrombocytopenia were dose-limiting. The serum level achieved with the 0.75 dose was 1.3×10^{-8}M.

Summary

In summary, the intracellular pharmacology of MTX has been investigated in detail, and studies in vitro suggest a potential role for the sustained high drug concentrations achievable with infusional therapy in the treatment of a variety of human carcinomas and hematologic malignancies. At present, clinical studies show good evidence for a dose-response relation in osteogenic sarcoma; however, clinical studies attempting to demonstrate an advantage to infusional therapy or a dose-response relation in other malignancies have not been rewarding. As new dose schedule regimens based on the leads provided by in vitro investigations are tested, we hope to achieve better responses in the treatment of clinically refractory tumors.

10

ANTHRACYCLINES

*Sewa S. Legha, M.D., Gabriel N. Hortobagyi, M.D., and
Robert S. Benjamin, M.D.*

Introduction

DOXORUBICIN (ADR) IS ONE OF the most useful of anticancer drugs, having a broad spectrum of antitumor activity. It is most effective in the treatment of acute leukemias, Hodgkin's disease, non-Hodgkin's lymphomas, breast cancer, and sarcomas. Other tumors where ADR has significant activity include lung cancer, thyroid cancer, gastric cancer, hepatoma, multiple myeloma, bladder cancer, testicular cancer, ovarian carcinoma, and endometrial carcinoma. The drug is commonly used as a single I.V. injection in a dose range of 60–75 mg/m² at 3-week intervals. Some treatment programs have used the drug in divided doses on days 1 and 8 and others on 3 consecutive days using the same total dose per course of treatment. Used in this fashion, ADR has side effects that include moderately severe nausea and vomiting, myelosuppression, alopecia, skin toxicity, and cardiac toxicity. The acute side effects are reversible, partially controllable, and rarely interfere with continued therapy. However, cardiac toxicity, which is dose-related, develops on repeated use of this drug and limits continued therapy beyond 6 to 9 months. The incidence of cardiac toxicity varies between 1% to 5%[1] when the cumulative ADR dose is limited to 450–550 mg/m². The clinical manifestations of cardiac toxicity during the early phase include cardiac arrhythmias that are generally reversible and rarely interfere with clinical use of the drug. The chronic cardiac toxicity generally manifests as congestive heart failure of varying degrees of severity, with a potential fatality rate of 20–40%.[2] Although there is a marked individual variation in the cumulative ADR dose causing significant cardiac toxicity, the lack of good predictive tests leads to interruption of therapy on an empirical basis and curtailment of the potential benefit of continued therapy in responding patients.

A number of investigations aimed at reducing the cardiac toxicity of ADR have been conducted during the past decade, but most of these have not been fruitful.[3,4] The most successful avenue has been a schedule of drug administration in which fractionation of the total dose, administered over a longer period of time than the standard rapid administration, has led to significant reduction in acute as well as chronic toxicity without compromising antitumor activity. The initial observations of reduced cardiac toxicity with dose fractionation, empiric in nature, were made in patients treated with the weekly schedule of ADR administration, which resulted in a considerable reduction in cardiac toxicity.[5,6] This result led to about a 50% gain in the cumulative ADR dose over that achieved with the bolus schedule, with a relatively low risk of cardiac toxicity. These observations have recently been confirmed in prospective studies proving that weekly administration of ADR is associated with an improved therapeutic index, with preservation of antitumor activity, and a clear reduction in cardiac toxicity.[7,8] More recently, continuous I.V. administration of ADR has been investigated; this approach has also proven to be associated with a marked reduction in cardiac and G.I. toxicity.[9,10] Details of continuous infusion schedules that have been investigated in the recent past will be described in this chapter.

General Considerations

There are several important considerations pertinent to the continuous I.V. infusion of doxorubicin. These include its solubility, the stability of the drug in solution under various conditions, compatibility with different I.V. fluids and other drugs, and the effect of drug on the veins and the perivenous tissues. ADR has excellent solubility—it can be dissolved in 5% dextrose in water or in normal saline in a concentration of 2 mg/ml or less. It has excellent stability in its powdered form as well as in solution, regardless of the concentration of the drug in the I.V. fluids. Decomposition of ADR in solution over periods of 7–10 days is less than 5%.[11] Once it is mixed in solution, the stability of the drug is not influenced by temperatures ranging from freezing to normal physiological temperatures.[12] Although limited, data on the compatibility of ADR with other cytotoxic agents have shown it to be incompatibile with 5-fluorouracil (5-FU), methotrexate (MTX), and heparin, but compatible with dacarbazine (DTIC) and vinblastine (VLB). Intravenous administration of ADR is commonly associated with varying degrees of phlebitis, and any extravasation of ADR into the perivenous tissues can lead to tissue necrosis, followed by ulceration and sloughing of the normal tissues. These vesicant effects make continuous venous infusion of ADR in the peripheral veins very hazardous. Accordingly, the infused drug must be delivered into the central veins by means of indwelling catheters of various types currently available. In our institution, we have used Silastic catheters inserted either via the antecubital veins (Intrasil) or by the subclavian vein (Centrasil), with the tip of the catheter placed in the superior vena cava. These catheters can be inserted percutaneously and left indwelling, with minimal local care in the form of weekly changes in dressing and daily heparin locks to keep the catheter from clotting with blood. The average duration of function of these catheters in our hands is about 1 year and sometimes as long as 2 years. Many other institutions have used implanted catheters of the Broviac or Hickman varieties, both of which require a surgical procedure for subcutaneous tunneling and placement of an externalized Silastic catheter into the cephalic or subclavian veins.[13] In addition, several other methods of venous access are currently under evaluation. These methods include a variety with a subcutaneous injection port connected to a Silastic central venous catheter (Infuse-A-Port), through which the drugs can be delivered via a specially designed Huber-point needle,[14] and subcutaneously implanted pumps of the Infusaid variety.[15] These latter devices have the advantage of not requiring any local care in terms of dressing changes and also minimize the risk of sepsis because of the closed nature of their operation. Depending on the method of venous access, ADR infusions can be accomplished with one of the several small-volume portable pumps currently available, or else the daily dose of the drug can be dissolved in a large bag of the standard variety and the drug delivered by means of a larger, nonportable pump in the hospital. The portable pumps generally hold 30–50 ml of solution, which can be delivered by the pump either daily or over several days, depending on whether the patient is being treated with the short-term venous infusion or the protracted infusion schedule described below. Because ADR is incompatible with heparin, a heparin lock is used only between ADR infusion periods.

Methods of Doxorubicin Infusion

Although the optimum schedule of continuous venous infusion of ADR has not been established, most current investigations can be grouped into two broad categories. The most experience has been accumulated with a schedule consisting of short-term venous infusions given over 1–4 days, with cycles repeated at 3–4 weeks. In more recent long-term infusion therapy, patients have received protracted infusions of ADR for several months or longer.

Short-Term Infusion Therapy

Our first study exploring the infusion of ADR started in 1977. Because of concern over the possibility of increased toxicity, initial patients were treated with shorter infusions beginning with 24 hours, gradually increasing the duration of infusion to 48 hours, and finally extending the period to 96 hours during subsequent cycles. Once the initial 3–4 patients at each of the different ADR infusion durations tolerated the therapy, all patients were subsequently started and maintained on 96-hour infusions. Accordingly, the most thoroughly investigated short-term ADR infusion duration has been the 96-hour cycle, which generally takes 5 days to complete. Since the 96-hour infusions provided excellent gain in therapeutic index of ADR, subsequent studies explored shorter infusion durations in order to determine the optimum infusion duration that would provide good cardiac protection and be most practical. Data on the antitumor activity and toxicity of various infusion schedules are described below.

Antitumor Activity

In order to determine the antitumor activity of ADR when given as a continuous infusion, a phase 2 study was conducted among 27 patients with metastatic breast cancer who had previously received chemotherapy with drugs other than doxorubicin. ADR was used in a dose of 60 mg/m^2 given over periods varying from 24 to 96 hours, the majority receiving the 96-hour infusions. Thirteen of 26 (50%) patients achieved objective response (1 CR, 12 PR), 6 improved, and 7 failed to respond.[9] The median duration of response in these patients was 7 months (range 3–21 months). Although these were highly selected patients, the 95% confidence limits (30%–70%) on this response rate indicate that the antitumor activity of ADR given by infusion was well preserved and possibly enhanced. Based on this experience, the continuous venous infusion method of ADR administration was incorporated into the various combination chemotherapy regimens in the treatment of solid tumors. The use of infusion ADR in patients with sarcomas and breast cancer resulted in response rates quite similar to those observed when the agent was used in the bolus schedule in combination with established drug regimens. In soft tissue sarcomas, ADR was combined with cyclophosphamide and dacarbazine; the results of this regimen (CyADIC) in 51 patients showed CR in 7 patients and a PR in 20, for an overall response rate of 53%. This compares favorably with our previous experience with the CyADIC regimen, in which a response rate of 50% was achieved in a large group of patients in our institution.[16] Data on response duration and survival of patients in this study so far appear to be comparable, although further follow-up is necessary before the data are mature. In patients with metastatic breast cancer, we have used ADR in combination with 5-FU and cyclophosphamide (CTX) in a triple-drug regimen, FAC, in which the doses of individual drugs used were similar to those in the standard FAC regimen used in our institution in the recent past. In these patients, ADR has been administered over 96 hours; in a subsequent study, infusion duration was reduced to 48 hours. In a total of 96 evaluable patients treated on these two infusion schedules, a complete and partial response rate of 76% was observed.[17] This compares very well with our previous experience with this triple-drug regimen with ADR used as a bolus, in which an objective response rate of around 70% has been observed. The median duration of response with the infusion of FAC is 16 months — slightly longer than the FAC regimen using bolus ADR.[18] Furthermore, we observed that 65% of the patients continued on ADR until their tumor became refractory to chemotherapy, whereas 70% of the responders on bolus FAC had been taken off ADR because of the empiric cumulative ADR dose limit of 450 mg/m^2. This study requires further follow-up for final results, but meanwhile it appears to show a prolongation in the duration of complete responses compared to our historical data in patients who achieved complete response on standard FAC chemotherapy with ADR administered by the bolus schedule. Based on these data, which clearly demonstrate equivalent antitumor activity when ADR is given by continuous infusion, nearly all of our patients with breast cancer currently receive their treatment with ADR given as a continuous infusion over 48 or 96 hours.

Toxicity Associated with Doxorubicin Infusions

ACUTE TOXICITY

In our first study using ADR as a single agent, we were impressed with a marked reduction in nausea and vomiting experienced by patients receiving the drug by infusion. Among the 27 patients, 12 patients had no nausea or vomiting, 11 had mild nausea with occasional vomiting, and only 4 patients (15%) had significant nausea and vomiting requiring antiemetic therapy. Patients who experienced nausea and vomiting did so predominantly during the time they were receiving 24-hour infusions; the 96-hour infusions were rarely accompanied by nausea. There did, however, appear to be some increase in the incidence of stomatitis, which was observed in 15–30% of patients treated with the infusion schedules. Stomatitis was more common with the 96-hour infusions than with the 24- and 48-hour infusions. In patients with severe stomatitis, reduction in the duration of infusion to 48 hours — and if necessary to 24 hours — generally reduced the severity or eliminated the problem altogether. Similarly, ADR used as infusion in combination chemotherapy regimens for sarcomas and breast cancer has resulted in significant reduction of nausea and vomiting. Because DTIC and ADR are compatible, both drugs have been mixed and infused over 96 hours, with a resultant marked reduction in nausea and vomiting experienced from the combined use of these two drugs.

The myelosuppressive toxicity and alopecia associated with infusion ADR appear to be similar to these effects expected from the standard schedule of ADR administration. With the single-agent ADR dose of 60 mg/m^2 in our breast cancer study, the median nadir WBC count was 2,000/μl, with a range of 500–5,000/μl.[9] The median nadir granulocyte count was 900/μl, with a range of 100–3,000/μl. These counts appear to be similar or somewhat more depressed with the continuous venous infusions as compared to the standard ADR schedule. Alopecia was nearly complete after 1 to 2 courses of infusion ADR.

In addition to some increase in the incidence of stomatitis, the infusion schedule of ADR has associated problems related to the use of indwelling catheters for drug administration. In some ways, the delivery of drugs through the indwelling catheters reduced the discomfort and pain associated with repeated needle insertions used for each course of standard chemotherapy. On the other hand, catheter-related problems such as catheter occlusion or leakage and venous thrombosis have been observed in some patients. Thrombosis of the subclavian vein and sometimes the superior vena cava has been observed in 2–5% of our patients on ADR infusions. This is a much lower incidence compared to that reported by Lokich et al.[19] Because the average duration of catheter function in our studies has been about 1 year, with a range of up to 2 years,[20] a majority of our patients on infusion therapy have had well-preserved arm veins. This benefit made it easier for them to tolerate repeated venesection for blood drawing in comparison to the difficulties experienced by patients who have received chemotherapy through the peripheral veins by the standard techniques.

Cardiac Toxicity of Infusion Doxorubicin

When used in the standard bolus schedule, ADR causes significant cardiac toxicity, mostly subclinical, in approximately 50% of patients treated with cumulative dosage of 200–550 mg/m². These are the findings of 2 separate studies, one conducted at Stanford University and the other at the M.D. Anderson Hospital.[21,22] In the Stanford study of a group of patients with various solid tumors and hematologic malignancies, 19 of 30 patients treated with ADR in the dose range of 240–550 mg/m² developed pathologic changes of grade 2 to 3 severity.[21] Further, among 23 patients who had no prior mediastinal irradiation, 13 (56%) showed grade 2 to 3 changes in their endomyocardial biopsies. Similarly, in our group of 52 patients with a variety of solid tumors, 29 (55%) patients developed evidence of grade 2 changes or congestive heart failure after receiving a median cumulative ADR dose of 485 mg/m².[22] The cardiac toxicity of ADR administered by infusion is markedly reduced. In the first infusion study in breast cancer patients, 7 of 19 patients responding to ADR received cumulative dose of 600–1,500 mg/m². Only 1 of the 7 showed significant evidence of cardiac toxicity in the cardiac biopsy specimen.[9] On the strength of this pilot study, the use of ADR as a continuous infusion has been expanded to several studies in combination with other drugs in the treatment of various solid tumors. In the initial studies, infusions of ADR were given over 96 hours, and later on, shorter infusions were evaluated. The most extensively evaluated infusion schedule to date is 96 hours; it has involved 200 patients treated with doxorubicin alone or in combination with other drugs. From this group, 55 patients have received a cumulative doxorubicin dose in excess of 500 mg/m² (range 500–1,900 mg/m²), and a total of 6 patients (11%) have developed clinical (9%) or grade 2 biopsy (2%) evidence of cardiac toxicity.[23,24] Clinical cardiac toxicity was observed only among the 34 patients who received cumulative ADR doses in excess of 800 mg/m², generally occurring in the dose range of 1,200–1,300 mg/m² (table 1). Therefore, although the 96-hour ADR infusions are not free of cardiac toxicity, the median cumulative dose to significant cardiac toxicity is two- to three-fold higher than that of the bolus schedule of doxorubicin administration.

To define the duration of ADR infusion that will be most efficient in reducing the cardiac toxicity, we have investigated the effects of infusion durations

Table 1. Cardiac Toxicity of Doxorubicin Used by 96-Hour Continuous Venous Infusion

Characteristic	Cumulative doxorubicin dose mg/m²				
	240-600	601-800	801-1,000	1,001-1,200	1,201-1,900
Number of patients	12	16	20	20	11
Mean biopsy grade	0.6	0.7	0.8	1.0	1.1
Percent patients with biopsy grade ≥ 1.5*	8	6	16	16	27

*Patients with cardiac biopsy grades of ≥ 1.5 are at high risk for developing congestive heart failure. Accordingly, further ADR administration in such patients is not safe.

of 48 hours in one group of patients and of 24 hours in another group.[17,22] When data on 96-hour infusions are compared to those of the 48-hour infusions, the degree of cardiac protection is nearly as good with the 2-day infusions versus the 4-day infusions. However, the best protection was achieved with the 96-hour infusions, which should be the best schedule to use in patients who are at high risk for cardiac toxicity, such as those with organic heart disease and those who have received previous mediastinal irradiation. When infusion durations were shortened to 24 hours, the degree of cardiac protection was not as good as that achieved with 48- and 96-hour infusions, but there was definitely reduced toxicity compared to that of the standard bolus schedule.[22] The median dose to significant cardiac toxicity with the 24-hour infusion schedule was approximately 850 mg/m^2, nearly twice the cumulative dose of the standard schedule, for a similar degree of cardiac toxicity. Other investigators have explored shorter durations of infusion over 6–10 hours, but these have not offered a significant degree of cardiac protection.[25]

Our data indicate that for the routine use of ADR as a continuous venous infusion, the optimum duration of infusion is 48 hours. In patients who are at high risk for cardiac toxicity or have any evidence of impaired cardiac function, the duration of infusion should be lengthened to 96 hours. On the contrary, when dealing with patients with malignancies where the duration of therapeutic response from ADR is expected to be less than 6 to 9 months, the duration of ADR infusion could be shortened to 24 hours, at least for the initial phase of treatment. If the patient achieves a good response, the infusion duration can subsequently be lengthened to 48 hours or to 96 hours in order to allow continued therapy.

Long-Term Infusions of Doxorubicin

Based on the marked reduction in the cardiac toxicity of ADR with short-term venous infusions, a number of investigators have recently initiated studies with low-dose ADR given as a continuous infusion on a more protracted basis.[11,26-28] Starting with a daily dose of 1– 2mg/m^2, the maximum tolerated daily dose has varied between 3 mg/m^2 and 5 mg/m^2/day for periods of several weeks to several months in the responding patients. Some investigators have used higher daily doses for 2-week cycles on therapy, followed by 2 weeks of no chemotherapy, to allow for recovery from side effects. These long-term infusions have been made possible by the availability of portable pump devices that can hold a 1- to 2-week drug supply. The remarkable stability of ADR under ambient conditions has made it unnecessary to refill the pumps more than once a week. Long-term venous studies have shown excellent tolerance to ADR, with stomatitis being the common dose-limiting toxicity. There is no significant nausea or vomiting with these schedules. The myelosuppressive toxicity and alopecia appear to persist, although the alopecia may be less severe compared to that observed with short-term venous infusions and with bolus schedules of ADR administration. Preliminary data on cardiac toxicity appear to be encouraging, but the number of patients treated with cumulative ADR in excess of 500 mg/m^2 are still low. However, several investigators have reported small numbers of patients receiving cumulative ADR doses of

500–1,000 mg/m² without any evidence of cardiac toxicity. Similarly, the anti-tumor activity of the drug seems to be well preserved in these long-term infusions, but whether it is enhanced or not remains to be proven. Whether long-term venous infusions are superior in terms of efficacy or reduced toxicity compared to the short-term venous infusions remains to be proven in further studies.

Therapeutic Implications of Continuous Venous Infusion of Doxorubicin

Data at hand make it quite clear that the cardiac toxicity of ADR is markedly reduced when the drug is administered in fractionated doses rather than the single bolus every-3-week schedule commonly used in the past. Dose fractionation has been accomplished in a number of different ways, initially in the form of small weekly doses, later with continuous venous infusion over the short term of 1–4 days, and most recently with long-term, continuous venous infusions indefinitely. In general, all of the fractionated schedules have resulted in marked reduction in nausea and vomiting and a significant reduction in cardiac toxicity. Interestingly, myelosuppressive toxicity and alopecia have not been altered by the schedule manipulations, and there is a clear increase in the incidence of stomatitis.

In terms of cardiac toxicity, the incidence and severity is reduced, but this undesirable side effect is not completely eliminated. The reduction in cardiac toxicity with the weekly schedule has been modest, but it has made it possible to increase the cumulative ADR dose to the 700–800 mg/m² range. The reduction in cardiac toxicity with the short-term venous infusion schedules is substantially greater, especially with the 48-hour and 96-hour schedules. The cumulative dose to significant cardiac toxicity on the 96-hour schedule is 1,200–1,300 mg/m², and a cumulative dose of 800 mg/m² is essentially free of serious cardiotoxic effects. When the infusion duration is limited to 24 hours, the gain in the cumulative ADR dose without significant toxicity is similar to that achieved with the weekly schedule. Whether the long-term venous schedules of ADR delivery would completely eliminate cardiac toxicity remains to be seen. Whether the long-term infusion schedules will further increase the therapeutic index beyond that achieved with the 96-hour infusion is also unclear. It appears that long-term infusion schedules do avert nausea and vomiting and result in lesser degrees of alopecia compared to other methods of ADR administration. In terms of therapeutic effects, ADR given by the fractionated schedules appears to maintain its antitumor activity. Despite several possible advantages of infusion ADR, there are some practical constraints in its wider application. The vesicant nature of the drug requires its delivery in the central venous system with the aid of indwelling catheters; slow infusions require either hospitalization or the use of a portable pump, each of which add to the costs of achieving this form of drug delivery. Additional risks are associated with the use of these catheters, including venous thrombosis and catheter-related infections. Although the ultimate cost/benefit ratio for general use of ADR infusions is yet to be defined, the following applications appear to be justified with the knowledge at hand about the reduced toxicity of this drug:

- A fairly significant number of patients with cancer who also have cardiac diseases should no longer be denied the therapeutic benefit of ADR therapy if their cancer is the more life threatening. In this regard, unless they are in frank congestive heart failure, most patients can be treated with infusion ADR with minimal risk of additional cardiac dysfunction up to modest cumulative doses.

- The reduced cardiac toxicity of infused ADR has also allowed renewed use of the drug in patients who previously responded to the drug used in the standard fashion but later developed tumor recurrence. Because second-line therapy for most human cancers is nonexistent, a majority of such patients have been able to achieve second useful remissions and have tolerated ADR doses in a cumulative dose range sometimes higher than that they had received with the standard mode of administration.[29] This has been particularly useful in patients with more responsive tumors such as lymphomas, leukemias, breast cancer, and sarcomas.

- Increasingly, ADR is being used for adjuvant therapy in high-risk patients with tumors such as breast cancer and sarcomas. In the past, the cumulative dose was generally kept low in order to avoid cardiac toxicity, which had the potential to be fatal in patients who were potentially free of disease. Using the infusion schedule, we are currently using ADR more liberally and in higher cumulative doses in such patients.

- The most difficult aspect of ADR infusion therapy is to demonstrate whether continued ADR therapy in the responding patients provides a gain in disease-free or overall survival. The most significant disease where this is important is metastatic breast cancer, where approximately 60–70% of the patients have to be taken off the drug while still responding to this chemotherapy as given in the standard bolus schedule. Currently, we are continuing ADR therapy in responding patients as long as the tumor is responding and the patient is free from cardiac toxicity. Although the overall median durations of response in patients treated with FAC chemotherapy by the infusion schedule appear to be only minimally prolonged, patients who achieved complete remissions on the infusion schedule appear to have longer duration of response compared to our past experience with using ADR by the bolus schedule. A longer follow-up of these patients will be required before the ultimate impact of infusion therapy with ADR can be determined.

Anthracycline Analogues

The broad-spectrum antitumor activity of ADR has led to a large-scale attempt to develop new analogues with a superior therapeutic index. The goal of the new analogues is either to improve efficacy or to diminish the cardiac toxicity associated with the use of ADR. Although several hundred anthracycline analogues have been synthesized and tested in preclinical systems, the expense and the time involved in screening for experimental antitumor activity and cardiac toxicity have been the limiting factors for their entry into clinical trials. Nevertheless, more than a dozen anthracycline analogues have made it to the level of clinical trials currently ongoing around the world. A brief summary of these analogues will be presented here; their clinical status is summarized in table 2.

Daunorubicin (Daunomycin)

This was the first anthracycline to enter clinical trials; it has been used almost exclusively in the treatment of acute leukemias, both in adults and in children. It was discovered almost simultaneously in France and Italy. Daunomycin is commonly used in a dose range of 30–60 mg/m² daily for 3 days, usually in combination with other antileukemic drugs. Because Daunomycin is clearly cardiotoxic, a cumulative dose limit of 550 mg/m² should not be exceeded when the drug is used in the standard fashion of short I.V. infusions. Although daunorubicin has been used as a continuous infusion in a phase 1 trial in previously treated patients with acute leukemia in our institution, no phase 2 evaluation was conducted because of somewhat limited antileukemic activity in patients who had previously received other anthracycline therapy. The activity of daunorubicin in solid tumors, although not thoroughly investigated, appears to be less than that of ADR.

Rubidazone (Zorubicin)

Rubidazone is a semisynthetic analogue of daunorubicin that proved superior to the parent drug in several animal tumor systems. It has shown remarkable antileukemic activity, both as a single agent and in combination with other antileukemic drugs. However, the drug has not shown significant activity

Table 2. Anthracyclines in Clinical Trials: Present and Past

	Drug	Current status in U.S.	Country of origin
1.	Daunorubicin	Phase 4, comercially available	Italy/France
2.	Adriamycin	Phase 4, commercial	Italy
3.	Rubidazone	Phase 2, investigational*	France
4.	Adriamycin-DNA	Phase 1-2, investigational*	Belgium
5.	AD-32	Phase 1-2, investigational	United States
6.	Carminomycin	Phase 2, investigational**	U.S.S.R.
7.	Aclacinomycin	Phase 2-3, investigational	Japan
8.	4'-Epi-Adriamycin	Phase 3, investigational	Italy
9.	Detorubicin	Phase 2, investigational	France
10.	Demethoxydaunorubicin	Phase 2-3, investigational	Italy
11.	4'-Deoxydoxorubicin	Phase 2, investigational	Italy
12.	Marcellomycin	Phase 1-2, investigational**	United States
13.	4'-Tetrahydropyranyl-Adriamycin	Phase 1-2, investigational	Japan
14.	Menogaril	Phase 1, investigational	United States

*IND, discontinued
**IND on hold, further development halted

against solid tumors; also, it has been limited by cardiac toxicity, resulting in diminished interest in its further development.[30] The optimum dose of rubidazone in patients with solid tumors was 200 mg/m^2, and in patients with acute leukemia, a 400-mg/m^2 single dose at 3-week intervals.[30,31]

Carminomycin (Carbucin)

Carminomycin, the anthracycline developed in the Soviet Union, was originally isolated from *Actinomadura carminata*. This drug was in common use in the Soviet Union for many years before it was evaluated in the United States and Europe. The major attractive features of the drug were its excellent absorption from the G.I. tract and a purported lack of cardiac toxicity. In addition, the drug caused minimal nausea and vomiting, only mild alopecia, and was free from skin toxicity on extravasation. The I.V. form of carminomycin has recently been evaluated in the United States using a dose of 20 mg/m^2 once every 3 weeks. Although the drug was better tolerated in terms of reduced nausea and vomiting and alopecia, the dose-limiting toxicity was myelosuppression. It clearly showed activity against breast cancer comparable to that of ADR. However, in the phase 2 trial of carminomycin in 21 patients with breast cancer, one patient developed clear evidence of congestive heart failure after receiving a cumulative dose of 188 mg/m^2, and two other patients showed marked reduction in cardiac ejection fraction, indicating that carminomycin was indeed cardiotoxic.[32] Consequently, there appears to be little additional interest in further clinical use of this drug in the United States.

Aclacinomycin-A (Aclarubicin)

Aclacinomycin-A is a trisaccharide anthracycline isolated from *Streptomysis galilaeus* by Japanese investigators. The compound is one of the class 2 anthracyclines, which mainly inhibit RNA synthesis; class 1 anthracyclines, such as ADR and carminomycin, mainly inhibit DNA synthesis. In various experimental animal tumors tested, aclacinomycin-A demonstrated antitumor activity superior to that of doxorubicin in several solid tumors, although it was less active in mouse leukemias. Furthermore, the drug demonstrated less cardiac toxicity in a hamster model compared to the cardiac toxicity of ADR or daunomycin. Phase 1 studies demonstrated the maximal tolerated dose to be 100–200 mg/m^2 repeated at 3-week intervals.[33] The dose-limiting toxicity was myelosuppression. Other side effects included mild nausea and vomiting; hair toxicity; and EKG changes in the form of ST-T wave changes, believed to be nonspecific. Extensive clinical trials in Japan and Europe have shown a broad spectrum of antitumor activity, most significantly against acute leukemias, lymphomas, breast cancer, ovarian cancer, and gastric cancer.[34] Dose schedules used in acute leukemia patients were either 120 mg/m^2 daily for 3 days or a daily dose of 15–25 mg/m^2 for 10–14 days before complete remission was achieved. Clinical data on the cardiac toxicity of aclacinomycin are limited in terms of the cumulative dose levels of drug reached in early trials. Congestive heart failure has, however, been observed in at least 2 patients who earlier had received Adriamycin in a European trial.

N-Trifluoroacetyladriamycin-14-valerate (AD-32)

This ADR analogue was synthesized at the Dana Farber Cancer Institute in the United States. In several experimental tumors, it has antitumor activity superior to that of doxorubicin. In comparison to ADR, AD-32 is lipid-soluble and only minimally soluble in aqueous media. The drug is thus formulated in a lipid-based vehicle, which has resulted in side effects related to the vehicle, including chest pain, bronchospasm and hypotension. These side effects were preventable with concomitant administration of hydrocortisone. Biochemically, AD-32 does not intercalate with DNA — a major departure from most other anthracyclines. In phase 1 studies, the dose-limiting toxicity was leukopenia; the maximal tolerated dose was 600 mg/m^2 repeated every 21 days.[35] Because of the solubility problems, the drug had to be dissolved in a large volume of fluid and given as a 24-hour continuous infusion. The toxicity of AD-32 included mild nausea and vomiting and partial alopecia, but there was no skin ulceration on extravasation of the drug. In limited phase 2 trials, antitumor activity has been observed in patients with solid tumors, but the patient sample was too small to evaluate efficacy of AD-32 compared to ADR. Similarly, the data on cardiac toxicity are limited, although a few patients have received cumulative dose levels of 3–16 gm/m^2 without clinical evidence of cardiac toxicity. Further development of this drug has been halted because of solubility problems, and efforts are under way to modify the compound to make it more soluble.

4'-Epidoxorubicin (Epirubicin)

4'-Epidoxorubicin is a stereo isomer of ADR. It has an identical molecular weight and similar antitumor activity against animal tumors. However, it has shown less toxicity in mice, where 25% more drug is required to reach a toxicity comparable to ADR. In phase 1 studies, epidoxorubicin showed a toxicity spectrum similar to that of ADR but with a lower incidence of vomiting and alopecia. At dose levels equivalent to the MTD of doxorubicin, epidoxorubicin is only mildly myelosuppressive; to reach the myelosuppressive level equivalent to 75 mg/m^2 of ADR, the dose level of epidoxorubicin is 90 mg/m^2.[36] The dose schedule of epidoxorubicin used against solid tumors has been 75–90 mg/m^2, and the antitumor activity appears to be the same with either of the dose levels. The spectrum of antitumor activity of epidoxorubicin is similar to that of ADR, with consistent activity observed against breast cancer, sarcomas, hematologic malignancies, and various other solid tumors. This analogue is clearly less cardiotoxic then ADR, although definite evidence of clinical cardiomyopathy has been observed in several studies when the cumulative dose level of 1,000 mg/m^2 or more is reached. The cumulative dose of epidoxorubicin that causes cardiomyopathy appears to be 25–50% higher than ADR using equally myelosuppressive dose levels.[37] The pharmacokinetics of this drug reveal extensive metabolism, significant biliary excretion, and a long half-life similar to that of ADR. There are only limited data on the effects of schedule on the cardiac toxicity of epidoxorubicin. One small study using this drug in a continuous infusion schedule in patients previously treated with ADR produced clear evidence of cardiac failure at cumulative dose levels of 400–1,150 mg/m^2. The median dose of epidoxorubicin that resulted in cardiac toxicity was 485 mg/m^2 in patients who had previously received a median cumulative ADR dose level of 400 mg/m^2 in our institution. These data are similar to those reported with continuous infusion delivery of ADR.

4-Demethoxydaunorubicin (IMI-30, Idarubicin)

This new daunorubicin analogue lacks the methoxy group at the C-4 position in the aglycone. In addition to having significant antitumor activity, Idarubicin is active by the oral route, although to reach similar myelosuppression the optimum dose is 4 times higher than the optimum I.V. dose. The toxicology studies revealed a better therapeutic index with significantly less cardiac toxicity. In patients, the acute toxicity pattern is typical of anthracyclines, with myelosuppression being the dose-limiting toxicity. Gastrointestinal intolerance and alopecia are milder, although nausea and vomiting were increased when the drug was used orally. The maximal tolerated dose of Idarubicin is 15 mg/m^2 I.V. and 60 mg/m^2 p.o., repeated at 3-week intervals.[38,39] Besides its myelosuppressive effects, the drug causes mild nausea and vomiting, alopecia, stomatitis, and nonspecific, transient EKG changes. No clinical evidence of cardiac toxicity has been observed in early phase 1 and phase 2 trials. Although the full antitumor spectrum of this drug is still under evaluation, significant antileukemic activity has been observed in previously treated patients.[40]

4'-Deoxydoxorubicin (Esorubicin)

Esorubicin differs from ADR in the lack of hydroxyl group in position 4 of the amino sugar moiety. The experimental antitumor activity of this drug is equal to that of doxorubicin, with a broad spectrum of activity against leukemias and solid tumors. The main reason for the introduction of Esorubicin into clinical trials is its very low cardiac toxicity, if any, in experimental studies in mice, rats, rabbits, and dogs. In phase 1 studies of the compound, different schedules have been tested. On the single-dose schedule, the maximum tolerated dose was 25–40 mg/m^2 in 3 different studies. The recommended dose for phase 2 trials is 30 mg/m^2 at 3-week intervals.[41] The dose-limiting toxicity has been leukopenia, and other side effects include mild nausea and mild to moderate alopecia. Some evidence of antitumor activity has been observed in several solid tumors in the 3 phase 1 studies reported so far. Phase 2 studies of Esorubicin that are currently under way should provide data on the antitumor activity of this drug in the near future.

Marcellomycin

This drug, which is closely related to aclacinomycin-A, has demonstrated experimental antitumor activity comparable to that of aclacinomycin. The drug was introduced into clinical trials because of its potential for reduced myelosuppression. In a limited phase 1 trial, the drug was used in a single-dose schedule ranging from 5 mg/m² to 60 mg/m². The drug caused significant nausea and vomiting and stomatitis. In addition, it caused significant phlebitis and myelosuppression, which proved to be the dose-limiting factor. Thrombocytopenia was more prominent than leukopenia, and the myelosuppressive toxicity was cumulative and unpredictable. The maximum tolerated dose is about half that reported for aclacinomycin, and the recommended dose for phase 2 trial is 50 mg/m². Interest in the further development of this drug has waned, primarily because of the unpredictable and cumulative myelosuppressive toxicity.[42]

Detorubicin

This drug, which is structurally related to ADR, was developed in France, where it has recently had a broad clinical evaluation. Although it showed some clinical activity, the drug appeared to have no particular advantage over doxorubicin except for demonstrated activity against malignant melanoma. The maximal tolerated dose of detorubicin was 120–150 mg/m² at 3-week intervals.[43] Our recent evaluation of this drug in the treatment of malignant melanoma demonstrated that it has significant activity against this otherwise anthracycline-resistant tumor. Unfortunately, detorubicin clearly has cardiac toxicity; in our trial, one patient developed congestive heart failure and other patients revealed endomyocardial biopsy evidence of cardiac toxicity.[44] Accordingly, further development of this drug is in jeopardy.

4'-O-tetrahydropyranyl Adriamycin (THP-adriamycin)

This drug was discovered by Umezawa and associates in 1979 from a culture filtrate of a daunomycin-producing strain. The compound demonstrated greater antitumor activity than ADR in L1210 leukemia, and for further development the drug has recently been synthesized. The mode of action is by inhibition of DNA synthesis similar to that of ADR and daunomycin. Based on reduced cardiac toxicity of the drug against animals, it has recently entered clinical trials in Japan. The maximal tolerated dose of THP-adriamycin in phase 1 trials has been reported to be 40-50 mg/m² at 3-week intervals.[45] Acute toxicity included mild nausea, vomiting, and minimal hair loss. The dose-limiting toxicity was leukopenia, thrombocytopenia being a minimal problem. In early phase 2 trials reported from Japan, the drug has shown activity against acute leukemia and non-Hodgkin's lymphomas and hints of activity against ovarian carcinoma, breast cancer, and cancer of the cervix.[46] Data on cardiac toxicity of this drug so far are limited. The drug is being studied in both Japan and France and will be introduced in the United States very soon.

Menogarol, 7-OMEN (Menogaril)

Menogaril is a new anthracycline that was selected for clinical trials based on broad spectrum of antitumor activity against a spectrum of murine tumors in a pattern similar to that observed with doxorubicin. Furthermore, the drug showed significantly less cardiac toxicity than ADR in the chronic rabbit model. Biochemically, Menogaril does not appear to inhibit DNA or RNA synthesis at cytotoxic concentrations. In phase 1 trials using a single-dose schedule, the maximum tolerated dose of Menogaril appears to be 200–250 mg/m^2, with myelosuppression and phlebitis being the dose-limiting toxicities.[47,48] Menogaril has also been used in a 72-hour continuous I.V. infusion schedule for which the MTD was substantially lower than that seen with I.V. bolus, and a recommended phase 2 dose was 125 mg/m^2 over 72 hours.[49] This drug is about to enter phase 2 trials in the United States.

11

CISPLATIN, PLATINUM ANALOGUES, AND OTHER HEAVY METAL COMPLEXES

Stephen P. Ackland, M.B., B.S., F.R.A.C.P. and
Nicholas J. Vogelzang, M.D.

Cisplatin

THE BIOLOGIC ACTIVITY OF platinum (Pt) coordination complexes was first observed in 1965 when Rosenberg et al fortuitously observed inhibition of *Escherichia coli* growth in a medium subjected to electrolysis.[1] The similarity of this inhibition to that produced by radiation and alkylating agents ultimately led to the discovery of the active antineoplastic agent cis-dichloro-diammine platinum II (cisplatin, DDP).[2]

DDP was almost discarded in the early 1970s when trials showed marked G.I. toxicity and nephrotoxicity. Interest was rejuvenated when responses were seen in testicular malignancies, and nephrotoxicity was reduced by hydration.[3,4,5,6] Over the past decade, there has been a proliferation of information regarding the pharmacology, toxicity, and clinical applications of DDP. The drug is dramatically effective in germ cell,[7,8,9] ovarian,[10,11] and head and neck tumors[12,13] and has modest efficacy in lung,[14,15,16] bladder,[17] cervical,[18] esophageal,[19,20] and gastric[21,22] cancers when used alone or in combination chemotherapy programs and given by I.V. bolus or I.V. short-term infusion.

Like most antineoplastic drugs, however, DDP has a low therapeutic index given by these schedules. In an attempt to improve the therapeutic index,

Acknowledgements: The authors thank Shirley A. Perry for secretarial assistance and Harvey M. Golomb, M.D., for sectional support. Supported in part by the Jazz and Blues Fund and a grant from Medtronic Inc.

variations on the method of drug delivery have been employed, including continuous infusion.

Mechanism of Action

The DDP molecule has two potential leaving ligands, the chloride (Cl⁻) ions, which can be displaced in an environment of low Cl⁻ concentration (e.g., in intracellular fluid) to yield a number of positively charged aquated complexes (see figure). These complexes can then interact with a nucleophilic site on DNA, RNA, or protein to form bifunctional covalent links analogous to alkylating reactions.[23,24,25] Interstrand and intrastrand cross-links are thought to be the major cytotoxic lesions, as cytotoxicity is most closely related to extent of DNA binding.[26] The formation of cross-links is a slow process, taking several hours, and is opposed by excision repair mechanisms.[26,27] Cross-links result in conformational DNA changes and inhibition of DNA synthesis.[26]

DDP cytotoxicity is unusual in its cell cycle phase-dependence. Some cell types are more sensitive in G_1-phase than in S-phase, possibly as a result of the time delay inherent in DNA cross-linking.[28] A dose-related delay in transit through S-phase and the succeeding cell cycle occurs, with larger doses blocking cell traverse in G_1 as well as S and G_2 phase.[29,30] Changes in cell cycle kinetics, however, did not predict for therapeutic benefit, suggesting that at low doses, cells were able to overcome sublethal damage.[30] Cycle specificity has been described in 2 studies in which exponentially growing cells were less sensitive to DDP than were stationary cells.[27,31]

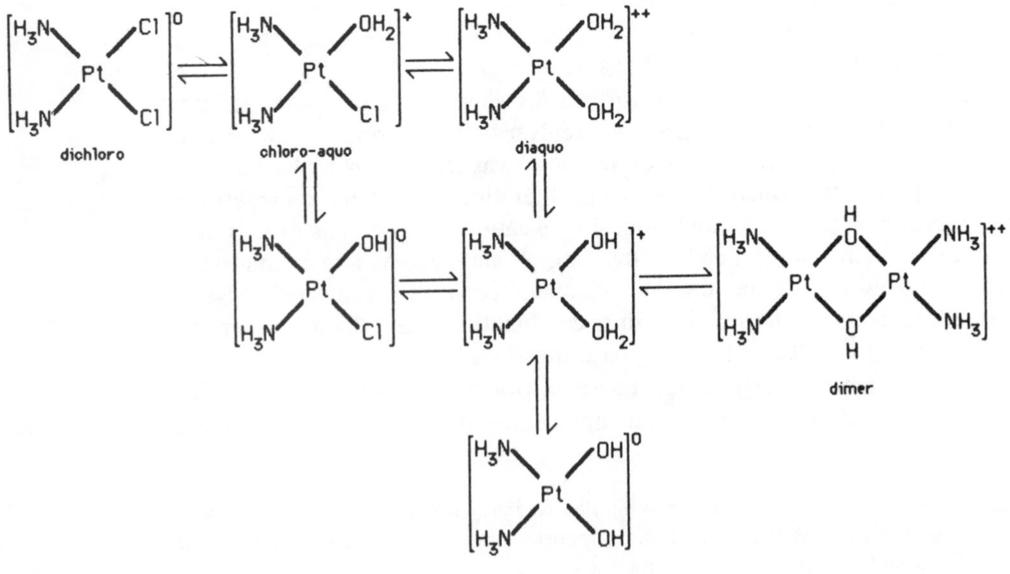

Figure 1.   Reactions of cisplatin with water.

Pharmacokinetics

The inorganic nature of DDP makes it difficult to measure in biologic fluids because the usual methods of radiolabeling of organic compounds ($^{14}C, ^3H$, etc.) are inapplicable. Radioactive forms have been used in pharmacologic studies, but the half-lives of isotopes are only about 4 days.[32] Pt analysis is commonly done by flameless atomic absorption spectrophotometry, which involves measuring absorbance after atomization at 2,300–2,700° C.[33] Detection limits of 10 ng/ml are possible with this technique.[34] Free plasma Pt complexes can be separated from protein-bound Pt complexes using centrifugal ultrafiltration.[35,36] Recent applications of high-pressure liquid chromatography (HPLC) techniques have allowed partial analysis of the various DDP transformation produces (see figure 1).[34,37,38]

Binding of DDP to plasma protein is of considerable importance in the pharmacokinetics of the drug. Binding to plasma protein has been shown to occur with a half-life ($t^1/_2$) of 2.7 hours.[39] However, due to tissue distribution and renal clearance of unbound Pt species, greater than 90% of total plasma Pt is protein-bound 2 hours after administration.[32,34,40,41] Proteins involved include gamma globulin and transferrin as well as albumin.[41] Binding is felt to be covalent and irreversible and renders the drug no longer cytotoxic to cells.[39,42,43,44] Unbound DDP undergoes a number of chemical transformations in aqueous media or plasma (see figure). The high Cl^- concentration of plasma retards the aquation reactions and tends to maintain the drug in the dichloro form. However, recent investigators have indicated that unchanged DDP may be almost completely eliminated from plasma within 3 hours of dosing, and that the predominant forms are hydrolysis products, presumably chloro-aquo and diaquo species.[34] Also, a significant amount of Pt appears to be converted to methionine complexes.[34]

Plasma levels of total Pt were initially reported by DeConti et al to show a biphasic mode of decay with an initial $t^1/_2$ of 25–49 min. and a terminal $t^1/_2$ of 58–73 hours after bolus injection.[32] More recent investigators have demonstrated a triphasic plasma disappearance curve after bolus injection, consisting of an initial rapid distribution phase; a secondary phase with $t^1/_2$ of 17–54 min., caused predominantly by renal excretion of unbound Pt; and a tertiary phase with $t^1/_2$ of 1.2–8.5 days due to slow disappearance of protein-bound Pt.[32,40,43,44,45,46,47,48,49]

Plasma levels of filterable (nonprotein-bound) Pt species after bolus injection decline in an apparent biphasic mode, with a terminal $t^1/_2$ of 17–54 min.[40,41,44,45,46,48]

Neither mannitol nor forced diuresis affects either peak plasma levels or the $t^1/_2$ of total or filterable Pt.[40] A recent study also demonstrated a lack of effect of hypertonic saline on pharmacokinetic parameters.[50]

Very little is known about the transport of Pt species into cells. On physicochemical grounds, it is generally believed that the uncharged species can enter the cell by passive diffusion and that charged species are excluded. However, the finding that the drug enters the CSF to only a small extent argues against free diffusion of any of the major species.[39,43]

Elimination and Distribution

During the first few hours after bolus dosing, elimination of Pt species from the body is mainly by renal excretion. The rate of renal excretion is inversely proportional to the extent of plasma protein binding,[43] which would be expected if only nonprotein-bound species were excretable. In rats, 30–40% of the administered dose can be excreted in the first 4 hours, and 75% by 30 days.[51] In humans, 15–27% can be excreted in 3–6 hours, and 27–45% by 5 days.[32,43,49] Excretion occurs by filtration, and probably also by active tubular secretion.[52,53]

A small percentage of Pt excretion occurs into bile,[54,55,56] mainly late after administration. This may indicate that only chemically or metabolically altered species are excreted by this route. DDP species rapidly enter tissues after I.V. administration, and a fraction is retained in tissue for long periods.[39,40,54] Litterst noted that 25–100% of the Pt content in various tissues of the dog was still present after 4 days.[39] Highest concentrations appear in kidney, liver, ovary, uterus, and lung.[43,54] Third spaces can also accumulate Pt and have been postulated to be potential Pt reservoirs.[46] Significant concentrations are also achieved in tumor tissue, especially liver metastases.[57]

Pharmacokinetics of Cisplatin Infusion

The above pharmacokinetic data pertain to DDP given by I.V. bolus or rapid infusion. Patton et al[45] found that the $t^{1/2}$ of filterable Pt after a 6-hour infusion is substantially shorter than after bolus injection (26 min. versus 44 min.). Furthermore, the fraction of administered Pt excreted in the urine in the first 24 hours is substantially greater with infusion (75% versus 49%). An explanation for this phenomenon is unclear; perhaps the higher plasma levels of free Pt attainable with I.V. bolus administration cause saturation of renal clearance mechanisms.

Williams et al[47] measured total Pt in 30 patients randomized between I.V. bolus, 24-hour, and 48-hour infusion of DDP. Peak levels were recorded at the end of administration; levels after infusion were 20% and 10%, respectively, of levels after I.V. bolus. The secondary plasma $t^{1/2}$ was 3–4 days in each case. With bolus injection, 20% was excreted in the urine in the first 24 hours and 30% in the first 48 hours; with infusion, excretion rates were not significantly different—14% was excreted at 24 hours and 21% at 48 hours.

Vermorken et al[48] compared filterable Pt levels in patients treated with I.V. bolus, 3-hour, and 24-hour infusions of DDP. The alpha and beta half-lives of serum Pt were not significantly different, but the shorter administration was associated with a shorter half-life, contrary to the findings of Patton. With I.V. bolus, all the Pt present in the serum at the end of administration was filterable; with 24-hour infusion, the peak total Pt was 27% of the peak level after I.V. bolus, and only 10% was filterable. Posner et al[58] compared 30-min. DDP infusion with a 5-day continuous infusion and found that although peak free Pt levels were only 10% of those in rapid infusion, the $t^{1/2}$ (40–206 min. versus 25–36 min.) and the plasma concentration × time factor (C × T) (6.4–15 versus 0.4–1.7 mcg/ml-hr) favored improved efficacy for long-term infusion DDP.

Toxicity

Nephrotoxicity remains incompletely understood, but until recently it was the predominant dose-limiting toxicity. In animals, various pathologic changes involving proximal tubules have been described, but in humans, distal tubular and collecting duct abnormalities predominate.[59-63] Hypomagnesemia associated with renal tubular magnesium wasting has been observed frequently.[64,65] Nephrotoxicity may be reduced effectively by diuresis or mannitol[66,65] apparently without altering pharmacokinetic parameters or antineoplastic activity.[40,46,70,71] The Pt species responsible for nephrotoxicity is not known. A recent study showed that in rats, injection of DDP metabolites was more nephrotoxic than injection of parent DDP at equal doses of Pt, suggesting that some of the Pt transformation products may be the responsible agents.[34] Reduction of nephrotoxicity by concomitant administration of sodium thiosulfate or diethyldithiocarbamate (DDTC)-derivatives lends further support to the impression that reactive species formed in plasma are the likely causes.[72-78] One group of investigators have demonstrated a circadian influence on renal toxicity, with less toxicity occurring if the drug is given when the normal circadian maximum in urinary volume occurs.[79,80] The significance of this finding to scheduling of drugs is yet to be fully determined.

Nausea and vomiting is a severe toxicity often causing poor patient compliance.[81] Numerous trials have shown partial alleviation of these side effects using phenothiazines, butyrophenones, cannabinoids, metoclopramide, benzodiazepines, steroids, and combinations of these agents.[82] Subclinical ototoxicity is common, but tinnitus and deafness are infrequently seen; this effect appears to be age- and dose-related.[83] Myelosuppression and peripheral neuropathy are infrequently seen but can be cumulative.[81,84,85]

Rationale for Continuous Infusion DDP

The rationale for continuous infusion (CI) DDP is based on cytokinetic, pharmacologic, and preclinical studies. Cytokinetically, various investigators have observed that DDP preferentially kills cells following exposure in the G_1 phase, although the drug is active in all phases.[87,88] Continuous infusion theoretically allows more cells to be exposed during the most sensitive phase of their cycle. Cytokinetic studies of DDP scheduling in L1210 leukemia in mice, however, have favored pulse doses over CI.[30]

Sparse pharmacologic data exist to support the use of CI DDP. Levels of total and filterable Pt after infusion are 10–20% of those after I.V. bolus.[40,45,47,48,58] If the area under the $C \times T$ curve is the important parameter in determining cytoxicity rather than the peak dose, then long-term infusions may be more effective.[58] Whether a sufficient extracellular fluid concentration of Pt species capable of crossing the cell membrane can be obtained to allow cytotoxic intracellular levels is not known.

In preclinical studies, Drewinko et al[81] showed that exposure of human lymphoma cells in culture to DDP for 8 hours gave a similar killing effect as a 1-hour exposure using 10 times the concentration. The $C \times T$ factor was lower for the long exposure. The same group[31] also showed that long-term exposure of colon carcinoma cells in culture to 2 mcg/ml of DDP produced a 3-log cell kill, similar to high concentration (10 mcg/ml) exposure for short periods. However, in this case, the $C \times T$ factor marginally favored the short exposure. No preclinical data for exposure longer than 24 hours are currently available.

Stability in IV Fluids

Stability of DDP in I.V. fluids is an important technical consideration in the clinical application of infusion chemotherapy. Chloride on concentration is the most important element in maintaining DDP in the intact state. In one study, less than 5% of DDP was lost over a 48-hour period in 0.45% saline at 25°C.[89] However, in 0.1% NaCl up to 10% degradation occurs within 40–60 min.[83] LeRoy et al[42] found about 15% loss of parent DDP after 4 hours incubation in 0.45% saline and 5% dextrose at 25°C, which was 10% higher than predicted by theoretical computations based on known and estimated rate constants for Pt transformation reactions. In contrast, a comprehensive study by Mariani et al showed good stability in a variety of solutions and conditions.[90]

In view of these uncertainties, DDP should not remain in solutions of low chloride concentrations for long periods. Despite these reservations, clinical studies using infusional DDP have described administration in 0.45% saline over periods as long as 24 hours after reconstitution.[91] Whether a loss of activity had occurred in these cases is not known.

Bicarbonate has little effect on the rate of loss of DDP, but a precipitate was observed to form within 8–24 hours.[89] Neither exposure to light nor the presence of 5% dextrose or mannitol has an effect on the rate of loss of DDP.[89,90]

Clinical Studies

The few studies performed to date have mostly involved 24 to 120–hour venous DDP infusions (see table 1). Only 3 studies have concurrently involved pharmacokinetic analysis.[47,92,58]

Williams et al[47] randomized 28 patients with ovarian carcinoma to receive DDP by I.V. bolus, 24-hour infusion, or 48-hour infusion. No difference in toxicity or antitumor effect was noted. Vomiting appeared more prolonged with infusion. Mean peak plasma levels of 10 mcg/ml total Pt were achieved for I.V. bolus, compared to 1–2 mcg/ml for infusion. The terminal half-lives of total Pt appeared similar.

Jacobs et al[92] treated 18 patients with advanced squamous cell carcinoma of head and neck with 24-hour I.V. infusions of DDP in doses of 50–130 mg/m². Moderate to severe nausea and vomiting was observed in only 9 of 34 courses and was dose-related. Five courses were associated with mild serum creatinine elevations, and 2 high-dose (mean 120 mg/m²) courses with severe elevations. Mild hematologic toxicity was observed. The mean peak total plasma Pt level was 1.4 mcg/ml in 9 patients examined. Fourteen percent of the administered

Table 1. Intravenous Infusion of Cisplatin

Study/Reference	Tumor (No. of patients)	DDP Dose/Duration	Other treatment	Outcome
Williams[47]	ovarian (28)	80 mg/m^2 a. I.V. bolus b. 24 hours c. 48 hours	none or doxorubicin and cyclophosphamide	no difference in toxicity or response
Jacobs[92]	head & neck (18)	80 mg/m^2 24 hours (hydration)	none	39% response rate; nephrotoxicity, N&V appeared lower
Bozzino[94]	ovarian (22)	60 mg/m^2 24 hours (hydration)	none	63% response rate; no nephrotoxicity
Amrein[93]	head & neck (70)	80 mg/m^2 24 hours (hydration)	5-FU	N&V grade 2+ – 28% nephrotoxicity (CR>2) – 16%
Salem[96]	various (34)	100 mg/m^2 5 days (no hydration)	none	nephrotoxicity similar to bolus; reduced N&V
Salem[97]	various (96)	100 mg/m^2 5 days (hydration)	none in 20 patients	N&V grade 2+ – 22% nephrotoxicity (CR>2) 5%
Lokich[91]	various (30)	20 – 40 mg/m^2/day 5 days (hydration)	none	myelosuppression dose-limiting at 30 mg/m^2/day; N&V grade 2+ – 24% (cumulative & dose-related); nephrotoxicity 11% (dose-related)
Tisman[98]	various (14)	20 mg/m^2/day 5 days escalated hydration	none	mild N&V in 4 patients; severe V in 1 patient; no nephrotoxicity; responses in 8/14
Posner[58]	various (22)	25 mg/m^2/day 5 days (hydration)	none	nephrotoxicity (CR>2) – 1 patient; N&V minimal; neutropenia dose-limiting
Sand[99]	various (15)	1 – 7 mg/m^2/day 5 – 6 weeks (no hydration)	radiation	no nephrotoxicity; no ototoxicity; nausea at 7mg/m^2/d; responses in 8/15
Loh[100]	squamous lung (8)	5 mg/m^2/day 5 days for 2 weeks ea. 4 weeks (no hydration)	radiation	>5 mg/m^2/d caused N&V; myelosuppression in all 4 patients; responses in 6/8
Lokich[101]	various (14)	5-10 mg/m^2/day 7 – 40 days (no hydration)	none	dose-limiting nausea at greater than 5 mg/m^2/d; minimal nephrotoxicity (none at 5mg/m^2/d)
Richardson[95]	testicular (28)	25 mg/m^2/day 5 days (hydration)	etoposide bleomycin	no significant nephrotoxicity; moderate neurotoxicity; moderate gastrointestinal toxicity; 86% complete response rate

N&V = nausea & vomiting, CR = serum creatinine, 5-FU = 5-fluorouracil dose was excreted in urine in the 24-hour infusion period. The response rate using standard criteria was 39%; most patients had had prior radiotherapy and surgery. Nephrotoxicity and nausea and vomiting were considered to be reduced by 24-hour infusion compared to bolus doses, allowing greater total doses of DDP to be given. Reduced toxicity using this schedule in head and neck carcinoma patients was also noted by Amrein et al.[93]

Richardson et al[95] gave DDP 25 mg/m²/day in 3 liters of N-saline as a continuous infusion for 5 days, in conjunction with bleomycin and etoposide, to patients with metastatic testicular carcinoma. Nineteen of 22 evaluable patients were rendered free of disease, a response rate comparable to that achieved with conventional combination chemotherapy. However, no significant renal toxicity was encountered.

Posner et al[58] treated 22 patients with a variety of tumors using a 5-day continuous infusion of DDP. Myelosuppression was the predominant toxicity; reversible creatinine elevation occurred in only 2 patients, and nausea and vomiting were minimal. Responses were seen in 29% of patients. Pharmacokinetic data have been cited above.

Bozzino et al[94] treated 22 patients with ovarian carcinoma using 60 mg/m² of DDP in a 24-hour infusion. A total of 82 infusions were given. No nephrotoxicity was observed. Fourteen of the 22 patients responded. This method of giving DDP was safe, but the diuresis induced by 5 liters of N-saline given in 24 hours could have been at least partially responsible for the lack of nephrotoxicity.

Salem et al[96] treated 34 patients with various solid tumors, using a continuous infusion of DDP 100 mg/m² given over 5 days. The incidence of nephrotoxicity, similar to that in I.V. bolus administration, may have been due to suboptimal diuresis. Nausea and vomiting were reduced compared to I.V. bolus, and no hematologic toxicity was observed. A more recent larger study by the same investigator in a different institution yielded similar results, with the exception that only 5% of patients had mild or moderate reversible hypomagnesemia. The therapeutic efficacy of this dose schedule could not be assessed, as most patients received other cytotoxic agents concomitantly.

Lokich et al[91] treated 30 patients with various solid tumors using a 120-hour cisplatin infusion. Starting doses of 20 mg/m²/day were escalated toward 40 mg/m²/day. Dose-limiting toxicity, manifested as myelosuppression, especially thrombocytopenia, was observed beyond 30 mg/m²/day. Eleven percent of courses were associated with nephrotoxicity despite hydration and diuretics, mostly with higher doses. Significant antitumor effects were observed in 6 patients. The dose of 30 mg/m²/day by continuous infusion was recommended for further trials of this dose schedule.

Tisman et al[98] used a technique in which DDP was given as 20 mg/m² in 50 ml 3N-saline with 10 mg dexamethasone as a 24-hour infusion on day 1 and the dose was progressively escalated daily by 5 mg/m² for 5 days so that 150 mg/m² per course was delivered. Additional hydration and diuretics were also given. With a variety of tumors so treated, responses were observed in 8/14 patients, mainly with nonsmall-cell lung cancer. Gastrointestinal toxicity was minimal, and nephrotoxicity was not seen.

In summary, although there are few preclinical data to support or refute an hypothesis that continuous infusion may improve the therapeutic index for DDP, clinical studies using infusions up to 5 days have demonstrated that this schedule allows larger total doses of DDP to be given safely and effectively, provided that adequate hydration and diuresis are maintained.

There are no reports concerning preclinical exposure of tumor cells to DDP, either in vitro or in vivo, for periods longer than 5 days. Continuous DDP infusion at a rate of 1–7 mg/m^2/day for 5–6 weeks as a radiosensitizer resulted in little toxicity in 15 patients and appeared to be useful with minimal toxicity when given in this way.[99,100]

Lokich et al[101] studied long-term continuous infusions for up to 30 days in 14 patients at daily doses of 5–10 mg/m^2/day. Nausea and vomiting limited dosage, resulting in early cessation of treatment on all patients receiving greater than 5 mg/m^2/day. Despite the absence of hydration, clinical nephrotoxicity was rare and was not seen at 5 mg/m^2/day. The cumulative dose of DDP delivered by this schedule was comparable to intermittent high-dose treatment but with less toxicity. A high incidence of catheter-related thrombosis has been noted by these investigators when other chemotherapeutic agents are delivered by continuous infusion.[102] Insufficient numbers of patients have been studied to date to ascertain whether this complication will occur with DDP infusion.

Intra-Arterial Cisplatin

Another means of theoretically improving the therapeutic index for DDP is by regional arterial perfusion for locally confined malignancies. This approach offers the potential advantages of greater total drug exposure for the tumor and a possible reduction in systemic toxicity. Theoretical principles dictate that a proportional increase in local drug concentration is conditional upon a low blood flow rate through the infusing artery and a high systemic drug elimination rate.[103] Furthermore, reduction in systemic drug delivery depends upon the ability of the infused region to eliminate the drug,[103,104] or the ability to give an antidote for the drug downstream of the infused region.[73]

With one exception, comparisons of the pharmacokinetics of I.V. and intra-arterial (I.A.) DDP have demonstrated minimal differences in the various parameters. The exception is hepatic arterial infusion, where some first pass extraction of total Pt by the liver is apparent.[105] An elegant study by Campbell et al[104] made direct comparisons of steady-state reactive (nonprotein-bound) Pt concentrations during I.A. and I.V. infusions in the same subject. No significant difference was found for either intrahepatic or femoral artery infusions at several different dose rates — the plasma clearance associated with I.A. infusion averaged only an insignificant 19% greater than that associated with I.V. infusion. Contrarily, Stewart et al,[57] in analyzing tissues collected at autopsy, found that Pt concentrations tended to be higher in areas of I.A. DDP infusion.

Despite a lack of preclinical data to support the concept, several phase 1 and phase 2 studies have been conducted to analyze the clinical value of I.A. DDP (see table 2). In primary and metastatic brain tumors, intracarotid infusions over a 1-hour period have resulted in remarkable response rates of 47% (14 of 30 patients) with primary brain tumors and 70% (16 of 23 patients) for metastatic tumors.[106,107] However, these response rates need to be considered in the context of recent reports of similar high response rates of brain tumors to DDP when the drug is given I.V.[108,109] Some severe neurologic toxicities were encountered, including seizures, deafness, and deterioration in vision,[106,107] all of which may be minimized by microfiltration of the infusion solution[106] or selective arterial cannulation to avoid vital structures where appropriate.[110,112] Despite these drawbacks, various investigators are now applying I.V. combination chemotherapy including DDP to brain tumors, with promising early results.[111-114]

Recent studies of regional perfusion for head and neck squamous cell carcinomas have demonstrated response rates marginally better than I.V. DDP.[115,116] Toxicity was generally acceptable, but unusual local toxicities of hemifacial alopecia and ischemic injury to the tongue were reported.[116]

Calvo et al[117] studied I.A. DDP administration in various regionally confined malignancies and demonstrated toxicities comparable to those in I.V. infusion. However, responses were achieved in 5/19 patients with melanoma, 4/10

Table 2. Regional Intra-Arterial Cisplatin (Alone)

Study/Reference	Tumor	Dose/Route	Response rate	Toxicity
Lehane[106]	brain − 1° −2°	100 mg carotid	8/10	deafness; visual/CNS – 10%
Feun[107]	brain − 1°	60 – 120 mg/m² carotid	6/20 5/10	seizures, agitation, transient hemiparesis, retinal, encephalopathy
Kapp/Vance[110,112]	glioma	150 – 200 mg supraophthalmic	83%	no neurologic deficit; lower doses→lower response rate
Frustaci[115]	head & neck	100 mg/m²/5 days regional	50%	as per I.V. administration
Mortimer[116]	head & neck	100 mg/m² carotid	14/20	unilateral alopecia, transient facial palsy, blurred vision, tongue infarction; others as per I.V.
Calvo[117]	various	120 mg/m²	overall 45% 5/19 melanoma 4/10 sarcoma 2/9 breast 3/11 others	as per I.V., local pain, erythema, edema
Jaffe[118]	osteosarcoma	150 mg/m²	12/18	local erythema & induration; others as per I.V.

N&V = nausea & vomiting
CR = serum creatinine

patients with sarcoma, 2/9 patients with breast carcinoma, 2 patients with squamous cell carcinoma of the cervix, and 1 patient with neuroblastoma.

Gratifying responses to I.A. DDP have been attained in patients with osteosarcoma. Jaffe et al[118] observed responses in 11/15 patients (67%), 9 of which were complete responses. Benjamin et al,[119] in a study confined to adults with osteosarcoma, demonstrated a 77% response rate in 35 patients using I.A. DDP and protracted I.A. doxorubicin infusion. Transient local cutaneous discoloration and erythema were common; otherwise, toxicities were comparable to those in I.V. DDP.

Thus, I.A. infusion of DDP appears to be efficacious in certain circumstances. In spite of preclinical evidence suggesting that DDP does not diffuse into normal brain or CSF to a significant extent,[39,43] high concentrations have been found in intracerebral tumors after both I.V. and I.A. infusion,[120] and effects not achieved by any other chemotherapeutic agent have been observed. Furthermore, in certain tumors not considered sensitive to DDP given I.V., I.A. infusion may have a role.

Whether these reponses are due to delivery of low concentrations of drug to poorly perfused areas of tumor or to achievement of higher peak concentrations of active DDP species at the tumor cell membrane than can be attained by I.V. DDP is unclear and needs further study.

Platinum Analogues

Clinical success with DDP and awareness of its narrow therapeutic index have led to the development of a vast number of analogues, with the hope of identifying drugs with less nephrotoxicity and emetic potential and with equal or greater antitumor effect. A number of these compounds have been evaluated in clinical trials,[121] and two in particular appear to have a clear advantage over DDP in these respects: CBDCA (JM-8, Carboplatin, cis-diammine 1, 1-cyclobutane dicarboxlato Pt II) and CHIP (JM-9, Iproplatin, cis-dichloro-trans dihydroxyl-bis-isopropylamine Pt IV).

CBDCA

This compound has demonstrated activity comparable to DDP against B16 melanoma, colon 26, and P388 leukemia[122-124] and has superior activity against PC6A plasmacytoma and against human tumor xenografts P246 epidermoid carcinoma and colon CX-1.[125,126] It is less effective than DDP against L1210 leukemia, CD8F1 mammary carcinoma, and murine osteocarcinoma.[122,123] It is inactive against Lewis lung carcinoma, lung LX-1 xenograft, mammary MX-1 xenograft, and DDP-resistant L1210.[122] The mode of antitumor action of CBDCA is not known, but is thought to be similar to that of DDP.

In animal and human toxicity studies, CBDCA has demonstrated comparable hematologic toxicity to DDP, manifest primarily as thrombocytopenia, but little or no nephrotoxicity, ototoxicity, or neurotoxicity,[121,127-138] even in the absence of diuresis. It is also less emetic than DDP.[127-145]

Pharmacokinetic studies have demonstrated a much lower rate of plasma protein binding of CBDCA compared to DDP; in one study, 20–40% of total plasma Pt was present as ultrafilterable (UF) Pt after 1 hour,[140] and in other studies, 35–45% at 4–6 hours.[127,129,146] Most of the ultrafilterable Pt present within the first 4 hours or more after administration is unchanged CBDCA.[146] As a consequence, the rate of renal excretion of Pt is much higher, accounting for the relatively higher molar dose required for the same biologic activity. Rates of disappearance of UF Pt from plasma have been reported to be triphasic with half-lives of 1–7 min., 25–87 min., and 100–354 min., respectively.[127-129,139,140,146] Considerable interpatient variability is apparent with respect to half-lives, protein binding, and renal excretion rates, some of which is accounted for by variations in glomerular filtration rate.

In clinical phase 1 and 2 studies, CBDCA has demonstrated activity against ovarian cancer,[128,132,135,137,138,142] squamous cell carcinoma of the head and neck,[137,138] small-cell lung carcinoma,[138,144,147] and DDP-resistant germ cell tumors.[141]

The in vivo antitumor activity spectrum of CBDCA seems similar to that of DDP, but responses have been seen in some DDP-resistant tumors.[128-132]

These data suggest that CBDCA may be a potential candidate for further continuous infusion studies of Pt analogues. Its lack of nephrotoxicity would obviate the need for the hydration and diuresis required for DDP. Furthermore, its low rate of protein binding and high rate of renal excretion of free drug would predict a much greater area under the C × T curve for UF Pt when given by I.V. infusion compared to I.V. bolus. This relationship has already been demonstrated in patients with impaired renal function given I.V. bolus CBDCA, where CBDCA clearance is reduced and the area under the curve and hematologic toxicity are inversely related to creatinine clearance.[145,146] Whether these pharmacokinetic differences will translate into an improved therapeutic index for continuous infusion is not yet known.

To date, little or no data are available in regard to continuous infusion CBDCA. One preliminary report comparing 24-hour infusion to I.V. bolus administration could not demonstrate a difference in toxicity between these 2 schedules, but the numbers of patients were prohibitively small.[130] In another study, a 48-hour continuous infusion of 800 mg/m² produced responses in 2 of 8 patients with DDP-resistant ovarian carcinoma; the only toxicities observed with this schedule were nausea, vomiting, and myelosuppression.[142]

CHIP

CHIP is a quadrivalent Pt complex with an octohedral rather than a planar configuration. As such, it may have an antitumor spectrum different from those of DDP and other divalent platinum analogues. It has demonstrated activity against L1210 leukemia, P388 leukemia, B16 melanoma, Lewis lung carcinoma, colon CX-1 xenograft, lung LX-1 xenograft, mouse mammary tumors, Walker carcinosarcoma, and Murphy-Sturm lyphosarcoma.[122,123,148] Superior activity of CHIP over DDP has been shown against PC6A plasmacytoma and alkylating agent-resistant Yoshida sarcoma.[125] It has little or no activity against CD8F1 mammary carcinoma, osteosarcoma, mammary MX-1 xenograft, epidermoid P246 xenograft, colon 38 carcinoma, and DDP-resistant L1210 leukemia.[122,123,125]

The spectrum of clinical toxicity of CHIP when given by I.V. bolus was predicted from rat and dog toxicity data. Myelosuppression is dose-limiting, with thrombocytopenia being more severe than neutropenia. Nausea and vomiting is mild to moderate, and there is little or no nephrotoxicity, ototoxicity, neurotoxicity, or alopecia.[149-152]

The pharmacokinetics of CHIP were originally studied in dogs and rats. In dogs, the decay of total Pt after administration of CHIP was biphasic, with a $t^{1}/_{2}\alpha$ of 0.6 hours — similar to that of DDP[153]. However, the $t^{1}/_{2}\beta$ was only 39.4 hours, a much shorter period than that reported following DDP administration in the dog.[39] Similar results have been observed in the rat.[154] CHIP does not bind to plasma protein in vitro, in contrast to DDP.[153] These data, coupled with the finding that most unchanged CHIP is excreted by the kidneys early after administration, lead to the supposition that the long $t^{1}/_{2}\beta$ is due to retention of nonprotein-bound metabolites.[153]

In humans, filtered Pt decay after single I.V. bolus doses was biexponential, with half-lives of 0.4–2.0 hours and >24 hours.[155] Total Pt half-lives of 0.4–2.2 hours and 58–103 hours have also been reported.[155] Urinary excretion was 15–61% of the administered dose by 24 hours and 16.5–63% by 48 hours.[155] Unchanged CHIP in plasma showed a $t^{1}/_{2}$ of 0.7–1.2 hours. These parameters have been described as being remarkably similar to those of DDP.[151] However, further study is required to confirm these impressions.

Because CHIP is dissimilar to DDP in its toxicity, preclinical antitumor spectrum, and, to some extent, pharmacokinetics, it may be expected to display different effects from DDP when administered by I.V. bolus or infusion. Phase 1 and 2 trials of I.V. bolus have not demonstrated any clear superior efficacy for CHIP compared to DDP, but studies are continuing. However, as with CBDCA, some patients with tumors resistant to DDP do respond to CHIP, and CHIP is less toxic.[152] Compared to CBDCA, CHIP seems more active in nonsmall-cell lung cancer.[156] Clinical trials of CHIP by continuous infusion are awaited.

Gallium Nitrate [Ga(NO$_3$)$_3$]

The clinical utility of DDP, coupled with the ability of gallium to localize in tumor tissue,[157,158] led to investigations of gallium nitrate and several other group III-A metal salts as potential antitumor agents.[159] Gallium nitrate [Ga(NO$_3$)$_3$] was shown to be active against Walker 256 carcinosarcoma, fibrosarcoma M-89, adenocarcinoma 755, lymphosarcoma P1798, and osteosarcoma 124-F experimental tumor systems.[160] This activity led to further studies in animals and humans.

The mechanism of cytotoxic action of gallium nitrate is unknown. Data suggest that it may impair calcium- or magnesium-dependent processes that are vital in rapidly proliferating cells.[161]

Following I.V. injection, gallium nitrate is rapidly bound to plasma protein, especially transferrin,[162] and may enter cells via transferrin receptors.[163]

In one study, a colorimetric technique was used to determine the pharmacokinetics following a short-term I.V. infusion of gallium nitrate in 8 patients.[164] In patients with normal renal function, total plasma gallium disappearance was biphasic with a $t^{1}/_{2}\alpha$ of 0.5–1.8 hours and $t^{1}/_{2}\beta$ of 10–50.4 hours. Urinary excretion rates of 15–72% in the first 24 hours were found. In patients with acute renal dysfunction or prior heavy metal therapy, gallium kinetics were altered, with a prolonged $t^{1}/_{2}$ and reduced urinary excretion rate. Krakoff et al,[165] using a flameless atomic absorption spectrophotometry technique, found similar kinetic parameters: $t^{1}/_{2}\alpha = 87$ mins, $t^{1}/_{2}\beta = 24.5$ hours, 65% urinary excretion in first 24 hours. Furthermore, most renal gallium excretion occurs in the first 4 hours.[165]

Kelsen et al[166] compared gallium kinetics following rapid I.V. infusion and continuous infusion. Following rapid infusion, a biphasic curve was found with $t^{1}/_{2}$ of 8.3–26 min. and $t^{1}/_{2}\beta$ of 6.3–196 hours. The $t^{1}/_{2}\beta$ was significantly affected by the onset of acute renal impairment, as was the urinary excretion rate, similar to the findings of Hall et al.[164] With continuous I.V. infusion over 7 days, steady state plasma levels were attained within 18–24 hours; following termination of infusion, they fell slowly, with substantial interpatient variability. Minimal nephrotoxicity was seen with continuous infusion compared to rapid infusion.[166]

Phase 1 studies of gallium nitrate have reported dose-limiting nephrotoxicity when the drug is administered by rapid I.V. infusion. This was manifest as proteinuria and azotemia. Other reported toxic effects include mild to moderate nausea and vomiting, diarrhea, mild myelosuppression, hypocalcemia, and hearing loss. A low incidence of nephrotoxicity has been reported with continuous infusion.[164,167–171] Responses have been observed in lymphoma[168,169,172,173] and in rare patients with small-cell lung carcinoma,[174] sarcoma,[175] and prostatic carcinoma,[176] but not in breast[177] or head and neck cancer.[178]

A study by Warrell et al[168] has focused on 7-day continuous I.V. infusion of gallium nitrate in patients with lymphoma. A total of 64 patients were treated, with a response rate of 34% — similar to the single-agent response rate for other drugs of proven efficacy in this disease. In the absence of attempts at hydration, nephrotoxicity, manifest as increased serum creatinine, was seen in 27% of patients, some of whom received other nephrotoxic agents concurrently. No cumulative nephrotoxicity was seen when serum creatinine, enzymuria, and β_2-microglobulinuria were monitored.[170] Hypocalcemia was observed, predominantly during infusion in two-thirds of patients, several of whom became symptomatic. This may be due to inhibition of calcium resorption from bone.[179] Pulmonary complications that may have been related to the drug or intercurrent infections occurred in 9 patients. Nausea was rare and vomiting was not observed.

Subsequently, the same group incorporated continuous I.V. gallium nitrate into combination chemotherapy with etoposide and methyl-GAG for relapsed lymphoma. A 51% response rate in 35 patients has so far been observed. However, toxicity, predominantly myelosuppression and, to a lesser extent, renal insufficiency, has been considerable.[169]

This schedule of administration of gallium nitrate appears relatively safe and effective for patients with lymphoma, but whether the therapeutic index is increased over that of short-term I.V. infusion remains to be clearly demonstrated. However, maintenance of a modest diuresis by oral hydration may reduce nephrotoxicity to more acceptable levels and allow achievement of this goal.

Spirogermanium

Spirogermanium is a unique new azaspiran antitumor agent, with the metal germanium substituted for a 1-carbon moiety in the heterocyclic ring structure. It is active against a variety of animal and human tumor models.[180,181] The mechanism of cytotoxic action of spirogermanium is unclear, but of all cell processes, protein synthesis is most readily interrupted.[181] Lack of phase specificity has been demonstrated, but logarithmically growing cell cultures are more sensitive than those in stationary phase.[181]

Limited pharmacokinetic data are available. In one study using a gas chromatographic method, plasma levels fitted a 2-compartment model with a $t^1/_2\,\alpha$ of 10–20 min. and a $t^1/_2\,\beta$ of 60–200 min. Considerable interpatient variability occurs. This study suggested an interval of 2–3 days between doses.[182]

Phase 1 studies have demonstrated dose-limiting neurologic toxic effects, manifest as lethargy, dizziness, ataxia, parasthesiae, and hallucinations, all of which are generally short-lived and fully reversible.[183-186] These effects are clearly related to the rate of drug administration. Nausea and vomiting are mild, and hematologic toxicity has been reported rarely, but there is no evidence of renal or hepatic toxicity.

In phase 1 trials, spirogermanium demonstrated antitumor activity against lymphoma, ovarian carcinoma, and breast carcinoma,[183-185] but subsequent phase 2 studies have not confirmed these expectations for breast or ovarian carcinoma in heavily pretreated patients,[184,187-192] in renal cell carcinoma,[193] or in nonsmall-cell lung carcinoma.[194-195] However, modest activity against lymphoma in a small number of heavily pretreated patients has been demonstrated.[183,184,196]

Spirogermanium as a continuous I.V. infusion has been compared to a short I.V. infusion by Legha et al.[184] This study demonstrated that larger total doses could be administered by continuous infusion over 5 days than by short I.V. infusion daily for 5 days. However, extension of continuous infusion for periods longer than 5 days was associated with a reduction in the maximum tolerated dose per day. Nonetheless, the only significant toxicity encountered was neurologic, with mild gastrointestinal and possible pulmonary toxicity. There was no clear evidence of cumulative toxicity. Responses were seen only in 3 patients given continuous infusion. In another study, continuous infusion for 5 days was well tolerated, with neurologic toxicity again being dose-limiting.[197]

These data, coupled with in vitro data indicating that the drug effect on tumor cells is enhanced by increased dose and time of exposure,[181] suggest that the therapeutic index of spirogermanium should be considerably improved by continuous infusion compared to short I.V. infusion. Further studies of continuous infusion of this promising new agent are therefore warranted. Moreover, the apparent complete lack of bone marrow, renal, and hepatic toxicity makes this drug an ideal agent to study in future combination chemotherapy programs.

12

CYTOSINE ARABINOSIDE

Gregory A. Curt, M.D., Carmen J. Allegra, M.D., and
Bruce D. Cheson, M.D.

Background

CYTOSINE ARABINOSIDE (ARA-C) IS a synthetic antimetabolite that functions as a structural analogue of cytidine. The drug differs from the physiologic nucleoside by the presence of a β-hydroxyl group at the 2'-position of the sugar moiety. Because ara-C cytotoxicity is S-phase specific and correlates with the rate of DNA synthesis,[1,2] clinical use of the drug has been restricted to treatment of rapidly dividing tumors such as the leukemias. Recent interest has focused on ara-C as a potential differentiating agent when given in low doses over a prolonged infusion.

Ara-C enters a variety of human tumor cells via carrier-mediated facilitated transport.[3] At drug concentrations achievable during both standard and high-dose regimens (1–10 µM), intracellular ara-C levels are fourfold higher in myeloblasts as compared to lymphoblasts,[4] providing one explanation for the relative sensitivity of the myeloblastic leukemias to this drug. The parent compound, however, is inactive. Once having entered cells, ara-C must be converted to its triphosphate, ara-CTP, to inhibit synthesis of DNA.

The activation pathway requires that ara-C first be converted to its monophosphate (ara-CMP) by deoxycytidine kinase, then to ara-CDP by the enzyme dCMP kinase, and finally to ara-CTP by the enzyme nucleoside diphosphate kinase.[5] Of these three separate activation steps, the first is rate-limiting, and decreased deoxycytidine kinase activity has been described as a mechanism of drug resistance in both murine models and human myeloblasts.[6,7]

The precise mechanism whereby ara-CTP inhibits synthesis of DNA remains speculative. Ara-CTP is a known competitive inhibitor of DNA polymerase α (involved in DNA synthesis)[8] and DNA polymerase β (involved in DNA repair).[9] Recent studies have shown that ara-CTP can be incorporated into DNA as a fraudulent base and that the extent of substitution correlates well with cytotoxicity.[10] Not only does incorporation of ara-CTP lead to increased strand breakage[11] but also to premature DNA chain termination[12] and blockage of initiation.[13] In whole cells, ara-C treatment causes accumulation of small segments of single-stranded DNA, suggesting defective ligation or interruption of DNA synthesis.[14]

In addition, ara-C and its metabolites can be inactivated by degradative enzymes: cytidine deaminase, which catabolizes ara-C to inactive ara-uracil (ara-U); and dCMP deaminase, which catabolizes ara-CMP to ara-UMP. Formation of ara-CTP is thus regulated by both anabolic and catabolic pathways. For example, high levels of cytidine deaminase have been reported in leukemia cells derived from patients refractory to ara-C treatment.[15]

The cycle specificity of ara-C makes dose scheduling a critical determinant of toxicity. The drug is rapidly cleared in man, with an initial half-life of 7–20 min. and a terminal half-life of 30 min. to 2.5 hours.[16]

Within a half-hour after bolus administration, most of the drug has been converted to ara-U as a result of deamination of parent compound in the plasma and liver.[17] Thus, inhibitors of endogenous plasma deaminase such as tetrahydrouridine must be added to patient specimens to prevent degradation prior to processing for determination of blood levels.

Because of its short half-life and rapid clearance, prolonged administration of ara-C provides a larger area under the concentration × time (C × T) curve and causes significantly greater cytotoxicity. This was elegantly demonstrated by Skipper and co-workers in early studies of murine leukemia. Ara-C administered in low doses 3 times daily proved consistently more effective than larger doses administered once a day.[18] As might be expected, the drug is significantly more toxic in man when administered as a prolonged infusion. In early clinical phase 1 studies, a single intravenous bolus dose of 4 gm/M^2 was virtually nontoxic, whereas the maximally tolerated dose administered as a 48-hour constant infusion was 1 gm/M^2.[19]

Ara-C has reproducible clinical activity in the treatment of acute leukemia[20] and non-Hodgkin's lymphomas,[21] although the drug has demonstrated only marginal activity against solid tumors.[22] When given at a standard dose of 100–200 mg/M^2/day for 5–7 days, ara-C alone will induce complete marrow remission in 33% of patients with acute myelogenous leukemia (AML)[23] and 25% of patients with acute lymphocytic leukemia.[24] Because of its rapid total body clearance and S-phase specificity, continuous drug infusions are now routinely used and appear to be more therapeutically effective.[25,26] In order to achieve steady-state concentrations rapidly, a loading dose of 3 times the hourly infusion dose may be given prior to beginning the infusion.[4] Drug levels attainable within the CSF are 40% of concomitant plasma levels, and because CSF is devoid of deaminase activity, cytotoxic drug concentrations (4–5 × 10^{-7}M) are maintained for more than 24 hours.[27]

Clinical Research

Because of the considerable amount of background information on the pharmacokinetics and pharmacodynamics of ara-C, much clinical research has focused on in vivo modeling in an effort to improve the drug's therapeutic index. Rustum and co-workers have demonstrated a direct correlation between ara-CTP formation and retention by leukemic blasts and likelihood and duration of complete clinical response.[28] However, even for standard doses of ara-C, there was an eightfold variation (40–320 ng/ml) in steady-state plasma concentrations between individual patients. Importantly, there appeared to be no correlation between drug plasma levels and intracellular ara-CTP formation, suggesting that drug transport is not an important determinant of response, at least in murine models.

While transport may not be a determinant of tumor cell resistance in murine tumors, this may not be the case for leukemia cells derived from patients. Capizzi and co-workers have demonstrated that whereas the number of nucleoside carriers present on tumor cell lines is substantial (63,000–197,000 sites/cell), cells isolated from leukemia patients express an average of only 10,000 binding sites/cell.[29] Because of limited membrane nucleoside binding sites, ara-C transport by human leukemia cells is a low affinity process (K_m = 362 μmol/L) with a high capacity (V_{max} = 71.1 pmol/million cells/min.). These parameters predict that for drug levels achievable during standard infusional therapy (0.5 μmol/L), transport will be the rate-limiting step to drug accumulation.[29]

These observations serve as a rationale for the administration of high-dose ara-C infusions. Steady-state plasma concentrations achieved during a 3-hour infusion of 3 gm/M[2] average 100 μmol/L, approximately 200 times that achievable during standard infusional regimens.[30] Importantly, ara-C elimination following high-dose short-term infusion is considerably prolonged. In addition to the α half-life of 7–20 min. and the β half-life of 30 min. to 2.5 hours, there is an additional γ terminal half-life of 6 hours.

The reasons for these dose-dependent pharmacokinetics are uncertain, although it is likely that high systemic levels of the catabolite, ara-U, are able to interfere with parent compound elimination.[30] Overall, high-dose short-term infusion of ara-C leads to a greater area under the C $\times$ T time curve than would be expected from the kinetics of the drug given at standard doses.

In addition, ara-U itself exhibits independent cytostatic effects and prolongs the S phase of murine cells.[31] This synchronization effect would theoretically enhance ara-C cytotoxicity.

Although most AML induction regimens use ara-C in conventional doses, the results of high-dose ara-C are encouraging, particularly in patients with refractory disease or secondary leukemia. In these particularly poor-prognosis patients, complete responses of 22–73% have been reported.[32-35] More recently, high-dose ara-C has been used as initial treatment with other agents in patients with acute leukemia.[36-38] Although these regimens are clearly active, it remains uncertain whether the considerable toxicities justify this approach as initial treatment. Induction deaths can be as high as 30–40%[39] and other toxicities (gastrointestinal, ocular, and cerebellar) are considerable. Prospective clinical trials comparing conventional high-dose with high-dose ara-C in induction therapy are warranted to address the question. Perhaps high-dose ara-C will prove most appropriate as a consolidating regimen following complete remission with standard agents. In such studies there may be a survival plateau.[38] This approach is currently being tested prospectively in a National Cancer Institute-supported trial, performed by Cancer and Acute Leukemia Group B, of intensive postremission therapy in adults with AML.[40]

Because of the considerable toxicity of high-dose ara-C infusion and the fact that leukemic blast cell kill can be correlated with intracellular formation of ara-CTP and incorporation into DNA,[41] Plunkett and co-workers at M. D. Anderson Hospital have developed a rationale for pharmacologically directed infusional ara-C.[42] Although a hundred-fold interpatient variation between intracellular ara-CTP formation by human leukemic blasts was found, drug half-life, peak drug level, and area under the C × T curve were all significantly higher in patients achieving complete remission after a 3 gm/M² bolus dose. Importantly, trough levels of intracellular ara-CTP in circulating blasts from patients treated with intermittent high-dose ara-C (3 gm/M² I.V. over 2 hours every 12 hours for 4 doses) correlated with likelihood of attaining a complete remission. For patients in whom trough ara-CTP levels were in excess of 75 µmol/L, the complete remission rate was 44% (8/18). However, in patients in whom trough levels were less than 75 µmol/L, the CR rate was only 13% (3/23). These differences were statistically significant.

These observations led to a series of studies in which dose intervals were shortened to raise trough intracellular ara-CTP levels between doses.[43,44] This approach did not improve overall response rates, perhaps because the contracted dose scheduling necessarily reduced total duration of drug exposure. However, this strategy has been reworked to use infusional ara-C, individualizing the dose rate to achieve intracellular blast levels of ara-CTP of 75 µM/L.[44,45] Patients first receive a dose of 3 g/M² ara-C to determine individual clearance rates of drug. The equation that determines the constant infusion dose necessary to maintain intracellular blast levels of ara-CTP at 75 µM/L can then be expressed as:

$$\text{infusion rate} = \frac{75 \ \mu\text{mol/L} \times 3 \ \text{gm/M}^2}{\text{ara-CTP AUC}}$$

where AUC is the area under the ara-CTP C × T curve generated by the test dose, expressed in hours × µmol/L. The infusion is continued for 96 hours; 4 patients received a second continuous infusion course that was extended to 120 hours.

This pharmacologically directed continuous drug infusion has achieved target intracellular ara-CTP levels of 95% of patients and early evidence of improved remission rates. The authors present a rational case that such individualized dosing, based on intracellular active metabolite accumulation and retention, may be the treatment of choice for patients with unfavorable ara-CTP pharmacologic profiles.

At the opposite end of innovative approaches to ara-C high-dose infusional therapy has been the considerable interest in protracted courses of low-dose treatment (20 mg/M²/day continuous infusion for 10–14 days) for patients with AML and myelodysplastic syndromes (MDS). This method is predicated on the in vitro observation that exposure to low doses of ara-C can induce terminal differentiation in human leukemia cell lines (46–49).

In the HL-60 model, ara-C in concentrations of 10^{-6} to 10^{-8}M/L for up to 72 hours results in loss of granulation, increased morphologic maturity, and expression of nonspecific esterase and MY4,[47] the differentiation markers in this cell line. Exposure to concentrations of ara-C greater than 10^{-6}M/L did not increase the absolute number of differentiated cells. Similarly, low-dose ara-C is capable of inducing hemoglobin synthesis in human K562 erythroblasts.[48] This irreversible effect is maximal at drug concentrations of 5×10^{-7}M and is accompanied by loss of clonogenic capacity.

Because administration of low-dose continuous infusion ara-C results in plasma concentrations of $1.8–6.9 \times 10^{-8}$M/L,[50] it is conceivable that these in vitro phenomena could be induced in vivo. Maloney and Rosenthal[51] and Housset and co-workers[52] demonstrated in the early 1980s that low-dose ara-C administered subcutaneously every 12 hours was capable of inducing complete remissions in patients with acute myelogenous leukemia and suggested that these effects could be attributed to the differentiating capacity of the drug.

More recently, workers at the Dana-Farber Cancer Institute in Boston have utilized continuous infusions of low-dose ara-C (20 mg/M^2/day for up to 21 days) in patients with preleukemic syndromes.[53,54] Eleven of 16 patients demonstrated marked improvement in peripheral counts and transfusion requirements. Myelosuppression was significant. Bone marrow biopsies in all responding patients demonstrated hypocellularity, and all of these patients required hematologic support with red cell and platelet transfusions. Although the median duration of response was short (3.5 months), the median survival in responding patients was 1 year. By comparison, median survival in nonresponding patients was 9 months.

At present, it is uncertain whether the clinical activity of low-dose ara-C infusion in preleukemia is due to cytotoxicity (clonal selection) or specific differentiation effects. In an attempt to address this issue, chromosomal markers before and after therapy have been studied. In the Dana-Farber series, these analyses were performed in four patients;[54] 3 patients demonstrated evolution to a new clone, while a fourth showed persistence of the original abnormal clone. Recently, a single patient with hypoplastic AML and trisomy for chromosome 8 was treated with low-dose continuous infusion ara-C.[55] Treatment induced a complete remission with a normal cellular karyotype. Additional data studying premature chromosome condensation in several patients, however, have provided evidence for differentiation.[56] Nevertheless, the weight of current evidence is that clonal selection rather than specific differentiation of abnormal clones may be the mechanism of action for low-dose continuous infusion ara-C.

The above data must be considered preliminary, however, because in the world literature, only 27 patients can be identified who have been treated with low-dose infusional ara-C.[57] Eighteen of these patients had AML, and 10 achieved a complete response. This compares with more than 500 patients who have been treated with intermittent low-dose subcutaneous drug, a regimen that, although convenient, does not achieve sustained ara-C exposure. Although infusional low-dose ara-C is still experimental, the approach deserves further exploration. There is no significant difference in ara-C pharmacokinetics given in high doses as an intravenous or subcutaneous infusion.[58] Outpatient therapy with infusion pumps might therefore be a feasible treatment option.

Intracavitary and Infusional Therapy

The rapid total body clearance of ara-C makes this agent an attractive candidate for site-directed therapy. However, the data in this area are limited. Canellos and co-workers reported using splenic arterial infusion of ara-C in 5 patients with massive splenomegaly associated with chronic myelogenous leukemia in blast crisis.[59] Ara-C was administered at standard doses (40–200 mg daily for 5–11 days), and all patients responded by reduction of spleen size. Interestingly, systemic toxicity in these heavily treated patients was minimal, suggesting rapid drug inactivation in spleen, liver, or peripheral blood.

The high specific activity of cytosine deaminase in liver makes peritoneal administration of ara-C an attractive investigational approach. Peritoneal drainage occurs predominantly via portal circulation,[60] and clearance of ara-C through the liver would theoretically provide a first-pass effect that would spare both the systemic circulation and bone marrow. Pharmacokinetic modeling predicts for as much as a 1,000-fold advantage for peritoneal to systemic ara-C exposure.[61] Although solid tumors have not been reproducibly responsive to ara-C, the pharmacokinetic advantage of intraperitoneal instillation could conceivably overcome innate ara-C resistance, particularly for tumors (e.g., ovarian) restricted to the peritoneal cavity. Indeed, in vitro clonogenic survival studies on ovarian cancer cells derived from patient ascites predict cytotoxicity only at ara-C levels that can be achieved via intraperitoneal administration.[62]

Phase 1 trials of patients instilled with intraperitoneal dialysates of 10^{-5} ara-C demonstrated undetectable systemic drug levels.[61] Ten patients with refractory ovarian cancer were subsequently treated in the phase 2 setting with 20 exchanges of 6×10^{-5}M ara-C over 5 days.[63] Myelosuppression was minimal. Two patients with minimal residual disease experienced a complete remission and 2 patients with positive peritoneal washings became cytology negative. Current intraperitoneal approaches to ovarian cancer are now exploring the use of combination regimens including ara-C as well as improved catheter delivery systems.[64] Clinical trials using interperitoneal ara-C with both melphalan and cisplatin have confirmed theoretical pharmacologic advantage and have suggested early evidence for clinical response in heavily pretreated patients with refractory ovarian cancer.[65]

13

PERIWINKLE ALKALOIDS I:
VINBLASTINE AND VINDESINE

Mark J. Ratain, M.D., Nicholas J. Vogelzang, M.D., and
Gerald P. Bodey, M.D.

Background

Mechanism of Action

VINBLASTINE (VLB) AND VINDESINE (VDS) are vinca alkaloids, a class of drugs in widespread clinical use. VDS (desacetyl vinblastine amide sulfate) is a semisynthetic derivative of VLB. The mechanism of action of these drugs has been extensively reviewed elsewhere.[1] These drugs have a very high affinity for tubulin and inhibit its polymerization. This leads to mitotic arrest and subsequent cell death. The vinca alkaloids are most active against premitotic cells and thus are cell cycle phase-specific agents.

Pharmacokinetics of Bolus Injection

The development of a sensitive radioimmunoassay for the vinca alkaloids has made detailed pharmacokinetic analysis feasible.[2] The assay has been modified by subsequent investigators to provide greater sensitivity.[3-5]

The initial pharmacokinetic studies of VLB and VDS were performed by Owellen et al.[6,7] Using an open three-compartment mammillary model, they demonstrated that there is a rapid initial distribution phase, a variable second phase, and a relatively prolonged terminal phase. There have been multiple other studies (see table 1) of the pharmacokinetics of VLB and VDS. Although the terminal half-lives are very similar, the clearance of VLB is about 2–3 times greater than the clearance of VDS.

Rahmani et al[10] recently studied the plasma concentration decay kinetics in 12 patients receiving VDS. Noting a consistent rebound between 1–4 hours after a bolus injection, they therefore felt that a linear 3-compartment model was inappropriate. They also observed statistically different pharmacokinetics between treatments in 4/6 patients. This was interpreted as evidence of time-dependent pharmacokinetics, although there was no consistent pattern in the deviations from linear pharmocokinetics.

Elimination of the vinca alkaloids is assumed to be predominantly hepatic, inasmuch as the renal excretion is less than 20%[6,7,9,10,13] and large quantities of drug can be detected in bile.[13,14] There may be large interpatient variations in clearance,[8-12] even in patients without obvious hepatic dysfunction. It remains to be determined whether the variations are due to subclinical hepatic disease or to genetic differences in vinca alkaloid metabolism and elimination.

Clinical Use of Bolus Injections

The toxicity and recommended doses of bolus VLB and VDS have been extensively reviewed.[1] Both of these drugs commonly cause transient dose-related neutropenia and peripheral neuropathies (including constipation and paralytic ileus). The latter can be disabling.

Phase 1 studies indicated that the appropriate bolus dose of VDS was 4–5 mg/m^2, repeated at 2-week intervals.[15,16] VLB has been in clinical use since the early 1960s, but thorough phase 1 testing of various drug schedules was not performed. Based on the initial clinical studies, the maximal tolerated bolus dose is approximately 0.3 mg/kg/week.[17]

Rationale for Infusion

Early preclinical studies with VLB (and vincristine [VCR]) in lymphoma bearing mice demonstrated a 20-fold increase in cytotoxicity when the duration of treatment was increased from 24 hours to 48 hours.[18] The drug was given every 8 hours rather than continuously, but use of a mathematical model for phase-specific agents applied to this study[19] suggests an increase in

Table 1. Review of VLB and VDS Bolus Pharmacokinetics

| Study/Reference | Compartments | VLB | | | VDS | | |
		Initial t½ (hrs)[a]	Terminal t½ (hrs)	Clearance (L/min/m^2)	Initial t½ (hrs)	Terminal t½ (hrs)	Clearance (L/min/m^2)
Owellen[6,7]	3	.065±.025	19.6±1.1	.63±.36	.054±.019	20.2±8.2	.24±.13
Nelson[8]	3	.062±.040	24.8±7.5	.49±.21	.037±.016	24.2±10.4	.17±.97*
Jackson[9]	3	———	———	———	.04±.04	15.0±21.1	.11±.10
Rahmani[10]	¶	———	———	———	———	22.7±5.7	.32±.11
Ohnuma[11]	3	———	———	———	.23±.14	40.5±20.2	.076±.041†
Ratain[12]	2,3**	———	25.2±11.1	.57±.19	———	———	———

*Converted ml/kg/min to L/min/m^2 (40/kg/m^2)
†Calculated from other pharmacokinetic parameters
¶Did not use linear compartment model
**Used best model for each patient
[a]Mean ± S.D.

cytotoxic effect with increasing number of divided doses. Thus, the maximal cytotoxic effect would occur with infinitely small doses, or with continuous infusion.

In vitro studies also demonstrate increased cytotoxic effect with prolonged exposure to the vinca alkaloids. Hill and Whelan[20] demonstrated that the in vitro survival curve is time-dependent rather than dose-dependent, although only for VDS concentrations of 100 ng/ml or more.

More recently, Ludwig et al[21] compared the in vitro cytotoxicity of a 200-hour VLB exposure to the standard 1-hour exposure, using 77 tumor specimens (clonogenic assay). For example, in fresh human melanoma, prolonged low VLB concentrations (1 ng/ml for 200 hours) yielded 97% inhibition, while a concentration of 10 ng/ml for 1 hour yielded only 55% inhibition. The IC_{50} (concentration required for 50% inhibition) was determined for all 77 tumors. The IC_{50} ratio (IC_{50} for 1 hour exposure divided by IC_{50} for 200-hour exposure) was greater than 200 in most tumors, suggesting an advantage for prolonged exposure. In addition, 42% of tumors sensitive to VLB were only sensitive to a 200-hour exposure.

Similar studies have been performed by Matsushima et al[22] comparing 24-hour and 1-hour exposures to VLB and VDS for PC-7 cells (adenocarcinoma of the lung). The IC_{50} ratio for VDS was 36, but the IC_{50} ratio for VLB was only 18. This suggests an advantage for prolonged exposure only for VDS. However, only 1 cell line was treated in this study.

Studies of the cellular pharmacology of the vinca alkaloids support the use of continuous infusion, at least for VLB. Lengsfeld et al[23] demonstrated that VLB is quickly and readily released from cells when placed in drug-free medium, while VCR is tenaciously retained by the cells. Ferguson et al[24] also compared the cellular pharmacology of VCR to VLB. For a 4-hour exposure (to L1210 and HL-60 cells), the IC_{50} of VLB was up to 40 times the IC_{50} of vincristine. However, for a 24-hour exposure, the IC_{50} was approximately equal. They suggest that with short exposure, VLB partitions in the membrane because of its higher lipid solubility.[25] Ferguson and Cass[26] have recently shown that VLB is rapidly released from HL-60 cells by processes that are not coupled to metabolism.

Gout et al[27] have also demonstrated the rapid release of VLB by malignant cells (Nb 2 lymphoma) in vitro. In addition, they demonstrated that prolonged exposure leads to increased cellular retention, which was highly correlated with the degree of growth inhibition. They suggest that the efficiency of VLB could be increased by continuous administration, noting that a simultaneous increase in toxicity could be expected.

Vinblastine (Phase 1 Trials)

Two schedules have been used for phase 1 trials of continuous infusion VLB: 5-day infusions[28-30] and prolonged (>30 days) infusions.[12,31]

5-Day Infusions

Yap et al[28] were the first investigators to use 5-day VLB infusions, as part of a phase 1 and 2 trial in 34 patients with advanced breast cancer. The maximal tolerated dose (MTD) was 1.6 mg/m^2/day) although 15 patients were treated at 2 mg/m^2/day with a mean granulocyte nadir of 600/mm^3. Mild to moderate nausea and vomiting also occurred in 14% of the 5-day courses.

Young et al[29] treated 10 patients with refractory malignancies at doses of 1.25–2 mg/m^2/day. Their recommended dose for phase 2 studies was 1.5 mg/m^2/day because of the marked leukopenia at higher doses. They also noted a 30% incidence of peripheral neuropathies.

Zeffren et al[30] treated 28 patients with a variety of tumors. The doses ranged from 0.75–2.0 mg/m^2/day. Fifteen patients received the highest dose, with only a 24% incidence of leukopenia, although there was a 40–50% incidence of leukopenia at 1.50–1.75 mg/m^2/day. Two patients also developed paralytic ileus. These authors recommended a starting dose of 2 mg/m^2/day for untreated cases and 1.75 mg/m^2/day for patients with prior treatment.

In summary, 5-day VLB infusions are well tolerated at doses up to 2 mg/m^2/day. Leukopenia is the dose-limiting toxicity, sometimes accompanied by thrombocytopenia, although severe peripheral neuropathies may occur unpredictably. Starting doses of 1.6 mg/m^2/day appear to be safe for most patients, many of whom may tolerate dose escalations to 2 mg/m^2/day.

Prolonged Infusion

The development of external[32] and implantable [33,34] infusion pumps has made prolonged infusion of antineoplastic agents a feasible option. Lokich et al[31] treated 26 patients at doses of 0.25–1.0 mg/m^2/day for a median duration of 30 days (range 7–89 days). Most (80%) of the patients were treated at 0.5 mg/m^2/day, which was extremely well tolerated, with only a 14% incidence of leukopenia and virtually no extramedullary toxicity. At higher doses (0.75–1 mg/m^2/day), there was a 50% incidence of leukopenia.

Ratain et al[12] recently reported preliminary results of an ongoing phase 1 study. The first 16 patients were treated with doses of 0.5–0.9 mg/m^2/day. The mean infusion duration was 10 weeks, although one patient received VLB for more than 6 months. Eight patients developed major toxicity (WHO grade 3 or 4), and 8 patients were withdrawn because of progressive disease. The dose-limiting toxicity was leukopenia in 7 patients and peripheral neuropathy in the other patient. Two minor responses were seen, one in a patient with renal cell carcinoma and the other in a patient with refractory breast carcinoma. However, both responses were transient (less than 2 months). There appears to be a wide range of tolerable doses with prolonged VLB infusions. One (of 14) patients had grade 4 leukopenia at the lowest dose (0.5 mg/m^2/day), while 2/3 patients at the highest dose (0.9 mg/m^2/d) had no toxicity. The steady-state VLB concentration (determined at biweekly intervals) may be useful in predicting toxicity, as the WBC was significantly decreased ($p < .0001$) at VLB concentrations of >1.4 ng/ml.

Pharmacokinetics of VLB Infusion

Pharmacokinetic studies were performed in conjunction with several of the phase 1 studies discussed above (see table 2). Lu et al[35] studied the pharmaco-kinetics of 5-day VLB infusions in 12 patients with breast cancer. There was a wide range in the serum clearance, from .052–2.45 L/min./m^2. The 4 patients with the lowest clearance were the only responders. However, it is not apparent why the VLB clearance was so depressed in these 4 patients.

The data of Zeffren et al[30] suggest that the elimination of VLB may be nonlinear, as the VLB clearance (calculated from infusion dose and plateau VLB concentration) was much decreased at the highest dose studied (see table 2). However, other investigators[29] found no change in clearance with increasing dose.

Ratain et al[12] suggest that the VLB clearance may decrease with duration of infusion. Analysis of 9 patients receiving VLB for more than 1 month demonstrates a significant decrease in VLB clearance with increased duration of infusion (see figure 1). This appears to be independent of the infusion rate (by multivariate analysis), but may be simply a manifestation of subclinical deterioration in hepatic function associated with progressive malignancy (hepatic metastases and/or cachexia).

Vinblastine (Phase 2 Trials)

Both schedules of VLB infusion discussed above have been tested in a variety of malignancies in phase 1 and 2 trials (see table 3).

Breast Carcinoma

Since the initial trial of 5-day VLB infusion,[28] much of the investigation into the use of VLB infusions has focused on this common tumor. However, the efficacy of 5-day VLB infusions in breast carcinoma is controversial, as

Table 2. Pharmacokinetic Studies of VLB Infusion

Study/Reference	Duration (days)	Dose (mg/m^2/d)	Clearance (L/min/m^2)[a]
Lu[35]	5	1.0–2.0	.11 ± .05 (responders)* .42 ± .15 (stable) 1.65 ± .85 (progression)
Young[29]	5	1.25–2.0	.63 ± .30
Zeffren[30]	5	1.25 2	.43 † .17 ± .28 †
Ratain[12]	> 30	0.5–0.9	.68 ± .12 (month 1) .54 ± .16 (month 2)

*Calculated from stated dose and AUC
†Calculated from VLB concentration and dose
[a]Mean ± S.D.

response rates have ranged from 0–40%, with an overall response rate of 22% (see table 3). Both Tannoch et al[37] and Ingle et al[38] have performed adequate negative phase 2 trials, with no responses in a combined total of 32 patients. However, in the former study, 14/17 patients received an initial dose of less than 1.6 mg/m²/day, as recommended by Yap et al.[28] It is quite possible that the dose-response curve of VLB infusions is very steep, inasmuch as Chacon et al[36] obtained a 33% response rate using higher daily doses (2–3 ng/m²) and 15 of Yap's patients received an initial dose of 2 mg/m²/day.

Yau et al[40] recently reported the results of a randomized phase 2 trial in advanced breast cancer that compared 5-day VLB infusions to 5-day VDS infusions and 5-day vincristine infusions. The latter arm was replaced by bolus VDS injections because of poor activity. A total of 131 patients were entered into the study, 31 of whom received VLB. Patients received initial doses of 1.4 or 1.7 mg/m²/day, depending on their predicted risk of toxicity. The response rate to 5-day VLB infusion was higher than in any of the other arms (5-day VLB 31%, 5-day VDS 19%, 5-day vincristine 0%, bolus VDS 17%). In addition, 2 of the 23 evaluable patients were complete responders. These investigators did not assess response by dose, which, as noted above, may be quite important.

Other Tumors

Adequate negative phase 2 trials have been performed in ovarian carcinoma[42] and metastatic soft tissue sarcoma.[44] One response was seen in a patient with a fibrosarcoma by Chacon et al[36] using a higher infusion rate.

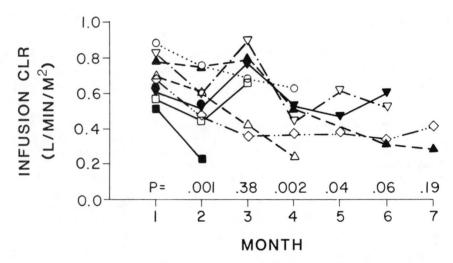

Figure 1.   Changes in clearance with duration of infusion. The infusion clearance significantly (p values as shown) decreased with increased duration of infusion. Multiple regression analysis of infusion clearance showed that infusion duration (p = .001) was significant while infusion dose was not significant (p = .47). (From poster presentation by Ratain et al[12] at American Association for Cancer Research Annual Meeting, 1985).

The use of 5-day VLB infusions in malignant lymphoma is quite promising. There have been only 5 reported cases treated with VLB infusions, of which 2 have responded. No large-scale phase 2 trials have been completed, although VCR infusions are now being used as part of initial treatment regimens (see next chapter).

There has been at least one response to VLB infusions in bladder carcinoma, gastric carcinoma, nonsmall-cell lung carcinoma, malignant melanoma, and renal cell carcinoma. With regard to the last, 5-day VLB infusions have some activity (0–16%), although probably are not superior to bolus VLB.[43] A phase 2 trial of prolonged continuous infusion VLB in advanced renal cell carcinoma is in progress (Ratain and Vogelzang).

In summary, phase 2 trials of 5-day VLB infusions are indicated in Hodgkin's disease, non-Hodgkin's lymphoma, bladder carcinoma, gastric carcinoma, nonsmall-cell lung carcinoma, and malignant melanoma. Phase 2

Table 3. Responses to VLB Infusion by Tumor

Tumor	Schedule	Dose $(mg/m^2/d)$	Reference	Responses/Patients (%)			
Bladder	5-day	2–3	Chacon (36)	1/1	(100)	1/3	(33)
		1.25–2.0	Zeffren (30)	0/2	(0)		
Breast	5-day	1.4–2.0	Yap (28)	12/30	(40)	28/125	(22)
		1.2–1.8	Tannock (37)	0/17	(0)		
		1.6	Ingle (38)	0/15	(0)		
		2–3	Chacon (36)	4/12	(33)		
		1.6	Shah (39)	5/21	(24)		
		1.7	Yau (40)	7/23	(30)		
		1.25–2.0	Zeffren (30)*	0/7	(0)		
Gastric	5-day	2–3	Chacon (36)	0/3	(0)	1/4	(25)
		1.25–2.0	Zeffren (30)*	1/1	(100)		
Lung (nonsmall-cell)	5-day	1.25–1.75	Young (29)	1/1	(100)	1/11	(9)
		2–3	Chacon (36)	0/9	(0)		
		1.25–2.0	Zeffren (30)*	0/1	(0)		
Lymphoma	5-day	0.5–1.5	Paschold (41)	1/3	(33)	2/5	(40)
		1.25–2.0	Zeffren (30)*	1/1	(100)		
		1,25–1.75	Young (29)*	0/1	(0)		
Melanoma	prolonged	0.25–1.0	Lokich (31)*	2/11	(18)		
Ovarian	5-day	1.0–2.0	Kavanagh (42)	0/16	(0)		
Renal	5-day	1.5–1.9	Keubler (43)	3/19	(16)	4/36	(11)
		1.25–2.0	Zeffren (30)*	0/10	(0)		
		1.25–1.75	Young (29)*	1/7	(14)		
Sarcoma	5-day	1.5	Yap (44)	0/15	(0)	1/18	(6)
		2–3	Chacon (36)	1/2	(50)		
		1.2–2.0	Zeffren (30)*	0/1	(0)		

*Phase 1 study

trials of prolonged continuous VLB infusion are also indicated in these tumors as well as in breast carcinoma, renal carcinoma, and soft tissue sarcoma.

High-Dose VLB Infusions

Logothetis et al[47] recently reported the use of high-dose (3 mg/m^2/day) 5-day VLB infusion in combination with multiple other agents as part of a pilot study of alternating cross-resistant chemotherapy regimens in advanced non-seminomatous germ cell tumors. The combination appears quite promising (92% actuarial survival), although there was severe hematologic and nonhematologic toxicity associated with high-dose VLB. The latter was significantly correlated with the peak serum VLB concentration.[48]

Further phase 1 and phase 2 trials of this high-dose regimen are indicated, as there may be a steep dose-response curve (discussed above in reference to breast carcinoma). It is possible that marked responses can be achieved in relatively refractory patients who can tolerate the higher dose. Possibly, this subset of patients may be determined by monitoring serum VLB concentrations.

Vindesine (Phase 1 Trials)

Despite the through phase 1 testing of VDS by bolus injection in the late 1970s and early 1980s, there have been few traditional phase 1 trials of VDS by infusion.

24-hour Infusion

Ohnuma et al[49] conducted a phase 1 study of vindesine in which patients with advanced malignancies were randomly assigned to receive bolus injections (2-5 mg/m^2) or 24-hour infusions (1-7 mg/m^2) at weekly intervals. The major toxicities included anemia, leukopenia, peripheral paresthesias, decreased deep tendon reflexes, and generalized muscular weakness. Neurological toxicity was more severe in patients with impaired liver function. The investigators concluded that both the quantitative and qualitative toxicities were similar with both regimens. The MTD was 4 mg/m^2 by both schedules. No significant therapeutic benefits were observed in this phase 1 trial.

Gilby[50] also compared the toxicity of VDS by bolus injection and 24-hour infusion, using a fixed dose of 3 mg/m^2. Patients were assigned to a schedule by randomization, 15 patients in each arm. Leukopenia was less marked in the infusion schedule, although the incidence of phlebitis was increased.

48-hour Infusion

Hande et al[13] administered VDS by weekly bolus injection and biweekly 48-hour infusion to 17 and 9 patients, respectively. The dose was 3 mg/m^2 in both schedules, but the selection process was not specified. One patient with bronchogenic carcinoma who received bolus injection therapy achieved a partial remission. Leukopenia, the most common side effect, occurred with equal frequency with both schedules. Paresthesias occurred in 8/17 patients who received bolus injections, but in none of 9 patients who received continuous infusions. However, the former patients received twice as much drug in a 2-week interval as the latter patients. Pharmacokinetic studies were conducted in a few patients. High peak serum concentrations (8–100 ng/ml) were observed in one patient who received a bolus injection of 3 mg/m², but the serum concentration had decreased to 2–20 ng/ml by 24 hours. Patients receiving the same dose by 48-hour infusion achieved maximum serum concentrations of 5–10 ng/ml, which were maintained throughout the infusion.

5-day Infusion

Because there has not been a phase 1 trial of VDS by 5-day infusion, data on the MTD of VDS by this schedule are limited. Yap et al,[51] the first investigators to use 5-day infusions, found a dose of 1.4 mg/m²/day to be excessively myelosuppressive in their first 5 patients.

Pharmacokinetics of VDS Infusion

Bodney et al[52] conducted pharmacokinetic studies in 10 patients who received VDS by the continuous infusion schedule in conjunction with their clinical trials. The average terminal half-life of unchanged VDS in the plasma on day 1 was 93 hours, and the plasma clearance was 277 ml/kg/hour (.185 L/min./m²). By 72 hours, 5.1% of the dose of VDS was excreted in the urine. However, in one patient with abnormal liver function, the terminal half-life of VDS was 138 hours. In patients studied on day 5, the average terminal half-life was 26 hours, and the clearance was 4,197 ml/kg/hour (2.80 L/min./m²). One of these patients had abnormal liver function and also had a prolonged terminal half-life (82 hours).

Ohnuma et al[11] studied the pharmacokinetics of 4 mg/m² VDS in cancer patients when administered by bolus injection or by 24-hour continuous infusion. Following the 24-hour infusion, the serum concentrations followed biexponential decay. Both the $t^1/_2\ \alpha$ and $t^1/_2\ \beta$ were similar to those following bolus injection (see table 1). The peak serum concentrations after continuous infusion were only 6% of the peak following bolus injection. However, the area under the curve (AUC) for the 2 schedules was identical.

Jackson et al[9] compared the pharmacokinetics of 3 schedules of VDS administration: 3 mg/m² bolus, 1.2 mg/m²/day × 5, and 2 mg/m²/day × 2. As expected, the highest peak levels (0.5µM) occurred with the bolus schedule. The AUC was highest with the 5-day infusion schedule: 35% higher than the bolus schedule, and 8% higher than the 48-hour schedule. The calculated clearance was approximately the same in all 3 schedules: bolus .11 ± .10, 48-hour .09 ± .06, and 5-day .13 ± .09 L/min./m². Because most patients received only one schedule, it cannot be determined whether these minor pharmacokinetic differences are patient-specific or schedule-specific.

Vindesine (Phase 2 Trials)

Both the 48-hour and 5-day schedules have undergone phase 2 testing in a variety of malignancies.

Breast Carcinoma

Many investigators have studied the efficacy of VDS infusions in advanced breast carcinoma, both in single-arm and randomized phase 2 trials. Sixty patients with advanced breast carcinoma who were refractory to combination regimens including doxorubicin (ADR) were entered on a prospective randomized study of VDS, administered by two different schedules.[51] Patients were randomly assigned to receive either 4 mg/m^2 as a single bolus injection at approximately 10-day intervals, or 1.2 mg/m^2/day by continuous infusion for 5 days at 3-week intervals. For patients receiving the continuous infusion regimen, VDS was dissolved in 1,000 cc of 5% dextrose or normal saline solution and administered via a central silicone elastomer venous catheter. A constant infusion pump was used to maintain the continuous infusion. The initial dose was reduced (3 mg/m^2 or 1 mg/m^2/day, respectively) for patients with impaired liver function or poor bone marrow reserve. The dosage of subsequent courses was adjusted based upon the toxicity from the previous course.

Sixty patients were entered in the study, 30 in each arm, but only 51 could be evaluated. There were no significant differences in the distribution of patients with respect to age, disease-free interval, number of organ sites involved, dominant disease site, performance status, number of prior treatments, or duration of prior therapy (see table 4). Seven (28%) of the 25 patients who received continuous infusions achieved a partial response (PR) compared to 2 (8%) of the 26 patients who received bolus injections ($0.05 < p < 0.1$). Sixty-nine percent of those receiving bolus VDS experienced progressive disease during therapy, compared to only 28% of those receiving the continuous infusion regimen. Eleven patients whose disease progressed while receiving bolus VDS injections were subsequently given continuous infusion VDS therapy, and 4 achieved a PR. Hence, a total of 11 (30%) of 36 evaluable patients who received continuous infusion VDS achieved a PR. The median time to disease progression was 6 weeks (range, 4–43 weeks), for all patients who received

Table 4. Characteristics of Patients with Breast Carcinoma Treated with Vindesine

	Continuous infusion	Bolus injection
Patients entered/evaluable	30/25	30/26
Median age (range)	54 (30 – 75)	55 (33 – 75)
Premenopausal/postmenopausal/unknown	2/20/3	3/21/2
Median prior treatments (range)	3 (1 – 17)	3 (1 – 7)
Dominant disease		
Soft tissue/osseous/visceral	3/6/16	2/6/18
Performance status 0 – 1/≥ 2	14/11	15/11

bolus injections, compared to 12 weeks (range 4–40+ weeks) for all patients who received continuous infusions (p = 0.004).

The toxicities observed in these patients appeared to be dependent upon the schedule of VDS administration (see table 5). Myelosuppression was moderate and transient with the bolus injection schedule and was not cumulative. The first 5 patients assigned to the continuous infusion schedule received 1.4 mg/m²/day, complicated by severe myelosuppression. When the dose was reduced to 1.2 mg/m²/day, neutropenia was tolerable but was still more frequent and severe with this schedule.

Other toxicities are listed in table 6. Nausea and vomiting and constipation were observed more often in patients receiving bolus injections, but stomatitis, paralytic ileus, and peripheral neuropathy occurred with equal frequency in both groups. Fever occurred in 32% of the patients who received VDS as a continuous infusion but in only 7% of patients who received it by bolus injection.

The results of this study suggest that continuous infusion therapy with VDS may be more effective in breast carcinoma than bolus injection therapy. Over a 3-week interval, patients assigned to bolus injection therapy received a total of at least 8–12 mg/m² VDS, whereas patients assigned to continuous infusion therapy received only 6–7 mg/m². Because both the toxicity and response rates were higher in the infusion arm, it is not clear whether the therapeutic index has been increased. Further studies are necessary comparing the activity of VDS infusions to equitoxic bolus injections.

Hansen and Brincker[53] treated 35 patients with refractory advanced metastatic breast carcinoma with VDS at 1.5 mg/day for 5 days. The lower dose used in this study was reflected in a low response rate (0% CR, 11% PR).

In total, 91 patients have been treated with VDS infusions in the 3 large phase 2 trials[40,51,53] reported to date (see section on VLB phase 2 trials for details of study of Yau et al). There have been no CR, but 17/91 (19%) have obtained

Table 5. Hematologic Toxicity in Patients with Breast Carcinoma

	Continuous infusion	Bolus injection
WBC count nadir*		
Median	2.0	2.9
Range	0.9–4.7	1.0–8.9
Absolute granulocyte count nadir*		
Median	0.9	1.5
Range	0.1–3.0	0–6.3
Absolute platelet count nadir*		
Median	185	156
Range	51–475	14–378
% of courses with absolute granulocyte counts ≤ 1,000/mm³	61	30
% of courses with absolute granulocyte counts ≤ 500/mm³	29	10

*cells/mm³ × 10³

PR. VDS is an active agent in advanced breast carcinoma, but it is not clear that infusion schedules are more efficacious than bolus injections.

Bronchogenic Carcinoma (Nonsmall-Cell)

Gralla et al[54] reported a 22% response rate with VDS alone, given by bolus injection (3–4 mg/m^2) at weekly intervals in 46 patients with nonsmall-cell carcinoma of the lung. Bodey et al[55,56] attempted to duplicate this result by using the continuous infusion schedule. Twenty-three patients with nonsmall-cell carcinoma received this regimen as initial therapy. Only 1 patient achieved a PR, and 11 had stabilization of previously progressive disease. As a consequence of these poor results, M. D. Anderson Hospital abandoned further trials of continuous infusion VDS therapy in patients with bronchogenic carcinoma. Dirks et al[48] gave 31 patients with nonsmall-cell carcinoma infusion VDS as initial therapy. The dosage schedule was 1–1.4 mg/m^2 over 8 hours daily for 3 days, repeated at 3-week intervals. None of the 25 evaluable patients showed any response to therapy, although all of them had a poor performance status. The results of these studies are hardly conclusive, but there is nothing to suggest that continuous infusions of VDS offers any advantage to patients with nonsmall-cell lung cancer.

Table 6. Nonhematologic Toxicity in Patients with Breast Carcinoma

	Continuous infusion	Bolus injection
No. of evaluable patients	25	26
No. and (%) of patients with		
Nausea	8 (32)	21 (80)
Vomiting	6 (24)	18 (69)
Stomatitis	5 (20)	5 (20)
Fever with infusion	8 (32)	2 (7)
FUO with neutropenia	4 (16)	2 (7)
Phlebitis	–	2 (7)
Alopecia	1 (4)	1 (3)
Neuropathy		
Constipation	6 (24)	15 (57)
Ileus	1 (4)	1 (3)
Paresthesia	5 (20)	7 (27)
Loss of deep tendon reflexes	2 (8)	2 (7)
Muscular weakness	2 (8)	0
Inappropriate ADH secretion	4 (16)	0
Catheter-related		
Pneumothorax	1 (4)	0
Thrombosis	2 (8)	0
Extravasation	1 (4)	2 (7)

*FUO = Fever of unknown origin
ADH = Antidiuretic hormone

Sarcoma

Patients with metastatic soft tissue or bony sarcomas who had failed to respond to other regimens, including an ADR-dacarbazine regimen, were entered in a study of continuous infusion vinca alkaloids.[44] Patients were randomly assigned to receive either VLB (1.5 mg/m^2/day) or VDS (1.2 mg/m^2/day) as a 5-day continuous infusion. A total of 33 patients were entered in the study, but only 30 could be evaluated. There were no significant differences between the 2 groups with respect to number of prior treatments and response and number of metastatic sites, although the VLB group was younger (median 29 versus 45 years) and had a larger proportion of females (60% versus 13%). No complete or partial responses were observed with either drug. Myelosuppression was limited to neutropenia, with mean nadirs of 700/mm^3 with VDS and 1,300/mm^3 with VLB. Nausea and vomiting were the most common nonhematologic side effects, occurring in 33% and 20% of the patients, respectively.

Magill et al[58] reported an overall response rate of 16% with VDS given at a dose of 3–5 mg/m^2 as a bolus injection every 1–2 weeks in adults with advanced sarcomas. Hence, VDS has little activity as a single agent for the treatment of sarcomas in adults, regardless of the schedule of administration.

Squamous Cell Carcinoma of Head and Neck

Popkin et al (59) treated 16 patients with advanced squamous cell carcinoma of the head and neck with 48-hour VDS infusions at 1.5 mg/m^2/day. Nine patients had had prior chemotherapy. There were 4 (25%) major responses, including 1 patient with a clinical complete remission for 15+ months. There have been no other studies of VDS infusions in head and neck cancer.

Other Tumors

Pilot studies of continuous infusion therapy with VDS have been conducted in patients with malignant melanoma and renal cell carcinoma.[56] Of 22 patients with melanoma, 2 achieved PR lasting 6 and 10+ months. Additionally, 6 patients had minor responses of short duration. However, 2 larger phase 2 trials of VDS infusion in metastatic melanoma have been disappointing. Mayol et al[60] treated 15 patients with 1.5 mg/m^2/day for 5 days, and Wagstaff et al[61] treated 18 patients with 3–6 mg/m^2 over 24 hours. No responses were seen in the combined 33 patients.

Three of 12 patients with renal cell carcinoma achieved PR lasting 3+, 6+, and 6+ months.[56] One additional patient experienced a minor regression. These preliminary results suggest that further investigations of this schedule of VDS administration should be conducted in renal cell carcinoma.

Bayssas et al[62] evaluated VDS therapy in patients with hematological malignancies. Twelve patients initially received 2 courses of VDS by bolus injection (2 mg/m^2/day $\times$ 2 days at weekly intervals). There were no PR or CR. Subsequently, they were given 48-hour infusions of VDS (4 mg/m^2 total dose); 6

responded to this change in schedule. Three patients received initial VDS therapy by continuous infusion and 1 achieved a PR.

A significant portion of the data on different schedules of VDS administration are fragmentary. However, in some diseases such as the hematological malignancies, head and neck cancer, and renal cell carcinoma, the initial results are sufficiently encouraging to justify further clinical trials. The data in breast carcinoma are more extensive and conclusive, but additional studies should be conducted to confirm the initial trials. Continuous infusion therapy with VDS does not appear to be effective in lung cancer, malignant melanoma, and saracomas, and further studies should not be attempted.

Conclusions

There is considerable preclinical evidence to support the use of VLB and VDS infusions. However, the results of clinical trials to date have not established any definite role for the infusion of these drugs. The use of 5-day VLB infusions in advanced breast carcinoma appears promising, and further trials are definitely needed. Thorough phase 1 testing with pharmacokinetic analysis, which should be performed for all new schedules, is particularly lacking for VDS. Because preclinical studies suggest that some apparently resistant tumors may be sensitive to prolonged exposure, disease-oriented phase 2 trials should be performed using 5-day VLB and VDS infusions against a multitude of tumors. These trials should be given the same priority as other drugs completing phase 2 trials. However, because continuous infusion chemotherapy is more difficult and expensive to administer, it is justified only if it is more effective or less toxic than conventional bolus therapy.

14

PERIWINKLE ALKALOIDS II: VINCRISTINE

Don V. Jackson Jr., M.D.

DURING THE PAST 2 DECADES, vincristine (VCR), an alkaloid obtained from the plant *Vinca rosea* Linn, has been one of the most frequently used chemotherapeutic agents because of its wide spectrum of antitumor activity and its lack of myelosuppression.[1] Although its mechanisms of action may be multiple, the major effect appears to be related to its high affinity binding to the basic protein subunit of microtubules, tubulin, which results in disruption of the mitotic spindle apparatus and arrest of cells in metaphase.[1]

The principal side effect limiting the use of VCR in cancer treatment is neurotoxicity.[1] It is age- and dose-related and is usually manifested by a peripheral mixed sensory-motor neuropathy with symmetrical neurological signs and symptoms. Central neurotoxicity may occur, but is uncommon, probably relating to the poor penetration of vincristine and its products into the CSF.[2,3] Peripheral neuropathy is frequently encountered in patients receiving repetitive doses of VCR, perhaps owing to neurotubular binding and damage of a cumulative nature associated with an enterohepatic circulation of the agent and its metabolic and degradation products. The principal route of its excretion in man appears to be the biliary system,[4] and its products have been measured in the bile of dogs for up to 2 weeks following a single I.V. injection.[5,6]

Acknowledgements: The assistance and support in these studies by the following individuals is deeply appreciated: Richard Bender, Bruce Chabner, Sagar Sethi, Mickey Castle, Deborah Rosenbaum, Tony Long, Hyman Muss, Charles Spurr, Robert Capizzi, Ellen Pope, Doug Case, Renet McMahan, Brad Wells, Davie Jackson and the oncology nurse specialists of the Oncology Research Center, Bowman Gray School of Medicine, Wake Forest University. These investigations were supported in part by CA-12197, CA-33499, and CA-24740 from the National Institutes of Health and Forsyth Cancer Service, Winston-Salem, NC.

In vitro cytotoxicity studies have demonstrated that the antitumor effect of VCR is critically dependent on both concentration and exposure interval.[7] Figure 1 depicts a steep dose-response curve for VCR in L1210 murine leukemia cells cloned in a soft agar system. The results of variable periods of drug exposure in this system are shown in figure 2. Whereas a 50% cell kill occurred following a 3-hour exposure to 10^{-7} VCR, a 6–12-hour period was required to

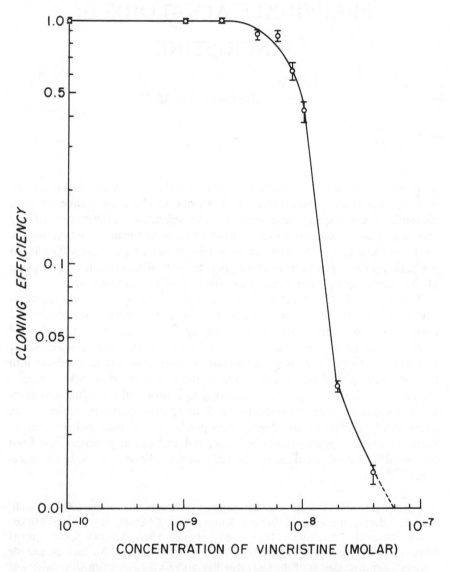

Figure 1.   Survival of L1210 murine leukemia cells constantly exposed to VCR. Cells were cloned in soft agar as previously described (7). Each point represents the mean ± SEM of 3 experiments. (From Jackson DV, Bender RA. Cytotoxic thresholds of vincristine in a murine and a human leukemia cell line in vitro. Cancer Res 1979; 39:4346 – 49.)

achieve this degree of cytotoxicity on exposure to 10^{-8}M vincristine. Further-more, exposure of this cell line to a concentration of 10^{-9}M VCR for up to 2 weeks resulted in no appreciable cell death; no evidence of cytotoxicity was observed until VCR concentrations of $>2 \times 10^{-9}$M were employed. Similar results were observed in cell growth of CEM human lymphoblastoid cells in suspension culture.[7]

Pharmacologic studies of I.V. bolus VCR have demonstrated a rapid blood decay curve with a β-half life of 23.7 ± 8.5 minutes.[8] Vincristine concentra-tions of 10^{-7} –10^{-8}M in the blood are clinically attainable following I.V. bolus injection, but these levels are not sustained (see figure 3). Blood concentrations usually fall below 10^{-8}M within only a few hours after administration and rapidly approach the cytotoxic threshold observed in the aforementioned tumor cell lines in vitro.[7] These data suggested that the effectiveness of VCR

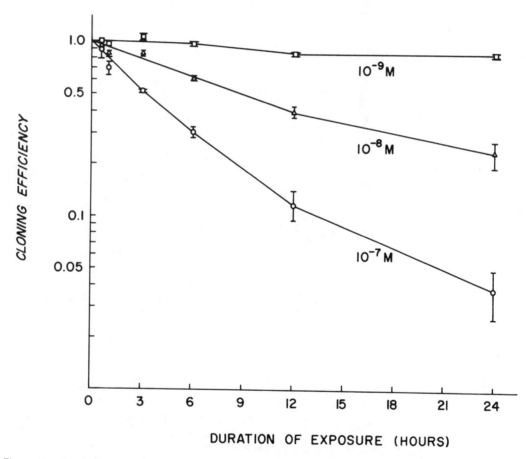

Figure 2.   Survival of L1210 murine leukemia cells exposed to VCR for variable time intervals and cloned in soft agar as previously described (7). Each point represents the mean ± SEM of 3 experiments. (From Jackson DV, Bender RA. Cytotoxic thresholds of vincristine in a murine and a human leukemia cell line in vitro. Cancer Res 1979; 39:4346 – 49.)

might be enhanced by infusion for a protracted period and led to the development of the clinical trials discussed herein. The earlier reports of antitumor responses observed by Ferreira[9] and Weber et al[10] in a small number of patients with leukemia, lymphoma, breast cancer, and melanoma also encouraged the evaluation of this technique.

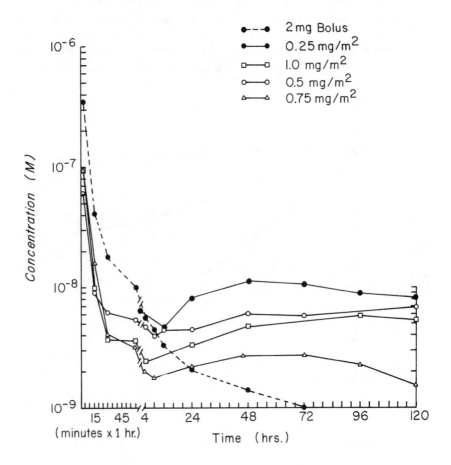

Figure 3.   Comparison of serum concentrations of VCR (and its metabolic and decomposition products) following I.V. bolus injection or infusion. Blood samples were analyzed by radioimmunoassay as previously described (8). Each curve is generated from data obtained in 4 patients with the exception of the 0.25 mg/m² infusion in which one patient was examined. (Modified from Jackson DV Jr, Sethi VS, Spurr CL, et al. Pharmacokinetics of vincristine infusion. Cancer Treat Rep 1981; 65:1043 – 48, and Jackson DV Jr, Chauvenet AR, Callahan RD, et al. Phase 2 trial of vincristine infusion in acute leukemia. Cancer Chemother Pharmacol 1985; 14:26 – 29.)

Clinical Trials

Phase 1-3 trials of I.V. vincristine infusion have been performed. Additionally, a phase 1 trial of hepatic intra-arterial infusion has been done. Each trial will be considered separately.

Intravenous Vincristine Infusion: Phase 1 Trial

From September 1979 to May 1980, 30 patients with advanced malignancies (see table 1) refractory to conventional chemotherapy were evaluated.[11] Patients were excluded from entry into the trial in the presence of primary neurologic disease or neurologic deficits or if there was evidence of renal or hepatic dysfunction unless due to metastatic disease. Treatment consisted of an initial 0.5 mg I.V. bolus injection of VCR followed immediately by continuous infusion of the drug using 1 of 3 doses (0.5, 0.75, or 1.0 mg/m²) given daily for 5 days. Infusions were repeated every 3 weeks in the absence of severe toxicity or progressive disease. The infusate, prepared daily, consisted of the appropriate dose of VCR, in 1,000 ml 5% dextrose and water to which was added 3,000 units of heparin and 50 mg of hydrocortisone to reduce phlebitis. The stability of vincristine in this solution at room temperature was established by high-pressure liquid chromatography.[11] Peripheral veins were generally used for infusion. Three groups of patients (by dosage) were evaluated: 0.5 mg/m², N = 15; 75 mg/m², N = 7; and 1.0 mg/m², N = 10 (see table 2).

The pharmacokinetics of VCR infusion were evaluated during this phase 1 trial.[8] A sensitive radioimmunoassay with the lower limits of detectability at ≅ 1×10^{-9}M was employed.[12]

Table 1. Phase 1 Trial of Intravenous VCR Infusion:[11] Response

Disease	No. Patients	Response (dosage, no. patients)[a]	Prior VCR[b] in responding patients
non-Hodgkin's lymphoma	6	4 PR (0.5,3;1.0,1)	4/4
Acute nonlymphoblastic leukemia	5	2 CR (0.5,1;0.75,1)	2/2
Acute lymphoblastic leukemia	1	0	−
Chronic granulocytic leukemia in blast crisis	5	1 CR (0.75,1)	0/1
Breast cancer	5	3 PR (0.5,1;1.0,2)	2/3
Small-cell lung cancer	3	1 PR (0.5,1)	1/1
Gynecologic cancer	3	0	−
Multiple myeloma	2	0	−

[a]Following a 0.5 mg I.V. bolus, patients were given infusions with 1 of 3 daily doses for 5d:0.50 mg/m², 0.75 mg/m², or 1.0 mg/m².
[b]Prior VCR implies previous treatment with VCR given by bolus injection.

Intravenous Vincristine Infusion: Phase 2 Trials

From August 1980 to December 1984, 120 patients with advanced metastatic malignancies no longer responsive to standard treatment programs were evaluated. Exclusion criteria for entry into the study were the same as for the phase 1 trial. Patient characteristics, including age, performance status, prior chemotherapy, prior VCR, and infusion dosage, are listed by tumor type in tables 3–9. The following types have been evaluated: leukemia,[13,14]

Table 2. Phase 1 Trial of Intravenous Infusion:[11] Nonhematologic Toxicity[a]

	0.50 mg/m^2/d		0.75 mg/m^2/d		1.0 mg/m^2/d	
	No. events	% of courses	No. events	% of courses	No. events	% of courses
Ileus	1	5	3	43	7	58
Hyporeflexia	5	26	2	29	6	50
Myalgias	3	16	3	43	4	33
Hyponatremia	1	5	2	29	4	33
Urinary retention	–	0	–	0	2	17
Phlebitis	–	0	2	29	1	8
Diarrhea	–	0	–	0	1	8
Nausea, vomiting	–	0	–	0	–	0

[a]Toxicity is listed as the number of events and percentage of courses in which the event occurred according to dosage. The number of courses by dose was as follows: 19 (0.50 mg/m^2); 7 (0.75 mg/m^2); and 12 (1.0 mg/m^2).

Table 3. Intravenous VCR Infusion in Acute Leukemia[13] (Phase 2 Trial)

	Total	Percent
Patient characteristics		
No. patients	21	100
Median age (range)	46 (15 – 64)	–
Performance status		
0 – 2	20	95
3 – 4	1	5
Prior chemotherapy	21	100
Prior VCR	19	90
Infusion dosage		
0.25 mg/m^2/d × 5d	17	81
0.50 mg/m^2/d × 5d	4	19
Response		
No. CR[a]	1	5
No. PR[b]	2	10

[a]Complete response was observed in 1/14 patients with ANLL (acute nonlymphoblastic leukemia) who received 0.25 mg/m^2 infusion.
[b]Partial response was observed in 1/14 patients with ANLL who received 0.25 mg/m^2 infusion and 1/2 with ALL who received 0.50 mg/m^2 infusion.

non-Hodgkin's lymphoma,[15] breast,[16], small-cell lung,[17] multiple myeloma,[18] and gynecological.[19]

Performance status was defined as follows: 0, fully active without symptoms; 1, ambulatory with symptoms; 2, bedridden <50% of the time; 3,

Table 4. Intravenous VCR Infusion in Chronic Lymphocytic Leukemia[14] (Phase 2 Trial)

	Total	Percent
Patient characteristics		
No. patients	7	100
Median age (range)	62 (45 – 76)	–
Performance status		
0 – 2	7	100
3 – 4	0	0
Prior chemotherapy	7	100
Prior vincristine	4	57
Infusion dosage		
0.25 mg/m^2/d × 5d	6	86
0.50 mg/m^2/d × 5d	1	14
Response		
No. CR	0	0
No. PR	0	0

Table 5. Intravenous VCR Infusion in Non-Hodgkin's Lymphoma[15] (Phase 2 Trial)

	Total	Percent
Patient characteristics		
No. patients	25	100
Median age (range)	55 (20 – 72)	–
Performance status		
0 – 2	23	92
3 – 4	2	8
Prior chemotherapy	25	100
Prior VCR	24	96
Infusion dosage		
0.25 mg/m^2/d × 5d	25	100
0.50 mg/m^2/d × 5d	0	0
Response		
No. CR[a]	1	4
No. PR[b]	8	32

[a]Complete response was observed in 1/2 patients with DML (diffuse mixed lymphoma).
[b]Partial response was observed in 4/10 patients with DPDL (diffuse poorly differentieated lymphocytic lymphoma), 2/7 with nodular PDL, 1/1 with nodular ML, and 1/3 with a diffuse large-cell lymphoma.

bedridden >50% of the time but capable of self-care; 4 bedridden 100% of the time and incapable of self-care.

Treatment consisted of an initial 0.5 mg I.V. bolus injection of VCR followed immediately by continuous infusion of the drug using doses of either 0.25 and 0.50 mg/m^2 daily for 5 days. An infusion dosage lower than that recommended from the earlier phase 1 trial (0.5 mg/m^2) was used because of lack of correlation of infusion dosage with serum concentrations and areas under the serum concentration curve.[8,13] Infusions were repeated every 3 weeks in the absence of prohibitive toxicity (grade 3–4) or disease progression. There were

Table 6. Intravenous VCR Infusion in Breast Cancer[16] (Phase 2 Trial)

	Total	Percent
Patient characteristics		
No. patients	18	100
Median age (range)	54 (33 – 68)	–
Performance status		
0 – 2	9	50
3 – 4	9	50
Prior chemotherapy	18	100
Prior VCR	7	39
Infusion dosage		
0.25 mg/m^2/d × 5d	18	100
0.50 mg/m^2/d × 5d	0	0
Response		
No. CR	0	0
No. PR	0	0

Table 7. Intravenous VCR Infusion in Small-Cell Lung Cancer[17] (Phase 2 Trial)

	Total	Percent
Patient characteristics		
No. patients	15	100
Median age (range)	61 (39 – 74)	–
Performance status		
0 – 2	13	87
3 – 4	2	13
Prior chemotherapy	15	100
Prior VCR	14	93
Infusion dosage		
0.25 mg/m^2/d × 5d	15	100
0.50 mg/m^2/d × 5d	0	0
Response		
No. CR	0	0
No. PR	0	0

no dose modifications. Preparation of the infusate was the same as for the phase 1 trial.

Response to treatment was confirmed by actual measurements. A complete response (CR) was a 100% reduction of all demonstrable tumor and no new area of malignancy. A partial response (PR) was indicated by a 50% or greater

Table 8. Intravenous VCR Infusion in Multiple Myeloma[18] (Phase 2 Trial)

	Total	Percent
Patient characteristics		
No. patients	18	100
Median age (range)	61 (34 – 76)	–
Performance status		
0 – 2	9	50
3 – 4	9	50
Prior chemotherapy	18	100
Prior radiotherapy	18	100
Prior VCR	7	39
Infusion dosage		
0.25 mg/m^2/d × 5d	7	39
0.50 mg/m^2/d × 5d	11	61
Response		
No. CR	0	0
No. PR	2[a]	11

[a]Both responding patients received 0.50 mg/m^2 infusions.

Table 9. Intravenous Vincristine Infusion in Gynecologic Malignancies[19] (Phase 2 Trial)

	Total	Percent
Patient characteristics		
No. patients[a]	16	100
Median age (range)	58 (25 – 70)	–
Performance status		
0 – 2	14	88
3 – 4	2	12
Prior chemotherapy	14	88
Prior VCR	1	6
Infusion dosage		
0.25 mg/m^2/d × 5d	16	100
0.50 mg/m^2/d × 5d	0	0
Response		
No. CR	0	0
No. PR	0	0

[a]Types of refractory gynecologic malignancies included the following: cervix (11), ovary (3), and endometrium (2).

reduction of the product of the longest perpendicular diameters of indicator lesions since first measured and no new area of malignancy. In leukemia, both the peripheral blood count and the marrow criteria were used to document response.[14] In multiple myeloma, a PR was indicated by a 50% or greater reduction of the monoclonal protein and/or product of the longest perpendicular diameters of plasmacytomas. Duration of response was calculated from the day an objective response was first noted.

Intravenous Vincristine Infusion: Phase 3 Trial

Continuous infusion of VCR in the primary treatment of non-Hodgkin's lymphoma is currently being evaluated in a combination chemotherapy program.[20] It has been substituted for vincristine given by bolus injection in a previously reported modified CHOP program to which was added the nitrosourea CCNU.[21] Twenty patients with stage 3-4 diffuse large-cell lymphoma have been enrolled into this study. Exclusion criteria for VCR infusion duplicate those previously given for the phase 1-2 trials. Patient characteristics are listed in table 10. Treatment consisted of 0.5 mg VCR I.V. bolus injection followed immediately by VCR 0.25 mg/m²/day for 5 days in combination with CCNU, cyclophosphamide, doxorubicin, and prednisone. Chemotherapy was given every 3 weeks. Infusions of VCR were given every 3 weeks for 2 cycles, every 6 weeks for 2 cycles, and every 9 weeks thereafter until completion of therapy (week 45). Standard response criteria were used as previously defined in the description of the phase 2 trials.

Table 10. Intravenous VCR Infusion in Large-Cell Non-Hodgkin's Lymphoma[20] (Phase 3 Trial)[a]

	Total	Percent
Patient characteristics		
No. patients[a]	20	100
Median age (range)	53 (19 – 76)	
Performance status		
0 – 2	17	85
3 – 4	3	15
Prior chemotherapy	0	0
Infusion dosage		
0.25 mg/m²/d × 5d	20	100
0.50 mg/m²/d × 5d	0	0
Response		
No. CR	10	50
No. PR	6	30

[a]Vincristine 0.25 mg/m²/d for 5 days was given after an initial 0.5 mg bolus and was combined with CCNU, doxorubicin, cyclophosphamide, and prednisone. See Clinical Trials section for further details of treatment.

Hepatic Intra-Arterial Vincristine Infusion: Phase 1 Trial

Six patients with refractory metastatic hepatic cancer were evaluated.[22] The types of metastatic cancer and patient characteristics are given in table 11. All patients had one or more abnormal serum liver function test and scan evidence of metastatic disease. Patients were not excluded from entry into the trial because of extent of metastatic disease in the liver. All patients with adenocarcinoma of the colon had eventually failed to respond to intra-arterial (I.A.) infusion of FUDR, and most had also received mitomycin-C intra-arterially.

Treatment consisted of VCR 0.4 mg daily by continuous hepatic I.A. infusion for 5 days. The infusate consisted of a heparinized solution of VCR in 5% dextrose in water. Catheter position was determined prior to treatment, generally with a radiolabel (99mTc macroaggregated albumin).

Results

Intravenous Vincristine Infusion: Phase 1 Trial

Objective responses occurred in 11 of 30 (37%) patients (see table 1) and were observed after infusions at each dose level. Responses were noted in patients with non-Hodgkin's lymphoma, acute leukemia, breast cancer, and small-cell lung cancer. Durations of response tended to be brief. Noteworthy was the fact that of the 11 patients in whom a response was noted, 9 had previously received VCR given by conventional bolus injection.

Toxicity was unacceptable with infusions given at the 0.75 and 1 mg/m^2 dose level and consisted primarily of neurotoxic complications (see table 2).

Table 11. Intra-Arterial VCR Infusion in Hepatic Metastatic Carcinoma[22] (Phase 1 Trial)[a]

	Total	Percent
Patient characteristics		
No. patients	6	100
Median age (range)	61 (34 – 76)	–
Performance status		
0 – 2	4	67
3 – 4	2	33
Prior chemotherapy	6	100
Prior VCR	1	17
Infusion dosage		
0.4 mg ($\cong$ 0.23 mg/m^2)/d × 5d	6	100
0.50 mg/m^2/d × 5d	0	0
Response		
No. CR	0	0
No. PR	0	0

[a]Types of metastatic cancer included 5 patients with adenocarcinoma of the colon and 1 patient with a poorly differentiated lymphocytic lymphoma.

Autonomic neuropathy manifested by ileus accounted for the greatest morbidity. Intravenous infusions of sincalide, a synthetic analogue of cholecystokinin capable of stimulating bowel motility, were often helpful in ameliorating the symptoms and signs of VCR-induced ileus.[23] Myalgias sometimes requiring analgesics, the syndrome of inappropriate antidiuretic hormone secretion (SIADH), muscle weakness, and urinary retention were also bothersome neurotoxic side effects and were most often observed at the 0.75 and 1 mg/m^2 dose levels. Myelosuppression also occurred and was dose-related. Leukopenia, frequently observed at the 1 mg/m^2 dose level, was often severe.

The degree of neurologic and hematologic toxicity was generally mild to moderate with 0.5 mg/m^2 infusions; this dosage was recommended as a maximum dosage for phase 2 trials. Of interest was the complete lack of nausea and vomiting observed at each of the 3 infusion dose levels.

Pharmacologic investigations during this trial revealed the ability of infusions of VCR at each of these dose levels to consistently sustain serum concentrations in excess of 10^{-9}M (see figure 3). However, in comparison, bolus injection of the agent was associated with rapid decline of blood concentrations. Similarly, areas under the blood concentration curve were greater in patients receiving infusion compared to bolus injections.[8]

Intravenous Vincristine Infusion: Phase 2 Trials

ACUTE LEUKEMIA

Objective responses occurred in 2 patients with acute nonlymphoblastic leukemia following 0.25 mg/m^2 infusion (see table 3). Following a single 5-day infusion, a CR occurred in one patient whose pretreatment WBC was 47,500/mm^3. One week after completion of the infusion, the WBC and differential were normal, and marrow blasts had fallen from 84% pretreatment to normal. The response lasted 2.5 months. A PR was observed in the other patient after 3 infusions, and relapse occurred after a fourth infusion. Neither patient had previously received VCR. Of 2 patients with acute lymphoblastic leukemia, 1 had progressive disease and the other had a partial response lasting 2.5 months, during which time 3 infusions (0.5 mg/m^2/day) were given. Progressive disease occurred in all 5 of the patients with blast crisis of chronic granulocytic leukemia. In one patient, however, marrow blasts decreased from 83% to 27% after 2 infusions (0.25 mg/m^2/day) and were associated with symptomatic improvement.

Toxicity was acceptable and manageable. Neurologic toxicity was generally mild or nonexistent, but most patients received only 1 course of infusion as a consequence of failure to control the leukemia. A sense of weakness and easy fatigability or depression occurred in 4 patients. Constipation (without ileus) and mucositis occurred in 1 patient each. No nausea or vomiting was observed.

Thrombocytopenia, the major hematologic toxicity, was generally mild. A marked fall in platelets along with progressive disease occurred in 2 patients.

Blood concentrations of VCR were determined during a 0.25 mg/m^2 infusion in 1 patient with acute nonlymphoblastic leukemia.[13] The serum concentrations attained at this dose level were quite similar to those attained with the larger infusion doses (0.5–1 mg/m^2/day) evaluated earlier during the phase 1 trial[8] (see figure 3).

CHRONIC LYMPHOCYTIC LEUKEMIA

Objective responses were not observed in any of the 7 patients (see table 4). Stable disease was observed in 3 patients for 1, 2.8, and 3 months. Six patients were treated with 0.25 mg/m^2 infusions and 1 received a 0.50 mg/m^2 infusion.

Toxicity was generally mild (paresthesias and constipation in 1 patient each), although severe paresthesias occurred following a single 0.25 mg/m^2 infusion in 1 patient. Hematologic toxicity was minimal (occasional mild reduction of platelets).

NON-HODGKIN'S LYMPHOMA

Objective responses were observed in 9 of 25 (36%) patients, all of whom received 0.25 mg/m^2 infusions (see table 5). A CR occurred in a patient with a diffuse mixed lymphoma. The duration of response was 16.2 months, during which time the patient received a total of 9 infusions. Partial responses were observed in 8 patients, including 4 with diffuse poorly differentiated lymphocytic lymphoma, 2 with nodular poorly differentiated lymphocytic lymphoma, 1 with diffuse mixed lymphoma, and 1 with diffuse large-cell lymphoma. The mean duration of response was 2.9 months in the patients with a PR.

All of the responding patients had previously received VCR by bolus injection, and all but 2 of these had previously experienced progressive disease while receiving a VCR-containing regimen. An analysis of variables in relation to response to VCR infusion revealed that prior response or toxicity to conventional vincristine treatment was not predictive of the outcome of VCR infusion. However, a comparison of responders and nonresponders to VCR infusion showed a significantly greater interval of time lapse between the last bolus injection of vincristine and start of VCR infusion in responders (12.5 months versus 5.6 months, p = .046). Also, the cumulative dosage of VCR (prior to infusion therapy) was less in responders than nonresponders (mean, 13.7 mg versus 25.1 mg, p = .056).

Neurotoxicity was observed in 48% of patients, most of whom had reduced deep tendon reflexes. Disabling neurotoxicity occurred in only 2 patients, both of whom had paresthesias causing difficulty with buttoning clothes. Paresthesias were noted in 24% of patients, constipation in 20%, myalgias in 8%, and decreased muscle strength in 4%. No cases of ileus, urinary retention, or SIADH were observed.

Hematologic toxicity was generally mild. Following 71 courses of VCR infusion, a leukocyte count of <2,000/mm^3 was observed in only 1 patient who had not had a pretreatment count at that level. Similarly, a platelet count of <50,000/mm^3 was observed in only 1 patient who had not had a pretreatment count of <50,000 mm^3.

Nausea and vomiting did not occur in any patient. Despite peripheral vein infusion in most patients, phlebitis was not observed.

BREAST CANCER

No objective responses were observed in 18 patients, all of whom received 0.25 mg/m^2 infusions (see table 6). Vincristine by bolus injection had previously been given to 7 of the patients.

Toxicity was primarily neurologic and generally was mild and reversible. Paresthesias and/or reduced deep tendon reflexes were observed in 44% of the patients, and constipation (without ileus) occurred in 28%. Transient urinary retention occurred in 2 patients. Phlebitis, observed in 1 patient, was not associated with ulceration.

SMALL-CELL LUNG CANCER

Objective responses were not observed in any of 15 patients, all of whom received 0.25 mg/m^2 infusions (see table 7). Prior VCR by bolus injection had been given to all but 1 of the patients.

Toxicity was minimal in general, consisting of mild to moderate constipation in 2 patients and myalgias in one patient. Confusion and shortness of breath of unknown cause occurred on the second day of infusion in 1 patient and persisted until his death 1 week after the start of therapy. No nausea and vomiting or phlebitis was observed.

MULTIPLE MYELOMA

Partial responses occurred in 2 of 18 (11%) patients, both of whom had received 0.5 mg/m^2 infusions. The M-protein, an IgA in both patients, decreased to $< 50\%$ of baseline following VCR infusion, and 1 patient also experienced marked reduction in the size of the plasmacytomas. However, the response durations were brief (1.2 and 2.2 months).

Toxicity consisted of neurotoxicity and myelosuppression. In addition to the occurrence of paresthesias (3 patients) and myalgias (2 patients), ileus developed in 2 patients who received 0.5 mg/m^2 infusions. Moderately severe reduction of muscle strength occurred in 2 patients who received 0.5 mg/m^2 infusions.

Following VCR infusion, a WBC of $< 2,000$/mm^3 was observed in 6 patients and platelets $< 50,000$/mm^3 were noted in 8 patients. The lowest mean WBC $(\times 10^3$/mm$^3)$ was 2.69 (range, 0.5–5.2) versus a mean pretreatment WBC of 3.69 (1.4–8.2), p = .002. The lowest mean platelet count was 79.1×10^3/mm^3 (5–176) versus a mean pretreatment platelet count of 111.7×10^3/mm^3 (17–229), p = .01. In general, patients receiving the higher infusion dosage incurred the greatest hematologic toxicity. Nausea was observed in one patient, but vomiting did not occur in any.

GYNECOLOGIC MALIGNANCIES

Objective responses were not observed in any patient. Patients received from 1 to 6 infusion of VCR (mean, 2).

No severe neurotoxicity occurred, but 1 patient developed severe myalgias requiring analgesics and muscle relaxants. This patient refused further treatment because of the severity of the myalgias. There was no major myelosuppression, even though all patients were heavily pretreated.

Intravenous Vincristine Infusion: Phase 3 Trial

Objective responses to the combination CCNU-CHOP, with the substitution of vincristine infusion for bolus injection of VCR, were observed in 16 of 20 (80%) patients. Complete response occurred in 10 (50%) patients. As of a November 1984 analysis, only 2 patients had relapsed (at 14 and 20 months). No CNS relapses had been observed. Eight (40%) of the total group of patients were alive and disease-free more than 2 years from initiation of therapy.

Neurotoxicity encountered during this trial was generally mild. Two patients who exhibited moderately severe toxicity developed disabling paresthesias after the fourth infusion of VCR; 1 had juvenile diabetes mellitus and no predisposing factor was present in the other.

Intra-Arterial Vincristine Infusion

No objective responses were observed in 6 patients who had metastatic liver disease. Thirteen courses were administered.

Transient but life-threatening toxicity that principally involved the nervous and gastrointestinal systems occurred in 5 patients, requiring discontinuation of therapy. Toxicity in each patient was encountered after 1 infusion. Neurotoxicity generally was either central or involved the autonomic system. Confusion and weakness occurred in 3 patients; urinary incontinency, postural hypotension, and ileus occurred in 1 patient each. Paresthesias developed in 1 patient.

Gastrointestinal toxicity, observed in 4 patients, consisted of anorexia and nausea and vomiting. Profuse watery diarrhea occurred in 1 patient, rapidly producing dehydration.

Blood concentrations of VCR (and its metabolic and degradation products) were measured in 3 patients. Serum concentrations approximated the lower range of sensitivity of the assay ($\cong \times 10^{-9}$M)[12] in one patient and were undetectable in 2 other patients examined.

Discussion

In these phase 1–2 trials of I.V. VCR infusion, objective antitumor responses have been observed in patients with acute leukemia (lymphoblastic, nonlymphoblastic, and blast crisis of chronic granulocytic leukemia), non-Hodgkin's lymphoma, breast cancer, small-cell lung cancer, and multiple myeloma. No objective responses occurred in a small number of patients with chronic lymphocytic leukemia or gynecologic malignancies (including cancers of the cervix, ovary, and endometrium). The toxicity incurred during hepatic I.A. infusion for metastatic malignancies prevented an adequate trial in order to assess response. The greatest antitumor activity has been seen in non-Hodgkin's lymphoma, and a current phase 3 trial incorporating VCR infusion has shown encouraging results. Complete responses in patients with untreated diffuse large-cell lymphoma appear to be quite durable, but further follow-up and ultimately randomized trials are needed to assess the value of VCR infusion in primary treatment regimens.

The phase 2 trials of VCR infusion have shown only minimal activity (<20%) in refractory multiple myeloma and acute nonlymphoblastic leukemia. There appears to be some activity in acute lymphoblastic leukemia, but further trials with a greater number of patients will be required to assess the value of VCR infusion as a potential salvage therapy. Ferreira[9] and Weber et al[10] reported responses in 1 patient each with acute lymphoblastic leukemia following VCR infusion (see table 12).

Information about VCR given as a single agent and as a bolus injection in the treatment of acute nonlymphoblastic leukemia and multiple myeloma is sparse. In acute nonlymphoblastic leukemia, the reported trials largely include children who were refractory to agents such as 6-mercaptopurine, steroids, and methotrexate. Among 46 such patients in 5 clinical trials, the overall objective response rate was about 40%, with a CR rate of about 25%.[13] Single-agent data for the treatment of multiple myeloma is virtually nonexistent. In a total of 635 patients involved in 4 early clinical trials of vincristine, only 1 patient who had multiple myeloma was mentioned, and there was no response in that patient.[24-27]

The antitumor activity in refractory breast cancer, small-cell lung cancer, and blast crisis of chronic granulocytic leukemia seems to be dose-dependent, inasmuch as responses were observed only during the phase 1 trial, in which larger infusion doses were employed. Responses were noted in 3/5 patients with refractory breast cancer following infusions with 0.50 mg/m^2 (1 patient) and 1.0 mg/m^2 (2 patients) during the phase 1 trial; no responses occurred with 0.25 mg/m^2 infusion in the phase 2 trial. The possibility of dose-dependent activity in breast cancer is further supported by a review of the literature (see table 12). Weber et al reported a PR in 1/3 patients following an infusion of 2.0 mg/m^2 given over a 24-hour period.[10] Bachmann et al noted objective responses in 2 of 4 patients who received 0.50 mg/m^2 infusions daily for 5 days; this dosage had been immediately preceded by a 0.5 mg/m^2 bolus injection.[28] Lower infusion doses used by Bodey et al ($\cong$ 0.12–0.23 mg/m^2/day for 5 days) were not associated with any responses among 15 patients with refractory breast cancer (none had previously received vincristine by bolus injection).[29]

In the phase 1 trial, 1 of 3 patients with small-cell lung cancer had a PR following 0.5 mg/m^2. However, no responses were observed among 15 patients who received 0.25 mg/m^2 infusions in the phase 2 trial. Bachmann and co-workers reported a single patient whose small-cell lung cancer responded to a 0.50 mg/m^2 5-day infusion.[28] These data suggest the possibility of a dose-response relationship for VCR infusion in the treatment of refractory small-cell lung cancer.

Treatment results were disappointing in chronic lymphocytic leukemia, especially when one would have predicted a better outcome in light of the responses observed in another lymphoid neoplasm, non-Hodgkin's lymphoma. Additionally, a comparison with the effectiveness of VCR given as bolus injection is difficult because there is a paucity of such information upon review of the early clinical trials. In 7 clinical trials of VCR involving a total of 732 patients with a variety of neoplasms,[24-27,30-32] 7 patients with chronic lymphocytic leukemia are mentioned,[24,30-32] of whom 1 had a response.[30] The likelihood that chronic lymphocytic leukemic cells would be sensitive to VCR was suggested by an early in vitro investigation demonstrating a greater susceptibility of the leukemic cells than normal lymphocytes to the cytotoxic effects of the drug.[33]

Infusion of VCR for the treatment of refractory gynecologic malignancies has been unimpressive in a small number of patients investigated. There does

Table 12. Objective Responses to VCR Infusion in Phase 1–2 Trials

Disease/Study	No. Patients	Response CR	Response PR	Prior VCR[a] in responding patients CR	Prior VCR[a] in responding patients PR
Acute leukemia[b]					
Ferreira[9]	7	1	2	?	?
Weber et al[10]	2	0	?2	–	?2/2
BGSM-POA[c]	32	4	2	2/4	1/2
Chronic lymphocytic leukemia					
BGSM-POA	7	0	0	–	–
Non-Hodgkin's lymphoma					
Ferreira	2	0	1	–	?1/1
Weber et al	1	–	1	–	1/1
Bachmann et al[28]	2	–	1	–	0/1
BGSM-POA	31	1	12	1/1	12/12
Breast cancer					
Weber et al	3	0	1	–	?1/1
Bachmann et al	4	0	2	–	0/2
Bodey et al[29]	15	0	0	–	–
BGSM-POA	23	0	3	–	2/3
Lung cancer (small-cell)					
Bachmann et al	1	0	1	–	0/1
BGSM-POA	18	0	1	–	1/1
Multiple myeloma					
BGSM-POA	20	0	2	–	0/2
Gynecologic cancer					
Weber et al	3	0	0	–	–
Bachmann et al	2	0	0	–	–
BGSM-POA	19	0	0	–	0
Melanoma					
Ferreira	1	0	0	–	–
Weber et al	3	0	1	–	0/1
Sarcoma					
Bachmann et al	6	0	2	–	2/2

[a]Prior VCR implies VCR given by I.V. bolus injection.
[b]Acute leukemia includes lymphoblastic, nonlymphoblastic, and blast crisis of chronic granulocytic leukemia.
[c]BGSM-POA - Bowman Gray School of Medicine, Wake Forest University—Piedmont Oncology Association.

appear to be minimal single-agent activity from review of the early clinical trials of vincristine given by bolus injection, particularly for carcinoma of the cervix. In 5 clinical trials involving a total of 512 patients with a variety of malignancies, 48 cases or carcinoma of the cervix were investigated in which there were 8 (17%) responses; there were no responses among 19 patients with ovarian cancer or in a single patient with endometrial cancer.[24,27,34-36] Cumulatively, infusion of VCR has resulted in no responses in 12 patients with carcinoma of the cervix,[11,19] in 6 patients with ovarian cancer,[11,19,28] and in 5 patients with carcinoma of the endometrium.[10,19]

Other malignancies in which infusion of VCR has been investigated in a small number of cases include melanoma (1 PR in 4 patients)[9,10] and sarcoma (2 partial responses in 6 cases).[28]

The toxicity of I.V. infusion of VCR using a dose of 0.25–0.50 mg/m^2 daily for 5 days has principally involved the neurologic system. The type, frequency, and degree of neurotoxicity have generally been no greater than that reported in review articles dealing with I.V. bolus injection of VCR.[27,37-39] Myelosuppression has generally been nonexistent or mild if present. Higher infusion dosages as explored in the phase 1 study (0.75 and 1.0 mg/m^2) were associated with unacceptable neurologic toxicity, with ileus occurring frequently ($\cong$ 40–60% of courses). Furthermore, hematologic toxicity of a dose-dependent nature, encountered during the phase 1 trial, was severe at the 1.0 mg/m^2 infusion level.

The severity of both neurotoxicity and myelosuppression appeared to be somewhat greater in patients with refractory multiple myeloma and was more severe in patients receiving 0.50 mg/m^2 infusions than among those treated with 0.25 mg/m^2 infusions. Perhaps there was some interaction of VCR with the myelomatous protein; this has been observed with albumin during in vitro cell uptake and cytotoxicity studies[40] resulting in an alteration of the drug's pharmacodynamics.

A different spectrum of toxicity was observed after hepatic I.A. infusion from that noted with I.V. infusion. Central rather than peripheral nervous system toxicity predominated and was manifested by prolonged periods of confusion. Also, G.I. symptoms of nausea, vomiting, and diarrhea were observed, whereas they were distinctly lacking during trials of I.V. infusion. Perhaps these complications relate to an alteration of the hepatic metabolism and biliary excretion of the agent upon its direct intrahepatic injection.

The ability of vincristine I.V. infusion to produce an antitumor response even after exposure to VCR given by bolus injection has been observed in a number of types of malignancies (see table 12). This suggests the possibility that infusion of VCR might enhance the clinical effectiveness of this agent beyond that seen with conventional bolus injection. Preclinical cytotoxicity studies showing a critical dependence on both drug concentration and exposure interval[7] support this possibility; and pharmacologic investigations have shown the ability of 5-day infusions to prolong potentially cytotoxic drug concentrations in the serum for days beyond those typically observed with bolus injection.[8,13] Further investigations of this promising technique appear to be warranted.

Two major drawbacks associated with trials of I.V. infusion of VCR remain:

(1) prolonged periods of treatment, perhaps associated with lengthy periods of hospitalization with the attendant expense and inconvenience to the patient; and (2) continued problems with neurotoxicity similar to those observed with conventional bolus injection. Outpatient venous access[41] and delivery systems[42,43] in an ever-increasing variety may allow assistance with the first problem. The second problem is more difficult, and no proven antidotes or ameliorating agents exist to deal with the frequent neurologic complications associated with VCR administration. It is hoped that pursuit of potential antagonists of VCR neurotoxicity in laboratory investigations[44-47] and clinical trials[48,49] will identify the means to allow an improvement in both patient comfort and therapeutic efficacy of this agent.

15

BLEOMYCIN

Robert B. Catalano, Pharm. D., and Robert L. Comis, M.D.

Introduction

BLEOMYCIN (BLM) IS A glycopeptide antitumor antibiotic that has been employed in anticancer chemotherapy for more than 2 decades. It is active in a variety of human tumors, most notably testicular cancer, lymphomas, and squamous cell carcinoma of the head and neck. Its lack of myelotoxicity led to its early use in combination chemotherapy programs. The primary dose-limiting toxicity of bleomycin is pulmonary fibrosis.

Data favoring the use of continuous infusion BLM include its mechanism of action, clinical pharmacology, pharmacokinetics, and, to some extent, the results of several uncontrolled clinical trials. This discussion is designed to present the rationale for studying bleomycin administered by continuous infusion and the status of the existing data.

Mechanism of Action

The primary mechanism of action of BLM is the production of single- and double-strand DNA breaks. Bleomycin is capable of intercalating with DNA, presumably through interaction between DNA and the bithiazole moieties.[1] DNA cleavage is produced when intracellular Fe^{2+} is bound in the metal binding site of the BLM molecule and an electron shunt is produced between $Fe^{2+} \rightarrow Fe^{3+}$, leading to the generation of highly reactive oxygen-free radicals.[2]

Presently, it is not known whether the same interaction between the drug and iron and oxygen is responsible for pulmonary damage. Bleomycin-related cytotoxic effects are cell cycle phase-specific. For most cell types, BLM produces a block in the early G_2 phase of the cell cycle. In spite of this preferential cytokinetic effect, there are conflicting data concerning the effect of BLM on plateau versus exponentially growing cells.[3]

Drewinko et al studied the effect of BLM on asynchronous human lymphoma cells (T_1) in culture.[4] The sensitivity of these cells to the drug was expressed as a biphasic dose-response survival curve. This suggests that the initial steep part of the curve represents a large cell kill of a sensitive cell fraction followed by a flat portion representing the response of the less sensitive fraction of cells. The effects on survival of a single dose of 50 µg/ml of BLM was a function of the duration of treatment. Survival decreased from 10% after 4 hours of treatment to ultimately 0.06% after 35 hours of exposure, a period slightly longer than the cell cycle time of T_1 cells (27 hours). This suggests that extending the duration of treatment allows the majority of the cells to progress through the sensitive stages of the cellular life cycle, thereby reducing the surviving fraction 1,000-fold. These findings have been used to support human studies investigating continuous infusion schedules of BLM.

Barranco et al[5,6] presented evidence that at low doses approximating those obtainable in vivo, bleomycin is cell cycle-specific, inhibiting cell progression at the S-G_2 boundary and in the mitotic period. Cells in other stages of the cell cycle are less affected. Therefore, for optimum activity in vivo, BLM might theoretically be required to be present throughout the cell cycle. In nonmitotic cells, BLM has been shown to produce preferential breaks in the linker regions between nucleosomes.[7] Maximum DNA damage occurs during the first 6 hours of drug exposure. Repair of DNA damage induced by BLM can occur.

Pharmacology

Preclinical pharmacology studies performed in rodent species using radiolabeled drug showed preferential uptake of bleomycin in the lung and the skin. These sites correspond to the primary toxicity target organs in both rodents and man. An enzyme termed bleomycin hydrolase, which was found to be present in large amounts in the liver and kidneys of rodents, was found to be decreased in the lung and skin.[8] Bleomycin hydrolase has not been consistently found in human tissues.

Human pharmacokinetic studies have generally employed radioimmunoassay techniques for measuring plasma BLM concentrations. The drug has an elimination half-life of about 2 hours after rapid I.V. injection.[9] The primary route of elimination is the kidney. Approximately 65% of the administered dose is excreted in the urine within the first 24 hours. Significant increases in the elimination half-life of BLM occur when the creatinine clearance is below 25–30 ml/min.[10] Studies performed in essentially anephric patients have shown that the elimination half-life is extended to about 20 hours, with drug levels being undetectable by 48 to 72 hours. Thus, in the absence of renal excretory capability, the drug is eliminated by other routes.[10]

A few studies have evaluated the pharmacokinetics of BLM administered by continuous infusion. As expected, steady-state levels are achieved within the first several hours of continuous administration. There is rapid disappearance of BLM from the plasma after infusion is discontinued. A study by Broughton and Strong had shown that the elimination half-life is significantly prolonged after termination of a continuous BLM infusion (about 9 hours); these data suggest that continuous exposure may saturate some undetermined deep compartmental binding site.[11] Studies employing continuous low-dose BLM infusions have not revealed this phenomenon,[11] possibly because of the inadequate level of sensitivity of the assay systems employed.

Bleomycin Toxicology

In humans, the primary dose-limiting chronic toxicity of BLM is pulmonary fibrosis.[12] Overall, the incidence of lethal toxicity is approximately 1–2%, with an additional 2–3% of patients developing irreversible pulmonary fibrosis. The precise incidence of pulmonary toxicity as a function of total dose is extremely difficult to determine because the treated groups are tremendously heterogeneous and the methods of detection vary from potentially sensitive pulmonary laboratory studies, such as the measurement of single-breath carbon monoxide diffusing capacity (DL_{CO}), to the physical examination. A number of factors appear to increase the risk of developing BLM pulmonary toxicity. These include a total cumulative dose of $\geq$ 450–500 units; age of $\geq$ 70 years; prior or concomitant radiotherapy to the chest and mediastinum; preexisting pulmonary function abnormalities; high intraoperative oxygen concentrations; combining BLM with other agents in the treatment of lymphomas; the presence of renal failure; and probably the route of administration.

All of the above factors complicate the precise definition of risk, particularly as it relates to total dose. It should be remembered that the dose/toxicity curve is not linear until a certain threshold dose is exceeded. Because of the sporadic nature of toxicity at lower doses, it is difficult to compare series employing different routes of administration as an attempt to alter the development of pulmonary toxicity.

In general, either randomized studies comparing administration routes and schedules or large numbers of well studied patients are required to detect a significant shift in this toxic effect.

Animal Studies

Peng et al compared the cytotoxicity of BLM given by continuous intraperitoneal (I.P.) infusion with the same dose administered by a daily I.P. bolus injection.[13] These 2 techniques were compared, using a spleen colony-forming unit assay (LCFU-S) for P388 leukemic cells. The continuous infusion of 8 units/kg/day × 6 days provided constant BLM plasma levels of 0.62 ± 0.03 mU/ml and a total plasma AUC (area under the plasma decay curve) of 89 mU/h/ml. Intermittent I.P. bolus injection of 8 units/kg/day × 6 days had a terminal phase plasma $T_{1/2}$ of 15 minutes and a total 6-day plasma AUC of 90.8 mU/h/ml; thus, the 2 administration schedules yielded equivalent bleomycin exposures as measured by AUC. The continuous infusion of bleomycin caused a 0.5-log greater reduction in LCFU-S than did the identical dose given by intermittent bolus administration. Although high-peak BLM plasma levels (32 mU/ml) were achieved with intermittent bolus administration, the greater inhibition of LCFU-S by BLM as a continuous infusion was most likely related to the drug's schedule-dependent cell cycle characteristics.

Mice implanted with Lewis lung carcinoma have been treated with equal doses of BLM by 7-day continuous infusion, twice daily injection, or twice weekly injection.[14] The continuous infusion regimen was superior to both intermittent injection schedules in antitumor efficacy, and it was also associated with significantly less pulmonary toxicity as defined by lung hydroxyproline levels. Osieka et al compared BLM administered by continuous I.P. infusion with daily I.P. bolus injections at various dosage levels in human embryonal testicular cancer xenographs implanted in nude mice.[15] Their data failed to support a superiority of continuous infusion BLM over daily intermittent injections in this tumor model, with both administration schedules yielding comparable results. Conflicting results have also been reported by other investigators who did not observe increased antineoplastic activity after fractionated or continuously infused doses of bleomycin.[16,17]

Taken as a whole, these data illustrate that the superiority of continuous infusion schedules may be heavily dependent upon the intrinsic characteristics of the tumor. Failure to improve the antineoplastic response using the continuous infusion technique may still result in an improved therapeutic index by reducing the potential for pulmonary toxicity.[15]

Pharmaceutical Data

Bleomycin is commercially available in vials containing a white or yellowish lyophilized powder equivalent to 15 units of sterile bleomycin sulfate. Intact vials of BLM have been shown to be chemically stable for 2 years at temperatures of 1–35°C. BLM should be reconstituted in 1–5 ml. of sterile water for injection, dextrose 5% water, or normal saline for injection. The diluent used should contain a bacteriostatic agent if prolonged storage is anticipated.[18] After dilution as above, the resulting solution is stable for at least 1 month if properly preserved and refrigerated or for 2 weeks at room temperature. Admixture compatibility shows that it is stable for at least 24 hours in dextrose 5% and water containing heparin 100 or 1,000 units per ml. final volume. BLM doses chelate various divalent and trivalent cations; therefore, the drug should not be admixed with solutions containing these ions (especially copper). BLM is also reported to be physically incompatible with ascorbic acid injection and to be inactivated by compounds containing sulfhydryl groups.

One of the principal considerations in the choice between continuous infusion, intermittent infusion, or I.V. bolus administration is the practical one of drug stability. Recent studies have been performed to establish the relative stability of BLM when prepared and administered in underfilled plastic and glass administration containers.[19]

In final solution, the drug was measured by HPLC. The results showed no significant loss of potency when bleomycin sulfate in 5% dextrose in water was administered in a glass container over 24 hours. When the same final solution was placed in plastic containers, there was a 10% loss of activity in 1 hour and 13.8% loss over 24 hours. These data suggest that prolonged infusion of BLM in plastic containers should be avoided.

Clinical Trials in Humans

The superiority of continuous infusion bleomycin in cell culture systems and in certain animal tumor models has led to the development of many therapeutic programs employing the continuous infusion schedule.[20,21]

Although there are no larger prospective controlled studies in humans comparing the efficacy and toxicity of continuous infusion versus bolus injection BLM therapy, several groups have reported either increased efficacy or decreased pulmonary toxicity when using a continuous infusion of BLM. Comparisons have been made to the result seen when using data derived from bolus injections in historical controls.[20,21]

Testicular Cancer

In 1970, Samuels et al initiated studies in the treatment of advanced non-seminomatous testicular cancer, using a 2-drug combination of vinblastine (VLB) and BLM.[22]

This initial study used dosages of 0.4 to 0.6 mg/kg of VLB on days 1 and 2, plus BLM $15\mu/m^2$ twice weekly. The study demonstrated 17/51 (33%) complete remissions (CR) with a relapse rate of 23%. In 1973, the BLM schedule was changed from intermittent to continuous infusion administration.[23] BLM was administered in a dose of 30 units in 1,000 ml of dextrose 5% in water over a 24-hour period daily for 5 consecutive days starting on day 2 of each cycle. VLB was given in a total dose of 0.4 mg/kg split into 2 fractions on days 1 and 2, but no less than 30 mg as the initial loading dose. Therapy was repeated every 28–35 days as toxicity permitted. A CR rate of 38% was reported. Although the CR rate is comparable with both methods of administration, the authors contend that there were more advanced patients in the infusion study. There was no difference in the incidence of pulmonary toxicity.

A second study used continuous infusion BLM in a group of patients with metastatic nonseminomatous testicular cancer who had been previously treated with combination chemotherapy that included BLM. Bleomycin was administered for 7–8 days followed by a single I.V. dose of cisplatin (DDP).[24] Eleven of 16 patients exhibited partial remissions (PR); 2 others had minor responses even though they had received previous BLM therapy. Although the author reported that these responses were evident before DDP was administered, the addition of the DDP confounds precise interpretation of the data.

Continuous infusion BLM is an integral component of the VAB-6 program for testicular cancer.[25] Although there are no direct comparisons available, there is no evidence to suggest that VAB-6 is superior to the more conventional treatment with VLB (or etoposide), DDP, and BLM administered by weekly bolus injection.[26]

Head and Neck Cancer

Several investigators have reported on the activity of high-dose cisplatin combined with a continuous infusion of BLM in previously untreated patients with advanced squamous cell carcinomas of the head and neck.[27,28,29] Randolph et al[27] reported a 71% objective tumor response in 21 previously untreated patients with unresectable disease. Hong et al[28] confirmed these results, using the same regimen in 39 patients; 8 achieved complete tumor clearance and 22 had partial responses, for a major response rate of 76% prior to the initiation of definitive radiation therapy and/or surgery. Glick et al[29] modified the above program by giving the DDP portion of the regimen via 24-hour continuous infusion in an attempt to decrease the G.I. and renal toxicity. The BLM was administered 15 units per m^2 I.V. push on day 3 and was followed by a 5-day continuous I.V. infusion of 15 u/m^2/day. Fourteen of 29 patients (48%) achieved an objective PR.

No studies are available that directly compare I.V. bolus to continuous infusion BLM in head and neck cancer. Considering the responsiveness of untreated stage 3 and 4 disease and the background of preexisting pulmonary disease in this patient population, a definitive study evaluating response and toxicity could be readily designed in this patient group.

Cooper and Hong have reported an extensive evaluation of pulmonary function tests in patients receiving continuous infusion of BLM (15 u/m^2 bolus followed by 15 u/m^2/day $\times$ 7 days) combined with DDP.[30] Thirteen of 15 patients had head and neck cancer, and 11/15 had documented preexisting pulmonary disease. Pulmonary function tests were performed prior to therapy and at 1, 3, and 6 months thereafter. No statistically significant abnormality in any parameter developed. Three of the 13 (23%) evaluable patients developed x-ray changes compatible with BLM pulmonary toxicity. None developed documented severe BLM pulmonary toxicty. The mean total dose administered was 227 units (range 165–289 units). The authors concluded that continuous infusion may be less toxic than intermittent bolus injection. However, it should be emphasized that definite BLM pulmonary toxicity occurs sporadically at total doses of 250–300 units,[12] which belies any definite conclusion concerning these uncontrolled results.

Cervical Cancer

Enhanced antitumor efficacy of BLM in patients with squamous cell carcinoma of the cervix has been claimed when BLM is administered by continuous infusion, with a 30% response rate in 32 patients, including 2 CR.[24] This 30%

rate was compared with reports of a 9% response rate for cervical carcinoma treated with bolus methods of BLM administration. With both methods of administration, the response duration is extremely short. Concerning toxicity, there was almost universal skin toxicity in patients receiving the infusional therapy. Also, the incidence of alopecia appeared significantly higher than that seen with bolus injection (71% vs 30%).

A comparison of 3 schedules of BLM (weekly, twice weekly, and a 4-day infusion) in combination with vincristine (VCR) and mitomycin (MIT) in the treatment of advanced carcinoma of the cervix showed a significantly longer median survival time with continuous infusion treatments than with weekly injections, although the overall survival time was short in both groups (6 months versus 4 months).[31] Twice weekly injections had a somewhat higher response rate than did infusions (60% versus 39%) but a shorter duration of response (9 weeks versus 16 weeks). Six of 53 patients treated with twice-weekly BLM developed severe pulmonary toxicity, but no severe pulmonary toxicity was seen among 42 patients treated by the infusion method. Unfortunately, there is no thorough description of the patient-related factors that might predispose to toxicity in each patient group.

Severe leukopenia was significantly less common in patients treated with infusion BLM as compared to those treated by bolus injection.

Lymphomas

Early studies with BLM infusional therapy established its effectiveness in several types of lymphomas.[32] When BLM is employed by bolus administration in the combination chemotherapy of non-Hodgkins lymphoma, it appears that low total doses of the drug result in a higher incidence of significant pulmonary toxicity than would be expected with similar doses and schedules employed in other diseases.[12,33,34] The incidence of pulmonary toxicity in non-Hodgkins lymphoma is substantially reduced by decreasing the dose of BLM employed.[33,34] Since no clear dose-response relationship for BLM has been established in lymphomas, this suggests that a low-dose continuous I.V. infusion of bleomycin may be as effective and less toxic than other methods of administration. Ginsberg et al[35] conducted a pilot study in which continuous I.V. infusions of 2 units of BLM per day for 5 consecutive days was given in combination with cyclophosphamide, doxorubicin, VCR, and prednisone (BACOP) for therapy of non-Hodgkins lymphoma.

The primary aims of the study were to assess toxicity and to investigate the pharmacokinetics of the low-dose continuous infusion of BLM. The pharmacokinetic data confirmed that detectable steady-state plasma concentrations of BLM can be obtained even with the administration of 2 u/day of the drug.

A therapeutic response frequency among 37 previously untreated patients was similar to that obtained using the same chemotherapy program employing the I.V. bolus administration of BLM. Neither clinical pulmonary toxicity nor subclinical pulmonary changes, as determined by serial measurement of the single-breath carbon dioxide-diffusing capacity, was observed. A recent update of this study revealed no therapeutic advantages to the BLM-containing program.[36]

Holister et al[37] examined the use of continuous infusion VCR and BLM with prednisone as a nonmyelosuppressive combination regimen for refractory non-Hodgkin's lymphoma. The program consisted of continuous infusion of vincristine at 1–2 mg per m²/day for 2 days followed by BLM at 0.25 units/kg given by bolus injection immediately followed by 0.12 units/kg infused daily for 5 consecutive days. Responding patients went on to receive a high-dose methotrexate regimen of 1,500 mg/m² with citrovorum rescue on days 15, 22, 29, and 36. Treatment cycles were repeated every 6 weeks in responding patients. Of 16 patients treated in this fashion, 3 had complete and 5 had partial responses, with a median response duration of 29 weeks. These occurred despite reported "resistance" to the standard bolus method of administration of VCR in all of these patients and to previous bolus BLM in all but 1 of the cases. The study design could not distinguish which agent administered by continuous infusion was responsible for this effect.

The implication of this study is that "resistance" to certain drugs may be schedule-dependent. This intriguing result has yet to be confirmed by other investigators.

Other Tumors

Kolaric et al, in testing BLM infusions combined with radiotherapy in inoperable squamous cell carcinoma of the esophagus, demonstrated a CR and PR rate of 52% in 25 patients.[38] The program consisted of BLM administered at a dose of 15 units/m² over 12 hours twice weekly, with concurrent radiation therapy, to a total dose of 3,600 to 4,000 rads. This trial did not involve a concurrent control group with BLM applied in the form of I.V. bolus injections. However, the same investigator found a response rate of 62% (15/24 patients) with 6 CR and 9 PR in a previous study using I.V. bolus BLM administration. Using this historical control group, one would conclude that BLM infusion combined with concurrent radiation therapy in the treatment of inoperable esophageal cancer presents no advantage over the conventional I.V. bolus method of bleomycin administration. On the other hand, the 12-hour infusion method used is theoretically less than optimal, inasmuch as a BLM infusion not preceded by an I.V. bolus dose would not be expected to reach steady-state levels until approximately 10 hours. One could argue that a 12-hour infusion administered twice weekly does not take full advantage of the potential for long-term BLM infusion. Nathanson[39] has investigated 2 regimens, both of which used continuous infusion BLM in combination with either VLB alone or with VLB plus DDP in the treatment of far advanced metastatic malignant melanoma. The initial regimen consisted of VLB 8 mg/m² given by I.V. bolus injection on days 1 and 2 followed by administration of BLM 20 u/m² by continuous 24-hour infusion for 5 consecutive days. The second regimen employed VLB 6 mg/m² on days 1 and 2, BLM 15 u/m² by continuous 24-hour infusion for 5 consecutive days, and DDP 25 mg/m² administered as a 1-hour

I.V. infusion with appropriate forced diuresis on days 4 and 5 of each regimen cycle. These investigations were prompted by the results reported by Mabel et al,[40] who evaluated the combination of BLM plus VLB in the murine B-16 melanoma model. The results demonstrated that the combination produced an increase in life span and cures when compared to either of the 2 agents used alone against both intraperitoneal and subcutaneous B-16 melanoma. When administered to humans with far advanced malignant melanoma, 4/9 evaluable patients receiving the 2-drug combination and 3/3 receiving the 3-drug combination demonstrated objective regression in this pilot project.

A more extensive evaluation of the 3-drug regimen was carried out by the same investigator[41] in 42 patients with advanced malignant melanoma. This study demonstrated a 47% partial response rate in evaluable patients treated. Severe hematologic and G.I. toxicity was encountered.

Pulmonary function, as measured by DL_{CO}, was frequently found to be impaired over the course of treatment, although no patient progressed to the point of life-threatening toxicity. The optimism generated by this positive pilot study prompted several confirmatory studies. The National Cancer Institute of Canada Melanoma Group[42] and investigators at Yale University[43] almost simultaneously initiated studies using the 3-drug combination described by Nathanson.[39,41] The Canadian study was a nonrandomized single-arm trial in which all eligible patients were registered to the 3-drug combination. The study conducted at Yale University was a randomized prospective trial comparing the 3-drug regimen as described above to what many regard as the standard treatment of advanced metastatic melanoma — dacarbazine in a dose of 2 mg/kg/day for 10 days by I.V. injection. The results of both studies were discouraging at best. The Canadian study demonstrated a response in 12/64 patients treated (19%), whereas the Yale group demonstrated only a 10% response for the 3-drug combination, which was similar to the 14% demonstrated for the single-agent treatment with dacarbazine. In addition, the dacarbazine responses were associated with a trend toward longer progression-free intervals and longer survival. The toxicity on both studies was significant for the 3-drug combination arm. Both studies conclude that the BVD combination is not as effective as previously reported and, because of major toxicity, cannot be recommended for initial treatment of metastatic melanoma.

Morantz has presented preliminary experimental data using the 9L gliosarcoma brain tumor model demonstrating that an intratumoral dose of BLM is more effective in prolonging survival than an I.V. dose 25 times as great.[44] A combination of intracerebrally administered BLM and radiation therapy was more effective than either modality alone. Furthermore, the combination of BLM delivered intracerebrally and BCNU given systemically was more effective than either agent used alone. Phase 1 clinical trials of BLM given via an Ommaya reservoir to 8 patients with recurrent malignant brain tumors demonstrated that individual doses of up to 7.5 units and cumulative doses of up to 255 units can be administered without significant toxicity. Based on this initial trial, a phase 1 study has been initiated in patients who, at the time of craniotomy for recurrent tumor, have an Ommaya reservoir and an Infusaid Model 400 pump implanted. BLM is administered by continuous infusion into the tumor cavity. Doses of BLM to date have ranged from 0.75–1.7 u/day at flow rates of 1.5–2.2 ml/day. Total dosage administered has ranged from 63 to 153 units. With the possible exception of cerebral edema, which has been well controlled with the use of corticosteroids, no untoward side effects of this method of drug delivery have been encountered.

Discussion

As stated above, evaluation of continuous infusion of BLM is supported by several characteristics of the drug, including its pattern of in vitro cytotoxicity, cell cycle phase specificity, pharmacokinetics after rapid I.V. injection, and preclinical data that indicate an increase in therapeutic index and a decrease in pulmonary toxicity in certain animal systems. Although the theoretical base for the continuous infusion schedule is sound, clinical data that would prove its advantage are presently lacking. Authors of certain small studies have claimed either an advantage in activity or a decrease in pulmonary toxicity with the continuous infusion schedule. None of these studies, however, conclusively support these contentions. Concerning pulmonary toxicity, a significant imbalance in any common factor such as age, significant preexisting pulmonary abnormalities, or prior chest radiotherapy could lead to erroneous conclusions based on small, uncontrolled trials. In addition, most uncontrolled studies employ different endpoints, a factor that can significantly alter the reported "incidence" of pulmonary toxicity.

Considering the rather narrow spectrum of activity for BLM , one would have envisioned trials in head and neck cancer, lymphoma, or testicular cancer that ultimately might have appropriately addressed the issues of increased antitumor activity as a function of bolus versus the continuous infusion schedule. No such studies currently exist.

On the other hand, data from uncontrolled trials indicate that there does not appear to be any significant disadvantage in terms of objective response with the use of the continuous infusion schedule. The need for further studies is emphasized by the fact that preclinical studies have shown that the advantage of continuous infusion may be disease-restricted; therefore, a positive result in one disease would not necessarily support its general application. The only controlled, randomized study comparing intermittent administration to continuous infusion BLM is, unfortunately, flawed in many respects.[31] This study was performed in patients with advanced cervical cancer, a rather chemotherapy-insensitive disease; important patient-related characteristics are not thoroughly presented; the data are derived from randomized and nonradomized patients; and an unexplained imbalance in the randomized portion of the trial is apparent. A modest improvement in response duration and survival was reported with the continuous administration schedule. Additionally, the incidence of "severe" pulmonary toxicity was reportedly lower when the continuous administration schedule (0/42 patients) was compared to the twice weekly schedule (6/53 patients). This apparently positive effect is somewhat clouded by the results in those patients receiving the weekly administration, where no such effect was noted.

In summary, the optimal mode of administration of BLM is currently not known. Theoretical considerations support the continued interest and investigation of the continuous infusion schedule, but additional studies should address the questions of activity and toxicity in controlled trials. Short of this, the next 15 years of research may yield data as inconclusive as those from the past 15 years.

16

THE EPIPODOPHYLLOTOXINS:
VP-16 AND VM-26

Nancy Phillips, R.Ph., and Robert L. Comis, M.D.

THE ROLE OF THE epipodophyllotoxins tenoposide (VM-26) and etoposide (VP-16) in the treatment of a variety of solid tumors and hematologic malignancies has been clearly established. This is particularly true of VP-16. Although both drugs possess comparable in vitro activities in human tumors,[1] the use of VM-26 has been somewhat limited to the treatment of childhood malignancies, and VP-16 has been primarily tested in adults. VP-16 has gained wide acceptance for the treatment of small-cell lung cancer and testicular cancer. Its activity is being further defined in other malignancies such as Hodgkin's and non-Hodgkin's lymphomas and in nonsmall-cell lung cancer, leukemias, and breast cancer.

A theoretical advantage may exist for administering the epipodophyllotoxins by continuous infusion as compared to the established method of intermittent dosing. Experimental evidence suggesting this advantage includes the mechanism of action, clinical pharmacology, and schedule dependency of both VP-16 and VM-26.

Clinical trials evaluating the effectiveness of continuous infusion VP-16 have been somewhat limited, particularly with regard to comparative trials. VM-26 administered as a continuous infusion is even less well studied.

Mechanism of Action

VP-16 and VM-26 possess similar mechanisms of action that relate to their ability to inhibit DNA synthesis. Their cytotoxic effects are believed to result from DNA strand breakage as first described for VP-16 by Loike et al[2] and subsequently for VM-26.[3] Further investigations have provided support for single- and double-strand DNA breakage as the primary mechanism of action.[4,5,6] On a molar basis, VP-16 is about 1/10th as effective as VM-26 in inducing DNA strand breakage.[7] Their ability to induce DNA breakage in vitro has been shown to be concentration-dependent. DNA breakage has been reported when cells have been exposed for 1 hour at concentrations as low as 1μM for VP-16[4] and 0.05μM for VM-26.[6] DNA breaks occur rapidly, with little increase after 30 min. of continuous exposure; repair of these breaks occurs rapidly once the drug is removed.

Recent studies suggest that the effects of VP-16 and VM-26 on DNA may be related to their ability to act as inhibitors of the DNA ligase activity of the type 2 topoisomerases.[8,9]

VP-16 and VM-26 are believed to be cell cycle-specific and phase-specific, with maximal cell death occurring between the S and G_2 portions of the cell cycle.[5,10,11]

Clinical Pharmacology

VP-16 (Short Infusion)

The disposition of VP-16 after I.V. infusion generally administered over 30 to 60 min. has been studied in adults and children using radiolabeled drug,[12,13] high-pressure liquid chromatography (HPLC),[14-19] and radioimmunoassay (RIA).[20,21] A biexponential plasma decay, with an elimination half-life generally in the range of 6–8 hours, as shown in table 1, was confirmed by all studies with the exception of the study by one group of investigators where there was triexponential plasma decay, with a terminal half-life ($t^1/_2$) of 20–46 hours.[15]

At typical plasma concentrations, 94% of VP-16 is protein-bound.[13] Distribution into the CSF is minimal, generally reported as < 10% of the concurrent plasma concentration.[12,21,22]

Recovery of a dose of I.V. VP-16, the majority of which is detected in the urine, is variable. Following the administration of a dose of radiolabeled VP-16, about 45% of the radioactivity has been recovered in the urine, which

Table 1. Plasma Kinetics of Etoposide*

Dose (mg/m²)	Terminal + ½ (hr)	Assay
70 – 290	11.06 ± 6.0	Radioisotopic
200	6 – 8(20 – 46)[a]	HPLC
100 – 200	7.05 ± 0.67	HPLC
80	5.95	HPLC
400 – 800	8.1 ± 4.3	HPLC
40 – 120/day	3 – 14	RIA
200[b]	6.5 ± 1.6[c]	HPLC
200[b]	5.7 ± 1.3[d]	HPLC

[a]triexponential plasma decay
[b]Study performed in children:
    [c]with solid tumors
    [d]with leukemia
*Adapted from Creavan[47] and Evans.[48]

presumably included some of the metabolites.[12] Using the HPLC assay, 20–46.5% of unchanged VP-16 has been found in the urine.[17,23] It should be remembered that HPLC assays using chloroform extraction do not allow the identification of water-soluble metabolites such as the cis-hydoxy acid. Biliary excretion of VP-16 is generally minimal (<1.5% of a dose), but up to 16% of a dose has been found in the feces of some patients.[12]

The major urinary metabolite of VP-16 is 4'-demethylepipodophyllic acid glucopyranoside (hydroxy acid).[21,24,25] Low levels of the picro lactone isomer have also been identified.[25] Although the hydroxy acid metabolite is devoid of cytotoxic effects, the picro derivative does produce G_2 phase arrest, but only at 100 times the concentration of VP-16 in vitro.[26]

VP-16 Bioavailability

We have recently completed a study evaluating the absolute bioavailability of VP-16.[27] The drug was administered orally, using the soft gelatin capsule, or intravenously at doses of 160 and 80 mg/m[2], respectively. Patients served as their own control, receiving the dose by the alternate route on 2 consecutive cycles of therapy. VP-16 was measured in plasma by HPLC, after chloroform extraction. The level of sensitivity of this assay is 0.1 µg/ml for plasma for 5 µg/ml for urine.

The median bioavailability was 48.4%, with a wide range among patients, 24.9–73.7%. The median $t^{1/2}$ was 6.8 and 5.3 hours, after oral and I.V. dosing, respectively, with significant variability in the half-life after both routes of administration. No significant difference in any important pharmacokinetic parameter was established when the oral and I.V. doses were compared.

The t max, or time to the maximal drug concentration (Cmax), was 1.12 hours (range 0.75–4 hrs.). T max was inversely related to bioavailability and Cmax was related to bioavailability in a linear fashion. The wide range in both parameters and the small numbers of patients in the study precluded using either as a predictive indicator of bioavailability.

High-Dose VP-16

The pharmacology of high-dose VP-16 has also been investigated.[28] After administration of 400–800 mg/m[2]/day for 3 days a bioexponential decay of VP-16 occurred, with a $t^{1/2}$ of 8.1 ± 4.3 hours. Although higher VP-16 plasma levels are obtained when compared to those achieved with conventional doses, the pharmacokinetics are similar for both high-dose and conventional-dose VP-16.

VP-16 (Continuous Infusion)[23]

Typical plasma levels of VP-16 after continuous infusion at 100 mg/m[2]/24 hours for 72 hours are shown in figure 1. Steady-state plasma levels in the range of 2–5 µg/ml are reached 2–3 hours after the start of the infusion. Following the end of the continuous infusion, the disposition of VP-16 is similar to that seen with rapid administration of the drug.

VM-26 (Short Infusion)

Few studies have been performed on the disposition of VM-26. Radiolabeled VM-26 was used in early pharmacokinetic trials performed in adult patients.[13,29] Plasma decay was triexponential, with a t¹/₂ of 21.2 hours.[29] More recent studies in children using a HPLC assay demonstrated a biexponential plasma decay, with a mean t¹/₂ of about 9 hours.[19,30]

VM-26 is more highly protein-bound than VP-16 (99.6% versus 94%),[29,13] and distribution into the CSF is generally <1% of the administered dose.[30,31]

Approximately 44% of radioactivity has been recovered in the urine when labeled VM-26 was administered, 21% of which was unchanged drug. Fecal recovery ranged from 0–10%.[29] Both the hydroxy acid metabolite and picro isomers have been detected.[19]

The systemic clearance of VP-16 is 3 times faster than for VM-26,[13,19] and so is the maximally tolerated dose.

VM-26 (Continuous Infusion)

The disposition of VM-26 given as a prolonged infusion has been reported.[32] Six ovarian cancer patients received a 1-hour intravenous infusion of 80 mg/m² followed by a 24-hour infusion of 120 mg/m². Plasma steady-state levels of 4–10 µg/ml were obtained at 4–9 hours during the continuous infusion. The mean t¹/₂ was 8.6 ± 1.1 hour. Only 6% of unchanged VM-26 was detected in the urine of patients up to 24 hours after the end of the infusion. The aglycone metabolite was found in the urine of all patients treated, corresponding to about 8% of the dose. This result is particularly interesting because this metabolite, which had not been identified in any previous studies, exerts its cytotoxic effect by inhibiting the microtubule assembly.[26,33]

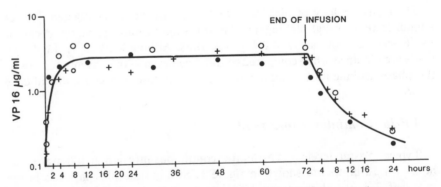

Figure 1.   VP–16 plasma levels in 3 patients receiving 72–hour continuous infusion (100 mg/m²/24 hr)*
*From D'Incalci et al[23]

Schedule Dependency

Preclinical animal studies in the L1210 leukemia system[34,35] and in Lewis lung carcinoma[36] have demonstrated that the activities of VP-16 and VM-26 are schedule-dependent. Repeated daily doses were superior to single-day treatments only. In addition, an advantage was found for administering VP-16 and VM-26 by divided injections every 3 hours.[34,35]

Although the evidence in humans for schedule dependency is not conclusive, an advantage for administering VP-16 over several days has been suggested.[37] In a randomized trial reported by Cavalli et al[38] using VP-16 for small-cell lung cancer, giving the drug over 3-5 consecutive days resulted in higher response rates than when administered once weekly.

Pharmaceutical Data

VP-16 and VM-26 are poorly soluble in water and are supplied for clinical use in nonaqueous parenteral formulations for I.V. administration. Early stability data suggested that VP-16 was incompatible with 5% dextrose injection USP. and therefore should be mixed with 0.9% sodium chloride injection USP.[39] In order to ensure stability for 6 hours, it was suggested that dilute solutions of at least 1 part VP-16 to 100 parts normal saline (volume to volume) be prepared. More recently, VP-16 has been shown to be stable in both 5% dextrose injection USP and 0.9% sodium chloride injection USP for 96 and 48 hours at concentrations of 0.2 to 0.4 mg/ml, respectively.[40]

VM-26 may also be diluted with 0.9% sodium chloride injection USP or 5% dextrose injection USP. When diluted with 5–20 volumes of diluent, VM-26 is stable for approximately 4 hours and with 50–100 volumes, for 6 hours.[41]

Clinical Trials

Continuous Infusion VP-16

Several trials of continuous infusion VP-16 have been performed, and the results have been reported over the past several years.

PHASE 1 STUDIES

Lokich et al[42] administered VP-16 as a continuous infusion for 5 days to 24 patients with advanced malignancy. A total of 30 courses were given. The maximally tolerated dose (MTD) was 60 mg/m^2/day, and the authors concluded that a reasonable starting dose for good-risk patients was as high as 80 mg/m^2/day, whereas for poor-risk patients the initial dose should be 50 mg/m^2/day. The dose-limiting toxicity in this study was myelosuppression; as shown in table 2, this was life-threatening in 3 patients, including 1 patient who had a septic death. The median duration of leukopenia and thrombocytopenia was 8 days. Stomatitis, which occurred in 17% of patients, was the only

G.I. toxicity noted. Dependent edema and congestive heart failure, which responded to treatment with cardiac glycosides and diuretics, was observed; this was attributed to the 1–2 L of normal saline necessary to deliver the VP-16 each day. It is important to point out that these investigators followed the early stability guidelines, which necessitated dilution of VP-16 with large volumes of normal saline. Partial responses were observed in 3 patients, 2 with lymphomas and 1 with an adenocarcinoma of the lung.

The MTD for VP-16 administered as a continuous 5-day infusion, as reported by Aisner et al,[43] was 125 mg/m^2/day. The dose-limiting toxicity was myelosuppression in this study also, consisting of both life-threatening leukopenia and thrombocytopenia. Median days to WBC nadirs and recovery occurred at day 15 and day 24, respectively; median days to platelet count nadirs and recovery were at day 12 and day 24. Other toxicities observed are shown in table 3. Once again, the normal saline believed necessary to dilute the VP-16 was implicated as a contributing factor for the cardiac effects. Of the 17 patients treated, 10 were evaluable for response. Two patients had partial

Table 2. Dose Escalation and Marrow Toxicity in Phase 1 Study of Continuous-Infusion VP–16†

Dose (mg/m^2/day)	No. patients	WBC count (cells/mm^3)		Platelet count (cells/mm^3)	
		< 1,000	1,000 – 3,000	< 50,000	50,000 – 100,000
20	3	0	0	0	0
30	2	0	0	0	0
40	2	0	0	0	0
50	2	0	0	0	0
60	7	3	3	3	1
70	7	2/4*	3/4*	1/4*	1/4*
80	2	0	1/1*	0	0

*Denominator = only patients for whom weekly blood cell counts were available
†Reprinted from Lokich et al[42] with permission

Table 3. Nonhematologic Toxicity from Phase 1 Continuous Infusion VP–16*

Type	Dose (mg/m^2/day × 5)			
	75	100	125	150
Nausea and vomiting	0	1	2	3
Mucositis (mild)	0	0	2	4
Diarrhea	0	1	0	2
Fever/granulocytopenia	0	0	2	5
Cardiac[a]	0	1[b]	1[c]	1[d]

[a]All patients "cardiotoxicity" had preexisting cardiovascular disease.
[b]One patient had anteroseptal infarction.
[c]Patient developed congestive failure and expired on day 8.
[d]Patient developed anteroseptal infarction on day 4 of course 2.
*Reprinted from Aisner et al[43] with permission

responses (PR), 1 with disseminated seminoma and 1 with renal cell carcinoma who had a response lasting 3 weeks.

PHASE 2 STUDIES

Schell et al[44] performed a randomized phase 2 trial in patients with refractory metastatic breast cancer, comparing equivalent doses of VP-16 administered as an intermittent 5-day bolus to a continuous 5-day infusion. Doses ranged from 50–70 mg/m^2/day. Of the 77 patients entered, 66 patients were evaluated for response. The results of this study, which included 35 patients on the intermittent schedule and 31 on the infusion schedule, are given in table 4. Although no advantage was demonstrated for the infusion group, patient characteristics were not considered to be equally distributed. Patients receiving continuous infusion VP-16 had a poorer performance status and a higher degree of tumor burden, both of which were described as marginal. A comparison of the toxicities reported in the 2 groups of patients is shown in table 5. Myelosuppression, the most common toxicity in both groups, was severe in about half of the patients. Gastrointestinal effects were more pronounced in the intermittent group, and heart failure secondary to saline administration was prominent in the continuous infusion group.

In another study reported by Steward et al,[45] VP-16 was administered at a dose of 600 mg/m^2 over 24 hours every 3 weeks to 35 patients with metastatic lung cancer; 14 had small-cell cancer (SCLC) and 21 had nonsmall-cell lung cancer (NSCLC). There were 3 PR, 2 in patients with NSCLC and 1 with SCLC. The toxicities reported with this 24-hour infusion schedule were minimal. There was no leukopenia or thrombocytopenia in 54% and 80% of patients, respectively.

PHASE 3 STUDIES

One randomized phase 3 trial comparing combinations of other agents plus VP-16 administered as a continuous infusion and as a short infusion has been reported. Aisner et al[46] treated patients with small-cell lung cancer with

Table 4. Response Rates in Refractory Metastatic Breast Cancer*

	Intermittent	Infusion	Total
CR	–	1 (3%)	1 (2%)
PR	5 (14%)	3 (10%)	8 (12%)
< PR	3 (9%)	3 (10%)	6 (9%)
SD	6 (17%)	5 (16%)	11 (17%)
PD	21 (60%)	19 (61%)	40 (60%)

Response duration

	Intermittent	Infusion	Total
Time to progression: Months (range)	4 (3 – 10)	5 (2 – 12 +)	5 (2 – 12 +)

*Reprinted from Schell et al[44] with permission

cyclophosphamide 1,000 mg/m^2, Adriamycin 45 mg/m^2, and VP-16 given either as 50 mg/m^2/day for 5 days over 1 hour or as 100 mg/m^2/day for 5 days by continuous infusion. The results of this study showed no significant difference in response or survival for either group (see table 6). A detailed comparison of adverse reactions was not included in this preliminary report.

Table 5. Toxicity in Refractory Metastatic Breast Cancer*

	Intermittent (%)	Infusion (%)
Total no. of patients	35	31
Alopecia	(29)	(23)
Nausea/vomiting		
(moderate to severe)	(29)	(3)
Anorexia	(29)	(19)
Diarrhea	(11)	(13)
Anaphylactoid reaction	(3)	(0)
Congestive heart failure		
(Reversible; secondary to saline)	(3)	(16)
Thrombocytopenia		
(< 100,000/mm^3)	(35)	(40)
Hemorrhage		
(life-threatening	(0)	(0)
Granulocytopenia		
(< 1,000 mm^3)	(60)	(50)
Infections	(11)	(19)

*Reprinted from Schell et al[44] with permission

Table 6. Response Rates in Patients with Small-Cell Lung Carcinoma Treated with Adriamycin, Cyclophosphamide and Etoposide (ACE)*

	ACE I[a]	ACE II[b]
Limited disease	N = 12	N = 15
	CR = 75%	CR = 53%
	PR = 8%	PR = 27%
	Total = 83%	Total = 80%
Extensive disease	N = 14	N = 15
	CR = 57%	CR = 47%
	PR = 21%	PR = 20%
	Total = 78%	Total = 67%

[a]Cyclophosphamide 1,000 mg/m^2, Adriamycin 45 mg/m^2, etoposide 50 mg/m^2/day over 1 h × 5 days
[b]Cyclophosphamide 1,000 mg/m^2, Adriamycin 45 mg/m^2, etoposide 100 mg/m^2/day × 5 days by continuous infusion
*Adapted from Aisner et al[46]

Continuous Infusion VM-26

To date, a single trial of VM-26 administered as a prolonged infusion to 6 patients with ovarian cancer has been published.[32] This investigation was instituted as a pharmacokinetic study as described earlier in this review. Treatment was described as being relatively well tolerated, with moderate leukopenia. None of the 6 patients responded.

Discussion

The potential value of continuous administration of an anticancer drug relates to the pharmacokinetics of the agent, its pharmacodynamics and cellular pharmacology, cell cycle phase specificity, and the effect of peak dose on antitumor effects or toxicity. The data presented above describe the differences in these various parameters for the two epipodophyllotoxins most often used in the clinic, VP-16 and VM-26.

On a pharmacokinetic level, VP-16 and VM-26 could be considered suitable for continuous infusion programs. Their elimination half-lives are generally on the order of 6–9 hours. Considering the pharmacodynamics and cellular pharmacology of these agents, it appears that both exert their antitumor effect by inducing single- and double-strand DNA breaks. Because rapid DNA repair occurs after removing the drug in vitro, one could speculate on the potential advantages for continuous exposure in vivo. Both agents appear to exert their maximal cytotoxic effect in the S and G_2 phases of the cell cycle. Usually administered by bolus, both drugs share myelotoxicity as their dose-limiting toxicity; neither agent has a major toxic end organ effect that continuous exposure might preclude. In summary, there are certain factors that favor the exploration of continuous exposure programs for the epipodophyllotoxins.

The pharmacology of VP-16 has been more extensively evaluated than that of VM-26. As noted above, several studies have evaluated VP-16 administered by continuous infusion. In general, these studies have shown that the maximally tolerated dose appears comparable when the drug is administered by bolus administration or continuous infusion. It is interesting to note that (in certain studies) the incidence of stomatitis appears higher after continuous administration. Studies performed at Vanderbilt have evaluated the pharmacokinetics of high-dose administration.[28] Doses of 400–800 mg/m² produce plasma drug levels within the potentially therapeutic range for 24 hours. Although the nature of these studies precludes the separation of an exceptionally high-peak drug effect from continuous exposure, this method of administration does produce a continuous exposure. In this setting, mucositis is the dose-limiting toxicity. Finally, it is conceivable that continuous exposure could be accomplished by repeated oral administration on a schedule of every 6–8 hours. Unfortunately, the wide range in bioavailability and absorption argues against the precision and reproducibility of this method.

Objective responses have been obtained with VP-16 administered by bolus, continuous infusion of conventional doses, and high-dose administration providing continuous exposure. Two randomized studies have shown no difference in antitumor effect in either breast cancer or small-cell carcinoma of the lung when VP-16 was administered by bolus or continuous infusion over 5 days. Studies in VP-16-responsive diseases such as lymphoma and testicular carcinoma have not been performed.

Far fewer data are available for VM-26 administered by continuous infusion. The recent study by Rossi et al,[32] if confirmed by other investigators, may be of considerable interest. Significant levels of VM-26 aglycone appear to be produced with continuous infusion. This compound is cytotoxic and exerts its effect through a mechanism different from that of the parent compound. Thus, 2 potentially different "drugs" may be involved. Such an approach could be of considerable interest and potential value in the future.

In summary, the data available for the continuous infusion of VP-16 do not show any striking toxicologic or therapeutic advantage for this method of administration. It should be noted, however, that at the present time, only 2 controlled studies have addressed efficacy in a randomized, controlled fashion: one in a minimally VP-16 responsive disease (breast cancer) and the other in small-cell lung cancer, a highly responsive disease. Further studies employing VM-26 administered by continuous infusion are indicated because data currently available are sparse. In addition, the preliminary evidence indicating that continuous administration of the parent compound may produce significant levels of the VM-26 aglycone, a mitotic spindle inhibitor, need to be confirmed and investigated further.

17

ALKYLATING DRUGS AND OTHER AGENTS

Jacob J. Lokich, M.D.

T HE ALKYLATING AGENTS AS a group have not been considered ideal agents for continuous infusion in spite of the fact that the pharmacology for most of the component drugs in the alkylating group is such that the plasma half-life and therefore tumor exposure time is relatively short. The hesitancy for performing infusion trials with alkylating agents has been related to the misconception that such agents are more effective in noncycling, or G_o cells. In fact, alkylating agents, like all antineoplastic drugs, are more effective in cycling cells relative to noncycling cells, and it is simply that the ratio of cell kill of cycling cells to noncycling cells is less for alkylating agents than, for example, the antimetabolities.

Other agents that may or may not have alkylation as a mechanism of action have not been administered by continuous infusion for other reasons. Some, such as streptozotocin, have such a limited spectrum of tumor activity and are relatively so active on standard bolus delivery that the infusion schedule has simply not been addressed. Nonetheless, it is conceivable that the infusion schedule could expand the tumor spectrum for these agents.

Table 1 shows the collective group of alkylating agents and miscellaneous other drugs that may be considered for a continuous infusion schedule. These agents generally have been administered for short intervals of 24-120 hours, and some have been delivered regionally on a pulse schedule. Each of the agents will be reviewed with regard to the rationale for a continuous infusion schedule based upon either experimental tumor data or pharmacologic data, and the existing clinical trails in which the infusion schedule has been applied will be analyzed.

Alkylating Agents

The alkylating agents represent a group of drugs whose cytotoxic effect is determined by the binding of alkyl groups with a variety of intracellular molecules, including enzymes and nucleic acids, with the major cytotoxic effect being inhibition of DNA synthesis. This group of compounds demonstrates clinical antitumor activity in a wide spectrum of tumors, although as with most antineoplastic drugs, the clinical usefulness of this class of compounds has been predominantly in hematologic malignancy.

The traditional schedule for administration has been on an intermittent bolus program, although the oral formulation for some of the agents (melphalan, chlorambucil and cyclophosphamide) has been a stimulus for their use in a chronic daily or intermittent daily dose schedule. A complicating issue in using oral formulations for these agents is the bioavailability of the drug related to absorption.

The fact that alkylating agents are actively transported across cellular membranes also suggests that high-dose pulse therapy, which may be necessary to promote diffusion across cell membranes for other agents, may be unnecessary for the alkylating drugs. In clinical trials in ovarian cancer, high-dose bolus

Table 1. Alkylating Drugs and Other Agents Delivered by the Infusion Schedule

Drug	t$\frac{1}{2}$ (min.)*
Alkylating agents	
Cyclophosphamide	240 – 390
Thio-tepa	60 – 240
Melphalan	40
Mitomycin-C	47
Antimetabolites	
6 Mercaptopurine	47
Hydroxyurea	180
Miscellaneous cytotoxic agents	
Dimethyltriazeno imidisole carboxamide (DTIC)	75
Streptozotocin	15
Actimomycin D	20
Biologic response modifiers	
Interferon	3 – 34

*t$\frac{1}{2}$ following bolus injection

alkylating agents are comparable to orally administered low-dose alkylating agents administered chronically.[1]

Cyclophosphamide

Cyclophosphamide (CTX) is a unique alkylating agent in that it is activated in the hepatic microsomes to eventually form phosphoramide mustard, the primary mediator of the biologic effect. Therefore, the pharmacology of CTX is complicated by the multiplicity of metabolites formed. Measuring the plasma level of alkylating activity has established the beta half-life $(t^1/_2 \beta)$ for the plasma alkylating activity as approximately 7 hours following bolus delivery.

CTX may be administered orally, as well as parenterally, either I.M. or I.V. The oral formulation provides for fairly complete absorption, so that clinical effects and toxicity are comparable dose-for-dose when the drug is administered by either route. Following reconstitution of the lyophilized preparation, CTX in solution is stable with less than 10% degradation at room temperature for at least 7 days.

In general, CTX is administered I.V. as part of combination chemotherapy programs, but it has also been used in the context of a single agent for bone marrow transplantation as a preparatory regimen. In standard clinical combination chemotherapy, the dose of I.V. CTX administered is 1.0–1.5 grams/m². For bone marrow transplantation, a dose of 60–80 mg/kg/day for 3–4 days is delivered. The oral formulation is often used in the context of immunosuppression in the treatment of collagen vascular diseases, as well as for malignancy in which either chronic daily or every-other-day dosing is the optimal schedule. Thus, for the oral formulation, doses of 50–100 mg/day in a chronic low-dose schedule or up to 200 mg/day in a short-term intermittent schedule are employed.

CTX may be associated with adverse effects that run the usual gamut of alopecia, nausea and vomiting, and bone marrow suppression. Some adverse effects have been related to specific metabolites of CTX that may induce hemorrhagic cystitis. This has prompted the use of neutralizing agents and optimal hydration to minimize this effect. Of some interest also has been the observation of bladder tumors developing in patients treated with CTX over long periods. Pulmonary toxicity has been observed in the context of the use of superlethal doses of CTX as a preparatory regimen for bone marrow transplantation.

The continuous infusion schedule for CTX has been employed in only 2 reported clinical trials using short-term infusion 24 hours a day for 3 or 5 days.[2,3] In a phase 1 study of 72-hour continuous infusion, CTX patients received 300 mg/m²/day to 750 mg/m²/day.[2] Dose-limiting toxicity was marrow suppression. Another study employed 5-day continuous infusions at a dose rate of 400 mg/m²/day.[3] In the latter study, of 42 patients with acute leukemia, 21 achieved complete remission (CR). Protracted infusion of CTX has been reported by Lokich et al[4] at doses of 50–100 mg/m²/day for periods of 28 days or more. Other than establishing the feasibility of this schedule, however, no other data have been reported.

Thio-tepa

Triethylene thio phosphoramide (thio-tepa) is one of the oldest-known alkylating agents, with initial clinical studies having been reported in 1953. The addition of sulfur to triethylene phosphoramide, or tepa, led to a more stable compound in a reconstituted solution and thereby was rendered more useful for clinical trials.

The lyophilized drug is reconstituted with sterile water to yield a concentration of 10 mg/cc; prior to administration it is diluted to a concentration of 1 mg/cc. It is generally administered as an intracavitary or intravesicle agent to control serous effusions and superficial bladder carcinoma, respectively. It has also been used in the treatment of carcinomatous meningitis, delivered via the intrathecal route and as part of combination chemotherapy for the treatment of breast cancer, ovarian cancer, and Hodgkin's disease.

The pharmacology of thio-tepa has recently been studied by Egorin et al[5] and by Kries et al.[6] In the study in patients with breast cancer, plasma concentrations of thio-tepa declined in a biexponential fashion following a bolus injection with a $t^{1}/_{2}\beta$ of 109 $\pm$ 21 min. These studies also demonstrated that the concentrations of tepa exceeded those of thio-tepa after a short time and persisted in plasma longer than the concentrations of thio-tepa, suggesting that thio-tepa may be converted to tepa over time and may represent a major mechanism for plasma clearance.

Continuous infusion of thio-tepa or tepa could be considered a reasonable schedule for this agent based upon the relatively short plasma half-life. A phase 1 trial of infusional thio-tepa over a 24-hour period was reported in 1983.[6] In that trial, patients received 15–35 mg/m^2 over a 48-hour period; the dose-limiting toxicity was myelosuppression. No therapeutic effects were observed in this group of patients.

Because of its instability, tepa has not been available for use in clinical trials for many years, although an early trial of the drug in malignant melanoma[7] suggested activity. In that study, 2/6 patients responded to tepa and 2/6 patients also responded to thio-tepa. The suggestion that thio-tepa may be converted to tepa as the active mediator of the biological effect possibly supports the rationale for an infusion schedule of delivery for thio-tepa. Ongoing phase 1 and 2 trials of short-term protracted infusion of thio-tepa may provide additional information on the clinical usefulness of such a schedule.

Melphalan

L-phenylalanine mustard (L-PAM), or MEL, is an alkylating agent that surfaced in the development of analogues for nitrogen mustard that might have clinical utility. The most common formulation of MEL is as an oral tablet, but parenteral formulations have been available for intra-arterial perfusion, particularly for the treatment of extremity melanoma. The oral formulation has been employed in clinical trials in the treatment of ovarian cancer, breast cancer, and multiple myeloma. Drug absorption studies, however, have demonstrated that the bioavailability of MEL following oral dosing is quite low and quite variable.[8] The use of oral dosing for chronic administration to simulate continuous infusion would therefore be unreliable.

The clinical pharmacology of I.V. MEL demonstrates a $t^1/_2\beta$ of 1.8 hours, suggesting that continuous infusion schedules may have some advantage for the delivery of this alkylating agent.

The delivery of systemic continuous infusion has not been studied in clinical trials to date. There is, however, a vast amount of literature on the regional delivery via the arterial route, generally confined to relatively short-term infusions. These studies have been extensively reviewed by Cumberlin et al.[9]

Mitomycin-C

The antibiotic mitomycin-C (MIT) is derived from *Streptomyces caepitosus* and has its primary mechanism of action an alkylating effect by covalent binding to DNA. The drug has been employed predominantly in combination chemotherapy for the treatment of gastric and pancreatic carcinoma, for which it was approved in 1974. Other tumor applications include administration in combination with vinblastine for breast cancer and as an intravesicle agent for superficial bladder carcinoma.

Initial clinical trials of MIT employed a daily regimen for 6 days at a dose of 50 μg/kg/day administered as an I.V. bolus, with the schedule continued on an every-other-day schedule thereafter to the point of toxicity. Subsequent schedules—particularly when the drug is administered in combination with other agents—have necessitated the use of a bolus at 6-week intervals as a consequence of bleeding disorders secondary to thrombocytopenia, which may develop in a delayed fashion and may accumulate over time.

Toxicity related to MIT include the usual bone marrow suppression and G.I. effects, but more recently, unusual effects including interstitial pneumonitis and fibrosis, renal failure, and microangiopathic hemolytic anemia have been identified. Tissue necrosis secondary to drug extravasation is comparable to that observed with doxorubicin.

The pharmacology of MIT has not been clearly developed because of limited assay systems. Recent studies, however, have suggested that MIT has rapid clearance like other alkylating agents, with a $t^1/_2\beta$ of 46 min.[10] The primary mechanism for elimination and metabolism of MIT is via the liver, with only a small amount of parent drug recovered in the urine.

Continuous infusion MIT has been studied in 2 clinical trials.[11,12] In a study by Miller et al, continuous infusion MIT was administered for 3–12 days, with an increase in the tolerated dose compared to the usual bolus schedule and with marrow suppression being dose-limiting.[11] The study by Lokich et al of short-term (5 days) and protracted (30-day) infusions of MIT suggest, however, that the cumulative dose may be decreased on the infusion schedule.[12] The optimal dose rate for the short-term infusion was 3 mg/m^2/day; for the protracted infusion, 0.75 mg/m^2/day was the maximum dose rate without developing marrow suppression.

Antimetabolites

Antimetabolites are a class of agents that interrupt cellular metabolic processes directed toward synthesis of DNA. Methotrexate, the antipyrimidines, and cytosine arabinoside have been reviewed in separate chapters. Two additional antimetabolites with relatively specific clinical indications are the antipurines and the inhibitor of ribonucleotide reductase, hydroxyurea.

Antipurines

6-mercaptopurine and 6-thioguanine are the 2 clinically available purine antimetabolites. 6-mercaptopurine (6-MP) is converted intracellularly to a ribonucleotide derivative that directly inhibits a variety of enzymatic processes in the de novo synthesis of purines. Thioguanine, which may be converted to 6-thioguanylic acid, also inhibits a variety of steps in purine biosynthesis in addition to being incorporated into DNA with consequent secondary effects.

The antipurines are generally available in an oral dosage form, but parenteral formulations exist as well. The $t^1/_2\beta$ for 6-mercaptopurine administered as an intravenous bolus is 47 minutes; for 6-thioguanine, the half-life is 80 minutes.[13] Renal excretion is the exception in terms of significance unless the drug is delivered at high doses I.V. For 6-MP, oral absorption is erratic, with approximately 16 percent bioavailability. Pharmacologic alteration of 6-MP may follow the use of concomitant allopurinol because the latter drug is an inhibitor of xanthine oxidase and the latter enzyme system is essential for metabolic inactivation of 6-MP.

Because of the lack of availability of parenteral preparations for 6-mercaptopurine and 6-thioguanine, the study of continuous infusion has been limited to a single report.[14] One might suggest that with an oral formulation, the infusion schedule could be reproduced by simply providing frequent oral dosing throughout a 24-hour period. The erratic absorption from the G.I. tract, however, would preclude establishing a meaningful steady-state infusion for these agents. In the phase 1 study of infusion 6-MP, an optimal dose rate of 50 gm/m^2/hour (1.2 mg/m^2/day) for 2 days was established. The dose-limiting toxicity was stomatitis, although hepatic toxicity and myelosuppression were also observed. Interestingly, allopurinal did not influence the plasma pharmacokinetics of 6-MP; importantly, tumor responses were observed.

Hydroxyurea

Hydroxyurea is unique in that it is the single drug in clinical use whose specific mechanism of action is the inhibition of ribonucleotide reductase. It is employed in an oral dose form using chronic administration over time on either a daily or every-other-day schedule to treat and control the WBC in patients with chronic myelogenous leukemia. It has also been used as a radiation sensitizer in the treatment of head and neck cancer and bladder cancer.

The pharmacology of hydroxyurea administered as an oral agent indicates that it is relatively completely absorbed; after intravenous administration, the

$t^1/_2\beta$ is approximately 3 hours.[15] The drug is well distributed in the extravascular spaces including effusions and in the CSF, and the major excretion pattern is via the kidneys.

The unavailability of a parenteral form of hydroxyurea for routine clinical use has limited clinical trials. An early trial using high-dose I.V. hydroxyurea with autogenous bone marrow transplantation did demonstrate objective responses in 4/8 patients with metastatic colorectal cancer and 4/12 patients with malignant melanoma.[16] A study of continuous infusion hydroxyurea delivered over a 72-hour period compared this schedule to oral administration.[17] This study was designed to look at blood levels and establish comparative bioavailability of the 2 schedules. The infusion schedule was clearly superior and also resulted in a complete response in 1 patient with a brain tumor. The dose rate delivered in this trial was 2.8 grams/m^2/day for 3 days.

Miscellaneous Cytotoxic Agents

Within the category of miscellaneous agents one may include the nonclassical alkylating agents: dimethyl trizeno imidazole carboxamide (dacarbazine, DTIC), procarbazine, and the nitrosourea streptozotocin, each of which has unique biologic effects and a unique spectrum of clinical activity. Other agents in the miscellaneous group include the antitumor antibiotic actinomycin D and the biologic response modifier interferon.

DTIC

This agent was originally developed as a potential antipurine, but it has been established that DTIC undergoes activation to an alkylating intermediate probably within the liver. Intratumoral conversion may occur as well, depending on the microsomal activity present within the tumor.

Based on the pharmacokinetic profile of DTIC, continuous venous infusion of the drug is rational; it has a plasma $t^1/_2$ of greater than 5 min. However, because the agent is apparently not stable for more than 8 hours, short-term or protracted infusion has not been reported for it. Regional delivery trials with DTIC, however, suggest that the drug may be active when delivered in this fashion.[18,19] In an early study by Savlov et al, 2/5 patients with extremity melanoma responded to intra-arterial DTIC administered as a bolus.[18] Also, Einhorn et al treated 17 patients with a regional delivery system in which patients received DTIC via an arterial catheter at a dose of 50–400 mg/m^2/day for 5 consecutive days, with the drug delivered over an 8–24 hour period.[19] Seven of 17 patients demonstrated an objective response to treatment with the regional infusion schedule.

Procarbazine

This agent also is not generally available as a parenteral formulation. In addition, like DTIC it requires activation to form free radical intermediates in order to achieve an alkylating effect. Activation may occur in the liver microsomal system and, as such, procarbazine activity may be influenced by the concomitant use of substances that induce microsomal enzyme systems. These issues obviously limit the clinical application of procarbazine for infusion trials.

Nonetheless, the pharmacology of this agent demonstrates a half-life of the I.V. preparation of 7 min., supporting a rationale for an infusion schedule. One clinical trial of a continuous infusion program employing procarbazine at a dose of 450 mg/m²/day did identify a response in a patient with a brain tumor.[20] Procarbazine, a drug that crosses the blood/brain barrier, has demonstrated activity in brain tumors, but its predominant if not exclusive role has been in the treatment of Hodgkin's disease as part of the multidrug regimen designated as MOPP.

Streptozotocin

This agent is one of a group of compounds designated as nitrosoureas, which function as alkylating drugs. As originally developed, the agents have the unique characteristic of being lipid soluble and have been promoted as agents which might cross the blood/brain barrier and be effective in brain tumors. Streptozotocin is a methyl nitrosourea with the unique features of affecting islet cells in animal systems and lacking bone marrow suppression. Because of the specific toxicity for beta cells, this agent has been predominantly employed in the treatment of human islet cell tumors, with substantial activity reported.

Streptozotocin has an extraordinary short plasma half-life of 15 min. and is stable at room temperature in glass for up to 4 days, making it a reasonable agent to be considered for continuous infusion.

Two clinical studies of continuous infusion streptozotocin have been reported.[21,22] In the phase 1 study of Seibert et al, a 5-day infusion schedule was employed at a dose rate of 0.5–1 gram/m²/day.[21] The CNS toxicity observed was probably related to the transport of the drug across the blood/brain barrier, but renal effects — the usual dose-limiting toxicity for this agent — were not observed, and 2 patients with non-Hodgkin's lymphoma demonstrated an objective response. Lokich et al[22] employed a similar schedule of 5 days of continuous infusion at a dose rate of 0.5 gram/m²/day, predominantly in patients with malignant melanoma. The toxicity pattern was generally limited to nausea throughout the infusion period, and renal effects or diabetogenic effects were not observed. Two minor responses were observed in this group of patients, but the study group was suboptimal. The rationale for considering phase 2 trials of streptozotocin in malignant melanoma is extrapolated from the fact that the best second-line agent for the treatment of islet cell tumors after streptozotocin appears to be DTIC. Because DTIC is the generally employed first-line agent for melanoma, streptozotocin would seem to be a reasonable agent to evaluate for this tumor. Five-day infusion of streptozotocin for islet cell tumors employing the same dose rate and schedule has been effective in a variety of islet cell tumors, including functional and nonfunctional tumors.

Actinomycin D

This agent represents one of the earliest antineoplastic agents developed. It has a long history of application, predominantly in childhood malignancies. It is an agent with a relatively long half-life following bolus intravenous injection (upwards of $1\frac{1}{2}$ days) and for that reason, as well as the fact that it is an agent with major sclerosing effects, a continuous infusion schedule has not been clinically practical or even rational. Nonetheless, the usual schedule of once daily injections for 5 days repeated at intervals suggests that such a schedule could be entertained.

A single clinical trial with a phase 1 design has been reported by Blumenreich et al.[23] In that study, a continuous 5-day infusion was employed at doses of 0.1 to 0.5 mg/m^2 for 24 hours. Although no responses were observed in 18 patients studied, the authors recommended a dose of 0.5 mg/m^2/day (total of 2.5 mg/m^2), with myelosuppression and stomatitis being dose-limiting. They concluded that a higher cumulative dose may be achieved with the infusion schedule when compared to the bolus schedule, which is generally in the range of 1.5 mg/m^2 delivered over 5 days.

Biologic Response Modifiers

Biologic response modifiers (BRM) represent an extension of the concepts of immunologic therapy in the treatment of malignancy. Recently, these concepts have involved the experimental application of interferons in the treatment of cancer. Interferons represent special antiproliferative substances that have some antineoplastic activity; they are currently undergoing clinical trials in the management of a variety of malignancies. Phase 1 studies evaluating the optimal dose and schedule for these agents have been severely restricted by the limited availability of the agent as well as by the cost in development. The schedule generally employed in clinical trials has involved a daily or 3 times weekly subcutaneous injection.

It is not within the purview of this chapter to review the details of the chemistry, current mechanism of action, and pharmacology of the various classes of interferons. Apropos to the concept of continuous infusion therapy, however, it is a fact that the pharmacokinetic patterns for the distribution and metabolism of at least gamma interferon is such that the agent has an abbreviated half-life, with a serum half-life of 3–34 min.[24] In the 2 reports of continuous infusion interferon (gamma and human lymphblastoid), substantial toxicity was observed.[24,25]

Further exploration of the infusion schedule for the biologic response modifers may not be practical, depending upon the intrinsic stability of the substance under consideration. In fact, the entire role of biologic response modifiers in the treatment of malignancy is yet to be determined, but an infusion schedule may be a potentially contributing factor to identifying activity.

Summary

Although a number of cancer therapeutic agents have been evaluated in the context of continuous infusion schedules, the alkylating agents as a group have been studied only exceptionally, and as a group the pharmacokinetic parameters for these drugs, which have a relatively short half-life in the plasma, suggests that an infusion schedule may in fact be preferable for such agents. The clinical studies to date have consistently demonstrated an alteration in the pattern of toxicity observed for all agents, and it is conceivable that for some drugs such as the antimetabolites, an expansion of the tumors for which these agents may be employed could be realized with an infusion schedule.

18

INVESTIGATIONAL AGENTS

Merrill J. Egorin, M.D., F.A.C.P.

Introduction

ADMINISTRATION OF INVESTIGATIONAL AGENTS by continuous infusion is a strategy commonly investigated in phase 1 clinical trials. Within the past 3 years, a majority of new agents whose phase 1 trials have been sponsored by the National Cancer Institute have had at least 1 trial by continuous infusion, although the duration of infusion has varied from 1–10 days, depending upon the agent (see table 1). The obvious goal of including continuous infusion therapy among the schedules of drug administration studied is to determine whether continuous infusion therapy will provide an increased therapeutic

Table 1. Investigational Agents Evaluated by Continuous Infusion in Phase 1
Studies (1983–1985 NCI-Sponsored Trials)

Agent	Infusion duration
Hexamethylene bisacetamide	120 hr
Caracemide	120 hr
Tiazofuran	120 hr
Taxol	24 hr, 120 hr
Acodazole	120 hr
Echinomycin	24 hr
Trimetrexate	24 hr
Fludarabine phosphate	120 – 168 hr
Pibenzimol	120 hr
Menogaril	72 hr
Carboplatin	120 hr
Bisantrene	72 hr
Diaziquone	120 hr
Homoharringtonine	120 hr, 168 hr, 216 hr, 240 hr
Tricylic nucleoside phosphate	120 hr
Dihydro-5-azacytidine	24 hr, 120 hr

index. This might be achieved either by decreasing the agent's acute or cumulative toxicity or by enhancing its activity, although the question of enhanced activity cannot be approached adequately in phase 1 trials. Unfortunately, reality does not always fulfill expectations, and recent phase 1 trials of several new agents have provided examples of all possible outcomes of the comparison of continuous infusion therapy with bolus schedules.

Certain agents, such as spiromustine and teroxirone, proved unsuitable for continuous infusion studies because of their great chemical reactivity and instability when formulated. Many other drugs proved no better by continuous infusion than by any other schedule of administration. Local toxicity made some agents, such as menogaril, unsuitable for continuous infusion therapy. In addition, at least 1 new drug, hexamethylene bisacetamide, has been tested only by continuous infusion based on preclinical studies of its mechanism of action. On the positive side, at least 3 new agents, spirogermanium, bisantrene, and homoharringtonine, have proven less toxic by continuous infusion than by bolus therapy. Unfortunately, and as discussed elsewhere in this book, the ability to deliver larger doses of spirogermanium has not improved the response rates of several tumors to this agent.[1,2,3,4] On the other hand, alteration of the schedule of administration of homoharringtonine has allowed documentation of this agent's antitumor activity,[5-12] which might not otherwise have been observed if the toxicities associated with bolus therapy had caused clinical trials to be stopped prematurely. Finally, continuous infusion studies of diaziquone have given promising results that do not reflect decreased toxicity and resultant increased amount of drug administered but may well represent a mechanistic advantage derived from prolonged exposure to the agent.[13,14] In this chapter, each of these cases will be addressed with an emphasis on the example of diaziquone because it represents a rational and mechanistic alteration in drug therapy rather than one based on empiric observations obtained in comparison to bolus administration.

Drugs Pharmaceutically Unsuitable for Continuous Infusion

The nature of some drugs proposed for phase 1 clinical trials by definition precludes their use by continuous infusion. Most recently, this has been the case with teroxirone[15-19] and spiromustine.[22-30]

TEROXIRONE

Teroxirone is a triepoxy derivative, also referred to in the literature as "Henkel's compound" and triazine triepoxide.[15-19] This agent has known alkylating ability and cytotoxic epoxide moities incorporated into its structure.[20] In preclinical studies, teroxirone showed good antitumor activity against both murine and solid tumors,[21] but the activity was schedule-dependent, with repeated daily administration for 5 or 9 days showing a great enhancement of activity as compared to single injection.[21] Clinical studies of teroxirone were limited to schedules employing bolus administration.[15,18] Studies using continuous infusion of this agent were viewed as impractical because of the severe phlebitis that was the dose-limiting toxicity of the agent.[15,18] This toxicity made administration of teroxirone on a prolonged basis by peripheral veins difficult, if not impossible, and to date, appropriate toxicology studies have not been published to warrant the risk of administration of this agent by centrally placed catheters.

SPIROHYDANTOIN MUSTARD

The second agent whose chemical nature has clearly precluded studies by bolus administration is the rationally synthesized alkylating agent spirohydantoin mustard.[22-30] This drug incorporates structural features intended to produce a lipophilic agent with known antitumor functional groups, i.e., an agent that might cross the blood/brain barrier and prove useful in the treatment of CNS neoplasms. Unfortunately, each of these structural features serves to make spiromustine impractical for continuous infusion therapy. Formulation of the compound proved difficult, and even in its current formulation the drug is highly unstable, requiring administration within minutes of preparation.[26]

Drugs Requiring Administration by Continuous Infusion

HEXAMETHYLENE BISACETAMIDE

Just as the knowledge of the pharmaceutical and preclinical pharmacological properties of certain agents have ruled out their evaluation by continuous infusion schedules, there also exists the case in which such knowledge has restricted a certain agent's clinical evaluation to continuous infusion schedules. An example of this is the differentiating agent hexamethylene bisacetamide, which was entered into clinical testing in early 1985. Despite the fact that HMBA's mechanism of action remains unknown, in vitro studies with a variety of solid and leukemic tumors have shown that continuous or prolonged exposure of cells to HMBA is required for the compound to manifest its differentiating action in vitro.[31-40] Moreover, because the concentrations of HMBA required for differentiation in vitro are clearly defined[31-40] and a suitable analytical method exists for determining concentrations of HMBA in plasma, a critical part of the ongoing phase 1 trials will be documenting and monitoring plasma steady-state concentrations of HMBA and defining the agent's pharmacokinetics.

PIBENZIMOL

Another new agent investigated only with a continuous infusion phase 1 trial is the water-soluble chromosome stain pibenzimol. This agent had moderate activity against I.P.-implanted P388 leukemia, although it was very schedule-dependent, with I.P. administration daily for 9 days producing the best results. The single phase 1 study reported to date used a 5-day continuous infusion schedule and determined unexpected drug-induced pancreatic injury as the dose-limiting toxicity.[41]

Drugs Shown in Clinical Trials to be Unsuitable for Continuous Infusion

The semisynthetic anthracycline analogue menogaril represents an agent that, after clinical testing, proved much less suitable for continuous administration than for bolus injection.[60-66] Unlike teroxirone and spiromustine, this result was not predictable because of menogaril's chemical structure or preclinical pharmacologic and pharmaceutical studies.[60] Rather, this fact was discovered during the course of a phase 1 clinical trial administering menogaril by 72-hour continuous infusion.[63] It should be mentioned, however, that this study used peripheral venous access, and to date, results concerning continuous infusion through a central line have not been published. In the case of menogaril, the inability to administer the drug successfully by continuous infusion is more than a clinical fact to be noted while the drug is explored further with bolus schedules. Rather, since menogaril is a member of the anthracycline antibiotic class of antitumor agents in which reduced cardiotoxicity has been documented when such agents are administered by continuous infusion, optimal utilization of this agent may be precluded by the inability to administer it over prolonged periods.

Drugs with No Apparent Advantage from Administration by Continuous Infusion

As might be expected, when phase 1 trials exploring varying schedules of administration have been completed, there have been a number of agents for which no clear-cut schedule dependence could be defined and no benefit of continuous infusion administration was documented. This has been the case for agents as diverse in structure and mechanism of action as the promising cisplatin analogue carboplatin,[41-48] the plant alkaloid taxol,[49-53] the cyclic peptide antibiotic echinomycin,[54-57] and the antimetabolite dihydroazacytidine.[58-59] In each case, the qualitative spectrum of toxicities associated with the agent was unchanged, and the cumulative amount of drug administered per course was no greater when given by any particular schedule.

Drugs with a Therapeutic Advantage When Administered by Continuous Infusion

For at least 2 other new agents, continuous infusion schedules may have resulted in an enhanced therapeutic index by amelioration of what appeared to be major or dose-limiting toxicities in phase 1 studies using bolus schedules.

BISANTRENE

Bisantrene is an anthracene bishydrazone derivative that was entered into phase 1 clinical trials based on its in vivo activity against a number of animal tumor models and its in vitro activity in the human tumor stem cell assay.[67-71] Initial trials of bisantrene employed bolus infusions, administered either weekly for 3 weeks, daily for 5 days, or once every 3 weeks.[72-74] In each case, although leukopenia proved the dose-limiting toxicity, local toxicities associated with drug infusion proved a major and frequent occurrence.[72-74] Careful investigation of the cause of bisantrene-associated phlebitis showed that the concentrations of drug infused in bolus studies resulted in drug precipitation and adherence to the walls of the infused vein.[75] Prolongation of the duration of drug infusion to 72 hours, dilution of the total dose of drug in 9 L of 5% dextrose in water, and administration of bisantrene by central venous catheter have not only ablated the vascular toxicity but also have allowed larger doses of drug to be administered.[76] Whether this enhanced ability to deliver more drug is translated into an actual therapeutic advantage still awaits confirmation from phase 2 and 3 clinical trials in which sufficient numbers of patients will document response rates adequately.

HOMOHARRINGTONINE

The alkaloid homoharringtonine is one of a group of cephalotaxine esters isolated from an evergreen of the genus *Cephalotaxus*.[77-79] The impetus for clinical trials of homoharringtonine in the United States came from clinical trials in China that claimed activity for a mixture for homoharringtonine and the structurally related alkaloid harringtonine.[80-81] Preclinical screening indicated good antitumor activity of homoharringtonine against murine P388 leukemia and colon 38 carcinoma and moderate activity against murine $CD8F_1$ mammary carcinoma and L1210 leukemia.[82-84] Homoharringtonine proved inactive against human colon, lung, and mammary tumors carried as xenografts in nude mice.[82-84] In these preclinical trials, the antitumor activity of homoharringtonine against P388 leukemia was highly schedule-dependent, with daily administration for 9 days proving more effective than therapy on days 1, 5, and 9 and much more effective than therapy by single dose administration.[82-84] Moreover, for any given schedule, therapy administered multiple times per day proved more effective than administration of the daily dose as a single bolus.[82-84] Initial trials in this country with a more highly purified pharmaceutical preparation of homoharringtonine used a schedule of daily bolus drug administration for 5 successive days.[85] In these studies, hypotension and myelosuppression were the major toxicities observed at maximally tolerated dosages of 3–5 mg/m²/day for 5 days.[85] In other phase 1 studies, hypotension and cardiovascular complications were major problems when homoharringtonine was infused on 10 successive days as a 6-hour infusion, but were greatly attenuated when the schedule was altered to a 10-day continuous infusion.[86] Although the severity of hypotension described at the various institutions ranged from mild, requiring only I.V. fluids for correction, to severe or fatal, requiring pressor agents for correction, all subsequent trials of homoharringtonine have employed continuous infusion schedules of drug administration.[87-91] Initial continuous infusion studies administering the drug over 5 days demonstrated myelosuppression as the dose-limiting toxicity at maximally tolerated dosages of 3.25–3.75 mg/m²/day.[88] Continuous infusion studies employing a 10-day schedule found myelosuppression to be the dose-limiting toxicity, but defined 4 mg/m² as the maximally tolerated dosage for solid tumor studies and 5–6 mg/m^2/day as the maximally tolerated dosage for leukemia studies.[86]

In a large phase 1 trial of continuous infusion homoharringtonine therapy that attempted to define the optimal dosage in adult patients with acute leukemia, homoharringtonine was infused at 3 dosage levels: 5 mg/m^2/day for 5 days, 7 mg/m^2/day for 7 days, and 5 mg/m^2/day for 9 days. These schedules and dosages had little effect on the bone marrow function of 8 patients with acute lymphocytic leukemia and 4 patients with chronic myelogenous leukemia in blast crisis. On the other hand, the lowest dosage produced marrow hypoplasia in 2/3 patients with acute nonlymphocytic leukemia. The 2 higher dosages caused marrow hypoplasia in 12/14 evaluable patients with acute nonlymphocytic leukemia; 3 of these patients eventually achieved a complete remission.[89] More recent studies[90,91] have continued to extend these observations and have concentrated on defining the optimal duration and dosage for continuous infusion administration of homoharringtonine. In the first of these studies, a phase 1–2 trial in patients with acute myelogenous leukemia, drug dosages of 5–7 mg/m^2/day were infused over 7–9 days.[90] Six of the 10 courses administered at 5 mg/m^2/day for 9 days had to be interrupted secondary to hypotension. This schedule also produced other nonhematologic toxicities such as hyperglycemia, diarrhea, mucositis, nausea and vomiting, and fluid retention that were noted in studies in which bolus administration of homoharringtonine was used. In the second recent continuous infusion study, homoharringtonine was infused by Cormed pumps and Hickman catheters to 48 outpatients.[91] The dosing regimen, altered in response to dose-limiting myelosuppression and hypotension, evolved from an initial 4 mg/m^2/day for 5 days to 2 mg/m^2/day for 13 days. Subsequently, a schedule of 1.5 mg/m^2/day for 13 days followed by 7 days of rest and retreatment produced dose-limiting myelosuppression but few other toxicities. The final modification by these authors of continuous infusion dosage involved an escalating scheme in which a daily dose of 1 mg/m^2/day was given for 13, 17, 21, 25, or 30 days. At 1 mg/m^2/day, only 3 of 26 patients treated experienced hypotension, and that which was observed was mild. At the longest duration of infusion, and therefore the greatest cumulative dose, cumulative myelosuppression was observed, and 3 of 9 patients had mild nausea, fatigue, or anorexia. These findings led to a recommended starting dose for phase 2 trials of 1 mg/m^2/day infused continuously for 25 days.

Careful consideration of the evolution of clinical trials of homoharringtonine shows that continuous infusion can produce a therapeutic advantage in this agent's use. At present, however, that advantage appears to rest primarily in the ability to reduce hypotension which, while clearly documented as a toxicity in studies with bolus injections, was quite variable in intensity not only among patients but also among institutions. It is still unclear as to how much, if any, more homoharringtonine can be safely administered to patients by continuous infusion as compared to bolus injection. Moreover, all of the studies published to date have been phase 1 studies devoted primarily to defining an acceptable and safe dosage and schedule for homoharringtonine. Although preclinical animal screening implies that repeated frequent dosing of homoharringtonine is the most efficacious way to give the drug, to date there exists no clear-cut evidence for continuous infusion schedules producing response rates any different from those that might be achieved in studies employing a bolus schedule and the appropriate maximally tolerated dosage.

DIAZIQUONE

Diaziquone, also referred to as "aziridinyl benzoquinone" or AZQ, is a diaziridinyl benzoquinone belonging to a group of compounds with well-known antitumor activity.[92-98] The exact structure of AZQ was rationally conceived in an effort to create a drug that also possessed chemical characteristics allowing it to cross the blood/brain barrier.[99-101] In preclinical testing, intraperitoneally injected AZQ demonstrated significant activity against intraperitoneal murine L1210 leukemia, P388 leukemia, and B16 melanoma.[99-101] More importantly, AZQ, injected I.P. on a day 1 through 9 schedule, showed great activity against intracerebral L1210 and P388. Injected intraperitoneally on a day 1 through 5 schedule, AZQ produced large numbers of cures of mice bearing an intracerebral murine ependymoblastoma.[99-101]

Based on these encouraging results, AZQ has been entered into phase 1 clinical trials at a number of institutions (see table 2). A variety of schedules, including 5-day continuous infusion, days 1 and 8 every 3 weeks, weekly for 4 weeks, and daily × 5 days, were investigated in solid tumors.[102-107] All studies described myelosuppression, with both leukopenia and thrombocytopenia, as the dose-limiting toxicity. There was no apparent advantage in any schedule with regard to the maximum tolerated dosage and the total amount of drug that could be administered per unit time. Similarly, there was no apparent difference in schedule with regard to the other toxicities associated with AZQ. To some extent, this was due to the infrequent and relatively mild nausea and vomiting and alopecia that comprised the nonhematologic toxicities resulting from AZQ therapy.

In addition to the phase 1 studies in solid tumors, pediatric[105] and adult[108,109] phase 1 evaluations of AZQ were performed in patients with acute leukemia. Each study used daily bolus therapy—the pediatric trials for 5 days and the adult trial for 7 days. In each leukemia trial, the tolerated doses of AZQ were much larger than those that would be acceptable in solid tumor patients, yet there were no qualitative differences in the spectrum of toxicity and there was no demonstrable quantitative difference in the severity or frequency of

Table 2. Phase 1 Studies with Diaziquone

Schedule/(reference)	Maximum tolerated dose
Bolus Q.D. × 5 (102)	4 mg/m²/d (poor risk)
	7 mg/m²/d (good risk)
Bolus weekly × 4 (103)	20 mg/m²
Bolus days 1 & 8 (104)	20 mg/m²
Bolus Q.D. × 5 (105)	9 mg/m²/d (pediatric)
Bolus day 1 (106)	30 mg/m² (poor risk)
	40 mg/m² (good risk)
Continuous infusion × 5 d (107)	4 mg/m²/d (poor risk)
	6 mg/m²/d (good risk)

nonhematologic toxicities that occurred. Rather, the only observed difference was more profound and prolonged marrow suppression, a pharmacodynamic consequence expected in chemotherapy of leukemia.

Based on the definitions of both an acceptable dosage and easily managed toxicity, AZQ progressed in phase 2 studies in a variety of tumor types. All of these studies were initiated with bolus administration of AZQ, although the schedules of therapy varied, i.e., once every 3 to 4 weeks, days 1 and 8 every 4 weeks, or daily for 5 days every 4 weeks[110-128] (see table 3). With the exception of a study of refractory lymphoma, the response rates for both CNS as well as non-CNS solid tumors have been disappointing. AZQ was not totally devoid of activity, but the responses observed were sporadic, without any large number in any tumor type except lymphoma, as mentioned above.

Such a disparity between preclinical screening and clinical results is in no way uncommon for investigational antineoplastic drugs, and the basis for such a difference often remains undefined. With time, however, a number of preclinical in vitro and in vivo studies provided data which, when combined with already published clinical pharmacologic and pharmacokinetic data, made a strong argument not only for the use of the AZQ as a continuous infusion but also for acute leukemia as the disease in which continuous infusion AZQ should be explored.

Although AZQ was known to possess both alkylating activity and a benzoquinone structure found in a number of antitumor agents capable of generating free radicals,[129,130] its mechanism of action was undefined, and there were no published studies of its in vitro cellular pharmacology. Subsequently, in vitro studies with murine L1210 and human HL60 leukemia indicated that AZQ required a long exposure to manifest its growth-inhibiting properties.[131] In growth curve experiments, AZQ not only reduced the rate of L1210 cell growth, but did so in a dose-dependent fashion. Although the inhibition of AZQ was apparent as early as 24 hours, evidence of the dose-dependent nature required several doubling times and therefore was not observed until 48 hours, after

Table 3. Phase 2 Studies With Diaziquone

Tumor Type/(reference)	Dose
Primary and metastatic CNS (110)	30 mg/m^2 bolus q 3 wks
High-grade gliomas (113)	20 mg/m^2 bolus d1 & d8 q 4 wks
Primary and metastatic CNS (126)	10 – 12 mg/m^2 bolus/d × 4 q 2 – 3 wks
Lung (118)	20.5 – 27.5 mg/m^2/bolus q 4 – 5 wks
Nonsmall-cell lung (111)	30 – 35 mg/m^2 q 3 wks
Small-cell lung (127)	20 mg/m^2/bolus d1 & d8 q & 8 d
Refractory lymphomas (112)	30 mg/m^2 bolus q 3 wks
Advanced genitourinary (116)	20 – 27.5 mg/m^2/bolus q 28 d
Colon (117,120)	5.5 – 7 mg/m^2/bolus/d × 5 q 28 d
Aerodigestive (119)	22.5 – 27.5 mg/m^2/bolus q 4 wks
Melanoma (121)	20.5 – 27.5 mg/m^2/bolus q 4 wks
Breast (123)	30 mg/m^2/bolus q 3 wks
Ovary (124)	25 – 30 mg/m^2/bolus q 4 wks
Renal (125)	27 mg/m^2/bolus q 4 wks
Multiple myeloma (128)	30 – 35 mg/m^2/bolus q 3 wks

which it became progressively more evident. The fact that this inhibition was due to AZQ and not the dimethylacetamide (DMA) vehicle associated with AZQ's administration came from control cultures where DMA at concentrations obligatorily included in AZQ experiments had no effect on L1210 cell growth until a small amount of inhibition was observed at the concentration of 0.1%, i.e., that DMA concentration associated with AZQ, 10 μM. The dose-dependent nature of the growth inhibition of AZQ was better assessed when cell concentrations achieved in AZQ-treated cultures after 72 and 96 hours of incubation were expressed as percentages of those in additive-free control cultures incubated for the same length of time. There was no inhibition of L1210 cell growth at AZQ concentrations of less than 0.3 μM.

As with L1210 cells, AZQ produced a dose-dependent decrease in HL60 cell growth. In these experiments, HL60 cells proved about as sensitive to AZQ as L1210 cells. Evidence for AZQ being cytotoxic as opposed to cytostatic was derived from experiments in which AZQ inhibited HL60 cell cloning in a dose-dependent fashion. As with cell growth, 0.3 μM was the lowest studied AZQ concentration at which cellular growth inhibitory effects were seen. Again, DMA had no effect on HL60 cell cloning.

Further investigation of exactly which cellular processes were inhibited by AZQ characterized the effects of the drug on incorporation of radiolabeled macromolecular precursors into trichloroacetic acid precipitable material. AZQ inhibited ^{3}H-thymidine incorporation by L1210 cells more than it did incorporation of ^{3}H-uridine and ^{14}C-valine. There were several notable aspects of this inhibition. As with the inhibition of cell growth and cloning, the drug reduced ^{3}H-thymidine incorporation in a dose-dependent fashion, with the first decrease noted at AZQ concentrations of 0.1–0.5 μM. Although AZQ inhibited ^{3}H-thymidine incorporation, the onset of this inhibition was slow, continuing to increase for at least 24 hours after addition of AZQ. AZQ had much less effect on ^{3}H-uridine incorporation by L1210 cells and, as with ^{3}H-thymidine incorporation, this effect was delayed in onset. No reduction of ^{3}H-uridine incorporation was observed with AZQ concentrations of less than 1 μM. Concentrations of AZQ as high as 5 μM had no effect on radiolabeled valine incorporation. DMA concentrations obligatorily added with AZQ had no effect on incorporation of any macromolecular precursor by L1210 cells.

Other in vitro experiments examining the accumulation of ^{14}C AZQ by leukemic cells provided further information as to the time requirements and nature of interaction of the drug with the cells. As with AZQ-induced growth inhibition, cellular accumulation of ^{14}C was a relatively slow process, requiring intact aziridine moieties to occur. In addition, AZQ is not highly concentrated in cells, achieving concentrations approximately 10 times those in the incubation media. When cell-associated radioactivity was examined more carefully, 2 radioactive species were observed: a very rapidly exchangeable portion, which was unaltered by temperature or metabolic inhibitors, and a progressively increasing nonexchangeable portion, the accumulation of which accounted for the progressive rise in cell associated ^{14}C. This production of nonexchangeable ^{14}C could represent an energy-dependent process, inasmuch as it was ablated by reduced temperature and the metabolic poison iodoacetate.

The potential clinical implications of these in vitro observations required their interpretation in the light of in vivo and clinical observations. The possibility that the poor clinical response rates observed with AZQ reflected the inability of the drug to reach tissue was ruled out by murine pharmacokinetic and tissue distribution studies that demonstrated wide distribution of AZQ in the tissue. However, these studies also demonstrated its rapid metabolic conversion to species, the exact nature of which remains undefined.[132] By 30 min., parent compound already represented less than 50% of the drug-related radioactivity present in plasma. Furthermore, careful clinical pharmacokinetic studies had already shown that AZQ disappeared from plasma with a terminal half-life of approximately 30 min., that the total body clearance of AZQ was approximately 500 ml/min., and that even with bolus injection of a maximum tolerated dosage, plasma concentrations of AZQ rapidly fell below those concentrations shown to inhibit growth in vitro.[104,113] Thus, the in vivo pharmacokinetic behavior of AZQ indicated that bolus administration of drug was incompatible with the data from in vitro studies of drug action. Moreover, the plasma steady-state concentrations of AZQ achieved in the 1 continuous infusion phase 1 study were known to be less than 0.05 μM, a fact not only determined by actual measurement of plasma steady-state drug concentrations[133] but also calculated from the pharmacokinetic theoretical relationship:

$$\text{plasma steady-state concentration} = \frac{\text{rate of infusion}}{\text{total body clearance}}$$

Consideration of these facts, along with the knowledge that bolus therapy for leukemia with AZQ doses 4 times greater than those used for solid tumors caused only more severe myelosuppression and no change in the qualitative spectrum of toxicities, led us to initiate phase 1-2 studies of continuous infusion AZQ therapy in adult patients with relapsed or refractory leukemia.[13,14] In this trial, AZQ was administered as a continuous infusion for 7 days by infusion pump. The total dose of AZQ was diluted in 1 L of 0.154 M NaCl and was prepared within 6 hours of use. Cohorts of 2-3 patients were treated at dosages ranging from 16-32 mg/m^2/day. The initial dosage was twice the maximum tolerated dose defined in the phase 1 continuous infusion trial of AZQ in solid tumor patients,[107] but two-thirds of the MTD in the phase 1 bolus leukemia study.[109] Dose escalations were 4 mg/m^2/day, and patients who failed to respond to their initial therapy were eligible to receive a second course at the next higher dose. The bone marrow response determined whether a second course of diaziquone was given. If the marrow revealed increasing cellularity with persistence of leukemia after day 15, then a second course of diaziquone was given. No further chemotherapy was given if remission was achieved. Patients who failed to respond to a second course were removed from study. As an integral part of this trial, plasma concentrations of AZQ were determined during and after the AZQ infusion.

A total of 49 patients with relapsed or refractory adult leukemia were entered into the study. These included 34 patients with *de novo* acute nonlymphocytic leukemia, 4 patients with secondary acute nonlymphocytic leukemia, 6 patients with chronic myelogenous leukemia in blast crisis, and 5 patients

with acute lymphocytic leukemia. All patients with acute lymphocytic leukemia had received standard induction regimen initially and received AZQ after
other second-line treatments were unsuccessful. Five of the 6 individuals with
CML and blast crisis received AZQ as their initial treatment. All patients with
secondary acute nonlymphocytic leukemia were treated initially with daunorubicin and cytosine arabinoside in conventional doses, and AZQ was the second
induction regimen used in each of these patients. Of the patients with *de novo*
acute nonlymphocytic leukemia, 11 patients had had 2 or more prior complete
remissions. AZQ represented the third to the tenth induction regimen given to
these patients. Eighteen patients with acute nonlymphocytic leukemia had had
a single prior complete remission. Of these, 11 received AZQ as their initial
treatment for relapse.

No patients with acute nonlymphocytic leukemia responded. Although all
became hypocellular, 2 were never aplastic, and all had regrowth of leukemia.
Similarly, no patient with chronic myelogenous leukemia in blast crisis or
secondary acute nonlymphocytic leukemia responded to continuous infusion
AZQ.

Thirty-four patients with relapsed (29) or refractory (5) *de novo* acute nonlymphocytic leukemia were treated at varying doses of AZQ. Six complete
remissions and 2 partial remissions were seen in this group of patients with
relapsed acute nonlymphocytic leukemia. All responders had very slow bone
marrow recovery. Two of these patients had remission durations from AZQ
that exceeded the length of their prior remissions.

Nonhematologic toxicity due to continuous infusion AZQ was mild, consisting of grade 3 gastrointestinal toxicity in 3 patients; mild hepatic toxicity was
observed in 21% of all courses. There were no drug-related toxicities involving
the CNS or the renal, cardiac, and pulmonary systems. One patient in this trial
did have an anaphylactic reaction to AZQ within minutes of starting the initial
infusion. This patient had a history of multiple drug allergies and had had an
anaphylactic reaction to vitamin K 2 weeks before institution of AZQ therapy.
Three courses of therapy were given at 32 mg/m^2/day for 7 days. Two of the 3
patients treated at this dosage developed bone marrow necrosis, although the
third patient had an uncomplicated but unsuccessful course of therapy. The
dose-limiting toxicity of AZQ was the duration of aplasia (median 49 days to
>500 neutrophils for responders, range 27–101 days). In view of this and the
occurrence of bone marrow necrosis in 2 of the 3 patients treated at 32
mg/m^2/day for 7 days, 28 mg/m^2/day × 7 days was established as the maximum tolerated dosage.

Steady-state plasma concentrations of AZQ in 11 patients treated with the
maximum tolerated dosage were 101 ± 10 ng/ml (mean ± SEM, range 54–150
ng/ml) and were achieved by 45 min. after initiating treatment. After cessation
of the infusion, plasma concentrations of AZQ declined by monoexponential
decay, with a mean half-life of 47.7 ± 11.4 min. The steady-state concentrations measured agreed quite well with those predicted from the relationship
described above for steady-state concentration, rate of infusion, and total
body clearance and are closely comparable with the concentrations of AZQ
required for inhibition of leukemia cells in vitro.[131]

The results observed in this study appear to confirm the theory upon which it was based. Previous studies of diaziquone, given as a bolus, had not demonstrated activity, inasmuch as no complete or partial responses were recorded among the 57 patients (36 with acute nonlymphocytic leukemia) treated. On the other hand, response rates observed with continuous infusion AZQ compare favorably with response rates for other new agents such as amsacrine, homoharringtonine, and mitoxantrone used in the treatment of relapsed or refractory leukemia. In addition to this documented activity, the lack of extramedullary or hepatotoxicity make AZQ an interesting drug to consider for combination with another agent of established activity in the treatment of acute nonlymphocytic leukemia. Such a trial examining the combination of AZQ and amsacrine is currently in progress. In addition, the demonstrated activity and mild nonhematologic toxicity associated with continuous infusion AZQ in the treatment of acute nonlymphocytic leukemia raises the question of using AZQ in the preparative regimen for bone marrow transplantation in patients with acute nonlymphocytic leukemia. To date, no such studies have been published; however, they would clearly be of considerable interest.

The studies with AZQ presented here have been presented in some depth because the decision to employ AZQ as a continuous infusion in the treatment of acute leukemia represented not merely an empirical exploration in a course of evaluating several schedules but rather was a rational decision based on both preclinical and clinical data. In addition, it represents a case in which use of continuous infusion does not allow administration of a higher dose of drug but results in enhanced response to similar doses of drug as given by bolus infusion. Why this should be the case with a potential alkylating agent such as AZQ is unclear.

19

PROTRACTED INFUSIONAL

CHEMOTHERAPY

Jacob J. Lokich, M.D.

THE CONCEPT OF EXTENDING the duration of treatment to maximize the "time" component of the concentration x time formulation is related to tumor cell kinetics and growth characteristics. Tumor cell killing is achieved with antineoplastic agents by means of disruption of active cellular or nuclear processes occurring during the G_1S, G_2, and M stages of the cell cycle. The major proportion of cells in a tumor mass, however, are in G_0, and transition from G_0 into the active phases of the cell cycle may occur randomly over time. The growth of a tumor mass follows a Gompertzian curve, with an exponential phase eventually achieving a plateau. A tumor doubling time reflects the exponential growth phase; in the plateau phase, the spontaneous cell loss rate is balanced by the cell expansion rate. Theoretically, providing cytotoxic drugs throughout the tumor doubling time or the potential exponential phase of tumor growth may allow the drug to interface with every cell destined to have clonogenic potential.

Based upon this concept and upon anecdotal clinical cases in which an interruption of chemotherapy may be followed by recrudescence of the tumor within 2 to 4 months but with the capacity for reinduction of response, the use of open-ended or protracted continuous infusion chemotherapy has been developed at the New England Deaconess Hospital. This type of infusional chemotherapy is distinct from short-term or intermittent continuous infusion and may be termed "continuous" continuous infusion chemotherapy. In this schema, patients receive 24-hour continuous infusion chemotherapy for extended periods, generally at a minimum of 30 days, but the open option is to extend treatment for months.

Phase 1 and 2 clinical trials of protracted duration infusional chemotherapy have focused on 8 individual agents. This chapter will review the individual phase 1 and 2 studies of protracted infusion chemotherapy that have been

243

previously reported and will develop the direction of ongoing and future clinical studies at the phase 3 level.

Preclinical Pharmaceutical Studies

A practical program for continuous infusion chemotherapy of protracted duration requires establishing the stability of the individual agents at room temperature and their compatibility with the drug reservoir—either plastic syringes or polyvinyl reservoir bags. Table 1 indicates the established data base for stability of a variety of chemotherapeutic agents reconstituted according to the manufacturer's recommendation with either bacteriostatic water or normal saline. For some agents such as cisplatin (DDP), a high salt concentration is essential to prevent aquation, which would render the drug inactive. For mitomycin-C (MIT), a buffered solution is necessary to prevent degradation of the drug over time as the pH decreases.

In the ideal circumstances for protracted infusion, drug reservoirs are exchanged at 5- to 7-day intervals according to the dose rates and volume delivered. Such a schedule allows for less patient responsibility and, therefore, more patient convenience. Drugs such as 5-fluorouracil (5-FU) and methotrexate (MTX) are extraordinarily stable over time for 30 days or more. For the anthracycline drugs, stability has been established for 14 or more days. For

Table 1. Stability of Drugs Reconstituted with Bacteriostatic Water or Normal Saline

Drug	Strength	Storage	Diluent	Amount	Concentration	Stability*
Adriamycin	10 mg	Room	NS	5 ml	2 mg/ml	14 d (RT)
	50 mg			25 ml	2 mg/ml	
Bleomycin	15 u	Refrig.	Bact. H_2O	5 ml	3 u/ml	28 d
			Bact. NS	15 ml	1 u/ml	
				3 ml	5 u/ml	
Cisplatin	10 mg	Refrig.	Bact. H_2O	10 ml	1 mg/ml	72 hr
	50 mg			50 ml		
Cytarabine	100 mg	Room	Bact. H_2O	5 ml	20 mg/ml	8 d
	500 mg			10 ml	50 mg/ml	
Cyclophosphamide	500 mg	Room	H_2O/NS	25 ml	20 mg/ml	6 d (RT)
Dacarbazine	100 mg	Refrig.	H_2O	9.8 ml	10 mg/ml	24 hr
	200 mg			19.7 ml		
Floxuridine	500 mg	Room	Bact. H_2O	5 ml	100 mg/ml	14 d (RT)
Methotrexate	100 mg	Room	None		25 mg/ml	filter
	20 mg (IT)		NS	10 ml	2 mg/ml	28 d (RT)
	20 mg (IT)		NS	20 ml	1 mg/ml	
Mitomycin-C	5 mg	Room	H_2O	10 ml	0.5 mg/ml	14 d
	20 mg			40 ml	0.5 mg/ml	4 d (RT)
Streptozocin	1,000 mg	Refrig.	H_2O	9.5 ml	100 mg/ml	4 d
Vinblastine	10 mg	Refrig.	Bact. NS	10 ml	1 mg/ml	30 d
						10 d (RT)

*All stabilities pertain to refrigerated storage unless (RT) designation, which indicates minimal stability duration at room temperature.

agents such as DDP, the parent compound is stable for only 3–6 days, necessitating frequent reservoir changes.

Another important issue with regard to pharmaceutical aspects of protracted infusion is drug solubility. The drug concentration and the optimal dose rate of delivery will determine the volume delivered over time and, therefore, will condition the optimal pump to be employed as well as the timing for exchanging reservoirs. Tables 2 and 3 summarize the volume of drug delivery based upon the optimal dose rate for short-term or prolonged infusion with a number of agents. The volume rates are categorized according to patient size defined by meter squared. These data have been designed to be employed in conjunction with the Cormed model ML4–6, which has a 60 cc reservoir and delivers 4–20 cc/day. Depending upon the drug, the volume delivered each day varies from 4 to a maximum of 12 cc.

Some drugs may not be logistically feasible to be delivered as a "continuous" continuous infusion. Bleomycin (BLM), for example, is unstable and requires fresh reconstitution at 8–12 hours. The epipodophyllotoxin etoposide (VP-16) requires large volumes in order to maintain the drug in solution. For practical reasons, these 2 agents therefore are not necessarily appropriate for continuous ambulatory infusion programs.

Phase 1 Studies

Phase 1 studies using a continuous infusion schedule have goals similar to traditional phase 1 studies in which the bolus schedule is used. The objective is to establish dose-limiting toxicity which, with the infusion schedule, is defined more precisely as a dose rate-limiting toxicity. In contrast to phase 1 studies in which the bolus schedule is used, the goal is to establish the dose rate that would permit continuous treatment and is therefore translated into a dose that is *not* associated with toxicity at all. The optimal dose from a phase 1 bolus trial is the one that induces consistent but tolerable toxicity that is not life-threatening.

Phase 1 studies involving infusion schedules are difficult, because identifying the initial or starting dose is problematic in that preclinical or animal toxicology studies are not available. The fact that the starting dose for phase 1 studies with the bolus schedule employs 1/3 the minimally toxic dose in large animal systems has proven to be an adequate guide for phase 1 studies in man. As a consequence of the limited preclinical studies of infusion, no guidelines are available; in some instances, our phase 1 studies selected a starting dose that was associated with toxicity at less than the projected study goal in terms of the duration of treatment. In those instances, a phase 1 infusional study proceeded with decremental dosage adjustments as opposed to incremental escalation.

5-Fluorouracil

The antipyrimidine 5-fluorouracil (5-FU) was administered as a continuous infusion as early as 1962 by Sullivan et al,[1] and short-term (5-day) infusions

Table 2. Volume of Delivery of Various Agents at Optimal Dose for Short-Term Infusion

Drug	Reconstituted dilution	Dose/m²/day			Patient size (meter squared)					
				1.5	1.6	1.7	1.8	1.9	2.0
5-FU	50 mg/ml	1 g	(A)	30 ml	32 ml	34 ml	36 ml	38 ml	40 ml
			(B)	30 ml	32 ml	34 ml	36 ml	38 ml	40 ml
			(C)	1,500 mg/30 ml [1 day]	1,600 mg/32 ml	1,700 mg/34 ml	1,800 mg/36 ml	1,900 mg/38 ml	2,000 mg/40 ml
ADR	2 mg/ml	15 mg	(A)	11.2 ml	12 ml	12.75 ml	13.5 ml	14.25 ml	15 ml
			(B)	11.2 ml	12 ml	12.75 ml	13.5 ml	14.25 ml	15 ml
			(C)	112.5 mg/56.2 ml [5 days]	120 mg/60 ml	51 mg/25.5 ml [2 days]	54 mg/27 ml	57 mg/28.5 ml	60 mg/30 ml
VLB	1 mg/ml	1.5 mg	(A)	1.5 ml	1.6 ml	1.7 ml	1.8 ml	1.9 ml	2 ml
			(B)	10 ml	10 ml	10 ml	10 ml	10 ml	10 ml
			(C)	7.5 mg/50 ml [5 days]	8 mg/50 ml	8.5 mg/50 ml	9 mg/50 ml	9.5 mg/50 ml	10 mg/50 ml
DDP	1 mg/ml	20 mg	(A)	30 ml	32 ml	34 ml	36 ml	38 ml	40 ml
			(B)	30 ml	32 ml	34 ml	36 ml	38 ml	40 ml
			(C)	30 mg/30 ml [1 day]	32 mg/32 ml	34 mg/34 ml	36 mg/36 ml	38 mg/38 ml	40 mg/40 ml
CTX	20 mg/ml	300 mg	(A)	22.5 ml	24 ml	25.5 ml	27 ml	28.5 ml	30 ml
			(B)	22.5 ml	24 ml	25.5 ml	27 ml	28.5 ml	30 ml
			(C)	450 mg/22.5 ml [1 day]	480 mg/24 ml	510 mg/25.5 ml	540 mg/27 ml	570 mg/28.5 ml	600 mg/30 ml
BLM	5 u/ml	10 u/m²/d	(A)	3 ml	3.2 ml	3.4 ml	3.6 ml	3.8 ml	4.0 ml
			(B)	10 ml	10 ml	10 ml	10 ml	10 ml	10 ml
			(C)	75 u/50 ml [5 days]	80 u/50 ml	85 u/50 ml	90 u/50 ml	95 u/50 ml	100 u/50 ml
Ara-C	50 mg/ml (500 mg vial) [20 mg/ml 100 mg vial]	100 mg	(A)	3 ml [7.5 ml]	3.2 ml [8 ml]	3.4 ml [8.5 ml]	3.6 ml [9 ml]	3.8 ml [9.5 ml]	4.0 mg [10 ml]
			(B)	10 ml	10 ml	10 ml	10 ml	10 ml	10 ml
			(C)	750 mg/50 ml [5 days]	800 mg/50 ml	850 mg/50 ml	900 mg/50 ml	950 mg/50 ml	1,000 mg/50 ml

A = minimum ml/day
B = Cormed ml/day
C = traditional Cormed concentration
[] = # days drug supply

5-FU = fluorouracil
ADR = doxorubicin
VLB = vinblastine
DDP = cisplatin
CTX = cyclophosphamide
BLM = bleomycin
Ara-C = cytosine arabinoside

Table 3. Volume of Delivery of Various Agents at Optimal Dose for Prolonged Infusion

Drug	Reconstituted dilution	Dose/m²/day		Patient size (meter squared)					
				1.5	1.6	1.7	1.8	1.9	2.0
5-FU	50 mg/ml	300 mg	(A)	9 cc	9.6 cc	10.2 cc	10.8 cc	11.4 cc	12 cc
			(B)	9 cc	9.6 cc	10.2 cc	10.8 cc	11.4 cc	12 cc
			(C)	2,250 mg/45 cc [5 days]	2,500 mg/50 cc	250 mg/50 cc	2,750 mg/55 cc	3,000 mg/60 cc	3,000 mg/60 cc ↑
CTX	2 mg/ml	0.75 mg	(A)	0.56 cc	0.6 cc	0.63 cc	0.67 cc	0.71 cc	0.75 cc
			(B)	7.5 cc					
			(C)	9 mg/60 cc [8 days]	9.6 mg/60 cc	10.2 mg/60 cc	10.8 mg/60 cc	11.3 mg/60 cc	12 mg/60 cc
ADR	2 mg/ml	3 mg	(A)	2.25 cc/day	2.4 cc	2.55 cc	2.7 cc	2.85 cc	3 cc
			(B)	7.5 cc/day					
			(C)	36 mg/60 cc [8 days]	38.4 mg/60 cc	40.8 mg/60 cc	43.2 mg/60 cc	45.6 mg/60 cc	48 mg/60 cc ↑
CTX	20 mg/ml	50 mg	(A)	3.75 cc	4 cc	4.25 cc	4.5 cc	4.75 cc	5.0 cc
			(B)	10 cc					
			(C)	450 mg/60 cc [6 days]	480 mg/60 cc	510 mg/60 cc	540 mg/60 cc	470 mg/60 cc	600 mg/60 cc
VLB	1 mg/ml	0.5 mg	(A)	0.75 cc	0.8 cc	0.85 cc	0.9 c	0.95 cc	1 cc
			(B)	7.5 cc					
			(C)	6 mg/60 cc [8 days]	6.4 mg/60 cc	6.8 mg/60 cc	7.2 mg/60 cc	7.6 mg/60 cc	8 mg/60 cc ↑
DDP	1 mg/ml	5 mg	(A)	7.5 cc	8 cc	8.5 cc	9 cc	9.5 cc	10 cc
			(B)	10 cc	10 cc	10.2 cc	10 cc	10 cc	10 cc
			(C)	45 mg/60 cc [6 days]	48 mg/60 cc	50 mg/60 cc	54 mg/60 cc	57 mg/60 cc	60 mg/60 cc ↑
MIT	1 mg/ml	0.5 mg	(A)	0.75 cc	0.8 cc	0.85 cc	0.9 cc	0.95 cc	1.0 cc
			(B)	7.5 cc					
			(C)	6 mg/60 cc [8 days]	6.4 mg/60 cc	6.8 mg/60 cc	7.2 mg/60 cc	7.6 mg/60 cc	8.0 mg/60 cc ↑
FUDR	100 mg/ml	0.1 mg/kg	(A)	50 kg / 0.05 cc	60 kg / .06 cc	70 kg / .07 cc	80 kg / 0.08 cc	90 kg / 0.09 cc	
			(B)	7.5 cc					
			(C)	40 mg/60 cc [8 days]	48 mg/60 cc	56 mg/60 cc	64 mg/60 cc	72 mg/60 cc	↑

5-FU = fluorouracil, CTX = cyclophosphamide, A = minimum cc/day, ADR = doxorubicin, B = Cormed cc/day, VLB = vinblastine, C = traditional Cormed concentration, DDP = cisplatin, [ ] = # days drug supply, MIT = mytomycin, FUDR = floxuridine have been employed commonly, particularly in conjunction with MIT delivered as a bolus for anal and esophageal cancer. The dose-limiting toxicity for short-term infusion has been stomatitis, with an optimal dose rate for 4- or 5-day infusion of 1.1 gram/m^2/day. A phase 1 study of protracted infusion of 5-FU was carried out at 5 dose levels involving 19 patients (see table 4).[2] Dose-limiting toxicity was uniformly manifested as stomatitis with neither leukopenia nor thrombocytopenia. At 200 or 300 mg/m^2/day, essentially all patients achieved a minimum treatment duration of 30 days, with a maximum of 180 days. Above 300 mg/m^2/day, all patients developed dose-limiting stomatitis at less than 21 days. The optimal dose rate for protracted infusion 5-FU, therefore is 300 mg/m^2/day, which permits a minimum duration of infusion of 30 days. This dose rate represents approximately 25% of the daily dose rate established for the short-term 5-day infusion.

In general, the daily dose rate that permits a minimum treatment duration of 30 days permits an extended duration of treatment beyond 30 days without cumulative drug effect resulting in stomatitis. However, an unusual cutaneous syndrome was observed in patients receiving protracted infusion 5-FU that had not been previously reported in patients receiving short-term infusion. The syndrome, designated as palmar plantar erythrodysaethesia, or the hand-foot syndrome, has been observed in conjunction with protracted infusion of doxorubicin (ADR) as well.[3] As suggested by the name, manifestations of the syndrome develop on the palms and soles, with paresthesias that progress to pain and erythema involving the entire surface, with swelling particularly of the distal phalanges. Periungual inflammation is also observed, and the distal phalanges subsequently develop a blister that progresses to desquamation. This syndrome is distinctive from Raynaud's type of cutaneous syndrome associated with high-dose MTX or the vinblastine-bleomycin-cisplatin combination.[4,5] It is also distinctive from the primary desquamation that is seen with severe 5-FU cutaneous sensitivity. The syndrome recedes with interruption of the infusion over a 7–10-day period. Reinstitution of the 5-FU infusion results in reappearance of the syndrome, generally at a shorter interval. In order to continue treatment in those patients who have an optimal tumor response, dose rate induction has been evaluated, but the syndrome will continue to appear. The 3 approaches to the syndrome are (1) to administer the infusional 5-FU on an intermittent schedule, interrupting at the first sign of development of erythema; (2) to employ the antipyrimidine analogue floxuridine (FUDR) on a continuous infusion schedule (see phase 1 study of FUDR); or (3) in those

Table 4. Phase 1 Study of Protracted Infusion of 5-Fluorouracil

Dose rate (mg/m^2/day)	No. patients	Treatment duration (days)	Toxicity
200	5	30 – 180	None
300	4	30 – 60	None
350	4	19 – 23	Stomatitis 3/4
400	4	8 – 12	Stomatitis 4/4
600	2	14	Stomatitis

patients with liver-dominant disease, to deliver the infusion via the regional route. Hepatic extraction minimizes host exposure and obviates the development of the syndrome.

The precise frequency of the syndrome is undetermined, but it may develop in the majority of patients in whom the infusion is delivered for more than 30 days. The pathophysiologic mechanism is unknown, and biopsy of the involved tissue has not been reported. The use of antiinflammatory drugs or corticosteroids has not been effective.

Floxuridine

This antipyrimidine is chemically distinctive from 5-FU in that it is more soluble and therefore is more amenable to regional arterial infusion, which has been the primary application for this agent. Sullivan and Di Conti et al, in separate phase 1 trials of continuous infusion of FUDR, confirmed the clinical efficacy of the drug delivered on this schedule and demonstrated that the tolerated dose decreased when the drug was delivered as an infusion compared to that dose delivered by bolus.[6,7]

In the phase 1 study of protracted infusion FUDR, the objective was to administer a minimum of 30 days of infusion; dose-limiting toxicity was predominantly manifested as gastroenteritis with consequent diarrhea (see table 5.)[8] This toxic manifestation of the disease may radiographically resemble regional enteritis.[9] Eighteen patients received FUDR at a dose rate of 0.1–0.2 mg/kg/day. At a dose of 0.15 mg/kg/day or greater, all patients experienced dose-limiting toxicity, and the median duration of the infusion varied from 9–16 days. In contrast, at 0.1 or 0.125 mg/kg/day, no patient experienced toxicity; the median treatment interval was 30 and 34 days, respectively, and the maximum treatment interval was 38 days.

This study established an optimal dose rate of delivery for protracted infusion of FUDR of 0.125 mg/kg/day for 14 days. This has served as a basis for selection of the dose rate of delivery employed in the prospective comparative trials of hepatic artery versus systemic venous infusion of FUDR.

Doxorubicin

Short-term doxorubicin (ADR) infusion studies employ the same bolus dose delivered over 24- to 96-hour period.[10] These studies established the comparable clinical efficacy of ADR infusion to bolus schedules in breast cancer and

Table 5. Phase 1 Study of Protracted Infusion of Floxuridine

Dose rate (mg/kg/day)	No. patients	Treatment duration (days)	Toxicity
0.1	4	18 – 78	None
0.125	2	30 – 38	None
0.15	5	9 – 28	Diarrhea 4/5
0.175	4	6 – 11	Diarrhea
0.2	3	8 – 14	Diarrhea/stomatitis 3/3

soft tissue sarcoma and identified the fact that a major reduction in cardiac toxicity was achieved by this schedule.

The protracted infusion schedule was employed in phase 1 studies by Garnick et al and by Vogelzang et al, employing an implanted pump system.[11,12] In a relatively small number of patients, dose-limiting toxicity was manifested as stomatitis, and a recommended dose level of 9 mg/m/day for 21 days was established. In these studies, cardiac toxicity was apparently reduced as judged by endomyocardial biopsy assessment in a small number of patients.

The study of protracted infusion ADR by Lokich et al (table 6)[13] was performed employing an external infusion pump with a standard subclavian venous access. A major difference of this study was the fact that patients were maintained on a single dose rate throughout their treatment. In contrast, the studies by Garnick et al and Vogelzang et al employed dose escalation within patient entries, and thus cumulative drug effect may have spuriously affected identifying the optimum dose rate for protracted infusion.

In 23 courses of continuous infusion ADR, the dose rates ranged from 2–5 mg/m^2/day. Dose rate-limiting toxicity was manifested as stomatitis. One patient developed the hand-foot syndrome at 59 days of continuous infusion. At 2 mg/m^2/day and 3 mg/m^2/day in a total of 14 trials, only 2 patients developed mild stomatitis at 30 days or greater. In contrast, at dose rates greater than 3 mg/m^2/day, 4 of 9 patients developed stomatitis associated with leukopenia. No G.I. effects were observed, and cardiac effects were assessed predominantly by standard clinical monitoring. Three patients who received 450 mg/m^2 cumulative dose underwent endomyocardial biopsy, and pathologic changes characteristic of doxorubicin-associated cardial biopsy were not observed. Pharmacologic studies in patients receiving the optimal dose rate of 3 mg/m^2/day failed to demonstrate detectable plasma levels of ADR or its metabolites in the circulation.

Mitomycin-C

This antibiotic alkylating agent has been administered as a short-term infusion for 5 days in 1 study and as a protracted infusion for 3–12 days in another study (see table 7).[14] In these studies, it was suggested that the cumulative dose achieved by infusion was higher than that deliverable by bolus delivery. In the

Table 6. Phase 1 Study of Protracted Infusion of Doxorubicin

Dose rate (mg/m^2/day)	No. patients	Treatment duration (days)	Toxicity
2.0	7	14 – 57	None
3.0	7	18 – 59	Stomatitis 2/7
3.5	3	23 – 35	Stomatitis 1/3 Leukopenia
4.0	5	10 – 28	Stomatitis Leukopenia 2/5
5.0	1	19	Stomatitis Leukopenia

5-day infusion, dose-limiting toxicity was manifested as bone marrow suppression, with major thrombocytopenia observed at day 25 to 33. Stomatitis was observed in only 1 patient. The recommended dose of 2 mg/m^2/day for 5 days was therefore considered the optimal dose rate.

In a protracted infusion study of MIT in 14 patients, the dose rate ranged from 0.75–3 mg/m^2/day and the treatment durations were maximal at the 0.75 mg/m^2/day. Above this dose, essentially all patients developed major leukopenia and thrombocytopenia, with a median nadir for WBC at 1,500 cells/dl at day 42 and a median nadir platelet count of 53,000 at day 36.

Concern regarding the stability of MIT for protracted infusion has been raised based upon the fact that in vitro studies indicate that with a falling pH over time, MIT is degraded to an inactive substance. In the phase 1 clinical studies, however, drug effect was observed in terms of bone marrow toxicity, suggesting that degradation of MIT may yield a substance that is cytotoxic and may be selective for the bone marrow.

Cisplatin

The relatively broad range of activity of DDP and its prominent G.I., neurologic, and renal toxicity have led to interest in the development of delivery schedules that might make this agent more tolerable. Short-term infusion studies have suggested that at a dose rate for infusion comparable to that delivered by bolus, a major reduction of the nausea and vomiting and possibly the renal failure effects may be modified.[15,16]

Protracted infusion DDP has been studied in 15 patients in a phase 1 study at doses ranging from 5.0 to 10.0 mg/m^2/day (see table 8).[17] Dose-limiting toxicity was manifested as nausea observed at dose rates of 6.5 mg/m^2/day or greater. In fact, the median duration of DDP infusion at doses of 6.5 or greater was 8 days, with all patients developing dose rate-limiting nausea. At 5 mg/m^2/day, the median duration of treatment was 21 days, but the range was 10 to 40 days, with essentially no patient developing significant toxicity. Renal failure was observed in 3 patients, possibly related to poor selection for patient entry, in that 2 of the 3 had a solitary kidney. The use of concomitant hydration, however, was not a part of the protocol, so that it is difficult to determine whether the protracted infusion schedule reduced nephrotoxicity. Thrombocytopenia was observed in 1 patient.

Table 7. Phase 1 Study of Protracted Infusion of Mitomycin-C

Dose rate (mg/m^2/day)	No. patients	Treatment duration (days)	Toxicity
0.75	2	30	None
1.0	9	16 – 30	Thrombocytopenia 6/6 Leukopenia 5/6
2.0	2	9 – 14	Thrombocytopenia and leukopenia 1/1
3.0	1	14	Leukopenia and thrombocytopenia

Methotrexate

The antifole compounds have been delivered by various routes and on various schedules, but in only 1 early study has continuous infusion been applied conceptually.[18] In that study, the agent was administered orally, and bioavailability of MTX administered in that fashion may be sporadic.[19] An earlier clinical trial of intermittent parenteral MTX demonstrated an advantage over daily oral administration in the treatment of leukemia and has been used as a basis for intermittent use of this agent;[20] however, the variable routes of administration may have contributed to the observed differences.

Protracted infusion MTX was studied in a phase 1 format by Lokich and Curt,[21] with parallel pharmacologic studies. In 26 courses of treatment, dose rates ranged from 0.75–3.0 mg/m^2/day (see table 9). MTX was detectable in the serum at all dose rates, with concentrations varying from 12.8 nanomolar at the lower dose rate to 140 nM in the higher dose rates. Dose rate-limiting toxicity was stomatitis at the higher dose rates and thrombocytopenia without leukopenia at the lower dose rates. The fact that doses of 2 mg/m^2/day or lower could be associated with cytotoxicity emphasizes the important component of exposure time for this agent in particular. The cumulative dose delivered by an infusion schedule is approximately 1/5 that deliverable by the bolus schedule excluding the concept of citrovorin rescue generally employed in high-dose MTX programs.

Table 8. Phase 1 Study of Protracted Infusion of Cisplatin

Dose rate (mg/m^2/day)	No. patients	Treatment duration (days)	Toxicity
5.0	5	10 – 40	None
6.5	2	6 – 28	Nausea 2/2
7.5	5	6 – 10	Nausea 5/5
10.0	3	4 – 15	Nausea 3/3

Table 9. Phase 1 Study of Protracted Infusion of Methotrexate

Dose rate (mg/m^2/day)	No. patients	Treatment duration (days)	Toxicity
0.75	6	13 – 28	Thrombocytopenia 1/6
1.0	3	6 – 42	Stomatitis 1/3
1.5	3	7 – 16	Anemia, pleurisy
1.75	3	7 – 35	Thrombocytopenia 3/3
2.0	4	17 – 43	Thrombocytopenia Stomatitis 2/2
2.5	3	8 – 28	Stomatitis 3/3
2.75	1	9	Stomatitis 3/3
3.0	3	8 – 12	Stomatitis 3/3

Vinblastine

The periwinkle alkaloids, which inhibit cell growth by arresting cells in mitosis, have a relatively short half-life. Thus, this class of agents would be appropriate for protracted infusion delivery. Vinblastine (VLB) has been studied in a phase 1 program for short-term continuous infusion in which the optimally tolerated dose rate of delivery was 1.2–2.1 mg per meter squared per day.[22]

A protracted infusion schedule for VLB was employed in 26 patients as a phase 2 study in malignant melanoma, but various dose rates were applied; these are presented in the phase 1 format in table 10. The dose rates evaluated range from 0.25–1.0 mg/m^2/day, and dose rate-limiting toxicity was manifested as leukopenia. The optimally tolerated and recommended dose is 0.5 mg/m^2/day, although even at this dose rate, 3/21 patients developed leukopenia.

Cyclophosphamide

As a class of drugs, the alkylating agents do not lend themselves to protracted infusion because of their relative instability. In addition, the concept that alkylating agents are effective against G_0 cells has suggested that the rationale for continuous infusion is marginal. However, as has been alluded to earlier, even alkylating agents are more optimally effective against cycling cells, and this group of compounds represents some of the oldest and the most effective of the antineoplastic drugs. Cyclophosphamide (CTX) was selected for phase 1 trial of protracted infusion because of its stability as well as its availability, parenteral melphalan being restricted to special applications. Thio-tepa, another unique alkylating agent, is presently being studied in a phase 1 trial of continuous infusion. Short-term infusion of CTX for 3 days identified an optimal dose rate of 600 mg/m^2/day, and a 5-day continuous infusion schedule employed a dose rate of 400 mg/m^2/day.[24,25]

The phase 1 study of protracted infusion CTX was carried out in 13 patients employing dose rates of 25–100 mg/m^2/day (see table 11.)[26] Dose-limiting toxicity, manifested as thrombocytopenia, was experienced by 4/13 patients at all but the lowest dose rate of delivery. Two of the 13 patients achieved cumulative durations of 50 and 30 days at dose rates of 25 and 100 mg/m^2/day, respectively.

Table 10. Phase 1 Study of Protracted Infusion of Vinblastine

Dose rate (mg/m^2/day)	No. patients	Treatment duration (days)	Toxicity
0.25	1	32	None
0.5	21	7–89	Leukopenia 3/21
0.75	3	12–30	Leukopenia 1/3
1.0	1	13	Leukopenia

The recommended dose rate of delivery for CTX as a single agent in a protracted infusion schedule was not precisely defined by this phase 1 study in that the majority of the patients did not develop dose-limiting toxicity but rather were removed from the study because of progressive disease or patient choice. In those patients developing thrombocytopenia, extensive prior therapy was identified as a possible contributing factor to the toxicity. The most reasonable conclusion for a recommended dose from the study would be: for good-risk patients, 100 mg/m^2/day; in poor-risk patients defined by age, marrow reserve, prior therapy, or performance status, a dose not exceeding 50 mg/m^2/day.

Summary of Phase 1 Trials of Protracted Infusion Chemotherapy

These phase 1 trials have achieved the following: (1) established the dose rate-limiting toxicity for each of the drugs; (2) identified a new type of toxicity in the form of the hand-foot syndrome; and (3) established the optimal dose rate of delivery defined as the dose rate that would permit a minimum treatment duration for continuous chemotherapy of 30 days.

The patterns of toxicity for each of the agents are shown in table 12. Gastrointestinal toxicity at *the optimal and recommended dose rate* was virtually eliminated for all of the agents. Similarly, marrow suppression was substantially diminished for 3 of the agents, although occasional leukopenia was observed with ADR even at the optimal dose rate. For 4 agents—MIT, MTX, DDP, and CTX—the development of isolated thrombocytopenia may be an unpredictable event, although in general at the optimal recommended dose rate these effects are not observed. Alopecia was inadequately assessed in most of the phase 1 trials in that patients were not monitored prospectively for this effect and, in some instances, insufficient time may have elapsed to permit any reasonable conclusions regarding alopecia. Organ-specific toxicity, particularly cardiac toxicity related to ADR, was substantially ameliorated. The effect of 3 agents known to induce renal failure—MIT, MTX, and DDP—was inadequately evaluated in the phase 1 trials, again related to the limited numbers of patients or duration of study. As a generality, renal effects were not a major complication, and those that did occur may have been obviated if adequate hydration had been employed. Pulmonary effects that have been reported with MIT were not observed in these trials, nor were such effects seen with MTX per

Table 11. Phase 1 Study of Protracted Infusion of Cyclophosphamide

Dose rate (mg/m^2/day)	No. patients	Treatment duration (days)	Toxicity
25	3	15–30	None
50	3	10–20	Thrombocytopenia 2/3
75	4	10–24	Thrombocytopenia 1/4
100	3	10–39	Thrombocytopenia 1/3

se, although some patients did develop a pleurisy syndrome. Finally, the hand-foot syndrome was observed with both 5-FU and ADR; it was not dose rate-limiting but may restrict the duration of treatment.

Dose rate-limiting toxicity in these phase 1 trials must be distinguished from toxicities that may be observed in the context of delivery of the optimal dose rate, which is defined as the dose that will permit delivery of at least 30 days without toxicity. Thus, dose rate-limiting toxicity is stomatitis for 5-FU and ADR; diarrhea for FUDR; marrow suppression for MIT; stomatitis for MTX at high dose rates and thrombocytopenia at low dose rates; marrow suppression for VLB; nausea for DDP; and unpredictable thrombocytopenia for CTX.

A detailed comparison of the cumulative doses delivered by infusion and those delivered by bolus for each of the agents studied in the protracted infusion Phase 1 trials is shown in table 13. The bolus dose rates are determined from the available literature, although the dose rates for VLB and MIT do not conform to the usual schedules in that they are administered, respectively, either weekly or at 4- to 6-week intervals, with relatively few trials on the traditional schedules of every 3–4 weeks. Nonetheless, as a generality, for at least 5 of the 8 studied, the cumulative dose delivered by infusion was comparable to that delivered by the bolus schedule. The 3 exceptions are unpredictable, yet confirm earlier trials in which there were similar findings. For 5-FU, the cumulative dose achievable increased by 400 percent with the infusion schedule, whereas for FUDR, the cumulative dose for the infusion was only 1/10 that achievable by bolus. For MTX, the infusion dose was only 1/4 that achieved by standard bolus schedules. It must be emphasized that toxicity was virtually absent for all the agents delivered by infusion and that for the majority of the patients receiving the same drugs by bolus, virtually all will develop

Table 12. Patterns of Drug Toxicity Observed for Protracted Infusion Chemotherapy at the Optimal Dose Rate

Agent	5-FU	FUDR	ADR	MIT	MTX	VLB	DDP	CTX
Toxicity								
G.I.	None	None	None	None	None	None	None	None
Marrow suppression	None	None	↓ WBC	↓ Plts	↓ Plts	None	↓ Plts	↓ Plts
Alopecia	None	None	+ +	None	None	None	+ +	None
Organ-specific								
Cardiac			Reduced					
Renal				Unknown	Unknown	Unknown		
Pulmonary				Unknown	Pleurisy			
Hand-foot syndrome	+ +	None	+	None	None	None	None	None

5-FU = 5-fluorouracil
FUDR = floxuridine
ADR = doxorubicin
MIT = mitomycin-C
MTX = methotrexate
VLB = vinblastine
DDP = cisplatin
CTX = cyclophosphamide

G.I. effects and bone marrow suppression at "optimal" doses. In comparing the cumulative dose delivered for short-term infusion for 5 days to that of protracted duration infusion for 28–30 days, the daily dose rate of the latter schedule is approximately 25% of the short-term infusion.

Nondrug-related toxicities such as subclavian vein thrombosis, subcutaneous infection, drug extravasation, or pump malfunction are uniquely associated with the mechanisms of the infusion delivery system. Subclavian vein thrombosis may occur in up to 40% of the patients, but is clinically significant in less than 15%.[27] Cutaneous infection, which occurs in less than 5% of the patients, is generally managed without obligate removal of the catheter. Drug extravasation is similarly infrequent and may occur as a consequence of such mechanical problems as needle displacement, catheter disruption or material failure, or central thrombosis with retrograde dissection of the drug. The efficiency and precision of the portable infusion pumps provides for a less than 3% underinfusion per week.

Phase 2 Studies

The phase 2 studies of protracted infusion chemotherapy for each of the 8 single agents have led to a tactical approach to patients as shown in figure 1. Eligible patients are defined by the presence of measurable disease and the conditions necessary for venous access. Patients are treated for an initial 4- to 6-week period and are then categorized as to response. Response criteria are those established for standard phase 2 trials, with standard definitions of progression or nonresponse, stable disease, partial response, and complete response. For patients developing progressive disease at 6 weeks, alternative treatment options are employed. For patients achieving stable disease, the protracted infusion is continued for 4 to 6 more weeks and the disease is

Table 13. Comparison of Cumulative Doses for Infusion Chemotherapy Delivered for 30 Days or Intermittent Bolus Projected for Same Interval Using Optimal Dose for Each Schedule

Agent	Infusion dose rate ($\times$ 30 days)	Bolus dose rate*	I/B‡ ratio
5-Fluorouracil	300 mg/m^2/day	400 mg/m^2/d $\times$ 5	4
Floxuridine	0.125 mg/kg/day	30 mg/kg/d $\times$ 5	0.1
Methotrexate	0.75 mg/m^2/day	40–80 mg/m^2†	0.25
Doxorubicin	3.0 mg/m^2/day	60–90 mg/m^2	1
Vinblastine	0.5 mg/m^2/day	16–20 mg	1
Mitomycin-C	0.75 mg/m^2/day	10–20 mg/m^2	1
Cisplatin	5.0 mg/m^2/day	100–120 mg/m^2/day 1,21	1
Cyclophosphamide	50–100 mg/m^2/day	1 gm/m^2/day 1,21	1

*Estimated dose delivered over 4 weeks
†Without CF rescue
‡Infusion/bolus

reassessed at that point. For patients achieving a minimum of partial response, protracted infusion is also continued in an open-ended fashion to the point of the development of toxicity or patient tolerance or progressive disease. In the latter group, interruption of the infusion for 1–4 weeks for a variety of reasons has often been necessary.

Of the 700 or more patients studied on the protracted infusion schedule with the 8 different single agents, approximately 25% were evaluated in the context of phase 1 trials. Some tumors have been treated with protracted infusion only exceptionally because of the high response rate to standard regimens. Such tumors include testicular cancer, Hodgkin's disease, and non-Hodgkin's lymphoma. This section will review the experience for protracted infusion according to the primary tumor.

Gastrointestinal Cancer

The 5 categories of G.I. cancer represent the most common tumor for which protracted infusion has been employed, and the most frequent agent has been 5-FU. For pancreas and esophagus cancer, the infusion of 5-FU has been combined with concomitant radiation therapy delivered following an initial interval in which the chemotherapeutic agent was administered alone for a 4- to 6-week period.[28]

COLORECTAL CANCER

More than 150 patients with advanced colorectal cancer have been treated with protracted infusion of 5-FU. Of this group, 55 who received treatment for a minimum of 30 days and had measurable disease parameters were evaluated. Of 21 patients with no prior 5-FU chemotherapy, 8 responded, for a response rate of 38%. For the 34 patients who had received prior bolus 5-FU and had not responded, 13 patients demonstrated tumor regression for a response rate of 38% as well, suggesting that infusion delivery schedules may overcome inherent resistance to 5-FU. The duration of responses varied from 3 to 12 months, and survival for the entire 55 patients was approximately 12 months (median),

Initial Treatment Interval

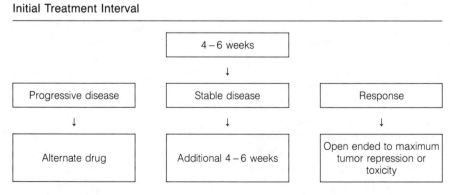

Figure 1.   Tactical approach to patients receiving protracted continuous infusion chemotherapy.

with a median survival of 16 months for responders versus 7 months for nonresponders. Survival times were measured from initiation of infusion chemotherapy.

An interesting aspect of this group of patients has been the subset in whom the liver was the solitary or dominant site of metastasis. Within this group, 15 patients subsequently received regional hepatic artery infusion following relapse after systemic venous infusion. There were no responses in patients receiving regional infusion after developing resistance to systemic infusion.

PANCREAS CANCER

In the group of patients with pancreas cancer receiving continuous infusion, the vast majority had received prior radiation; for the most part, this group did not have measurable tumor by classic criteria. Of 10 evaluable patients receiving protracted infusion 5-FU, there were no responders. Approximately half of this group of patients subsequently received ADR as a single-agent infusion, also without response.

GASTRIC CANCER

Patients with gastric cancer are included in 2 categories. In patients with advanced disease, single-agent protracted infusion 5-FU demonstrated objective responses in 6/13 patients. In addition, 9 patients with surgically removed gastric cancer and positive lymph nodes received postoperative radiation delivered concurrently with protracted infusion 5-FU. Within this group of patients, 6/9 remain disease-free at up to 2 1/2 years postsurgery.

HEPATOCELLULAR CARCINOMA

Protracted infusion chemotherapy for hepatoma has involved either 5-FU or ADR. In 1 of 5 patients receiving protracted infusion ADR, a sustained response was achieved for about 12 months, at which time brain metastases developed. In 1 of 3 patients receiving single-agent 5-FU as a continuous infusion, a transient objective response in pulmonary metastases was observed for about 4 months.

ESOPHAGEAL CANCER

The strategy of esophageal cancer has involved single-agent 5-FU administered for about 6 weeks, at which time a reassessment determines the role of concomitant free agent therapy. A general schema for this approach to esophageal cancer is shown in figure 2. This treatment program does not involve additional agents such as MIT or DDP, which have been employed in conjunction with short-term 5-FU infusion. In 6 of 8 patients with primary esophageal cancer (2 adenocarcinoma, 6 epidermoid carcinoma), regression of the primary tumor was observed, although the usual criteria for objective response were not applicable. All 6 patients improved symptomatically and maintained weight throughout their treatment. Three of the 8 patients had a complete regression following the addition of radiation and for various clinical reasons did not subsequently come to surgery. All 3 remain disease-free at 2 or more years since initial treatment.

Other Cancers

BREAST CANCER

All patients with breast cancer have received prior chemotherapy and in some instances hormone treatment as well. The initial chemotherapy in general was the standard 3-drug regimen consisting of CTX, MTX, and 5-FU. The primary agent evaluated in this tumor category was protracted infusion ADR, and responses were observed in 2/11 patients. At least half of the patients with breast cancer had received prior ADR by standard bolus delivery. In addition, 4 patients received infusion VLB as a single agent, and no responses were observed on the protracted infusion schedule.

LUNG CANCER

Nonsmall-cell lung cancer was approached with protracted infusion of 5 different single agents involving only 13 patients. No responses were observed. There were no patients treated with protracted infusion in the category of small-cell carcinoma of the lung. Although bronchogenic carcinoma is a common tumor, it was inadequately represented in the protracted infusion series for any of the agents; therefore, the role of chemotherapy infusion on this schedule remains undetermined.

OVARIAN CANCER

Although no responses were observed in the 11 patients receiving 1 of 4 different single-agent protracted infusions, all patients had received prior therapy; for many, tumor resistance to the agent had been established. Thus, for example, of the 4 patients treated with protracted infusion ADR, all had received standard bolus ADR as part of a combination regimen.

MALIGNANT MELANOMA

Of the agents administered to patients with advanced melanoma, the largest experience was with protracted infusion VLB. With this agent, 2/11 patients

Integrated Multimodality Therapy for Esophageal Cancer

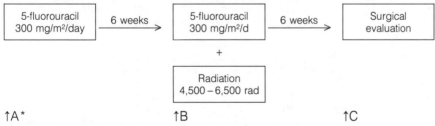

↑A*   ↑B   ↑C

*Pretreatment staging to include endoscopy, barium swall, CT scans of chest and abdomen. Increased reassessment points for tumor status and response to modality.

Figure 2.   Tactical approach to the management of esophageal cancer employing protracted infusion schedules.

demonstrated response in soft tissue and lymph node disease, respectively. VLB has been a known active (albeit marginally) drug in the treatment of melanoma. The responses observed were short-lived, lasting less than 3 months.

SOFT TISSUE SARCOMA

One of 14 patients treated with protracted infusion ADR responded in this tumor category, and 1 of 3 responded to VLB. There were no responses in small groups of patients treated with CTX, DDP, and MTX. For the most part, the last 3 drugs were administered to patients previously treated extensively with standard regimens as well as infusion regimens.

MISCELLANOUS TUMOR CATEGORIES

For head and neck cancer, only 2 patients have been treated: 1 patient receiving protracted infusion 5-FU demonstrated a complete response after not having responded to a regimen of BLM and DDP. In the category of non-Hodgkin's lymphoma, there were no responses observed in 3 patients who received protracted infusion ADR after extensive prior therapy including a minimum of 4 different regimens, at least 1 of which included standard bolus ADR. Finally, in the category of unknown primary tumor, one patient responded to protracted infusion 5-FU.

Summary

A summary of the total experience for the 7 single-agent protracted infusion phase 2 studies is shown in table 14. It is evident that many of the tumors are underrepresented in each of the phase 2 trials, and it should be emphasized that the groups were extraordinarily heterogeneous in terms of disease distribution and performance status; also, patient entries were heavily weighted on the side of extensive prior therapy. Thus, low response rates and even high response rates must be viewed with some circumspection. There are, in fact, no definitive conclusions that can be drawn from this experience except to state that antitumor activity is observed for most of the agents. The absence of any

Table 14. Summary of Observed Tumor Responses According to Infusion Agent and Tumor Category

Agent	5-FU	ADR	DDP	CTX	MTX	MIT	VLB
TUMOR							
Colorectal	21/55	–	–	–	–	–	–
Pancreas	0/10	0/2	–	–	–	–	–
Gastric	6/13	0/2	–	–	–	–	–
Hepatoma	1/3	1/5	–	–	–	–	–
Esophagus	6/8	0/1	0/1	–	–	–	–
Breast	–	2/11	–	–	–	–	0/4
Lung	–	0/8	0/2	0.3	–	–	–
Ovary	–	0/4	0/3	–	–	–	0/4
Melanoma	–	0/2	–	–	0/2	–	0/11
Sarcoma	–	1/14	0/2	0/1	0/2	–	1/3

activity whatsoever for MIT delivered by protracted infusion may be related to the small number of patients studied with generally resistant tumors. For the CTX and MTX trials as well as for the DDP trial, the data in table 14 are actually derived from the original phase 1 trial for these agents. Thus, these agents need to be explored further in the context of formal phase 2 trials.

In addition to indicating that there is in fact some measure of activity for the protracted infusion schedule, there is also a suggestion that the antitumor activity is consistent with the spectrum of tumors usually associated with the bolus schedule. Thus, 5-FU is active in the G.I. carcinomas and ADR is active in breast cancer and to some degree in sarcoma, but not in ovarian cancer. However, such a conclusion is not totally supported by an ideal data base. Evaluating protracted infusion for individual agents in tumors other than those for which the agent is usually employed is still reasonable.

Two clinical observations made in the context of these trials deserve mention. First, the concern that protracted low-dose infusion may lead to the development of early tumor resistance is an important issue – one that would only be reasonably addressed in the context of phase 3 trials. The rather short duration of responses observed in the above trials, however, does lead to some concern that low-dose protracted infusion may, in fact, lead to tumor cell resistance. Secondly, on an anecdotal level, patients achieving response and interrupting treatment for whatever reason, generally for personal preference, may have an early recrudescence of tumor that in some instances, at least, responds to reexposure to the initial treatment. Such observation suggests but does not definitively establish the fact that an extended drug exposure for long periods may maximize the antitumor effects.

Phase 3 Trials

Although the phase 2 trials have identified the fact that protracted infusion chemotherapy may induce tumor responses, there is at this point no definitive evidence that infusion chemotherapy is superior to standard bolus treatment. Furthermore, although it can be definitely established for most of the agents that infusion, either short-term or protracted, may substantially modify the acute and chronic toxicity patterns for these agents, it is not at all clear that the therapeutic index is substantively affected, particularly when all parameters involved in a cost/benefit analysis are considered. Thus, the critical importance of phase 3 trials comparing infusion schedules to standard bolus regimens is obvious.

Such trials are, by the nature of the practice of oncology, difficult to execute. The technology and cost involved in developing venous access programs and ambulatory infusion pump capability has impeded cooperative group trials from taking the initiative to evaluate infusion chemotherapy. Nonetheless, it is clear that because of the larger numbers of patients necessary to answer the questions of the relative effectiveness of bolus and infusion chemotherapy, such group trials are essential.

Single-agent phase 3 trials are ongoing in advanced colorectal cancer for 5-FU, but such trials would seem to be warranted also to assess ADR. The latter agent is more difficult to evaluate because it is generally included in multidrug regimens for breast cancer and soft tissue sarcoma; therefore, it would be necessary to compare (in a phase 3 experimental design) a 3-drug regimen using an infusion schedule for the study agent (ADR) in one arm and a bolus schedule for all component drugs in the second arm.

These phase 3 trials should address not only the relative effectiveness of the 2 schedules but also the relative cost-effectiveness. In addition, the important question of induction of tumor cell resistance as a consequence of bolus versus infusion may be identified if adequate patient accrual can be accumulated. An important question that has not been addressed in ongoing trials is a determination of what might be the optimal duration of infusion. Thus, if infusion chemotherapy should be established as superior to bolus chemotherapy, there may be an optimal duration of treatment. Future trials should therefore compare a variety of infusion schedules. The concepts of combination chemotherapy employing multiple drugs and the use of alternating noncross-resistant combinations will result in a variety of potential permutations for interdigitating the infusion schedule and, it is to be hoped, will result in an improvement in the effectiveness of cancer chemotherapy.

SECTION III

Systemic Infusion by Tumor Category

20

HEAD AND NECK CANCER

Efstathios Tapazoglou, M.D., and
Muhyi Al-Sarraf, M.D., F.R.C.P.(C), F.A.C.P.

Background

SQUAMOUS CELL CARCINOMA OF the head and neck, a rare (5% of all types of cancers) tumor in the United States,[1] represents a heterogeneous group of malignant tumors with a history of high morbidity and mortality. The cure rate is low despite the fact that most lesions are localized or have spread only to the regional lymph nodes at the time of presentation.[2] Squamous cell cancer is the most common tumor of the head and neck region. The standard therapies of surgery and radiotherapy have a high cure rate for patients with early stages (1 or 2) of disease, but have often failed for advanced tumors (stages 3 and 4). Local recurrence and persistent disease occur in 20–40% of the patients, and approximately 10–20% of all patients develop distant metastases.[3]

The treatment of advanced and recurrent head and neck epidermoid cancer remains a significant clinical problem. This group of tumors is associated with a very dismal prognosis and reported median survival of less than 6 months.[4,5] Several reasons account for this shortened survival, but the primary reasons are persistence and local recurrence of disease (despite optimal local treatment with surgery and radiation therapy) and the development of distant metastases. In addition, multiple primary cancers are observed quite often and can be synchronous or metachromous, thus having a high fatality rate. The most common sites for these tumors are other head and neck regions, lung, and esophagus. Finally, the high incidence of other medical problems, such as heart disease, pulmonary disease, and cirrhosis, account for the increased morbidity rate and impose difficulty in the treatment of these tumors.

Until recently, chemotherapy has been reserved for those patients with advanced or recurrent stages of disease. The value of its use in head and neck tumors was questioned[6] and its effective development was halted by several obstacles. The treatment of this disease was based totally on local therapy modalities such as surgery and/or radiation therapy. In addition, there was a lack of effective chemotherapeutic agents. Finally, the extensive prior therapy and declining performance and nutritional status of these patients has predictably resulted in poor responses and short survival.[7] Despite these obstacles, the development and evaluation of a number of newer agents active against head and neck squamous carcinoma and the encouraging results of adjuvant chemotherapy strategies in other solid tumors have provided rationale for the development of similar programs for head and neck carcinoma. Additionally, the grim statistical results for patients with advanced and recurrent head and neck cancer made such treatment programs a necessity.

A number of theoretical mechanisms would support the use of combined treatment modalities in head and neck tumors. Chemotherapy prior to definitive treatment (induction chemotherapy) may reduce the size of the tumor and allow a reduction in the field of surgery or radiotherapy, thus allowing surgery or radiotherapy that otherwise would not have been possible. The intact vascular supply to the tumor prior to surgery or radiotherapy may lead to better vascular access of the drug to the tumor. Further, reduction of the tumor size may increase vascularization and oxygenation, rendering tumors more sensitive to radiation therapy and thereby acting as a radiosensitizer and improving the response to radiation. The generally better nutritional and performance status of patients at the beginning of their disease may result in better responses. A reduction of local recurrences and perhaps of distant metastases from tumor cells spreading at the time of surgery would be expected using induction chemotherapy. The use of chemotherapy as induction or as classic "adjuvant" treatment early in the course of the disease would be expected to eradicate micrometastases and reduce distal spread.[7-9]

Multiple studies have now been performed using chemotherapy in the combined modality fashion, predominately in the induction role or concurrent with radiotherapy.[2,10,11] Prior to these studies, a large number of single cytotoxic agents have been tested in patients with metastatic head and neck cancers.[2,12,13] The use of these single agents has produced a wide range of response rates that were found to vary according to the primary site of origin, previous therapy, performance status and selection of the patients, response criteria, and methods of data collection[2,5,14-17] (the factors that may affect the response rate to systemic chemotherapy and the survival in recurrent and metastatic head and neck cancer are extensively outlined in reference 2). The three most investigated single agents that have consistently been shown to have antitumor activity are methotrexate (MTX), bleomycin, and cisplatin.

Methotrexate

The activity of MTX has been known for a number of years. It is the most studied agent and is regarded as the standard therapy for recurrent head and neck squamous cancer.[2,4,12,13,18,19] MTX has been administered in different dosages and schedules and by different methods with or without leucovorin rescue. The overall response rate ranged from 8–63% in evaluable patients.[2] In a large series of reports representing reports of single arm or randomized trials in which MTX was used, the response rate (complete [CR] and partial [PR]) was 31% (305/988).[2] The reported CR ranged from 0%–15%. At Wayne State University, we gave MTX at a dose of 40 mg/m² I.V. weekly without rescue in patients with adequate renal function. Our overall response rate (CR + PR) was 30% for all patients entered with evaluable and measurable lesion(s).[5,17,20] The results of the widespread experience with the use of MTX indicate that the response duration and the overall survival of these patients are short-lived (median 3 and 6 months, respectively).

Bleomycin

As a single agent, bleomycin (BLM) appears to be generally less effective than MTX, although no comparative study has been performed.[2,4,9,21] The drug has been mainly given I.M. or I.V. (bolus) on a weekly (22) or twice-weekly frequency as well as by I.V. infusion for 72– 100-hour schedules. The optimal method of administration remains to be determined. The overall response rate to this agent was 21% (73/347) and the complete response rate 2% (6/347).[2] Remissions generally have been of short duration. Although prolonged treatment is limited by cumulative pulmonary toxicity, the lack of severe myelosuppressive toxicity has led to the use of BLM with other chemotherapeutic agents for patients with recurrent head and neck cancer or as induction combined therapy before surgery and/or radiotherapy for locally advanced disease.

Cisplatin

Cisplatin (DDP) is the most recently introduced agent in the treatment of squamous cell cancer of the head and neck. Experience with this agent suggests that its antitumor activity is comparable to that of MTX with respect to both remission and duration of response.[2,23-26] It has antitumor activity even in patients previously treated with other chemotherapeutic agents. Prehydration and mannitol diuresis have minimized the nephrotoxicity of the drug without affecting its antitumor effect. The overall response rate of DDP as a single agent in patients with head and neck cancer was 28% (81/288), with a range of 14% to 41%.[2] Unfortunately, responses to single-agent DDP are of approximately 4 months' duration.

In addition to the above 3 most active agents, antitumor activity has been reported with the use of 5-fluorouracil (5-FU), cyclophosphamide (CTX), vinca alkaloids, doxorubicin, and the nitrosoureas.[2,27-29] These agents have been used mainly as part of combination chemotherapy regimens.

Combination Chemotherapy

The development of single active chemotherapeutic agents soon led to the use of combinations of these agents in the treatment of advanced and recurrent head and neck tumors.[2] Although many clinical trials have investigated the effects of combination chemotherapy in this type of disease, few prospective randomized studies have compared combination chemotherapy with single-agent therapy. The overall response rate does not seem any different when compared to single-agent therapy. Neither the complete response rate nor the overall survival was better with the use of combination chemotherapy versus single agents in head and neck cancer patients.[2,20] The use of combination chemotherapy was found to be tolerable, and the degree of toxicity varied according to the dose and schedule of each agent used in the combination. The combination chemotherapy trials have been extensively reviewed by Al-Sarraf for the reader interested in a detailed discussion.[2]

Only 8 randomized trials have been performed and reported so far.[2] We reported on the randomized study between MTX and DDP, oncovin, and BLM (COB), with stratification based on previous radiation therapy and the patients' performance status.[17,20] No differences were found in response rate, duration of response, or survival between the 2 groups. Deconti et al[16] compared MTX to high-dose MTX with leucovorin rescue to a combination of high-dose MTX with rescue, CTX, and cytarabine. They reported that the combination was not better than single-agent MTX for response rate and/or overall survival.

Induction Chemotherapy

Patients with locally advanced head and neck cancers (stages 3 and 4) have always presented a challenge in the management of head and neck tumors. The survival statistics for these groups of patients are grim at best. Surgery and radiotherapy have been used in combination, aiming at improving local control.[46] Unfortunately, the overall survival continues to be poor and unacceptable. Recent emphasis has been on the use of chemotherapy as initial treatment before surgery or radiotherapy in patients with locally advanced stage 3 and 4 head and neck tumors. The several theoretical advantages to using induction chemotherapy have already been mentioned. This rationale was influenced by the observations of higher tumor response rates and longer durations of response in previously untreated patients when compared to the effects in patients with recurrent tumors. In addition, the use of this type of treatment was supported further by experimental evidence in several animal tumor models.[30]

MTX, DDP, and BLM (either alone or in combination) have been used for induction chemotherapy.[2,31-42] The response rate observed with induction chemotherapy in previously untreated patients is clearly superior to the response rate in patients who have undergone prior surgery, radiation therapy, or both.[2,14,32] Several studies have confirmed that it is feasible to proceed to surgery, radiotherapy, or both after such induction chemotherapy without any obvious increase in morbidity. High rates of tumor regression have been achieved using multidrug combinations, primarily DDP, BLM, and MTX, and lately, 5-FU.[2] Recent combinations of DDP and 5-FU have achieved complete responses in the range of 30–54% and overall responses in the range of 80–100%.[2,43,77,96,101,109,112,116] Although some of these CRs were associated with histologic evidence of persistent tumor, the achievement of high numbers of complete responders and an improved survival for patients achieving a CR to chemotherapy prior to local therapy compared to partial- or nonresponders has been demonstrated.[44,45] Although results are very optimistic, it is unfortunate that they have not been translated into an increase in overall survival.[47] Further studies and detailed analysis of randomized trials with patient populations carefully balanced for prognostic factors will be required in the future.

Chemotherapy Combined with Radiotherapy

The very poor survival results of patients with stages 3 and 4 head and neck cancers prompted the investigators to initiate trials of combination chemotherapy and radiotherapy. The principal objectives of using this combination modality were to improve the therapeutic efficacy by controlling disseminated disease with the chemotherapy and simultaneously enhancing local control. In addition, cytoreduction of the tumor by radiation could enhance the cytotoxic ability of the chemotherapeutic agents. Further, simultaneous use of certain chemotherapeutic agents could potentiate the killing effect of ionizing radiation.[2,48]

Several studies have been performed in which various single agents and drug combinations have been used simultaneously with radiation.[2,4,49-51] BLM has been the chemotherapeutic agent most frequently used concurrently with radiotherapy for head and neck cancer. In addition, 5-FU, MTX, hydroxyurea, and recently, DDP were included in these kinds of trials. Most of these studies of single-agent and multidrug combination chemotherapy and concurrent radiotherapy have not demonstrated any significant survival advantage, even though the results of some of the studies have been contradictory. Most of the studies did demonstrate an enhanced loco-regional tumor control,[49,52] but local toxicities (other than DDP and radiotherapy) increased markedly; also, morbidity has been severe and patient tolerance very poor, necessitating the interruption of the radiotherapy. No evidence of decreased incidence of distant metastases has been demonstrated in these studies. The principal objectives of combining the 2 modalities (to obtain improved therapeutic ratio) have not been achieved at present.

Rationale of Infusion Chemotherapy

There is abundant evidence that differences in rate of drug administration may produce profound differences in biologic effect, among which may be differences in therapeutic response. The effects of a particular dosage schedule on the activity of an antineoplastic drug involve a complex interaction between the pharmacokinetic behavior of that drug, its actions on the various phases of the cell cycle, and the growth kinetics and drug sensitivity of individual tumors. Numerous studies with experimental animal tumors as well as human tumors have demonstrated the critical importance of drug scheduling in therapy.[53-59] An example demonstrating the effects of rate of drug administration is found in the experience with cytarabine, which is known to be a cycle-specific drug. When this compound is given by continuous infusion, it is far more effective than when given once daily in both murine and human leukemia.[56,57]

Another difference in the biologic effect of a chemotherapy drug, one that is produced by changes in the rate of drug administration, is the improvement in the therapeutic ratio or index of that particular drug. It is well known that the therapeutic index or ratio between therapeutic and toxic doses is low for most anticancer agents. Therefore, efforts to improve this low index have been directed toward modifying the schedule of drug administration using continuous drug infusions. Several such studies have been conducted, and the results have suggested that some anticancer agents demonstrate improved therapeutic index when administered by continuous I.V. infusion when compared to conventional I.V. bolus injections.[60-63] The toxicity of the anticancer drugs used in these studies was observed to be decreased. One additional advantage is the possibility of overcoming the resistance due to the low proportion of proliferating cells in a tumor that may be prominent when cell cycle or phase-specific drugs are administered by bolus injections.[64]

Continuous I.V. infusion chemotherapy has been incorporated into many different chemotherapy regimens. Many agents have been studied extensively, including those most commonly used in the treatment of advanced head and neck cancer—BLM, 5-FU, and DDP.

Bleomycin appears to affect cells by directly binding to and cleaving DNA and is considered cell cycle phase-specific.[53] BLM has a short half-life when I.V. bolus injection is used, with rapid renal excretion in both mice and man. It is believed that cells in the G_2 phase of the cell cycle appear to be most sensitive to the lethal effects of BLM.[65] Because of the cell cycle specificity and short half-life of the drug, it was speculated that its administration by continuous infusion would be more advantageous than by bolus injection. This hypothesis has been tested in experimental animal studies that revealed superior antitumor activity and simultaneously decreased pulmonary toxicity when BLM was administered by continuous infusion.[60,66] The effects on pulmonary function of 7-day continuous infusion of BLM were prospectively studied in 15 patients, 13 of whom had squamous cell cancer of the head and neck. None of the patients demonstrated clinically evident pulmonary toxicity.[64]

5-FU, a relatively S phase-specific agent, was initially used as an I.V. bolus injection. These initial studies demonstrated significant antitumor activities associated, however, with a relatively high incidence of toxicity. The short serum half-life of the drug and the high incidence of toxic side effects of the bolus schedule led to early trials using continuous infusion.[62,68-70] These studies showed decreased incidence of myelosuppression and nausea, but somewhat increased incidence of mycositis and diarrhea. When compared to bolus injections, the antitumor efficacy in most of the studies was not any different between bolus and continuous-infusion 5-FU.[62] In our own experience in a randomized trial, the combination of 96–hour continuous infusion 5-FU and DDP was superior to the combination of bolus 5-FU and DDP. (76% versus 20% response rate) in patients with recurrent head and neck cancer.[71] Recent experimental work at Wayne State University has demonstrated the superiority of continuous infusion over the bolus treatment.[76]

Cisplatin, a heavy metal compound that acts by cross-linking of DNA and is believed to have action similar to that of the alkylating agents, has been noted in clinical trials to have activity against several types of tumors, including head and neck cancer. Nephrotoxicity and severe nausea and vomiting are the limiting toxicities. In an attempt to modify their side effects, especially the renal toxicity, various doses and schedules have been used. Preclinical studies have shown that continuous infusion DDP therapy against malignant cell lines was not superior to bolus.[72,73] The clinical studies demonstrated that continuous infusion DDP resulted in less severe nausea and vomiting than the bolus and decreased nephrotoxicity when given with vigorous diuresis.[74,75]

In addition to the above-mentioned agents, MTX has been used in an intra-arterial infusion schedule, as a single agent and in combination with other agents.[4]

Clinical Trials

Continuous I.V. infusion chemotherapy recently has been incorporated into many different experimental chemotherapy regimens. Although a large number of single cytotoxic agents and combination chemotherapy have been tested in patients with head and neck cancer, and multiple studies have been performed using chemotherapy in the combined modality approach, studies using continuous I.V. infusion are limited. The 3 most investigated single agents used as a continuous I.V. infusion in head and neck cancer are BLM, 5-FU, and DDP. Because these 3 drugs have consistently been shown to have antitumor activity against head and neck tumors, it was only natural to test them first, using the continuous infusion mode. The advantages of their antitumor efficacy and therapeutic index have been demonstrated by their administration in a continuous infusion mode. In the treatment of head and neck cancer, these advantages have led the investigators to administer continuous infusion of these agents as part of combination regimens with other chemotherapeutic agents and radiotherapy.

Before addressing the results of these clinical trials, it is very important to emphasize the significance of factors that may affect the response rate to chemotherapy and the overall survival of patients with advanced and recurrent head and neck cancers. These factors have been extensively reviewed by Al-Sarraf for any reader interested in a detailed discussion.[2] Several prognostic factors (variables) that influence response rates to chemotherapy have been recognized. The most widely accepted ones are the primary site of involvement, the stage and particularly the nodal status, and the performance status.[2,5,14-17] Another factor is the previous therapy and further, the response to chemotherapy. Our results and the results of others do suggest that patients who have demonstrated a complete or partial response to chemotherapy are more likely to remain free of disease following definitive therapy with surgery and radiation.[77-79] Additionally, patients responding to chemotherapy have been far more likely than nonresponsive patients to respond to radiation therapy.[80] Because the several study results will be influenced by these variables, it is important to consider them when pilot studies are evaluated.

Infusion Chemotherapy for Recurrent Disease

SINGLE AGENTS

Although a large number of single cytotoxic agents have been tested and have shown antitumor activity in patients with head and neck tumors, studies of the use of these agents as a single continuous infusion are scant in the literature. The most investigated agents used in a palliative therapy of head and neck cancer have been MTX, BLM, and DDP. MTX, the most widely studied single agent in patients with recurrent disease, has been administered in different schedules and doses, with or without leucovorin rescue, but has not been used as a continuous infusion. BLM, the other active agent in head and neck cancer, has limited usefulness as a single agent in recurrent disease and has not been used in a single-agent continuous infusion mode. In an attempt to ameliorate renal toxicity and improve the therapeutic index of DDP, Jacobs et al[74] administered this agent as a 24-hour infusion. The most frequent dose used was 80 mg/m² repeated every 3 weeks. Eighteen patients participated in the study, but only 12 were treated for recurrent disease, following radiation and surgery and/or chemotherapy (4 patients). One complete, 5 partial (>50% regression), and 4 minimal (25–50% regression) responses were achieved. The overall response was 39% (50% for the recurrent disease patients). Mild renal and hematological toxicity was observed. Nausea and vomiting, which was mild and of short duration, was reported. The median duration of response was 6+ months for CR and 2–4+ months for PR.

Subsequently, Jacobs et al,[81] reporting for the Northern California Oncology Group, demonstrated an overall response rate of 18% in 40 evaluable patients with recurrent squamous cell cancer of the head and neck using cisplatin at a dose of 80 mg/m² delivered as a 24-hour infusion. Three patients (8%) achieved a CR and 4 patients a PR (10%). The median duration of the response was 7.5 months. The toxicity was tolerable.

A higher dose of DDP was used by Creagan et al,[82] who administered 90 mg/m² delivered by 24-hour infusion in 33 patients with advanced upper aerodigestive cancer. Twenty-three of these patients had squamous cell carcinoma of the head and neck. An overall response rate of 13% was achieved in these patients for a median duration of response of 5–8 months. No complete responses were achieved. Although the toxicities observed were comparable to those seen in the two studies by Jacobs et al,[74,81] these results were inferior. This study also included patients who were previously treated with radiation and surgery.

Prolonged DDP infusion was used by Lokich,[83] who treated 33 patients with metastatic malignancies of various types with continuous 120-hour infusion. Only 3 patients with squamous head and neck cancer were included in the study. The pattern of toxicity observed differed from that observed when the drug was administered by bolus or short-term infusion. The most striking difference was the dramatic reduction in G.I. toxicity. The author concluded that the recommended starting dose for continuous various infusion therapy with DDP was 30 mg/m²/day for 120 hours.

The administration of DDP in these studies was associated with vigorous pre-

and posttreatment hydration with normal saline,[74,81-83] the administration of mannitol,[83] and the supplementation of potassium and magnesium when necessary. The use of furosemide was individualized to the needs of the patients.

5-FU is another agent that has demonstrated activity in head and neck cancer, with overall response rates of approximately 15%.[2] This agent, because of its limited myelotoxicity when administered as a continuous infusion,[62] has been used extensively in combination with DDP for recurrent disease and in induction regimens for locally advanced disease. We have studied a group of 11 patients with recurrent and locally advanced head and neck cancer who, because of poor renal function, received 5-FU as a 96- to 120-hour continuous infusion as a single agent.[84,85] Seven patients had been previously treated with surgery and/or radiation, 3 patients had locally advanced disease, and 1 patient had disseminated cancer. The infusion dose was 1,000 mg/m²/24 hours for 4 days (previously radiated patients) or 5 days (for patients without previous radiation therapy). Eight of 11 patients (72%) demonstrated a response (7 partial and 1 complete). Responses occurred in 4/4 (all PR) in previously untreated epidermoid cancer and 4/7 in recurrent cancer not previously treated with chemotherapy. The predominant toxicities were stomatitis (55%) and mild leukopenia (18%).

COMBINATION INFUSION CHEMOTHERAPY

Continuous I.V. infusion chemotherapy has been recently incorporated into many different experimental chemotherapy regimens. Over the past few years, active combinations identified have included continuous infusion chemotherapy, many of them synergistic in action. Because extensive controlled trials have not been conducted and those that have been represent small numbers of patients from single institutions, no single regimen can be advocated as the superior regimen for patients with recurrent head and neck cancer. Nevertheless, some combinations have been used so extensively that investigators have become experienced with their use and toxicities.

Most infusion chemotherapy tested in recurrent head and neck cancer has included the use of BLM, 5-FU, and DDP infusion. Multidrug continuous infusion has been used in a limited numbers of trials (see table 1).

Costanzi et al[86] reported on the use of 48-hour continuous infusion bleomycin (7.5 mg/m²/24 hours in 5% dextrose and 0.45 NaCl saline solution), followed by a dose of either MTX or hydroxyurea in 36 patients with disseminated carcinoma. Although a 59% response rate was noted among 17 patients with recurrent epidermoid carcinoma of head and neck, the median duration of response was only 2 months. High response rates were achieved by Ervin et al[87] with DDP (20mg/m²/day I.V. days 1–5), BLM (10 units/m²/day I.V. continuous infusion days 3–7), MTX (200 mg/m² I.V. days 15, 22), and leucovorin (20 mg p.o. 96 hour × 48 hour). They reported on 11 patients with recurrent disease who achieved 100% overall response rate for a median duration of 4+ months. The toxicity of this regimen was tolerable.

At Wayne State University,[14,17,20] the combination of DDP, oncovin, and BLM produced a response rate of 50% (11/12) and 40% (11/27) in 2 consecutive trials. BLM was administered at a dose of 30 units/day continuous infusion

Table 1. Combination Infusion Chemotherapy in Recurrent Head and Neck Cancer

Study/Reference	Regimen	Evaluable patients	No./% CR	No./% PR	Overall Response (%)
Costanzi et al[86]	Bleomycin (I)* Methotrexate or Hydroxyurea	17	1 (4,5)	12 (4,5)	59
Ervin et al[87]	Cisplatin Bleomycin (I) Methotrexate Leucovorin	11	3 (27)	8 (73)	100
Amer et al[14]	Cisplatin Bleomycin (I) Vincristine	22	0	13 (50)	50
Al-Sarraf et al[20]	Cisplatin Bleomycin (I) Vincristine	27	3 (11)	8 (30)	41
Amrein et al[88]	Cisplatin (I) Bleomycin (I) Vincristine	33	1 (3)	9 (27)	30
Plasse et al[89]	Bleomycin (I) Cyclophasphamide Methotrexate 5-Fluorouracil	24	1 (4)	4 (17)	21
Gonzalez et al[90]	Cisplatin (I) Bleomycin (I) Vinblastine Methotrexate	15	3 (20)	8 (53)	73
Carey et al[19]	Cytoxan Methotrexate Bleomycin (I) Cisplatin (I)	23	5 (21)	9 (39)	60
Kish et al[15] [71]	Cisplatin 5-FU (I)	30	8 (27)	13 (43)	70
	Cisplatin + 5-FU (I) vs	17	4 (23)	9 (53)	76
	Cisplatin + 5-FU bolus	20	3 (15)	1 (5)	20
Rowland et al[94]	Cisplatin 5-FU (I)	21	5 (24)	10 (47)	71
Fosser et al[95]	Cisplatin 5-FU (I)	30	6 (20)	14 (47)	67
Amrein[96]	Cisplatin (I) 5-FU (I)	30	7 (13)	10 (28)	40
Spaulding[97]	5-FU (I) Vinblastine (I)	21	NA	NA	28

*Infusion

for 4 days to patients with adequate renal and pulmonary functions. In the second trial[17,20] the combination was prospectively compared to weekly administration of MTX. The overall response to MTX was 33.3%, not statistically different from the response to the 3-drug combination.

DDP, oncovin, and BLM were also administered by Amrein et al[88] to 33 patients on a different schedule. DDP was given at a dose of 80 mg/m^2 as a 24-hour continuous infusion, followed by vincristine (1 mg/m^2) and bleomycin at 15 units/day for 4 days as continuous infusion. The overall response rate was 30%, with a median duration of response of 4 months. The toxicity of those regimens was mild and without severe renal toxicity.

BLM as a continuous I.V. infusion has been administered in combination with CTX, MTX, 5-FU,[89] and in combination with continuous infusion DDP, vinblastine, and MTX and CTX.[90,91] The overall responses in these studies have been reported as 21%, 73%, and 60%, respectively.

Despite the response rates achieved by these combinations, many patients with carcinoma of the head and neck are not candidates for the above regimens because of their previous smoking history and age. Marginal pulmonary functions cannot withstand therapy with BLM, since its pulmonary toxicity is cumulative and irreversible. On this basis, at Wayne State BLM was replaced with 5-FU, which we found to have (as a single agent) good activity, producing a 31% overall response rate (5) in advanced, previously treated head and neck patients. Because of the increased myelosuppression associated with 5-FU bolus, we preferred the continuous 5-FU infusion.[62] We initially used 5-FU continuous infusion with DDP in previously untreated patients.[115] The excellent response rate (89%) obtained with this combination[92,115] encouraged us to use it for recurrent and/or disseminated squamous carcinoma of the head and neck.[15,93] DDP 100 mg/m^2 I.V. bolus was administered on day 1 with hydration and mannitol diuresis. 5-FU 1,000 mg/m^2/day for 96-hour infusion was started immediately after cisplatin on day 1. Of 30 patients, 8 (27%) achieved a CR and 13 (43%) a PR, for an overall response rate of 70%. The response rate in patients with recurrent loco-regional disease (89%) was observed to be superior to that in patients with disseminated disease (36%). The toxicities were mild and well tolerated by the patients.

In a subsequent study that attempted to minimize inpatient hospital days and evaluate bolus toxicities, we prospectively evaluated 5-FU infusion and DDP versus 5-FU bolus and DDP.[71] Among 37 evaluable patients with recurrent and/or advanced squamous head and neck cancer, 13/17 in the infusion arm (76%) and 4/20 in the bolus arm (20%) responded (p = 0.01). The bolus group developed more severe leukopenia, and the incidence of stomatitis in the infusion arm was 35%.

Rowland et al[94] also have reported on the use of 120-hour continuous infusion of 5-FU (1,000 mg/m^2/day) with DDP (100 mg/m^2 I.V. bolus). Studying 21 evaluable patients, they observed a similar response rate of 71% (5 CR and 10 PR), with median duration of response of 14 weeks.

Similar results were also reported by Fosser et al,[95] who observed an overall response rate of 67% in 30 evaluable patients with recurrent and disseminated head and neck cancer. The toxicity reported in this study was more severe, with stomatitis seen in 67% of patients. The mortality rate for severe renal and hepatic toxicity was 17%.

Sequential use of continuous 24-hour DDP infusion and 5-day 5-FU infusion has been recently reported by Amrein et al.[96] DDP was administered at 80 mg/m^2 on day 1 and 5-FU at 800 mg/m^2/day on days 2-6, repeated every 21 days. For 39 patients with recurrent disease, there were 7 (18%) complete responses and 10 (28%) partial responses, for an overall response of 46%. Toxicity was tolerable. The median duration of survival was 10 months.

5-FU infusion has also been combined with vinblastine infusion,[97] resulting in a 28% (6/21) overall response rate of 4-9 months duration in patients with recurrent disease.

Infusion Chemotherapy for Previously Untreated Squamous Cell Carcinoma of the Head and Neck

Surgery and radiation therapy, the standard primary therapies in head and neck cancer, usually fail to cure the majority of patients in stages 3 and 4, leading to disappointingly low cure rates. Because chemotherapy for recurrent disease is only palliative, major alternatives in the use of all available modalities in treatment of head and neck tumor had to be innovated. The incorporation of chemotherapy as induction therapy into combined modality therapy of head and neck cancer was the major step that changed our thinking of the treatment of this disease.

Numerous chemotherapeutic agents and combinations have been used, and many trials (mostly pilots) have been reported to date. In most of the studies, the combination of BLM and DDP has been used, as have regimens of DDP, BLM, and vincristine[2,98-99] and regimens that combine DDP and BLM with MTX and/or vincristine,[87,100] and finally, regimens of DDP and 5-FU[92,101,115,116] (see table 2). In most of these combinations, BLM has been used in a continuous infusion schedule at varying doses in different studies. A limited number of studies have used continuous infusion of DDP,[33,38] and all combinations of 5-FU and DDP have used continuous infusion of 5-FU.[92,101,115,116]

BLM, as a single 7-day continuous infusion used for induction in advanced head and neck tumors by Popkin et al,[102] gave a response rate of 30%, which was inferior to responses obtained from BLM in combination with other agents.

Response rates ranging from 66% to 90% have been produced by regimens that included BLM infusion, DDP, and other agents in a number of studies of induction chemotherapy.[31,88,98,103,104] These regimens have been well tolerated and have not compromised patients receiving definitive radiation therapy or surgery.

BLM infusion has been used in combination with DDP in several trials of induction treatment of head and neck tumors.[31,33,41,105-107] In most of these studies, a BLM bolus was given followed by continuous I.V. infusion of various doses and schedules. The number of chemotherapy courses prior to definitive treatment also varied. Although overall responses of up to 80% were achieved, complete responses were only in the range of 0 to 18%. Cisplatin was also administered at various doses and schedules, including 24-hour infusion.[33] The interpretation of these trials and the impact of this combination treatment on

Table 2. Infusion Chemotherapy for Previously Untreated Advanced Head and Neck Cancer

Study/Reference	Regimen	Evaluable patients	No./% CR	No./% PR	Overall Response
Popkin et al[102]	Bleomycin (I)*	20	1(5)	5(25)	30
Randolph et al[31]	Cisplatin Bleomycin (I)	21	4(19)	11(52)	71
Glick et al[33]	Cisplatin Bleomycin (I)	29	0	14(48)	48
Hong et al[9,36,41]	Cisplatin Bleomycin (I)	39	8(20)	22(56)	76
Baker et al[105]	Cisplatin Bleomycin (I)	113	8(7)	47(42)	49
Jacobs et al[107]	Cisplatin Bleomycin (I)	282	8(3)	95(34)	37
Spaulding et al[99,108]	Cisplatin Bleomycin (I) Vincristine	50 22	11(22) 1(5)	33(66) 19(86)	88 9
Amrein et al[88]	Cisplatin Bleomycin (I) Vincristine	37	2(1)	23(62)	67
Al-Sarraf et al[98]	Cisplatin Bleomycin (I) Vincristine	77	21(28)	39(52)	80
Ervin et al[79]	Cisplatin Bleomycin (I) Methotrexate Leucovorin	93	22(24)	59(64)	88
Tannock et al[100]	Cisplatin Bleomycin (I) Methotrexate Leucovorin	33	3(9)	17(52)	61
Laccourrey et al[104]	Cisplatin 5-FU (I) Bleomycin (I)	43	14(33)	22(51)	84
Al-Sarraf et al[115]	Cisplatin 5-FU (I)	26	5(19)	18(69)	88
Al-Sarraf et al[116]	Cisplatin 5-FU (I)	88	48(54)	35(39)	93
Ensley et al[113]	Cisplatin 5-FU (I) Methotrexate Leucovorin 5-FU	12	9(75)	2(16)	91
Greenberg et al[114]	Cisplatin 5-FU (I) Allopurinol	20	9(45)	11(55)	100

*Infusion

survival is a critical issue. Jacobs et al,[107] in a large, randomized trial involving 462 patients, randomized patients to standard therapy (surgery and postoperative radiation), induction chemotherapy (DDP 100 mg/m² on day 1, and BLM 15 units/m² I.V. bolus on day 3, followed by 15 units/m²/day by continuous infusion days 3 through 7), plus standard therapy, or induction chemotherapy, standard therapy and maintenance. The 2-year disease-free survival was similar for patients treated with standard therapy alone (55%) and for patients treated with induction chemotherapy plus standard therapy (57%). The 2-year survival was also similar for the 2 treatment arms. Because only a single course of chemotherapy was given prior to surgery, no conclusions can be drawn regarding the overall value of more intensive induction regimens.

In search of more active combinations, investigators added vincristine and/or MTX to the BLM-DDP combination. Beginning in 1978, Spaulding et al[38,99,103,108] administered 2 courses of DDP, vincristine, and BLM as induction prior to surgery in patients with advanced resectable disease. Their regimen included DDP at a dose of 80 mg/m² on days 1 and 22, vincristine 1 mg/m² on days 3 and 24, BLM 15 units/m²/day I.V. continuous infusion on days 3–7 and 24–28. An overall response rate of 88% was achieved in 50 evaluable patients (11 CR and 30 PR). With a minimum follow-up of 30 months, the disease-free survival was 61%. These investigators have also administered the same regimen in 22 patients with hypopharyngeal carcinoma,[108] achieving a 91% overall response rate (1 CR and 19 PR). Other investigators have confirmed these results using similar combinations. Amrein et al,[88] administering an identical combination of BLM, DDP, and vincristine, observed a 67% overall response in 37 evaluable patients. We have administered the same drugs in a slightly different schedule at Wayne State.[34,37,98] Seventy-seven patients with advanced head and neck cancer were treated with DDP (100 mg/m² I.V. on day 1), BLM (30 units/day I.V. continuous infusion, days 2–5), and vincristine (1 mg I.V. on days 2 and 5) for 2 courses. We observed an overall response rate of 80%, with a CR rate of 28%. Surgery was possible in 36 patients. The median duration of survival for all the patients was 18 months.

The combination of DDP, BLM (infusion), and MTX has been studied by Ervin et al[79,87] as well as others.[35,40,100] At the Dana-Farber Institute, 93 patients with advanced squamous cell carcinoma of the head and neck were given induction treatment with DDP (20 mg/m²/day I.V. on days 1–5), bleomycin (10 units/m² I.V. continuous infusion days 3–7), MTX (200 mg/m² I.V. on days 15,22), and leucovorin (20 mg q 6 h p.o. days 16–18 and 23–25) for 2 courses before standard local treatment.[79,87] An overall response rate of 88% (24% CR and 64% PR) was observed. Sixty percent of the patients were alive and free of disease at a median follow-up of 28 months.

Other investigators, using BLM, DDP, and MTX in different doses and schedules as induction for advanced head and neck cancer, achieved overall response rates of 48% to 73%[35,40,100] and complete response rates of 0 to 9%.

The combination of DDP (100 mg/m² I.V. infusion day 1), 5-FU (1 gm/m² I.V. continuous infusion days 1–4), and BLM (30 units/m² I.V. day 1, then 7.5 units/m² continuous infusion days 2–4) for 3 courses has been administered by Laccourrey et al.[104] An 84% overall response rate (33% CR and 51% PR) was achieved in 50 evaluable patients. The regimen was reported as being tolerable.

One of the most successful regimens, one that has produced excellent results in previously untreated patients with advanced head and neck cancer, is the combination of DDP and continuous infusion of 5-FU.[115] The previously used bleomycin was replaced by 5-FU in the Wayne State trials in an attempt to avoid the pulmonary toxicity of the former agent. Two courses of the combination of DDP (100 mg/m^2 I.V. day 1) 96-hour infusion of 5-FU (1,000 mg/m^2/day I.V.) were administered originally in 26 patients with stage 4 inoperable epidermoid head and neck cancer. The response rates we observed were 5/26 (19%) complete and 18 (69%) partial, for an overall response of 88%.[92] Six of the patients underwent surgery after induction and 6 after chemotherapy and radiation therapy. Because the toxicities were very tolerable and the preliminary results were promising, we started administering 3 courses of DDP and 120-hour 5-FU infusion in patients with advanced head and neck cancers.[101,109,110,116] The overall response rate achieved was 94% (54% CR and 39% PR). The complete response rate achieved in these studies was greater than those achieved by the use of DDP, BLM, and vincristine in previous trials at Wayne State. The 3-course DDP-5-FU combination produced tolerable and reversible toxicity not different from the toxicity in the earlier studies. The achievement of a higher complete response rate of 54% is very significant and very important.

We have demonstrated that superior survival is observed when a complete remission is achieved with chemotherapy alone rather than with both chemotherapy and radiotherapy.[45,111] Further, a superior histological complete response has been achieved with the use of this combination that resulted in prolonged survival and disease-free survival of more than 4 years.[45] The Wayne State studies and high response rates were confirmed in cooperative group trials.[112]

A 24-hour (DDP 80 mg/m^2/day) infusion and 120-hour 5-FU infusion have been used by Amrein et al.[96] Among 31 patients with no prior treatment, there was observed a 23% complete and 61% partial response for a total response rate of 84%.

In an attempt to increase the CR rate, we investigated the use of 5-course alternating combination regimens consisting of DDP and 120-hour 5-FU infusion (standard doses) (courses 1,3,5) alternating with MTX (250 mg/m^2) followed in 1 hour by 5-FU (600 mg/m^2) and leucovorin rescue 24 hours later. Among 17 studied patients with advanced head and neck cancer, 8 have completed therapy and all of them achieved clinical complete response. No increase in toxicity was observed in this preliminary trial.[113] Further continuation and study of this regimen is necessary.

The administration of higher dose 5-FU infusion (1.5 gm/m^2/24 hours for 5 days) with DDP and allopurinol (900 mg/day) has been recently reported as feasible and very effective.[114]

Summary

Recent studies have used continuous infusions of several active agents to decrease drug toxicity and increase antitumor efficacy in the treatment of patients with recurrent and advanced head and neck cancer. The continuous infusion of several agents has been tested as a single modality in combination with other chemotherapeutic agents for recurrent and/or locally advanced disease and for induction chemotherapy as part of a multimodality treatment approach in previously untreated advanced head and neck carcinoma. The feasibility and the antitumor effectiveness of the administration of continuous infusion chemotherapy have been clearly shown. This treatment modality generally has been well tolerated and, when used in combination with other chemotherapeutic agents, has resulted in high overall response rates and many clinical and histological responses. Despite these high responses, definitive conclusions cannot be made as to long-term value of infusion chemotherapy in improving survival and quality of the life of these patients because controlled clinical trials have not been conducted. Further, the majority of these studies are pilot trials that have included small numbers of patients. The follow-up has been short, and prognostic factors that may influence response have not been taken into consideration.

Until the long-term benefits of chemotherapy regimens that include agents administered by continuous infusion are established, other approaches to advanced head and neck cancer should be investigated. Such approaches would include simultaneous administration of chemotherapy and radiation therapy, the use of radiosensitizers and chemotherapy response modifiers, the use of local and whole body hyperthermia in association with chemotherapeutic agents, and/or radiation. While these approaches are investigated, special effort should be made for the initiation of controlled clinical trials using the most effective regimens available today. Furthermore, studies should be undertaken to investigate the timing of chemotherapy with other treatment modalities and the need for extensive surgery. Finally, new agents that demonstrate higher therapeutic index should be sought.

21

ESOPHAGEAL AND ANAL CANCER

Lawrence Leichman, M.D., Jacob J. Lokich, M.D., and
Cynthia G. Leichman, M.D.

MEDICAL, RADIATION, AND SURGICAL oncologists have been stymied in their efforts to produce meaningful changes in the natural histories of most cancers of the gastrointestinal tract. But new clinical strategies used in the treatment of squamous cell cancers at opposite ends of the G.I. tract have caused these tumors to yield to efforts. This chapter will outline the clinical data that have evolved from protocols developed at Wayne State University combining preoperative infusion chemotherapy and external beam radiation for epidermoid malignancies of the anal canal and esophagus. These data allow us to conclude that the natural histories of these malignant diseases have indeed changed. Furthermore, there is now reason to question the role of the time-honored method of treatment for these tumors—surgery—in terms of adding to the survival and comfort of patients with these cancers.

The combination of modalities to improve cure rates in solid tumors has been a rational goal for clinical oncologists since Powers et al produced markedly increased cure rates in mice with implanted tumors when treated with radiation after surgery.[1] Interdisciplinary cooperation has often been hampered, however, by petty rivalries and very real scientific disagreements among potential partners. It is no wonder, then, that efforts in combining modalities have been piloted at single institutions where the individual investigators were known to each other and mutual trust was at the highest. This serves as at least a partial explanation of why a group at a single institution with a fair-sized patient population could develop a series of preoperative protocols for relatively uncommon tumors.

Preoperative Versus Postoperative Therapeutic Concepts

Accurate staging of gastrointestinal malignancies can be accomplished only by surgical removal of the tumor. In most adjuvant clinical trials involving the

G.I. tract, only surgically staged patients are entered into study. In this way, only those patients with pathologically defined highest risk tumors receive adjuvant therapy. In the postoperative adjuvant setting, the modalities of radiation and chemotherapy are dealing with microscopic disease. By design, preoperative adjuvant strategies take on bulky tumors and tumors of advanced stages based on clinical criteria. In the preoperative setting, the tumor has an intact blood supply, and the treatment may have better vascular access to the cancer. An important aspect of preoperative therapy is to deliver a treatment that will not impede healing of the wound or render the patient too ill to tolerate the potentially curative surgery.

The decision to attack tumors of the anal canal and esophagus with preoperative chemotherapy and radiation was due, in large measure, to the development of the infusion schedule of 5-fluorouracil (5-FU) pioneered by Vaitkevicius and his co-workers. Their clinical and laboratory investigations were among the first to point out that the infusion of 5-FU leads to a far different toxicity than the bolus schedule.[2,3,4] In the era preceding the advent of aminoglycoside antibiotics, the absence of leukopenia with infusion therapy allowed 5-FU administration with far less risk to the patient and allowed it to be combined with other potentially bone marrow-toxic drugs or with radiation. Byfield and others have since suggested that 5-FU, especially when given as an infusion, acts as a sensitizing agent for radiation.[5] Thus, the combination of the 5-FU as an infusion (in which the total dose of the drug would be far greater than that obtained by the bolus administration of the drug) in combination with radiation was a rational and scientifically interesting preoperative approach to tumors of the G.I. tract.

Anal Canal Tumors

At Wayne State University, the combined modality therapy for tumors of the lower G.I. tract was initiated in 1971 based upon data from a variety of sources. Several retrospective reviews had suggested that preoperative radiation could potentially downstage tumors of the rectum,[6] and the efficacy of external beam radiation for inoperable squamous cell tumors of the anal canal had been established.

Two protocols were developed (see figure 1). For adenocarcinoma of the rectum, preoperative radiation (2,000 rad over 10 days) and infusion 5-FU with bolus mitomycin-C was administered. For squamous cell tumors of the anal canal, the chemotherapy remained the same, but the preoperative radiation dose was increased to 3,000 rad in 15 fractions. Both programs called for a rest period of at least 4 weeks after the last dose of chemotherapy before an abdominoperineal resection (APR) was carried out. The data for the adenocarcinoma patients have not been published in more than abstract form because they are difficult to interpret[7] and, although an apparent downstaging of tumor was observed with attendant improvement of survival, patient numbers were small, and no definitive conclusions could be reached. A subsequent randomized trial initiated by the Southwest Oncology Group was not completed because of accrual problems.

The preliminary report by Nigro and Vaitkevicius focused on the safety of the combined modality therapy.[8] Practically overlooked in this presentation was a patient who exhibited a dramatic and apparent complete response that was surgically documented. A similar complete response was offered by Stearns et al in describing the Memorial Sloan Kettering experience with this regimen.[9] The safety, especially the lack of bone marrow toxicity, was emphasized by these investigators. Ironically, the chemotherapy was dismissed as possibly a sensitizer to the radiation or perhaps not necessary at all in these initial reports.

Subsequently, the series from Wayne State was expanded, and from 1972–81, 45 patients with clinically localized epidermoid malignancies of the anal canal were treated with combined preoperative chemotherapy and radiation therapy with curative intent.[10] All patients had tumors greater than 2 cm, but all tumors were confined to the anal canal as shown by physical examination, routine liver function studies, chest X rays, and bone scans. All histologic subtypes — squamous, baseloid, and cloacogenic — were accepted. Tumors ranged in size from 2 cm to 8 cm. At the conclusion of radiation and chemotherapy, a deep biopsy of the anal canal was obtained with the patient under general anesthesia. This biopsy was designed to tell the investigators the results of their treatment before the surgical resection.

An APR was carried out on the first 6 patients. When 5 of the first 6 (83%) patients who underwent the operation after the preoperative combined therapy had no cancer in the posttreatment biopsy and no tumor was found in the full surgical pathology material from the APR, only patients with cancer in the posttreatment biopsy were mandated to undergo an APR. In practice, however, a number of surgeons in the Detroit Medical Center continued to perform the APR regardless of the posttreatment biopsy. Eighteen patients in this series underwent an APR.

Hematologic monitoring confirmed the lack of bone marrow toxicity using the infusion method of delivery for 5-FU. Only 5 patients (11%) had nadir WBC

5 – FU 1,000 mg/m² 24 h infusion	96 h			96 h	
Mitomycin-C 15 mg/m² bolus					*Surgery
Radiation 200 rad/fx	1,000 rad	1,000 rad[1]	1,000 rad[2]		
Day	1 – 5	8 – 12	14 – 19	29 – 32	56

*Local excision biopsy or abdominal perineal resection
[1]Rectal cancer (2,000 rad)
[2]Anal cancer (3,000 rad)

Figure 1.   Treatment schematic for combined 5-FU infusion, mitomycin-C, and radiation for anal or rectal cancer.

below 2,000/mm^3 or platelet counts below 50,000/mm^3. Although only 40% of patients underwent APR, no mortality from the operation was encountered. There was no protocol mortality. No permanent radiation stenosis of the rectum has been encountered for those patients at risk.

Of the 38 patients who had negative biopsies or negative surgical specimens following preoperative treatment, no patient has had recurrence of cancer. Of the 7 patients with tumor after preoperative treatment, no patient remains alive. All these latter patients expired because of recurrent cancer. Recurrence patterns, detailed in table 1, show treatment failure to be related to distant metastases and not to local recurrence, as suggested by the older literature. In fact, all 7 patients developed distant recurrence, with 2 patients experiencing local recurrence as well. At a median follow-up time of 6+ years, no recurrence has been recorded beyond 30 months after completion of treatment.

Interpreting the relative contributions of radiation, infusional 5-FU, and mitomycin-C (MIT) to the success of this treatment regimen for anal cancer is difficult. It is clear that the radiation dose of 3,000 rad is less than that which has been generally employed for this tumor. It is therefore suggested that the chemotherapy must be an essential if not critical component of the treatment program. Byfield et al have emphasized that MIT is probably not an important component and that the infusion schedule for 5-FU is the most substantive element, along with the radiation.[11]

The neoadjuvant preoperative approach to true epidermoid malignancies of the anal canal differs radically from earlier reports from series that treated patients with this tumor with surgery as the only modality. Although Stearns and Moertel had pointed out that true epidermoid cancers of the anal canal have a very high propensity for local spread, the Wayne State study revealed only 2/38 (5%) local treatment failures. This study suggests that surgery may be unnecessary and that cure may be achieved with tolerable chemotherapy along with the radiation and local surgical excision, precluding the need for colostomy. Others have confirmed this approach, with results very similar if not identical to the Wayne State study, although the length of follow-up and numbers of patients are quantitatively less.

Table 1. Recurrence Patterns in 7 Patients (of 38) with Cancer of the Anal Canal Following 5-FU Infusion, Mitomycin-C, Radiation, and Surgery

Patient	Local	Bone	Liver	Lung	Pericardium
1	+	+			
2				+	+
3	+		+		
4		+			
5		+			
6		+			
7				+	

A summary of the selected phase 2 trials in which infusional 5-FU with or without MIT is delivered in conjunction with radiation is presented in table 2.[10-15] The 6 trials comprise a total of 127 patients. In all trials, 5-FU was administered as a continuous infusion for 96 hours at a dose rate of approximately 1 gm/m^2/day. MIT was added in all trials except that of Byfield et al.[11] Radiation therapy was delivered at various dose rates and total cumulative dose. In the study by Michaelson et al, radiation therapy followed the initial chemotherapy regimen but in all other trials was administered concomitant with chemotherapy.[12] More than 90% of the patients achieved a response, with the vast majority demonstrating a complete response (CR) and local control. The report by Tiver and Langlands[15] reviews these trials as well as additional reports of smaller patient populations. The report emphasizes the critical contribution of chemotherapy as well as the ability of the combined modality approach to provide an alternative to abdominal perineal resection.

Squamous Cell Cancer of the Esophagus

The success with cancer of the anal canal no doubt allowed for a certain boldness in the approach to squamous cell cancer of the esophagus. This disease is seen far more often than anal cancer and is treated with far less success. During the 5-year period 1969–74, no patient treated for esophagus cancer at the Detroit Medical Center with operation alone or external beam radiation alone survived 2 years. As in cancer of the anal canal, radiation therapy as a single modality has a comparable role to surgery in terms of cure rate and palliation for patients with squamous cell malignancies of the esophagus. Drawing from the experience with cancer of the anal canal, the Wayne State group initiated a trial of infusion 5-FU and MIT with radiation.

The initial report by Franklin et al detailed 30 patients treated with infusional 5-FU infusion (1,000 mg/m^2 days 1–4 and 29–32), MIT 10 mg/m^2 (day 1) and radiation (3,000 rads in 200-rad fractions delivered in 15 sessions over 3 weeks).[16] The radiation port had a minimum width of 8 cm (4 cm to the left

Table 2. Selected Phase 2 Trials of Neoadjuvant Infusion 5-Fluorouracil (96 hours) with or without Mitomycin-C Concomitant with Radiation in Anal Cancer

Study/Reference	No. patients	MIT (+/−)	Radiation dose (rad)	Response	Local control (%)
Leichman et al[10]	45	+	3,000	38/45	95
Byfield et al[11]	11	−	3,000 – 4,750	11/11	100
Michaelson et al[12]	31	+	3,000	29/31	NS*
Cummings et al[13]	13	+	5,000	13/13	100
John et al[14]	22	+	NS*	20/22	100
Tiver and Langlands et al[15]	5	+	5,000 – 7,000	5/5	100
TOTAL	127				

*NS = Not stated.

and right of the oropharynx) and the vertical dimensions were 5 cm above the upper level and 5 cm below the lower level of the lesion as measured by the esophagogram.

At the conclusion of the preoperative therapy, each patient underwent endoscopy to judge lesion response to treatment. Every lesion responded, and more than 80% of the lesions disappeared, with endoscopic biopsies of the suspected lesions revealing no mucosal tumor. Twenty-three patients subsequently had surgery; all of them had negative biopsies after chemotherapy and radiation. Six of the 23 (26%) had no cancer in the resected specimen. Thus, 17 of the 23 patients with negative posttherapy biopsies had tumor under the mucosa, indicating that post chemoradiation biopsy does not accurately predict a CR. Six patients, however, were completely devoid of tumor at the time of the surgery.

In 1979, the Southwest Oncology Group completed a trial of cisplatin (DDP) for patients with advanced measurable epidermoid carcinoma of the esophagus.[17] These patients exhibited a 26% response, with a small group achieving a CR. The WSU protocol for patients with potentially curable cancer of the esophagus was thereafter modified, and DDP at 100 mg/m^2 on days 1 and 29 was substituted for mitomycin-C (see figure 2). Twenty-one patients were treated in this pilot trial, 19 having surgery. Five patients (27%) had no cancer in the resected esophagus.

This initial trial has spawned a number of reports of infusional 5-FU with MIT or with DDP with radiation, surgery, or both (see table 3).[16-25] The sequen-

Protocol 1. 5-FU + Mitomycin-C

5 – FU 1,000 mg/m² 24 h infusion	96 h			
Mitomycin-C 10 mg/m² bolus				Surgery
Radiation 200 rad/fx	1,000 rad	1,000 rad	1,000 rad	
Day	1 – 5	8 – 12	14 – 19	56

Protocol 2. 5-FU + CACP

5 – FU 1,000 mg/m² 24 h infusion	96 h			96 h	
CACP 100 mg/m²					Surgery
Radiation	1,000 rad	1,000 rad	1,000 rad		
Day	1 – 5	8 – 12	14 – 19	29 – 32	56

Figure 2.   Sequential treatment schematics for combined 5-FU infusion and radiation with either mitomycin-C or cisplatin for esophageal cancer.

tial studies by Franklin et al[16] and Leichman et al[18] using MIT or DDP, respectively, as the additional agents have been discussed previously. In the total of 177 patients, not all came to surgery. Complete responses represent those identified surgically.

In the study reported by Carey et al, preoperative chemotherapy was administered employing infusional 5-FU and DDP without radiation.[19] Radiation was given postoperatively, however, when adenopathy was demonstrated and in those patients achieving only a partial remission. Twelve of 20 patients (60%) had a response, 8 of which were clinically complete. Projected median survival is 16 months.

The study by Engstrom et al employed infusional 5-FU with MIT administered concomitant with radiation to a dose of 6,000 rad.[20,21] Clinical responses were observed in 13 of 15 evaluable patients. Six patients remained disease-free at the time of the report, with a median survival of 22 months.

Lokich et al employed protracted infusion 5-FU for 4–6 weeks without the addition of either MIT or DDP.[22] Patients subsequently received an additional 4–6 weeks of infusional 5-FU in conjunction with concomitant radiation therapy to a dose of 4,000–6,000 rad. Eleven of 12 patients demonstrated a major local response to therapy and 3 patients (25%) are disease-free beyond 3 years from completion of therapy without surgical intervention.

The report by John et al of infusional 5-FU with MIT and DDP administered as a multiagent regimen in conjunction with radiation has been reported in abstract form only, and the details of the radiation therapy are not known. However, 4 of 13, or more than 25% of the patients, are without evidence of disease.[14]

A recently reported study by Trillett et al in 47 patients employed infusional 5-FU with DDP and radiation therapy, with patients also receiving laser therapy following the first course of chemotherapy in order to optimize palliation and correct dysphagia early on.[23] Forty-nine percent of patients demonstrated

Table 3. Selected Phase 2 Trials of Neoadjuvant Infusion 5-Fluorouracil with Mitomycin-C or Cisplatin with or without Concomitant Radiation

Study/Reference	No. patients	Cisplatin	Dose or Mitomycin-C	Radiation dose (rad)	Response
Franklin et al[16]	30	0	10 mg/m^2	3,000	6/23 CR
Leichman et al[18]	21	100 mg/m^2	0	3,000	5/19 CR
Carey et al[10]	20	0	0	None	12/20 R
					8/12 CR
Engstrom et al[20,21]	15	0	10 mg/m^2	6,000	13/15 R
Lokich et al[22]	12	0	0	4,000 – 6,000	11/12 R
John et al[14]	13	DNS*	DNS*	DNS*	4/13 NED
Trillet et al[22]	47	80 mg/m^2	0	5,000 – 6,500	22/47 CR
Arbitbal et al[24]	9	10 mg/m^2	0	6,000	8/9 R
					5 CR
Hellerstein et al[25]	10	100 mg/m^2	0	0	8/10 R
					2 CR
TOTAL	177				

*DNS = Dose not stated

regression following the chemotherapy only, and in all patients, dysphagia was substantially improved following the combination of chemotherapy and laser. Forty-six percent of patients achieved a CR following radiation therapy. Although the mean survival time was only 8 months, 26% of patients had an actuarial survival in the T1 category of more than 2 years.

In the small study by Arbitbol et al involving 9 patients with either esophageal or gastric carcinoma, a regimen of infusional 5-FU and DDP was delivered in conjunction with radiation to a dose of 6,000 rad.[24] Eight of 9 patients responded, with 5 CR. Local failure was observed in only 2 patients.

Hellerstein et al, in a group of patients with advanced esophageal cancer, employed infusional 5-FU with DDP but without radiation; 8 of 10 patients responded, with 2 CR.[25]

The only other agent administered on an infusional schedule in esophageal cancer has been bleomycin (BLM). Although there are no clinical trials of single-agent BLM administered as an infusion for this tumor, at least 6 trials have used BLM as a short-term infusion in combination with bolus DDP, and a third agent has been added in 4 trials (see table 4).[25-31] In a study by Coonley et al, 43 patients with localized disease and 27 with extensive disease received BLM as a 4-day infusion in conjunction with bolus DDP.[26] The overall response rate was only 15%, and there was no apparent difference in the two groups. In the second generation trial from the same institution, vindesine (VDS) was added to the BLM infusion with DDP.[28] Of a total of 68 patients, 45 had regional disease and 24 extensive disease. The response rate to chemotherapy alone was 63% and 33%, respectively, in the 2 groups, and the overall response rate was 53%. No survival data were reported in this trial, but the median duration of response was 7 months, compared to 6 months for the 2-drug regimen.

Bosset et al employed BLM infusion in combination with infusion DDP in which each was administered for a 12-hour period.[27] The drugs were presumably administered on alternate 12-hour intervals for a total of 8 days. A response rate of 24% was observed, with 3 CR, but no survival data have been reported.

Table 4. Selected Phase 2 Trials of Neoadjuvant Infusion Bleomycin with Cisplatin with or without Additional Agents

Study/Reference	No. patients	Bleomycin dose	Cisplatin dose	Other agents	Response (%)
Coonley et al[26]	70	10 mg/m²/d × 4	3 mg/kg	Surgery* or Radiation	15
Bosset et al[27]	17	10 mg 12 h	20 mg 12 h inf	–	24
Kelson et al[28]	68	10 mg/m²/d × 4	3 mg/kg	Vindesine	53
Forastiere et al[29]	17	10 mg/m²/d × 4	80 mg/m²	Etoposide Surgery	31
Hermann et al[30]	23	10 mg/m²/d × 4	120 mg/m²	Vindesine	43
Marantz et al[31]	32	10 mg/m²/d × 5	60 mg/m²	5-FU + XRT	53
TOTALS	227				

*Selected patients

Forastiere et al administered infusion BLM for 4 days along with bolus DDP and added VP-16 to the 3-drug regimen.[29] The response rate was only 31% in a total of 17 patients treated, and remission durations were 5–11 months.

More recently, Hermann et al[30] administered BLM infusion along with high-dose bolus DDP to which was added VDS. The response rate was 43% in 23 patients, 21 of whom underwent surgery. The operative mortality of 20% was related in part to the preoperative BLM in conjunction with high oxygen concentrations during anesthesia.

Finally, Marantz et al reported on BLM infusion in conjunction with a lower dose of DDP in 32 patients.[31] Patients subsequently were treated with radiation administered in conjunction with bolus 5-FU. Responses were observed in 53% of the treated group (25% CR).

A number of other chemotherapeutic agents have been employed in the chemotherapy of esophageal cancer,[32-35] but in all such trials the agents are delivered on a bolus schedule. The most successful regimen has been the infusional 5-FU regimen administered in conjunction with DDP. The infusional BLM has not been combined with infusion of 5-FU and DDP, and such a regimen as well as other possibilities may be left for future exploration in this tumor, where chemotherapeutic response has been amply demonstrated.

Present and Future Status of Anal and Esophageal Cancer Therapy

For anal cancer, the extraordinary success of infusional 5-FU and radiation is evident in that virtually all patients respond to such therapy. The standard surgical approach has been changed from a radical APR to simple local excision. The important issues to be addressed in this tumor relate to those patients presenting with advanced disease or incompletely responding to initial therapy. For such patients, the role of DDP to replace MIT may be an important issue for investigation. Another direction to be explored is the use of drugs such as BLM or methotrexate; expansion of the combinations of 3- or 4-drug regimens; alternating noncross-resistant regimens; prolonging the duration of infusion of 5-FU; and delivery of more of the drug components on an infusion schedule. In addition, technological improvements in radiation therapy or intensification of the cumulative dose or dose rate can be considered.

The issues for esophageal cancer are different from those for anal cancer in that the surgical approach to this tumor has not substantially changed; this may be one of the most important questions to be addressed in future clinical trials. The initial clinical trials of infusional 5-FU and radiation were confounded by an unacceptable surgical mortality. For patients treated with 5-FU and MIT, immediate postoperative mortality was 13%; an additional 17% of the patients failed to leave the hospital after surgery. Therefore, almost 30% of the adjuvant patients expired on the basis of therapy. In the 5-FU and DDP trial, 5 of 19 patients (27%) did not leave the hospital after surgery. These data were confirmed in a national trial in which the Radiation Therapy Oncology Group and the Southwest Oncology Group independently tested the DDP and 5-FU regimen preoperatively. This trial has been preliminarily reported[36] and subsequently completed. A total of 180 patients were registered, and 130 have come to surgery; 32 (24%) had no cancer on pathologic examination of a resected esophagus. This result confirmed earlier data from Wayne State University and brought into sharper focus the question of the role of surgery following preoperative chemotherapy and radiation. Was the surgery a necessary part of the treatment, or did it serve as an invasive staging procedure? The issue is compounded when one considers the fact that only 2.5% of those patients who had tumor identified in the resected specimen achieved survival beyond 2 years. Furthermore, the mortality related to surgery was 10% in the cooperative group trial, and some patients died without microscopic evidence of cancer in the resected esophagus.

The surgical component to therapy is not the only part of combined modality approach to esophageal cancer that should come under scrutiny (see table 5). Should preoperative radiation be more intense? Should the chemotherapy be improved in some fashion as suggested for anal cancer by adding more drugs or prolonging the infusion period? Finally, the optimal interdigitation of the 3 modalities in terms of sequence of application should be considered in planning clinical trials to establish the most effective treatment plan for this tumor.

Table 5. Esophageal Cancer: Questions for Clinical Trials

Surgery	Comparison of surgery vs radiation
	Optimum time for surgery
	Potential role for laser surgery
Radiation	Optimum dose/rate cumulative
	Optimum timing (preop;postop)
	Use of radiation sensitizors
Chemotherapy	Expanded drug combinations
	Infusional schedule proglonged
	Duration extended

22

COLORECTAL CANCER

Jacob J. Lokich, M.D.

B Y VIRTUE OF BEING common (about 150,000 new cases annually), cancers of the colon and rectum represent a substantial focus for cancer chemotherapy in both the adjuvant setting as well as for advanced disease. In spite of the identification of an "active agent" in the form of 5-fluorouracil (5-FU) more than a quarter of a century ago, however, and in spite of the development of regional delivery systems for hepatic metastases for this tumor category, it is difficult to state that meaningfully effective chemotherapy is available.

Although 5-FU has become the "standard" chemotherapy approach to colorectal cancer, such a role must be ignominious in that translating the modest response rates achieved (at 8–15%) into significantly improved survival over that of patients unexposed to chemotherapy has not been possible. A variety of bolus schedules for 5-FU have been studied in prospective trials in an attempt to improve the track record for this agent. Various routes of delivery, including oral and hepatic arterial and the more recent intraperitoneal delivery, have been studied. The major thrust of clinical trials employs 5-FU-based multiple drug regimens. No unequivocal advantage or improved effectiveness for drug combinations has been demonstrable, however.

This chapter will review the data base for 5-FU delivered as a single-agent bolus and in combination with other agents in the treatment of colorectal cancer. The available literature on 5-FU delivered as a systemic infusion also will be surveyed. The infusion schedule for other agents in the antimetabolite class, as well as the alkylating agents, antibiotics, etc., can, for the most part, only be speculated upon in that such agents have demonstrated little or no activity when administered as a standard bolus. Agents that may be more optimally delivered as an infusion for pharmacokinetic reasons could potentially be reconsidered in phase 2 trials in colorectal cancer. Those possibilities will be reviewed as well.

Standard Bolus 5-Fluorouracil

Carcinomas of the colon and rectum traditionally have been treated with 5-FU since the introduction of this agent in 1957. Initial phase 1 studies with 5-FU employed a bolus schedule administering a dose of 15 mg/kg/day for 5 days followed by a 50% dose reduction for alternate days to the point of toxicity. Clinical antitumor activity on this dose schedule was modest, but this agent nonetheless became the "standard" therapy for metastatic colorectal cancer. Subsequently, a variety of dose schedules and routes were employed in uncontrolled trials, suggesting comparable activity for a weekly schedule delivered intravenously or even orally and for a schedule of 5-day bolus repeated at 4- to 5-week intervals.

In 1977 Ansfield et al, in a preliminary report of 462 patients, detailed the results of a prospective randomized trial comparing 4 bolus regimens for 5-FU.[1] The 4 regimens were defined as follows (see table 1): (1) bolus × 5 days at 12 mg/kg/day followed by 11 doses administered on alternate days at 6 mg/kg/day with treatment interruption at the development of drug-related toxicity; (2) weekly I.V. delivery at 15 mg/kg for 4 weeks with dose escalation to 20 mg/kg in the absence of toxicity; (3) 500 mg total dose administered for 4 consecutive days and weekly thereafter by I.V. bolus; and (4) oral delivery at 15 mg/kg/day for 6 days followed by the same dose delivered weekly. A total of 198 patients with colon or rectal cancer entered the trial. The response rate was highest for the most intensive treatment arm (33% response rate), and the remaining 3 arms yielded response rates of 13% and 14%. Although there were no significant differences with regard to the treatment arms and survival, there was an apparent tendency in the direction of an improved survival for the most intensive treatment. However, follow-up analysis has not been reported.

In spite of the reported results of this study, the standard regimen for 5-FU therapy as a bolus has been the delivery of 400–500 mg/m²/day for 5 consecutive days at 5-week intervals. Such a schedule optimizes patient as well as physician convenience and has also permitted (with the modification of the 5-FU dose) the introduction of additional agents for multiagent regimens. The 3 reported prospective randomized trials employing 5-FU in a standard bolus regimen as the control arm for comparison with a variety of combination

Table 1. Bolus 5-FU Schedules in Colorectal Cancer as Part of Prospective Randomized Trials

Study/reference	Dose schedule	Response rate (%)
Ansfield et al (COG)[1]	12 mg/kg/d × 5 then 6 mg/kg × 11	16/48 (33)
	weekly 15 mg/kg × 4 weeks	7/52 (13)
	500 mg (total)/d × 4 then weekly	7/50 (14)
	oral 15 mg/kg/d × 6 then weekly	6/48 (13)
Douglas et al (ECOG)[2]	oral or I.V. 600 mg/m² weekly	6/49 (11)
Presant et al (SEOG)[3]	400 mg/m²/d × 5	3/40 (8)
Windshill et al[4]	500 mg/m²/d × 5	4/29 (13.7)

regimens with and without 5-FU[2,3,4] have yielded consistent response rates (8–16%) that were comparable to the multidrug regimens.

The North Central Cancer Treatment Group employed 5-FU as a control arm in a prospective comparative trial in which 5-FU was administered at a dose of 500 mg/m^2/day for 5 days repeated at 5 weeks.[4] This arm was compared with 5 alternative treatments that included 5-FU with triazinate; 5-FU with ICRF 159; methyl CCNU with ICRF 159; methyl CCNU with triazinate; and ICRF 159 with triazinate. For this study, 187 patients were randomized, and response rates again were comparable across arms (5.8–16%). Median survival for the overall group was 8.5 months, but interestingly, the survival was significantly better for those patients receiving 5-FU-based combinations compared to those not receiving 5-FU in a treatment regimen.

In spite of the modest activity demonstrated for 5-FU in these prospective randomized trials, and in spite of the absence of substantive clinical evidence that multiple drugs are superior to single-agent 5-FU, combination chemotherapy regimens continue to be explored in advanced colorectal cancer. Throughout the decade of the 1970s, the nitrosoureas were added to 5-FU as a result of initial reports of response rates up to 43%.[5] Subsequent phase 2 studies demonstrated that the nitrosourea methyl CCNU added to 5-FU did not yield significant antitumor effects.[6] Phase 3 comparative trials have also addressed 5-FU combinations. Engstrom et al[7] reported the data of the Eastern Cooperative Oncology Group, with a total of 472 patients entered in 1 of 5 combination arms, all of which included 5-FU. Four of the treatment arms involved adding methyl CCNU to 5-FU with or without additional agents that included vincristine (VCR) and dacarbazine. The fifth arm employed hydroxyurea in combination with 5-FU. In the first 4 arms, 5-FU was given as a 5-day bolus at doses of 150–325 mg/m^2/day repeated at 5-week intervals. For the arm containing 5-FU in conjunction with hydroxyurea, a weekly regimen was employed at 600 mg/m^2/week, with the hydroxyurea administered orally at home. Response rates were essentially the same in all 5 arms, varying from 9–15%; survival was also comparable, varying from 26–38 weeks.

The thrust of combination chemotherapy in the decade of the 1980s has been guided by concepts related to biochemical modulation; clues have been developed from in vitro studies that may rationally relate to optimizing the effectiveness of 5-FU. The use of methotrexate (MTX) and of leucovorin as biochemical modulators has received the major emphasis in this area. For the most part, such studies have been at the phase 1 and 2 levels, but 2 prospective randomized trials are ongoing. In the preliminary report by Buroker, 5-FU was administered in a control arm at a dose rate of 500 mg/m^2/day for 5 days and was compared to combinations of 5-FU with the biologic modifiers thymidine or PALA (N phosphonacetyl 1 aspartate), or with levamasole, the last drug representing an immune rather than biochemical modulator. These 4 arms were compared to an arm in which MOF-STREP was delivered. In a total of 293 patients who were available for survival analysis in particular, there were no statistically significant differences among the 5 treatment arms.[8]

In an ongoing trial from the Gastrointestinal Tumor Study Group, patients with advanced colorectal metastatic cancer enter a comparative trial in which 5-FU is delivered in a control arm at a dose rate of 500 mg/m^2/day for 5 days and is compared to a weekly regimen of 5-FU and leucovorin delivered on a bolus schedule with various doses of each component drug. Interim data have not been reported for this study. However, preliminary results from Roswell Park of 5-FU delivered in conjunction with leucovorin have identified a relatively high response rate on a bolus schedule for 5 days with 5-FU and leucovorin, and studies employing a short-term infusion of 5-FU are ongoing.[9]

Another major 2-drug combination involved in the concept of biochemical modulation is that of MTX and 5-FU, and a host of clinical trials have been reported at the phase 2 level in advanced colorectal cancer.[10] In few of these reports is the delivery of 5-FU on a daily schedule for 5 days related to the potential additional cytotoxic effect induced by the modulator, in this case MTX, necessitating a 1-week interval to prevent untoward toxicity. Furthermore, a review of collected trials of MTX combined with 5-FU has suggested that there are complexities related to the duration of MTX preexposure that may be essential to optimizing the modulating effect and may be associated with substantial toxicity as well.[11] However, it is not at all clear that the interval between MTX and 5-FU at the clinical level is consequential. In fact, in a trial by Beck et al, patients with advanced colorectal cancer received 5-FU on a dose schedule of 300 mg/m^2/days 1 through 5 and in addition received MTX on days 1 and 5 along with vincristine and mitomycin-C on day 1 and VCR on days 1 and 5. The response rates in this series of 53 patients was 43%, but with a mean survival in responders of 15 months.[12]

Another recent 5-FU combination using the daily bolus schedule for 5-FU has been the 2-drug regimen that introduces cisplatin (DDP) as a second component drug. A preliminary report by Einhorn et al indicated that this combination in a bolus schedule system resulted in a response rate of 32%.[13] Because DDP is not active as a single agent in colorectal cancer, it may be that if functions as a biochemical modulator. Studies to confirm the activity of this combination are ongoing.

5-Fluorouracil and FUDR Continuous Infusion

The antipyrimidines are theoretically ideal drugs for delivery by continuous infusion, and of all the cytotoxic agents, the 2 analogues 5-FU and FUDR are the oldest to have been employed in such a dose schedule. Floxuridine (FUDR) in particular has been employed with an infusion schedule, as it represents the ideal agent for hepatic arterial infusion from a pharmaceutical standpoint because of its solubility. On the other hand, 5-FU, partly because of the relatively large volume necessary to achieve a therapeutic dose and partly because the tolerated dose increases with an infusion schedule, is a less practical agent to be used for infusion. There are, in fact, major physicochemical differences between FUDR and 5-FU, and earlier clinical trials have suggested that there may be major clinical differences as well.

5-Fluorouracil

As indicated earlier, infusion should be defined as a minimum of 24 hours of continuous administration of drug. Two early studies employed what may be termed ultrashort-term infusion of 5-FU, with delivery of the agent for either 2 hours or as an 8-hour infusion.[14,15] In the study by Reitemeier and Moertel reported in 1962, patients were randomized to receive an 8-hour infusion at a dose of 22.5 mg/kg/day for 5 days or a rapid bolus at a dose of 15 mg/kg/day for 5 days. Forty-five patients were randomized into each group, and the response rates were 11% for the "infusion group" and 20% for the rapid injection group. Toxicity was enhanced in the rapid injection group, but there were no significant differences in response rate. Similarly, Moertel et al reported a randomized study of bolus versus 2-hour infusion, with a 12% response rate in both arms. It is not unexpected that short-term infusions of less than 24 hours would be precisely comparable to the bolus delivery based upon pharmacokinetic considerations of this agent.

Short-term infusions of 2–5 days duration have been evaluated in 3 studies (see table 2). Seifert et al in 1975 reported the only prospective study in which 69 patients were randomized to receive either a 5-day infusion of 5-FU at a dose of 20–30 mg/kg/day or a 5-day bolus at a dose of 12 mg/kg/day.[16] The study demonstrated a doubling of the response rate in the group receiving the infusion, with a statistically significantly improved survival. The randomization, however, had failed to precisely balance the group with regard to sites of metastases. Additional prospective trials have not explored this seminal observation, although Kish et al in 1984 reported on a prospective comparative trial of 5-FU delivered by infusion versus a weekly bolus in patients with head and neck cancer. That study demonstrated a statistically significant advantage in terms of response rate for the infusion arm (72%) over the bolus arm (20%).[17]

In an uncontrolled study by Hartman et al, 58 patients were treated with 5-day continuous infusion 5-FU at 20 mg/kg/day.[18] A response rate of 23% was observed in the 36 patients who had received no prior therapy; in the 22 patients receiving the infusion as secondary therapy following bolus-5-FU, the response rate was 10%.

Table 2. Infusion 5-Fluorouracil in Advanced Colorectal Cancer

Study/reference	No. patients	Response rate (%)
Short-term:		
Seifert et al[16]	34	42
Hartman et al[18]	36	23
Shah et al[19]	30	30
Protracted:		
Lokich et al[21]	55	38
Benedetto et al[22]	9	33
Ausman et al[23]	36	36
Belt et al[24]	22	39
Leichman et al[16]	16	31

Shah et al reported on 48- and 72-hour infusion at a dose of 30 mg/kg/day administered at weekly (48-hour) or 2 or 3 weekly intervals. A total of 94 patients were evaluated, and the optimal treatment (although not a randomized study) was the weekly 48-hour schedule, which produced a response rate of 30% (9/30) and a median survival of 14 months. In the group receiving 5-FU infusions with the 3-week interval, there were no responses in 33 patients.[19]

Protracted infusions of 5-FU are based upon the rationale of maximizing the tumor cell exposure, which in slow-growing tumors with a small proportion of cells in cycle may necessitate long durations of delivery. Lokich et al established in phase 1 studies the optimal dose rate of delivery of a minimum duration of 5-FU by continuous infusion for 28 days of 300 mg/m²/day.[20] In a retrospective analysis of patients with colorectal cancer entered on such a regimen, a response rate of 38% was observed in 55 patients with advanced measurable colorectal cancer.[21] The response rate was similar in patients previously untreated or patients treated with prior 5-FU delivered as a bolus. Four additional studies have been reported employing long-term, low-dose continuous infusion 5-FU in colorectal cancer. In the study by Benedetto et al,[22] 3/9 patients responded, and in the study by Ausman et al,[23] a response rate of 38% was achieved.

In the studies of Belt et al, 22 patients with colorectal cancer were treated at 200–300 mg/m²/day, with a response rate of 39% in the overall group, which included other tumor sites.[24] Leichman et al treated patients at 200 mg/m²/day and achieved detectable blood levels at 5–17 ng/ml, with 31% of the 16 patients responding.[25] Finally, Faintuch et al treated 25 patients at 170–350 mg/m²/day and reported toxicity data, but no therapeutic information was available.[26]

These studies failed to demonstrate a major increment of success for protracted infusion compared to short-term infusion. However, the studies of protracted infusion have not been conducted in a rigorous experimental design. An ongoing trial within the Mid-Atlantic Oncology Group compares, in a prospective randomized design, protracted infusion 5-FU delivered at a dose of 300 mg/m²/day to "standard" intermittent bolus 5-FU delivered at a dose rate of 500 mg/m²/day for 5 days, repeated at 5-week intervals. There is no built-in crossover design, and the major parameters to be monitored are response rate and survival. A preferable design trial would be a 3-arm comparison in which short-term infusion could be compared directly with bolus in a repetition of the previous ciphered study, as well as with long-term infusion.

Combination chemotherapy employing 5-day infusion of 5-FU with a second agent delivered on a bolus schedule has explored the use of methyl CCNU, mitomycin-C (MIT), DDP, and leukovorin as the second agent (see table 3). In the prospective randomized trial by Buroker et al, 5-FU infusion was delivered with either MIT or methyl CCNU. The response rate achieved was similar to that observed in studies in which the 5-FU was infused for a short term without an additional agent.[27] DDP added to 5-FU infusion has been reported by Sheppard et al in a small group of 20 patients in which no responses were observed,[28] although Einhorn et al had observed responses in 3/12 patients on such a regimen.[29] The true role of DDP added to 5-FU in the context of the latter agent delivered as a short-term infusion will need to be addressed in prospective comparative trials. Leucovorin has been delivered in conjunction with a 4-day infusion of 5-FU, and in 13 patients, 4 responses were observed. A second group of patients received bolus 5-FU with leucovorin, and of 24 patients, 9 responses were observed.[30] This study suggests that leucovorin may add to the therapeutic efficacy of 5-FU, but the contribution of the schedule of delivery is unclear.

Combination chemotherapy using the protracted infusion schedule for 5-FU admixed with MTX has been reported.[31] In a phase 1 trial of delivery for the 2 agents, an optimal dose schedule was established in which MTX was administered combined with 5-FU for 14 days and 5-FU was delivered as a single agent for the subsequent 14 days. This schedule was established because of the identification of chemical hepatitis, leukopenia, and thrombocytopenia associated with the concomitant administration of MTX with 5-FU for more than 14 days. In fact, these effects were obviated in spite of continued 5-FU when the MTX compound was interrupted at 14 days. In the initial phase 1 study, responses were observed in 6/12 patients with advanced measurable colorectal cancer.

The combination of sequential MTX and 5-FU is based not upon the additive cytotoxic effects of the component drugs, but rather upon the concept of biochemical modulation. Other types of biochemical modulation that may include an infusion schedule include thymidine and PALA. Thymidine (TdR) blocks the degradation of 5-FU, providing a prolonged plasma half-life for the antipyrimidine and increased incorporation of 5-FU into RNA. In a phase 1 study of weekly bolus TdR and 5-FU, major CNS adverse effects were identified, although pharmacokinetic studies demonstrated a prolonged half-life for 5-FU.[32] However, in a pharmacologic study in which 5-FU was administered as a 5-day low-dose infusion with concurrent TdR, only 2 of 8 patients responded.[33] PALA inhibits aspartate transcarbamylse, thereby depleting intracellular pyrimidines and enhancing incorporation of 5-FU into RNA. PALA is a totally inactive cytotoxic agent, but when administered in conjunction with 5-FU in experimental tumor systems, it has a synergistic effect. Clinical trials employing PALA with 5-FU and TdR, with all agents delivered as a bolus on an every-4-weeks schedule, have yielded a response rate of 27% in 37 patients evaluated.[34] Of some importance is the potential for the effectiveness of this regimen in patients with anaplastic or rapidly progressing tumors, in which the response was 46%.

Table 3. Multidrug Regimens in which 5-Fluorouracil Is Delivered as a Continuous Infusion

Study/reference	5-FU infusion dose rate	Combined agent	Response rate (%)
Buroker et al[27]	1 gm/m^2/d × 5	MeCCNU	19/111 (17)
	1 gm/m^2/d × 5	Mitomycin-C	34/124 (19)
Shephard et al[28]	1,000 mg/m^2/d × 5	Cisplatin	0/ 20 (0)
Budd et al[30]	1 gm/m^2/d × 4	Folinic acid	12/ 53 (23)
Lokich et al[31]	300 mg/m^2/d × 28	Methotrexate	6/ 12 (50)
Lai-Sim Av et al[33]	7.5 mg/kg/d × 5	Thymidine	1/ 11 (9)

A modulator of 5-FU is provided by allopurinol. This agent is an inhibitor of xanthene oxidase as well as orotidylate decarboxylase. The toxicity of 5-FU is modified in that normal cells exposed to allopurinol develop a high intracellular concentration of orotic acid; this acid competes with 5-FU for the enzyme system, resulting in the formation of FDUMP. In a small series in which 5-FU was delivered by continuous infusion in conjunction with allopurinol, 5/10 patients with tumors of the G.I. tract responded to the combination.[35]

Floxuridine (FUDR)

FUDR is an antipyrimidine with clinical and pharmaceutical features distinct from those of 5-FU. Regional infusion trials have been relatively common with this antipyrimidine because of its solubility, which permits delivery of relative small volumes in a 24-hour period. Furthermore, the optimal or therapeutic dose on a continuous infusion schedule is less than that necessary on a bolus schedule, contributing to the small volumes that may be administered.

5-fluorouracil and FUDR may be distinctive in terms of clinical tumor response as well (see table 4). In the study by the Mayo Clinic Group,[36] 10/84 patients with advanced colorectal cancer responded to 5-FU and 19/84 responded to FUDR, but the difference was not statistically significant. In both groups, the antipyrimidine was administered on a bolus schedule. In the study from the University of Wisconsin, a more substantial difference was observed (17% for 5-FU and 43% for FUDR); the difference was statistically significant at the .001 level, but the patient entries were not randomized.[37] The dose schedule of delivery was comparable to that in the Mayo Clinic study.

Infusional delivery of FUDR systemically was first reported by Sullivan and Miller in 1965.[38] These investigators established that the continuous infusion schedule decreased the tolerated dose of FUDR to more than 1/30 of the bolus dose and suggested that the activity was enhanced. Responses were observed in 6/20 patients with colon cancer using a dose rate of 0.5 to 1.0 mg/kg/day for 5–10 days. Responses were also observed in 6/10 gastric cancers and 5/10 breast cancers as well as 3/10 lung cancers. In a prospective comparative trial of systemic FUDR delivered as a rapid injection or a short-term 5-day infusion, Moertel et al suggested that infusion therapy was "significantly" inferior to bolus therapy, with a response rate of 6.2% compared to 17.5%.[39] Sixty-eight patients with advanced measurable colorectal cancer were randomly allocated to receive either a rapid injection of FUDR at 40 mg/kg/day for 5 days compared with infusion of 1.5 mg/kg/day for 5 days. The latter dose was subsequently increased to 2.25 mg/kg/day for 5 days. On the infusion schedule, FUDR toxicity was manifested more frequently as stomatitis, and on the bolus

Table 4. Comparison of Clinical Effectiveness of 5-FU and FUDR in Advanced Colorectal Cancer

Trial/reference	5-FU	FUDR
Mayo Clinic (1965)[36]	10/84 (12%)	19/84 (23%)
University of Wis. (1962)[37]	24/141 (17%)	25/57 (43%)

schedule, toxicity was manifested predominantly as leukopenia. Ansfield et al also studied the continuous infusion schedule for FUDR using a dose rate of 3 mg/kg/day to the point of toxicity (average 5.5 days). The study group was small, but no responses were observed in 8 patients with colorectal cancer.[40] The 2 "negative" studies used high FUDR dose rates (2.2–3 mg/kg/day for short durations (5 days) compared to the lower dose rates (0.5–1.0 mg/kg/day) for longer intervals (5–10 days). This may not be the real reason for the differences observed, however. The decade 1960–70 represented an early period for chemotherapy trials, and criteria for patient selection and response were not as rigorous as those applied to more modern trials. Also, the diagnostic tools were more limited. In view of the apparent clinical differences between 5-FU and FUDR and the conflicting reports on the effectiveness of the infusion schedule for FUDR, it would seem reasonable to reevaluate the latter agent as a systemic infusion, possibly using the protracted infusion at a lower daily dose rate.

Two phase 1 trials of protracted continuous infusion FUDR have been reported. In the study reported by Lokich et al, and optimal dose of 0.15 mg/kg/day for 14 days was identified. No antitumor effects were observed in the small series of patients who had received extensive prior therapy. In the phase 1 trial by DiConti et al, the continuous infusion schedule used higher doses (1 mg/kg/day) for 2–16 days. Tumor responses in gastric and breast cancer were seen, but only 3/34 patients with colorectal cancer responded.[42]

Two prospective randomized trials of hepatic arterial infusion versus systemic venous infusion of FUDR are ongoing. In both trials, the venous infusion arm delivers a dose of 0.08 to 0.15 mg/kg/day for 14 days.[43,44] Both studies have demonstrated that systemic delivery of FUDR in colorectal cancer is active, achieving response rates of 30% or more and are comparable to those observed in the hepatic arterial infusion arms and superior to previous reports of infusion FUDR. Further suggestive evidence of the effectiveness of the systemic infusion of FUDR in these trials is reflected in the fact that the development of extra hepatic metastases has been markedly decreased in patients receiving the systemic infusion compared to patients receiving intrahepatic infusion.

Other Antipyrimidines

Ftorafur (tegafur) is a slow-release form of fluorouracil that can be administered orally and in essence leads to a pharmacologic pattern similar to that achievable by continuous parenteral administration of 5-FU. In a comparative study of oral tegafur and "standard" I.V. 5-FU, response rates in colorectal cancer were comparable (7/35 [20%] compared to 6/32 [19%]), but toxicity was minimized.[45] Doxifluridine is another fluoropyrimidine that has been in phase 2 trials in Europe. On a bolus schedule, measurable colorectal cancer responses were observed in 7/27 (26%) patients.[46] No studies of an infusion schedule for this agent have been reported.

Other Agents

As is the case for other tumors in the G.I. tract, agents other than the fluoropyrimidines have not been identified as having significant activity in colorectal cancer. One could speculate that drugs shown to be inactive in colon cancer could reasonably be reexamined, using a continuous infusion schedule. A listing of some agents that would be evaluated in the context of infusion schedules based on pharmacokinetic considerations or modest activity observed in bolus trials is given in table 5. The antimetabolites would be of particular interest.

Hydroxyurea is an oral agent that lends itself to the capability of chronic administration to emulate continuous infusion. In a series of trials reported by Livingston and Carter,[47] only 6/80 patients responded, and in 1 trial in which 8-hour infusions were administered daily for 5 days there were no responses in 23 patients.[48]

Cytosine arabinoside (ara-C) delivered on a standard bolus schedule has had modest activity in advanced measurable colorectal cancer, with 9/49 patients responding to an unpublished trial referred to in Carter and Livingston's compendium of single-agent activity.[47] The antipurine agents have been evaluated in modern clinical trials, but an infusion schedule has not been used.[3,47] Both agents have a short serum half-life.

A small number of patients have been studied using continuous infusion of mercaptopurine at up to 1 mg/kg/day for 6–10 days but only in the context of

Table 5. Agents Other Than the Fluoropyrimidines in Advanced Colorectal Cancer

Agents/reference	Bolus activity	Infusion activity
Antimetabolites		
Hydroxyurea[47,48]	+/−	ND*
Cytosine arabinoside[47]	+ +	ND
Antipurines		
6 – Thioguanine[3]	+/−	ND
6 – Mercaptopurine[49,50]	+/−	ND
Methotrexate[47,51]	+ +	+
Alkylating agents		
Mitomycin-C[52,53]	+ +	+
Cyclophosphamide[47]	+/−	
Vinblastine[47]	+/−	ND
Vincristine[47]	ND	ND
Anthracycline antibiotics		
Doxorubicin	0	0
Epidoxorubicin[54]	0	ND

*ND = no data

a toxicity study.[49] Chronic oral administration, however, also was not active in a large series of 45 patients.[50]

MTX, which has some activity in colorectal cancer, has been studied with an infusion schedule.[51] In 17 patients treated with 5 mg/24 hours for 5–10 days, 7 patients had tumor regression (41%), but except for protracted infusion studies at low doses (less than 1 mg/m²/day), no additional studies have been reported. In the protracted infusion studies, no responses were observed in 10 patients so treated.

The alkylating agents have similarly demonstrated only minor activity in colorectal cancer. MIT is a potentially active agent in colon cancer on a bolus schedule, and an infusion schedule is rational based upon the pharmacokinetic characteristics of this agent. A review of the Japanese literature in 1960 suggested that this agent may achieve a 28% response rate,[52] and Miller et al did administer MIT by continuous infusion,[53] with a 56% response rate in collected patients with G.I. tumors. Thio-tepa and cyclophosphamide (CTX) have had no meaningful clinical trials, although high-dose bolus CTX yielded occasional responses.[47] Streptozotocin, an agent that has been part of the MOF-STREP regimen, is another type of alkylating agent that could reasonably be delivered on an infusion schedule based upon pharmacokinetic information.

The periwinkle alkaloids vinblastine and vincristine have been employed in relatively small trials, with a total experience for vinblastine in collected trials of 71 patients and for vincristine only 13 patients.[47] These agents presently are being reexamined in continuous infusion schedules.

The antibiotics, particularly the intercalating agents such as the anthracycline analogues, have never demonstrated meaningful activity in colorectal cancer. Again, one could speculate that an infusion schedule could potentially expand the spectrum of tumors for which this class of agents may be active; therefore, clinical trials of doxorubicin or even the newer anthracine analogues could reasonably be reexamined in colorectal cancer using an infusion schedule. A trial of infusion epirubicin has suggested that this schedule will not improve the effectiveness of the anthracyclines.[54]

Infusional 5-FU Concomitant with Radiation

The combined application of chemotherapy and radiation for gastrointestinal cancer has been an active area of clinical investigation since the introduction of the concept of multimodality therapy for cancer. The earliest reported prospective randomized trial comparing radiation to radiation plus bolus 5-FU demonstrated an improved palliative effect for the combined modality approach in gastric, pancreatic, and colorectal cancer.[55] Subsequent studies by the Gastrointestinal Tumor Group, particularly for pancreatic cancer, have confirmed this observation, demonstrating an improved survival for combined chemotherapy and radiation.[56]

The schedule for the 5-FU delivered in the combined modality programs has generally been limited to administration of a bolus dose on the first 3 days of a 2–4 week period of radiation. It is difficult to conceive of the regional impact of such bolus treatment in the context of radiation sensitization, inasmuch as the radiation is delivered over a much longer period. Furthermore, clinical trials in which infusional 5-FU is delivered throughout the period of radiation in esophageal cancer and anal cancer have been extraordinarily successful compared to the bolus 5-FU trials in gastric, pancreatic, and rectal cancer. Trials in anal and esophageal cancer have involved short-term infusions, with radiation therapy.

Rich et al have established in a phase 1 feasibility trial that protracted infusion 5-FU at low daily dose rates can be delivered concomitant with sustained refractionation radiation for a variety of tumors, including colorectal cancer.[57] This regimen is designed to maximize radiation sensitization with the optimal dose of radiation. The tolerance to such a delivery system and the performance record in which chemotherapy always adds substantially to radiation in gastrointestinal cancers suggests that radiation therapy should always be administered in conjunction with infusional chemotherapy. However, prospective comparative trials are essential to establish such a clinical practice.

Another application of combined modality treatment for colorectal cancer has been in the palliation of biliary obstruction due to metastases to the portal lymph nodes with external compression of the biliary tract. The use of radiation therapy as a singular modality has had limited effect in such circumstances, and radiographically guided decompression with percutaneous catheters has generally been necessary. A recent report by Cochran et al on combined low-dose infusion with regional radiation for biliary obstruction established that 7 patients responded with resolution of jaundice and a mean survival of 1.5 years.[58]

Adjuvant Infusional Chemotherapy

The use of infusional chemotherapy in the adjuvant setting is reviewed in the chapter by Sugarbaker and Lokich. Ongoing trials of regional infusion employing the portal vein or hepatic artery, or both, represent the predominant clinical investigational effort. Smaller trials of intraperitoneal and of systemic infusion employing untreated controls have established the feasibility of such approaches. These trials also have provided provocative (although scientifically unanalyzable) information suggesting an advantage for infusion chemotherapy in the adjuvant setting. Definitive clinical trials, however, must await the results of ongoing comparative trials in advanced disease in which the bolus schedule is being compared to infusion schedules.

Summary

5-fluorouracil continues to be the "standard" chemotherapeutic approach to advanced measurable colorectal cancer. Data derived from prospective randomized trials suggest that the infusion schedule is superior to the standard bolus schedule for this agent, and prolonged infusion is being tested in an ongoing regional group trial. In the absence of newly identified agents, combination chemotherapy is being explored based upon the rationale of biochemical modulation rather than synergistic or additive cytotoxic effects of multiple drugs. Although the latter represents a most exciting and rational approach to clinical trials in colon cancers, a reexamination of older agents would seem in order, particularly for those drugs for which schedule dependency can be established in experimental tumor systems and in which the pharmacokinetic profile of the agent would support a rationale for continuous infusion.

23

GASTRIC, PANCREAS, AND
BILIARY TRACT CANCER

Geoffrey Falkson, M.D., and Baruch Klein, M.D.

INFUSION THERAPY REPRESENTS A treatment modality exposing tumor cells for longer periods of time. Infusion therapy includes the following modes of administration: (1) short-term continuous I.V. infusion, usually for 5 days; (2) long-term I.V. infusions for 30 days or more; and (3) intra-arterial infusions that may deliver systemic or regional infusions to the tumor bed.

In order to assess the efficacy of the various forms of infusion therapy, the results usually obtained with conventional systemic treatment must be reviewed. No prospective randomized stratified trials have shown an unequivocal survival advantage for patients with either advanced stomach, advanced pancreas, or advanced biliary tract cancer on any systemic treatment. Likewise, no survival advantage has been demonstrated for patients with these diseases who are randomized to receive infusion chemotherapy. The evaluation of treatment in these 3 diseases is therefore dependent on response evaluation.

Conventional Treatment

Gastric Cancer

Gastric cancer is more sensitive to chemotherapy than are the other gastro-intestinal malignancies.[1]

SINGLE ANTICANCER DRUGS

Single agents given by bolus injection or orally bring about low response rates of short duration. Among the single agents, the drug most adequately

This study was supported in part by a grant from the National Cancer Association of South Africa evaluated is 5-fluorouracil (5-FU). Falkson and co-workers[2,3] obtained a response rate of 17% in patients treated with 5-FU alone (15 mg/kg × 5 days) and a response rate of 55% with 5-FU plus radiotherapy. Similar results were observed by Moertel and co-workers.[4] The response rate to 1,3-Bis (2-chloroethyl-1-nitrosourea (BCNU) is 18% and to methyl-CCNU (MeCCNU), 8%.[5,6]

Various antitumor antibiotics show activity in stomach cancer. Mitomycin-C (MIT) (10–20 mg/m^2 every 5–8 weeks) gives response rates of 15–30%.[7] The anthracycline antibiotic doxorubicin (ADR) has response rates of up to 36%.[8] Using the standard dose of 60 mg/m^2 q 3–4 weeks, the Eastern Cooperative Oncology Group (ECOG) showed a response rate of 22% in previously untreated patients and a response rate of 15% in previously treated patients.[9] Similar results were observed by the Gastro-Intestinal Tumor Study Group (GITSG), with response rates of 24%.[10] Recently, new ADR analogues were tested in the hope that they might be less cardiotoxic. 4-Epi-doxorubicin (40–50 mg/m^2 I.V. every 2–5 weeks) gave a response in 4/15 patients[11] in one series and 1 minor response among 9 patients in separate series.[12] No objective response was seen in 6 patients using esorubicin (4-deoxydoxorubicin).[13] Likewise, mitoxantrone produced no objective response in stomach cancer.[14] More recently, in an evaluation of cisplatin (DDP), at a dose of 100 mg/m^2 I.V. bolus q 3 weeks, a response was observed in 5/14 patients in one series[15] and in 1/15 patients[16] in another.

COMBINATION CHEMOTHERAPY

Various combination chemotherapy regimens have been studied in advanced gastric cancer. In a double-blind study, the addition of ara-C did not enhance the activity of 5-FU.[17] Seventeen out of 31 patients treated with 5-FU + radiotherapy by Falkson et al[18] showed response, compared to 10 of 28 patients treated with 5-FU, DTIC, vincristine, (VCR), BCNU + radiotherapy (FIVB). In a randomized study, the response rate for 5-FU alone was 29%, for BCNU alone 17%, and for the combination 41%.[5] In an ECOG trial, MeCCNU gave a response rate of 8% compared to 40% for MeCCNU plus 5-FU, with survival benefit for patients treated with the combination.[6] Other studies failed to confirm this response rate for MeCCNU plus 5-FU. In a more recent ECOG study comparing ADR alone to MeCCNU plus 5-FU to 5-FU plus MIT, ADR gave a response rate of 22%, MeCCNU + 5-FU 24%, and 5-FU + MIT 32%, with no differences in survival.[9]

The current most popular drug combination is 5-FU + ADR + MIT (FAM) (5-FU 600 mg/m^2 day 1, 8, 29, 36; ADR 30 mg/m^2 day 1, 29; and MIT 10 mg/m^2 day 1, repeated every 8 weeks), first reported in 1979.[19] Eighteen of 36 patients (50%) achieved partial response (PR). The same group updated their results in 1980[20] in a trial including 62 patients. Twenty-six of 62 patients (42%) had a PR. Response rates in nonrandomized published series had varied from 8 to 55% (see table 1), with a mean response rate of 35%. In randomized multiinstitutional series where the number of patients studied is given, the median response rate is 30.5% (see table 2).

Several groups have studied a modification of the FAM regimen substituting

MeCCNU for MIT. The GITSG[21] compared 5-FU + ADR + MeCCNU (FAMe) to
5-FU + ICRF + MeCCNU (FIMe) to FAM to 5-FU + MeCCNU (FMe). Responses
were recorded in 3/10 patients (30%) on FAMe, 4/19 patients (21%) on FIMe,
3/12 patients (25%) on FAM, and 1/18 patients (6%) on FMe. Median survival
times were FAMe 34 weeks, FIMe 77 weeks, FAM 30 weeks, and FMe 23 weeks.
ECOG[26] compared 5-FU + MeCCNU (FIMe), FAMe, ADR + MIT, and FAM. Of 241
patients studied, 196 were evaluable for analysis. Response rates were: FIMe
17%, FAMe 26%, ADR + MIT 32% (no prior chemotherapy), and 25% (prior
chemotherapy) and FAM 40%. Median survival times were: FIMe 12 weeks,
FAMe 25 weeks, ADR + MIT 18 weeks (no prior chemotherapy) and 16 weeks
(prior chemotherapy), and FAM 27 weeks. Another study by GITSG[27] compared
FA (5-FU + ADR) to FAMe to FAM (modified regimen). Responses were recorded
in 1/19 (5%) for FA, in 4/16 (25%) for FAMe, and in 3/18 (17%) for FAM. The
North Central Cancer Treatment Group (NCCTG)[30] compared 5-FU with 5-FU +
ADR with FAM in stomach and pancreatic cancer. Of 301 patients randomized,
296 were evaluable. In 62 patients with measurable disease, response rates
were: 5-FU 26%, FA 24%, and FAM 23%. Median survival for stomach cancer
was 7 months and for pancreatic cancer 5 months. The authors conclude that
there is no therapeutic benefit for the combinations over 5-FU alone, and there
is increased toxicity.

Table 1. Stomach Cancer Treated with FAM: Nonrandomized Studies

Investigator/ reference	No. patients	No. (%) responses
McDonald[20]	62	26 (42)
Bitran[21]	11	6 (55)
Haim[22]	33	7 (21)
Beretta[23]	45	20 (44)
Biran[24]	25	2 (8)
Haim[25]	22	4 (18)
TOTALS	198	65 (33)

Table 2. Stomach Cancer Treated with FAM: Randomized Studies

Investigator/ reference	No. patients	No. (%) responses
[a]GITSG[26]	12	3 (25)
[b]ECOG[27]	44	17 (41)
GITSG[28]	18	3 (17)
[c]SWOG[28]	83	25 (30)
[d]SWOG[29]	81	19 (23)
TOTALS	238	67 (28)

[a]Gastro-Intetinal Tumor Study Group
[b]Eastern Cooperative Oncology Group
[c]Southwest Oncology Group
[d]Modified FAM

The synergism between DDP and ADR in model systems resulted in clinical trials with these drugs. Several studies are reported with ADR- and DDP-containing regimens. The results are shown in table 3. Woolley[31] reported on 35 patients treated with 5-FU (600 mg/m² I.V. day 1, 8) and ADR (40 mg/m² day 1) and DDP (75 mg/m² day 1, q 28 days) (FAP). Response was observed in 29%. Wagener,[32] using FAP (5-FU 300 mg/m² I.V. day 1–5), ADR (50 mg/m² I.V. day 1) and DDP (20 mg/m² day 1–5 q 21 days), documented response in 8/16 patients, with median survival of 10.5 months. Moertel[37] reported on 9/17 patients treated with FAP with DDP (given in a 3-hour infusion, q 5 weeks), with median survival of 10 months. A GITSG study[34] compared FAP (employing a lower dose of ADR 30 mg/m² but a higher dose of DDP 100 mg/m², q 4 weeks) to 5-FU + ADR + triazinate (FAT) (250 mg/m² day 22–24, q 5 weeks). Ten patients were entered on each arm. The authors did not report on response rates, but median survival was 17 months on FAP and 11 months on FAT. ECOG[35] reported 1 complete remission among 15 patients treated with FAP; only 3 patients were evaluable. Toxicity was marked. With these small numbers, no conclusion can be drawn.

Several workers have added further drugs to the FAM regimen. The Southwest Oncology Group (SWOG)[36] prospectively compared FAM to FAM + VCR (V-FAM). Responses were observed in 6/27 patients (22%) on FAM and in 6/38 patients (16%) on V-FAM. Median survival times of 22 and 20 weeks, respectively, were reported. Berreta[37] prospectively compared FAM to FAM + BCNU (FAMB). Five of 13 patients (38%) on FAM responded, compared to 5/18 patients (32%) on FAMB.

Combination chemotherapy gives better response rates than single agents, with a slight improvement in survival time claimed. The results obtained with the FAM regimen as tested in prospective randomized trials are inferior to those reported originally by MacDonald et al.[20]

Pancreas Cancer

SINGLE-AGENT THERAPY

5-FU has been extensively evaluated in the treatment of patients with pancreatic cancer. Moertel[8] studied 39 patients and reported a 15% response rate

Table 3. Stomach Cancer Treated with 5-Fluorouracil plus Adriamycin plus Cisplatin (FAP)

Investigator/ reference	No. patients	No. (%) responses
Woolley[31]	35	10 (29)
Wagner[32]	16	8 (50)
Moertel[33]	17	9 (53)
GITSG[34]	10	– (–)
ECOG[35]	15	1 (7)
TOTALS	83	28 (34)

(median duration of response 2.5 months). Carter et al[38] recorded a cumulative response rate of 28% in review of selected series.

BCNU and MeCCNU give response rates of 0 to 9%.[5,39] MIT gave a ±27% response rate (12/44 patients),[38] while streptozotocin gave a response rate of 31–50% in a small reported series[40,41,42] and ADR[43] produced responses in 2/15 patients. In a study of 4-epidoxorubicin by Nicoletto et al,[44] 1 of 8 patients responded. Hochster et al[45] found no responses in 10 patients on the same drug.

No response in 14 patients treated with DDP was reported by Ajani et al.[15] Melphalan was evaluated in an ECOG trial, with 1 response in 43 patients.[46] Ifosfamide was studied by Lochner et al.[45] The dose employed was 1.25–1.5 mg/m² day 1–5 combined with uroprotection with N-acetylcystine. Four of 21 patients treated responded, 1 with a complete response (CR).

COMBINATION CHEMOTHERAPY

5-FU + BCNU was evaluated by Kovach et al.[5] A response rate of 33% was observed in 10/30 patients treated. Survival benefit was not observed when compared to the survival of 5-FU or BCNU alone. Lokich et al,[48] employing 5-FU + BCNU, reported responses in 4/20 patients. In an ECOG study,[46] 4/41 patients (10%) treated with 5-FU + MeCCNU and 3/43 patients (7%) treated with 5-FU + MeCCNU + stz had an objective response.

5-FU + MIT + S(SMF) was evaluated by Wiggam,[49] and an objective response was claimed in 10/22 patients (43%). Bukowski[50] reported response in 7/22 patients (32%) treated with SMF. The FAM regimen was also studied in pancreas cancer. Bitran[51] observed objective response in 6/15 patients (40%), while Smith[52] reported response in 10/27 patients (37%). Sternberg et al[53] employed MIT (2 mg/m²), 5-FU (500 mg/m²) and ADR (20 mg/m² q 3 weeks) in 19 evaluable patients, of whom 15 had failed prior therapy. Preliminary results showed 4 patients had a partial response and 2 a minimal response. The GITSG[54] evaluated FAM combinations in a concurrent but not fully randomized study. The regimens compared 2 SMF schedules, FAM, and SAMe. Objective responses were recorded in 4/28 patients treated with SMF given weekly, 4/27 on SMF loading, 4/30 on FAM, and 0 of 25 patients on SAMe. They concluded that SMF and FAM have minimal activity in measurable pancreatic cancer.

Of greater significance than the above trial is a study by Oster et al[55] that compared FAM and SMF in a randomized controlled trial. Among the 58 patients on FAM, the response rate was 9.3%, while a 4.4% response rate was documented in 66 patients treated with SMF.

In 3 studies, other drugs were added to FAM. S-FAM[56] produced responses in 12/25 patients (40%), hexamethylmelamine + FAM (HexaFAM) resulted in response in 5/30 patients (17%),[57] and chlorozoticin (C) + FAM (C-FAM)[59] gave a response in 3/23 patients (13%).

The FAP regimen gave response in 3/15 patients (20%) in one study[59] and in 5/21 (24%) in another.[33]

The mean response rate for combination chemotherapy in nonrandomized studies is 29% (see table 4), whereas the mean response rate in randomized studies is 8% (see table 5). The chemotherapy of pancreatic cancer remains unsatisfactory except in uncontrolled and nonrandomized single-institution studies. The short duration of the responses seen in controlled studies is as poor as the response rate.

Table 4. Pancreas Cancer: Nonrandomized Combination Chemotherapy

Regimen/ reference	No. patients	No. (%) responses
5-FU + BCNU[5]	30	10 (33)
5-FU + BCNU[48]	20	4 (20)
SMF[49]	22	10 (43)
SMF[50]	22	7 (32)
FAM[51]	15	6 (40)
FAM[52]	27	10 (37)
MIFA[53]	19	4 (21)
S-FAM[56]	25	12 (41)
Hexa-FAM[57]	30	5 (17)
C-FAM[58]	23	3 (13)
FAP[59]	15	3 (20)
FAP[33]	21	5 (24)
TOTALS	269	79 (29)

F = 5-FU	=	5-fluorouracil
BCNU	=	1,3-Bis(2-chloroethyl-1-nitrosourea)
S	=	Streptozotocin
M = MI	=	Mitomycin-C
A	=	Adriamycin
Hexa	=	Hexamethylmelamine
C	=	Chlorozotocin
P	=	Cisplatin

Table 5. Pancreas Cancer Treated with Combination Therapy: Multi-Institutional Studies

Regimen/ reference	No. patients	No. (%) responses
5-FU + MeCCNU[46]	41	4 (10)
5-FU + MeCCNU + S[46]	43	3 (7)
SMF[55]	66	3 (4)
SMF[52]	28	4 (14)
FAM[55]	56	5 (9)
FAM[52]	30	4 (13)
SAMe[52]	25	0 (0)
TOTALS	289	23 (8)

F = 5-FU	=	5-fluorouracil
Me = MeCCNU	=	Methyl-CCNU
S	=	Streptozotocin
M	=	Mitomycin-C
A	=	Adriamycin

Bile Duct Carcinoma

Chemotherapy of bile duct cancer is rarely reported or adequately studied because of the small number of patients available for evaluation.[60]

5-FU was employed in 17 patients, with a 23% response rate.[61] MIT had a response rate of 42% in 7/15 patients.[61] FAM had response in 4/13 patients (31%) in 1 study and in 4/14 (31%) in another.[62,63] Falkson et al[64] recently reviewed the ECOG experience in gallbladder and bile duct cancer. Treatment arms were: oral 5-FU, oral 5-FU + streptozotocin (stz), oral 5-FU + MeCCNU, stz alone, and MeCCNU alone. In previously untreated patients with gallbladder cancer, 5/53 responded objectively to treatment, 2/18 oral 5-FU, 2/16 on 5-FU + stz, and 1/19 on oral 5-FU MeCCNU. Of 34 patients with previously untreated bile duct carcinoma, 3 responded objectively, 1/12 on oral 5-FU, 1/100 on 5-FU + stz, and 2/12 on oral 5-FU + MeCCNU. Among patients with prior chemotherapy, 1/14 patients responded to MeCCNU alone. There was no response among 17 patients treated with stz alone. There was no statistically significant difference in survival.

Chemotherapy by Infusion for Stomach, Pancreas, and Biliary Tract Carcinoma

The perfusion technique for local cancer chemotherapy was developed by Creech in 1958, and the arterial infusion technique with methotrexate (MTX) and systemic protection with leucovorin factor was developed by Sullivan in 1959. In 1960, Sullivan[65] employed continuous I.V. infusion of 5-FU lasting 3–36 days and found that the tolerated dose could be increased either because of an altered catabolic pathway or different pharmacological distribution. The short half-life of the cytostatic drugs, coupled with the relatively small proportions of tumor cells in the growth phase of the cell cycle sensitive to bolus injection, provided the rationale for the use of continuous infusion.

In a controlled comparison, Reitemeier[66] employed equal doses of 5-FU either by rapid bolus injection or by 8–hour infusion. With infusion, less toxicity was observed, but a corresponding decrease in objective response rate occurred. In 1976, Moertel[8] concluded that slow infusion adds no more than expense and nuisance to the treatment procedure. In a randomized but not blind or stratified trial, Serfint et al[67] in 1975 compared 5-FU given as a bolus injection (12 mg/kg I.V. × 5 days) to 30 mg/kg as continuous infusion for 5 days in patients with metastatic colorectal cancer. The infusion method resulted in a response rate of 44%, compared to 19% for the bolus method. Myelosuppression was rare in the infusion groups, but severe stomatitis occurred in 65%, compared to 16% in the bolus group.

Grillo-Lopez[68] studied 65 patients with G.I. cancer treated with 5-FU infusion. Twenty-one of these patients had stomach cancer, and the response obtained was encouraging.

Nixon et al[69] conducted a phase 1 study employing a 5-FU continuous infusion for 5 days + MTX + leucovorin + MeCCNU. One response was observed in 3 patients with stomach cancer and none in 1 with pancreatic cancer. Toxicity included bone marrow suppression and stomatitis.

Hartman et al,[70] in a retrospective study of G.I. neoplasms, compared infusion 5-FU (20 mg/kg/24 hours × 5 days followed by weekly 5-FU injection) to 5-FU weekly injections alone. Eight patients with stomach cancer were treated by infusion therapy and 8 patients by the weekly injections. Twelve patients with pancreatic cancer were treated with infusion and 12 patients with weekly injections. The median survival for gastric cancer patients in the infusion group was 3 months and in the bolus group 4 months. For patients with pancreas cancer, the median survival was 3 months with infusion and 5 months with bolus. The toxicity was similar. It must be noted, however, that these patients also received radiotherapy. Krauss et al[71] employed 5-FU as a continuous infusion plus MIT day 1 every 8 weeks. Four of 9 patients with stomach cancer had objective responses, with 1 CR; 4/8 patients with pancreas cancer had objective responses. The median survival time for patients with stomach cancer was 11 months and for patients with pancreas cancer 6 months. Toxicity was mainly hematologic.

A more scientific clinical basis was required for infusion treatment, and this was provided by Lokich and co-workers. In a phase 1 trial[72] of 5-day continuous infusion, 150 patients were studied with the following agents: DDP (55 patients), VP-16 (20 patients), vinblastine (VLB) (35 patients), MIT (20 patients), and 5-FU for 30–60 days (20 patients). The maximum tolerated dose of each drug was comparable to that of bolus therapy.

With the development of safe venous access via subclavian vein by Broviac and Hickman catheters and improvements in the portable infusion pumps, the way for studies using various drugs in ambulatory patients was further paved. A phase 1 trial of prolonged continuous I.V. infusion was reported by Lokich et al in 1981[73] The optimal dose of 5-FU was 300 mg/m^2/day and could be administered for up to 60 days without significant bone marrow suppression. Subsequently, experience in 124 patients was reported in 1983.[74] In addition to 5-FU, ADR, MIT, and VLB were studied. The dose-limiting toxicity for ADR was stomatitis; for MIT and VLB, stomatitis and leukopenia. Of 4 patients with stomach cancer, 1 had a CR. One patient treated with ADR did not respond.

Vaughn et al[75] compared 5-FU for 5 days by continuous infusion (25 mg/kg) plus MeCCNU 150 mg/m^2 po day 1, to 5-FU as above plus MIT 20 mg/m^2 8 weekly. Eleven patients with stomach cancer, 8 with pancreas cancer, and 2 with gallbladder and bile duct cancer were studied. Of 6 patients with stomach cancer treated with 5-FU plus MeCCNU, 1 was evaluable and had a CR. Of 2 evaluable patients with pancreas cancer on 5-FU plus MeCCNU, none responded. Of 3 evaluable patients with stomach cancer treated with 5-FU plus MIT, 2 had a partial response (PR). Among 4 patients with pancreas cancer, 1 had a PR. None of the gallbladder patients responded objectively to treatment.

Bruckner et al[76] employed 5-FU 30 mg/kg/day as continuous infusion for 5 days plus MIT 10 mg/m^2 on day 2 and HXM 150 mg/m^2 days 2–15 every 4–5 weeks. Among 21 patients with pancreas cancer, 6 responded (2 CR and 4 minor responses). Cazap[77] studied 5-day continuous venous infusion of bleomycin (BLM) (15 mg bolus followed by 15–18 mg/m^2 × 5 days) in 8 patients with stomach cancer. One patient had a PR. Of 6 patients with hepatobiliary and pancreas cancer, 1 had an objective response. Bukowski et al[78] studied 6 patients with stomach cancer with a 4-hour I.V. infusion of anguidene but documented no response.

Intra-Arterial Therapy

Intra-arterial (I.A.) treatment for stomach, pancreas, and biliary tract cancer was extensively employed by Watkins and Sullivan at the Lahey Clinic in the 1960s, with satisfactory response being recorded. Subsequently, various authors have reported on their longer term follow-up of I.A. treatment for stomach, pancreas, and biliary tract cancer. Unfortunately, none of the series has been prospectively stratified and randomized. The hope that agents with a short half-life would be of specific value when given by the I.A. route seemed promising 20 years ago. Despite positive results seen with short-acting agents such as epoxides given intra-arterially,[79] this approach failed to gain general popularity.

In the 1960s, I.A. MTX was shown to be superior to I.A. 5-FU in patients with primary liver cancer. Despite the fact that patients randomized to I.A. methotrexate or 5-FU were more carefully selected than those patients randomized to systemic treatment.[80] The survival time for I.A. 5-FU was similar to that for ineffective systemic treatment.

In gastrointestinal cancer, I.A. infusion has been more extensively studied than systemic infusion. Freckman[81] treated 50 patients with stomach cancer with I.A. infusion of 5-FU + cyclophosphamide + VLB; a response rate of 30% and survival of 13 months was observed. Davis[82] reported on 328 patients with stomach, pancreas, liver, and biliary tract cancer given fluoropyrimidine therapy. In 30 patients with stomach cancer with liver metastases, 24 patients were treated with I.V. 5-FU and 6 patients with I.A. 5-FU. Survival for more than 1 year was recorded in 21% on I.V. 5-FU and in 30% on I.A. 5-FU. In 60 patients with pancreas cancer and liver metastases, 40 were treated with I.V. 5-FU and 20 with I.A. 5-FU. Survival for more than 1 year occurred in 15% with I.V. 5-FU, compared to 10% with I.A. infusion. Despite the absence of improved survival rates, this treatment nevertheless remains in everyday use at the investigator's institution because of individual patient response and the subjective response obtained when expertise in administering this type of treatment is available. Yoshikawak[83] has reported his 10-year experience in 114 patients with G.I. malignancies, including 84 patients with stomach cancer. Theodor et al[84] employed FAM plus stz (FAM-s) in 19 patients with pancreas ampulary cancer. A catheter was placed in the celiac artery, patients were kept at complete bed rest, and infusion was given using an Imed volumetric pump. The catheter was removed after each treatment. Among 12 patients with measurable disease, total response rate was 65%, with 1 CR (8%) and 7 PR (57%). Survival in the 19 patients was 5.2 months.

Intra-arterial therapy with 5-FU in pancreatic cancer resulted in relief of pain in more than half of 63 patients treated in a series at St. George's Hospital in London,[85] but this was followed by slow but predictable recurrence of this symptom.

Discussion

The rationale for employing cell cycle-specific drugs by infusion therapy in contrast to conventional bolus treatment is attractive in view of a knowledge of cell kinetics, namely that only a relatively small proportion of solid tumor cells are in cycle.[86] Many of the currently available agents that have some therapeutic effect in stomach, pancreas, and biliary tract cancer are cycle-specific. The continuous exposure of cancer cells to agents that are not cycle-specific could also be of theoretical value. Additional effort should be made to take advantage of these facts.

The first issue to be addressed is the safety of the procedure. Of 124 patients studied by Lokich et al[74] using continuous infusion with tunneled versus catheters, catheter complications occurred in 20%, with 16 patients developing subclavian vein thrombosis. Although the complication rate declines with the development of technical proficiency within an institution, the same authors reported a 42% incidence of subclavian thrombosis (22 of 53 patients), with 7 patients having asymptomatic thrombosis.[87] With I.A. infusion therapy, complications occur in some 13% of patients.[88] With the conventional bolus system or short-term (less than 1 week) peripheral vein infusion, complications are virtually nonexistent.

The second issue is the relative toxicity of the drugs given by infusion as compared to bolus. Several authors have confirmed that when given as an infusion, the dose-limiting toxicity of 5-FU, ADR, MIT, and VLB is changed from G.I. toxicity and bone marrow suppression to stomatitis. This is important, as the usual dose-limiting toxicity for these cytotoxic drugs is hematologic. On the other hand, stomatitis can be debilitating. Hematologic toxicity is usually asymptomatic. The cumulative maximum dose that can be safely delivered with infusion therapy is comparable for most drugs. The exception is 5-FU: the cumulative dose that can be delivered by infusion is far greater than that by bolus. Claims that ADR in both short- and long-term continuous infusion decreases the incidence of cardiac toxicity have been made.[74] The use of infusion pumps makes feasible the treatment of patients on an ambulatory basis. This is of great importance for the patient. However, the substantial cost of the pump and the catheter insertion procedure must be born in mind.[74]

When these factors are taken into account, the main question is, How effective is the infusion treatment for patients with stomach, pancreas, and biliary tract cancer? The small numbers of patients treated by infusion therapy and the fact that in many studies 5-FU given in continuous infusion is compared to drug combinations given by injection obtund the comparisons. The median response rate obtained by infusion treatment for patients with stomach, pancreas, and biliary tract cancer has not been shown conclusively to differ from that obtained by conventional therapy. When the series of patients treated by infusion are larger, the response rate is found to be less. The response rate for pancreas cancer both by systemic and infusion therapy is less than that obtained in patients with stomach cancer, so that series considering these 2 diseases together are difficult to interpret. Tables 6 and 7 show the results of infusion therapy for patients with stomach and pancreas cancer. Although responses are observed, the number of patients is small compared to the number studied with conventional treatment. During the past few years, it has become abundantly clear that it is fallacious to compare the survival of responders with that of nonresponders.[89] It is equally important that this comparison not be used to incorrectly advocate any treatment, including long-term infusion and intra-arterial chemotherapy. It is hoped that stratified, randomized trials (proposed and ongoing) investigating the important biological principles involved in long-term infusion treatment will soon give results.

There is reason for optimism about the use of infusion chemotherapy for patients with stomach, pancreas, and bile duct cancer, but at present this approach remains fraught with problems. Some degree of patient selection tends to be unavoidable, and until such time as prospective randomized trials are available, more scientific evaluation of the results is not possible. With the development of the necessary expertise, the technical problems of continuous infusion are considerably decreased.

Table 6. Response Rate of Patients with Stomach Cancer Treated by Infusion

Investigator/ reference	Drugs and administration	No. patients	No. (%) responses
Nixon[69]	5-fluorouracil (VCI)[a] Methotrexate + Methyl-CCNU	3	1 (33)
Krauss[71]	5-fluorouracil (VCI) Mitomycin-C	9	4 (44)
Lokich[74]	5-fluorouracil (VCI) Adriamycin (VCI)	5	1 (20)
Vaughn[75]	5-fluorouracil (VCI) Methyl-CCNU Mitomycin-C	6	1 (17)
Cazep[77]	Bleomycin (VCI)	8	1 (13)
Bukowski[78]	Anguidine	6	0 (0)
Freckman[81]	5-fluorouracil (VCI) CTX[b] (IA)[c] Vinblastine	50	15 (30)
Theodor[84]	S-FAM[d](IA)	12	8 (65)
TOTALS		99	23 (23)

[a]VCI = Venous continuous infusion
[b]CTX = Cyclophosphamide
[c]IA = Intra-arterial
[d]S-FAM = Streptozotocin + ADR + MIT

Only institutions constantly using the technique have a low complication rate. Finally, although the longer exposure of the cancer cell to drug is laudable, the longer exposure of normal tissue to drug creates potential problems, especially as patients with better prognoses are included in future studies.

Table 7. Response Rate of Patients with Pancreas Cancer Treated with Infusion Therapy

Investigator/ reference	Drugs and administration	No. patients	No. (%) responses
Nixon[69]	5-fluorouracil (VCI)* Methotrexate Methyl-CCNU	1	0 (0)
Krauss[71]	5-fluorouracil (VCI) Mitomycin-C	8	4 (50)
Vaughn[75]	5-fluorouracil (VCI) Mitomycin-C Methyl-CCNU	2	0 (0)
Bruckner[76]	5-fluorouracil (VCI) Mitomycin-C Hexamethylmelamine	21	6 (29)
Cazep[77]	Bleomycin (VCI)	6	1 (17)
TOTALS		42	11 (26)

*VCI = Venous continuous infusion

24

BREAST CANCER

Sewa S. Legha, M.D.

CHEMOTHERAPY AGAINST BREAST CANCER is quite useful, playing an important role in the treatment of metastatic disease as well as in adjuvant therapy in patients with regional lymph node metastasis. The most effective chemotherapeutic agents against breast cancer include doxorubicin (ADR), cyclophosphamide (CTX), methotrexate (MTX), 5-fluorouracil (5-FU), vinblastine (VLB), and mitomycin-C (MIT). Combination chemotherapy is clearly superior to single-agent treatment, and the 2 most commonly used combination chemotherapy regimens include 3-drug combinations, 1 containing 5-FU, ADR, and cyclophosphamide (FAC) and the second containing CTX, MTX, and 5-FU (CMF). VLB and MIT are generally used as second-line drugs, either in combination or as single agents. Patients initially treated with CMF are commonly treated on relapse with combinations of ADR, either with VLB and/or MIT. Besides the drugs mentioned above, cisplatin (DDP) and etoposide (VP-16) also have a low order of activity and have been used when the other more active drugs have been used and are no longer effective.

Traditionally, the various chemotherapeutic agents listed above have been administered either in the form of I.V. injection over a period of several minutes or as short I.V. infusions. More recently, other modes of drug administration have been investigated, including continuous I.V. infusion or intra-arterial administration of some of these drugs. The rationale for continuous infusion of chemotherapeutic agents is based on certain pharmacologic and kinetic advantages to the use of anticancer drugs, which as a rule have low therapeutic indexes, and provides potential advantages in reducing the toxicity, increasing antitumor efficacy, or both.[1] Recent advances in infusion pump technology have also reduced the costs and inconvenience to patients, thus facilitating ambulatory infusion chemotherapy. Experiences with the I.V. infusion chemotherapy in the treatment of breast cancer are described in this chapter.

Infusion Studies of Doxorubicin

ADR is the single most active drug in the treatment of breast cancer; it is commonly used in combination with other cytotoxic drugs. The major limitation of this drug has been the development of a dose-related cardiomyopathy that prevents its use beyond 6–9 months of chemotherapy. When used as a bolus injection in a dose range of 50–60 mg/m^2, the risk of cardiac toxicity approaches 5 to 10% at cumulative ADR dose level of 550 mg/m^2. Clinical observations of reduction in cardiac toxicity when ADR was given on weekly fractionated doses led to the evaluation of continuous I.V. infusion of the agent several years ago. The observation that fractionation of the dose was less cardiotoxic in experimental animals, and the preservation of antitumor activity in experimental systems as well as clinically, encouraged us to explore the efficacy and toxicity of ADR in the treatment of breast cancer. Because ADR is a potent vesicant resulting in severe tissue necrosis on extravasation, infusion of the drug required placement of a central venous catheter. In the first trial in breast cancer, 27 patients with metastatic breast cancer who had previously received and failed CMF chemotherapy were treated with ADR at a dose of 60 mg/m^2 delivered over periods of 24–96 hours in a stepwise increase in duration of infusion. Among the 26 evaluable patients, 1 achieved a complete response (CR) and 12 patients had partial response (PR), for an overall response rate of 50%.[2] The median time to progression of disease from initiation of therapy was 7 months. There was a marked reduction in the nausea and vomiting associated with ADR infusion, although the incidence of stomatitis was slightly higher than that expected from the bolus schedule. The severity of alopecia and bone marrow toxicity was not altered by continuous infusion delivery of ADR. Most interestingly, 7 patients received a cumulative ADR dose level of 600 mg/m^2 or higher without developing clinical evidence of cardiac toxicity.

Encouraged by the results of this pilot study, ADR was subsequently evaluated in combination with other drugs active in the treatment of breast cancer. In one such trial, ADR administered as a continuous infusion has been used in combination with VLB. Forty-two patients with metastatic breast cancer who had previously received treatment with CMF were treated with ADR, 50 mg/m^2 administered over 48 hours followed by VLB, 1.4 mg/m^2, as continuous infusion over 24 hours for 4 days. Two patients achieved a CR and 16 achieved a PR, for a total response rate of 43%.[3] A similar study with continuous infusion of ADR and VLB has been reported by Bitran et al;[4] 13/20 patients had an objective response, for a response rate of 65%. The results of these 2 trials support the use of the ADR and VLB combination as the best salvage treatment in CMF-treated patients with metastatic breast cancer. Whether the infusion regimen described here is superior to the standard use of these 2 drugs remains to be proven. The excellent tolerance of this regimen and the reduced cardiac toxicity of ADR given as a continuous infusion provide added support for the use of the regimen for second-line chemotherapy. The experience with ADR infusion from the trials mentioned above, as well as its use in the treatment of other tumors, provided substantial data on its cardiac effects. The largest experience was gained with ADR administered over 96 hours. This experience clearly demonstrated a marked reduction in the drug's cardiac toxicity, which allowed its safe administration in the dose range of 800–1,200 mg/m^2.[5,6] Based on the evidence of reduction in cardiac and gastrointestinal toxicity of ADR used as an infusion, our current treatment program for metastatic breast cancer includes ADR as a continuous infusion in combination with CTX and 5-FU.

We have recently carried out a phase 3 study of FAC with ADR as a continuous infusion over 96 hours initially and subsequently over 48 hours. The dose of ADR was 50 mg/m^2 and the dose of 5-FU and CTX was similar to the standard dose FAC. In the initial 123 patients with metastatic breast cancer, 93 patients (76%) achieved a CR or PR, which is identical to our previous response figures with standard FAC regimen.[7] Whereas 68% of the patients treated with standard FAC went off ADR therapy upon reaching the dose limit of 450 mg/m^2, 64% of the patients treated with continuous infusion ADR went off therapy because of tumor progression. This allowed continued ADR beyond 450 mg/m^2, since no cardiac toxicity was observed until a cumulative ADR dose of 800 mg/m^2 was reached.[7] The median duration of response in patients treated with FAC containing infusion ADR was 16 months, which is similar to that with standard bolus FAC. However, patients who achieved CR with continuous infusion FAC had a longer duration of a remission compared to duration of response with the standard FAC regimen in the past. Although the results achieved with FAC with continuous infusion ADR appear to be superior to those with the FAC regimen used in the past, these data need to be confirmed with prospective comparative trials. We believe that a significant reduction in the toxicity of FAC given by the continuous infusion schedule with no compromise in its activity makes it a more attractive alternative to the standard FAC regimen. The reduction in cardiac toxicity of ADR infused over 48 hours was nearly equal to that observed with the infusion duration of 96 hours.

Encouraged by a significant improvement in the therapeutic index of ADR when given as a continuous infusion, we have recently introduced this method of ADR administration in FAC for adjuvant chemotherapy of high-risk stages 2 and 3 breast cancer. Although the cumulative dose of ADR in our previous adjuvant studies in breast cancer was limited to 300–400 mg/m^2, a small proportion of patients developed definite cardiac toxicity. We hope to avoid this result by using ADR as a continuous infusion, which will also allow us to raise the cumulative dose to somewhat higher levels. The duration of infusion of ADR in adjuvant breast studies should be no less than 48 hours and preferably longer, in order to achieve the best level of cardiac protection.

Another area in which ADR infusions have been useful is in the treatment of patients with metastatic breast cancer who had previously received ADR by short infusion schedule, either as adjuvant therapy or as a treatment for recurrent breast cancer, and the cumulative dose was limited to 450–550 mg/m^2. Because the options in therapy after failure of first-line chemotherapy for recurrent breast cancer are limited, reintroduction of FAC with ADR given as a 96–hour infusion has provided very useful palliation in approximately 50% of the patients who had previously responded to primary induction with FAC chemotherapy.[8] Although these patients are at high risk for cardiotoxicity, close monitoring of cardiac function has allowed continued therapy with FAC to cumulative dose levels of 300–450 mg/m^2 of ADR in addition to their prior ADR dose. In this situation, using ADR by the current bolus schedule carried a very high risk for heart failure, and the few patients we have treated in this fashion were not able to tolerate an ADR cumulative dose of more than 200 mg/m^2.

Continuous Infusion of Vinca Alkaloids

Vinca alkaloids, including VLB, vindesine (VDS), and vincristine (VCR), have been extensively used in the treatment of breast cancer. Both VLB and VDS have documented antitumor activity and are commonly used as second-line chemo-therapy in patients who have received and failed chemotherapy with FAC and CMF regimens. VCR, although definitely active in previously untreated patients, has no significant activity in previously treated patients and is clearly inferior to the other vinca alkaloids. All 3 drugs have been used by the continuous infusion schedule, and the results are as follows.

Vinblastine

The rationale for continuous infusion therapy with VLB is based on its cell cycle phase-specific effects. Like other vinca alkaloids, the drug is a potent vesicant and requires central venous access for continuous infusion delivery. In the first clinical trial with VLB in patients with refractory breast cancer, a dose schedule of 1.4 to 2.0 mg/m^2/day as a 5-day continuous infusion was used; this schedule resulted in a response rate of 40% in 30 evaluable patients.[9] Myelosuppression was found to be dose-limiting and unacceptable above the dose level of 1.8 mg/m^2/day. Six of the 12 patients who had previously received vinca alkaloids by the conventional dose schedule responded, includ-ing 2 who had progressed with bolus schedule of VLB. Another series using VLB in a dose schedule of 1.2–1.8 mg/m^2/day as a 5-day continuous infusion produced no responses in 17 patients with refractory breast cancer.[10] Although the results of the latter study questioned the value of VLB as a continuous infusion, further experience in a larger group of patients from the institution from which the first study was reported indicated reproducible activity, with 25 objective responses (36%) out of a total of 70 patients.[11] The median duration of response with VLB has been 5–6 months. Although VLB therapy is associated with intense myelosuppression, the period of myelosuppression is short and the response appears to be dose-related; for this reason, a relatively high dose must be administered to achieve the best therapeutic effect with this drug.

Vindesine

Vindesine is a semisynthetic vinca alkaloid derived from VLB. The spectrum of its antitumor activity is similar to that of VLB and the dose-limiting toxicity is myelosuppression, although the drug also causes significant peripheral neu-ropathy. When used in the standard bolus schedule at a dose of 3–4 mg/m^2 at

10- 14-day intervals, VDS induced partial regressions in approximately 20% of the patients with breast cancer. The improvement in the response rate of VLB when given by continuous infusion led to a similar trial in which patients were randomized to receive VDS either by the bolus schedule at a dose of 3–4 mg/m^2 I.V. or as a 5-day continuous infusion at a dose schedule of 1–1.2 mg/m^2/day for 5 days every 21 days. Among 26 evaluable patients treated with the bolus schedule, 2 patients achieved a PR (7%) compared to 7 PR (28%) among 25 evaluable patients treated with continuous infusion.[12] Furthermore, among the patients initially treated on the bolus schedule, 4/11 (36%) achieved a PR when given continuous infusions of VDS. Except for more intense myelosuppression with infusion, there was no significant difference in the other side effects, which included nausea and vomiting, stomatitis, and peripheral neuropathy. In an effort to further define the schedule-dependent activity of VDS, another randomized trial has recently been conducted in which patients received VDS either as a 5-day bolus injection of 1–1.2 mg/m^2/day I.V. repeated at 3-week intervals or as a 5-day continuous infusion at the same dose level. Of the 25 evaluable patients on the bolus schedule, 1 CR and 5 PR were observed, for a total response rate of 24%. This compares to 8 PR (31%) among 26 evaluable patients on the continuous infusion schedule.[13] Toxicity and time to progression of disease were similar with both schedules. The results of this trial indicate that fractionated treatments either by 5-day bolus or 5-day continuous infusion were equally efficacious.

Vincristine

Vincristine has also been studied in a continuous infusion schedule against breast cancer at a dose of 0.4–0.5 mg/m^2/day for 5 days.[14] No objective responses were observed among a total of 15 patients who had previously received standard chemotherapy. In this comparative trial, both VDS and VLB showed significant activity in the same group of patients.

Continuous Venous Infusion Trials with Other Drugs

Among the other drugs that are effective in the treatment of breast cancer, very limited data are available on their use as continuous infusion. MTX has been used in the form of continuous infusion over 24–36 hours without any demonstrated improvement in its therapeutic index compared to infusion periods of 2–6 hours. Among the alkylating agents, a phase 1 study of cyclophosphamide given as a continuous infusion revealed no particular advantage in terms of the spectrum of toxicity. The maximum tolerated dose was 600 mg/m^2/day for 3 days, and this dose was associated with severe nausea and vomiting. Significant myelosuppression also was observed.[15] The data on the efficacy of cyclophosphamide given in this manner in breast cancer are not available. Similarly, MIT has been given as a 5-day continuous infusion, and the maximum tolerated dose was believed to be 3 mg/m^2/day for 5 days. Among 17 patients with metastatic breast cancer treated in a phase 1–2 study of MIT, 1 patient achieved a PR. Although the data are limited, there appears to be no particular advantage in using this drug as a continuous infusion.[16] 5-FU has been used in several studies with the infusion schedule, but most of these were done in patients with metastatic colon carcinoma. When given as a continuous infusion, a marked reduction in the myelosuppressive toxicity of 5-FU allowed a doubling of the dose to a level of 1,200 mg/m^2/day $\times$ 5 days, and the dose-limiting toxicity was stomatitis.[17] In a randomized trial comparing the bolus schedule to continuous infusion in colon cancer, the response rate on the continuous infusion schedule was 44% versus 22% on the bolus schedule. The difference did not reach statistical significance because of small numbers. No detailed studies of 5-FU given as a continuous infusion have been carried out in breast cancer, although the drug was used in combination with high-dose CTX and ADR in 1 trial in which the dose of 5-FU was 500 mg/m^2/day for 5 days. Among 32 patients treated with this regimen, the response rate was 84% compared to 82% among 23 patients treated with the bolus schedule of 5-FU in combination with a standard dose of ADR and CTX.[18] It appears, therefore, that the toxicity of 5-FU is clearly reduced with the infusion schedule, although no significant improvement in antitumor activity was demonstrable in the limited experience to date.

Two other drugs having a low order of activity against breast cancer also have been investigated using the continuous infusion schedule. The first, VP-16, has been used against breast cancer in a randomized trial using a dose of 50–70 mg/m^2/day over 5 days by bolus versus continuous infusion schedule. In the intermittent group, 5/35 patients (14%) achieved a PR, compared to 4/31 evaluable patients (13%) who responded on the infusion schedule. Although there was slightly less nausea and vomiting on the infusion schedule, there was no clear advantage of infusion over bolus.[19] The second drug, DDP, has also been used in the treatment of breast cancer and has been shown to be active, especially when used in a high-dose schedule of 120 mg/m^2.[20] We have carried out a phase 2 study of DDP given as a continuous infusion of 20 mg/m^2/day for 5 days.[21] Among 26 patients with refractory breast cancer, no significant response was observed. There was, however, a significant reduction in nausea and vomiting when DDP was given as a continuous infusion.

25

INFUSION FOR

HEMATOLOGIC MALIGNANCIES

Murray M. Bern, M.D.

WITH THE DEVELOPMENT OF reliable, compact, and portable drug pumps and with the safe, prolonged use of I.V. catheters, it is now feasible to give continuous infusion chemotherapy. This technique opens the door to investigations of new therapy schedules using standard and new drugs in the treatment of hematologic neoplasms. Although there have been notable successes in the treatments of myeloma, leukemias, and Hodgkin's and non-Hodgkin's lymphomas, there is a continued need for further improvement in the treatment of those patients who fail primary induction therapy or relapse after successful primary induction therapy. In a recent report, Vogelzang[1] reviewed the broad questions created by this technique, including the pharmacologic variables of drug dose and distribution, drug metabolism and excretion, and host differences. These issues are reviewed elsewhere in this volume.

The goal of infusion chemotherapy is to improve the therapeutic index by delivering to the tumor an increased amount of drug, represented by serum concentration × time, or C × T. The technical capability of infusion chemotherapy has been accomplished.[2] Other techniques may be applicable as well, including the use of liposomes.[3] The latter technique has been applied in experimental systems, with a decreased cardiac uptake of doxorubicin (ADR) but with preservation of the antitumor activity.[4] The use of pharmacologic enhancers is another method of improving the C × T of antineoplastic drugs. For example, verapamil increases the intracellular accumulation and retention of daunorubicin. Unfortunately, when studied ex vivo using cells from acute nonlymphoblastic leukemia, there was no increase in cellular accumulation.[5] Another example of enhancement is the use of allopurinol which, when used with mercaptopurine, decreases drug clearance.

Carefully designed comparative studies are still needed to establish the true advantage of infusion therapy versus bolus therapy. Moreover, there needs to be a coordinated effort to investigate the myriad possible combinations and dose schedules available. It would also be advantageous to have in vitro assays with predictive capacity for in vivo sensitivity of single and combination agents administered by continuous infusion.[6] It would also be useful to monitor the serum concentrations — or, more specifically — the intracellular drug concentrations of the cytotoxic drugs.

This chapter will not review the basic concepts associated with continuous infusion therapy, but instead will deal with the results of clinical trials in hematologic malignancies. The individual single-agent infusion experience is analyzed, and the multidrug combinations in which infusion schedules have begun to be evaluated are reviewed briefly.

Vinca Alkaloids

Vincristine

Ferreira first gave vincristine (VCR) as an infusion at $2 \text{ mg/m}^2/\text{day}$ for 24–48 hours for advanced cancer.[7] Based upon the logic that prolonging otherwise short $t^1/2$ drugs could have increased tumoricidal effects, Jackson et al further studied the pharmacokinetics of VCR using infusion therapy.[8] Patients were given 0.5 mg I.V. bolus injections followed by infusions of 0.5 mg, 0.75 mg, or $1.0 \text{ mg/m}^2/\text{day}$ for 5 days. Heparin and hydrocortisone were added. A steady state of greater than 1×10^{-9} M/L was reached, with 21–28% of the drug excreted in the urine. After stopping the infusion, the $t^1/2$ for drug clearance was similar to that following I.V. bolus. As hoped for, there was an increased area under curve (AUC) using the infusion program, although this varied greatly across patients. Toxicities observed included neuropathy, muscle wasting, ileus, and hyponatremia. These were mild to moderate using 0.5 and 0.75 mg/m^2, but were severe at higher doses.[9] Similar toxicities were observed by Weber et al.[10] Importantly, patients who had failed previous treatments with I.V. vincristine responded to the drug when it was given by infusion.[9]

Jackson et al[11] then infused VCR for treatment of multiple myeloma. Eighteen patients with refractory multiple myeloma received 5-day continuous infusions of VCR at $0.5 \text{mg/m}^2/\text{day}$ preceded by I.V. bolus injections of 0.5. Therapy was repeated every 3 weeks. Most of the patients so treated had poor performance status, with 9 of the patients being performance status 3 or 4. Seven had received prior VCR therapy. Three patients with no prior exposure to VCR attained partial remissions (PR) with infusions alone. Complications included marrow suppression and neurotoxicity with ileus, paresthesia, and weakness.

Jackson et al[12] then applied this approach in treating 25 patients with advanced refractory non-Hodgkin's lymphoma. After an initial I.V. bolus of 0.5 mg, they received $0.25 \text{ mg/m}^2/\text{day}$ by infusion. One of the 25 patients attained a complete remission (CR) and 8 attained PR lasting 1.2–16.2 months. Twelve (48%) of the patients had mild to moderate neurotoxicity.

Paschold et al gave VCR as 0.5 mg bolus followed by $0.5 \text{ mg/m}^2/\text{day}$ by constant infusion, repeated every 3 weeks for refractory lymphoma.[13] There was 1 CR lasting 207 days and 4 PR.

Vinblastine

Lu et al reported the pharmacokinetics of vinblastine (VLB) when given at 1-2 mg/m^2/day for 5 days by infusion.[14] This approach has been applied in limited fashion to treat hematologic neoplasms. Yap et al studied continuous 5-day infusion VLB at 1.4–2.0 mg/m^2/day.[15] Myelosuppression was mild to moderate at the lower doses but was severe after 2 mg/m^2/day. In studies by Zeffren et al, neurotoxicity was also a major complication following the 5-day infusion of VLB.[16] Lokich et al found that marrow toxicity was dose-limiting when 0.5 mg/m^2/day was infused over more prolonged periods.[17]

In the study already referred to by Paschold, VLB was infused to treat refractory lymphomas.[13] It was given as 0.5 bolus followed by 0.5–1.5 mg/m^2/day infusions for 5 days and also repeated every 3 weeks. Three patients attained PR lasting up to 122 days.

Vindesine

Vindesine (VDS), an analogue of VLB, is another drug with short plasma half-life and thus is suitable for study by infusion. It has been given as continuous 5-day infusions for nonhematologic neoplasms. Sixty patients at the M. D. Anderson Hospital were treated with continuous infusions of 1.0–1.2 mg/m^2/day for 5 days every 21 days. Results were compared to I.V. bolus injections given every 10–14 days.[18] Myelosuppression appeared to be more severe in the infusion arm of this comparative study. Fleishman et al concluded that 5-day infusion of VDS is preferable to a single bolus VDS in the treatment of refractory breast carcinoma.[19] Vindesine by infusion has been used in the treatment of hematologic neoplasms. Maraninchi et al[20] gave 0.7 mg/m^2/day for 5 days to 21 patients with ALL (5 cases), CML in blast crisis (6 cases), and lymphoma (10 cases). Of the 18 evaluable patients, 13 had PR or minor regressions. Toxicity was not considered important. Thus, VDS is available for further study in hematologic disease.

Epipodophyllotoxins

Etoposide (VP-16)

Etoposide has a broad spectrum of activity against lymphomas and leukemias. A phase 1 infusion trial using etoposide (VP-16) at 20–80 mg/m^2/day for 5 days was conducted in 30 courses of therapy by Lokich and Corkery.[21] Major toxicity was encountered at 60 mg/m^2/day. Another trial indicated that continuous infusion of VP-16 did not improve the therapeutic ratio and may have been associated with cardiotoxicity.[22] Infusion therapy may enhance delivery of the drug to the CNS.[23] No clinical trials of infusion schedules have been reported in hematologic neoplasms.

Tenoposide (VM-26)

This derivative of podophyllotoxin, designated as VM-26, has a longer half-life than etoposide. The pharmacokinetics have been established using 24-hour continuous infusion.[24] This drug, using this delivery approach, has not yet been applied to hematologic neoplasms. Thus, both VP-16 and VM-26 are available for study by infusion in treatment of hematologic diseases.

Antibiotics

Doxorubicin

Doxorubicin (ADR) is an active antineoplastic antibiotic with significant activity in the treatment of the lymphomas, the leukemias, and myeloma. The pharmacokinetics of infused ADR were reported by Riggs et al using 45–75 mg/m² given over 96 hours by infusion to 6 patients during 10 courses.[25] The AUC was equivalent to that found using bolus therapy. Existing data indicate that the cardiotoxicity associated with bolus injection is diminished by continuous 96-hour or longer infusion therapy.[26-30] Cardiotoxicity is not reduced when infusion is given for only 6 hours at 50 mg/m².[31] Lokich et al reported that ADR infused up to 30 days at 4 mg/m²/day caused stomatitis and leukopenia in 50% of patients. However, there appeared to be less cardiotoxicity, alopecia, and gastrointestinal toxicity.[28,32] Garnick et al reported the pharmacokinetics of the drug when given by long-term continuous infusion,[33] and marrow suppression and mucositis were again dose-limiting toxicities. Legha et al confirmed these findings, reporting that ADR retained its effectiveness when given by long-term infusion. They also reported that when given by infusion, the drug could be given up to a cumulative dose of 1,000 mg/m² without encountering cardiotoxicity, although stomatitis was a significant problem.[34,35]

ADR infusion therapy has not been studied rigorously in humans comparing bolus to infusion in a single disease. In the L1210 mouse model, infusion therapy was compared to pulse therapy, and pulse therapy was associated with slightly increased life span. However, it appeared that tolerance was slightly better following the continuous infusion.[36]

Bleomycin

Bleomycin (BLM), a glycopeptide, has a serum t$^{1}/_{2}$ of just 2 hours following I.V. bolus and has activity in a wide variety of hematologic diseases. As duration of exposure increases, there is an improved cell lysis of cultured lymphocytes.[37] In a study involving 382 patients, I.M. BLM was compared to the I.V. infusion therapy.[38] Pulmonary toxicity was less common following the I.M. therapy. In 1977, Krakoff et al reported on 119 patients in a nonrandomized study who were given continuous infusion BLM. These patients responded better than did those treated once or twice per week by short infusions for treatment of nonhematologic neoplasms, including cervical and testicular carcinoma.[39] Other infusion studies, including animal studies, are available using several dose schedules. These indicate that pulmonary toxicity is reduced by continuous infusion.[40,41] Based upon these results, BLM infusion therapy has been incorporated into several combination drug studies for hematologic neoplasms.

Alkylating Agents

As with some of the antimetabolites, several of the alkylating agents are well absorbed through the intestinal tract and thus probably are not suitable for testing by infusion. Divided daily doses mimic the infusion concept. Among these are melphalan, busulfan, chlorambucil, and the nitrosoureas CCNU and methyl-CCNU. Studies of serum levels, as a reflection of absorption, have in some cases demonstrated that absorption of some of these drugs is not consistent. Other alkylating agents, including the recently introduced aziridinylbenzoquinone (AZQ), are suitable for study using infusion techniques. To date, the alkylating agents have not been extensively investigated using the continuous infusion approach.

Streptozotocin

Seibert et al reported on the 5- or 6-day infusion of 0.5–1.0 gm/m²/day of streptozotocin, a nitrosurea alkylating derivative with antiobiotic capacity.[42] There was less myelosuppression and renal toxicity following this route of therapy. Two of 8 patients treated with non-Hodgkin's lymphoma attained CR. There was, unfortunately, a newly recognized CNS toxicity manifested by confusion and lethargy. It is unknown whether these toxicities would be eliminated by reducing the amount of streptozotocin given each day.

Cyclophosphamide

Solidoro et al treated 42 patients with acute lymphoblastic leukemia by infusion of cyclophosphamide (CTX) at 400 mg/m²/day for 5 days.[43] Twenty-one of the 42 patients achieved CR. The mean duration of response was 18.5 weeks. Of the 42 cases, 23 had relapsed from prior therapy, and the remaining 19 were "high-risk" patients. Steuber et al earlier had given 1-hour infusions of CTX at 40–60 mg/kg/day for 4 days. In that study, remissions were obtained in 4/15 children with ALL, each lasting 4–6 weeks.[44] Patients who had been previously untreated had a 40% response rate (21/42 patients), whereas only 9% of previously treated patients responded. This drug, too, has potential for further investigation.

Thio-tepa

Thio-tepa pharmacokinetics have been reported when the drug was given by infusion at 15-35 mg/m²/day for 48 hours.[45] The use of this alkylating agent in Hodgkin's disease may provide a basis for clinical trials as part of a combination. Also, in multiple myeloma, combining alkylating agents may provide a basis for the use of thio-tepa.

Antimetabolites

Three of the most commonly used antimetabolites have not been studied by infusion for appropriate reasons. Because methotrexate (MTX) is absorbed by the G.I. tract, parenteral therapy is not essential, although recent studies question the bioavailability of this drug. Interestingly, when MTX is carried in liposomes it has increased antitumor activity against mouse lymphoma;[46] therefore, it may be interesting to study by infusion. Mercaptopurine and thioguanine have not been studied in the infusion schedule in phase 2 trials. The fact that these drugs remain unavailable in parenteral form makes organizing infusion studies difficult.

Cytosine Arabinoside

Cytosine arabinoside (ara-C) is a standard agent used in the treatment of acute leukemia and is active in the treatment of non-Hodgkin's lymphoma. Because of its very short plasma half-life, it is usually given at 100–200 mg/m^2/day for 5–7 days for 24-hour infusion in most leukemic regimens.[1,47] The indications for use of ara-C recently have been expanded to include resistant or relapsing lymphomas and leukemia, preleukemia syndromes, and some solid tumors. These additional indications for the drug are predicated upon changes in dose and schedule, using both low-dose infusion and high-dose boluses or infusions. These adjustments significantly alter the pharmacokinetics and possibly the primary antitumor activity of the drug.[48-52] There are large variations in serum concentrations observed following 20/mg/m^2/day by constant infusion, without apparent correlation with therapeutic responses. Most of the infused ara-C given in low doses is excreted in the urine as ara-U.[53]

Low doses of ara-C given at 10–20 mg/m^2 every 12 hours for 14–21 days were thought to have a differentiating effect in vitro upon tumor cells.[54,55] Wisch et al gave 20 mg/m^2/day for 7–21 days to treat preleukemic syndrome and found some clinical improvement.[51] Castaigne et al gave 10 mg/m^2/12 hours for 15–21 days and attained CR in 57% of 8 patients after 1 course. Marrow aplasia was not observed.[56] However, Beran et al, when treating 39 patients with myelodysplastic syndrome or untreated and relapsing AML and CMML, concluded that marrow toxicity was substantial.[57] Schiff et al compared subcutaneous injections of ara-C to infused ara-C, each given for 14 days.[58] They concluded that 20 mg/m^2/day of ara-C given by infusion for 14 days was preferable to 3–20 mg/m^2/day of ara-C given every 12 hours subcutaneously for 14 days. Whatever the mechanism, low doses of ara-C have been applied to patients with overt acute leukemia. For patients 70 years and older, this low-dose approach seems to offer remission rates and survival comparable to those available from some intensive chemotherapy programs.[59,60] The possible roles of this therapeutic approach are reviewed in greater detail elsewhere.[61,62]

Consideration recently has been given to infusing *very* high doses of ara-C. With 3-hour infusions given every 12 hours, previously unobserved toxicities have appeared, including cerebellar failure, conjunctivitis, and retinopathy. Plunkett and Liliemark presented evidence that infusion of high-dose ara-C maximizes the accumulation of ara-CTP by blast cells when it is given by continuous infusion at 2–4 gm/m^2/day.[63] High doses infused from 12 to 36 hours at 250 mg/m^2/hour quickly reached steady-state, with widely ranging plasma levels (mean 19.6 μM). Myelosuppression was the dose-limiting toxicity.[64]

Several groups have used high-dose ara-C to achieve remissions in patients with refractory or relapsing leukemias and lymphomas. The dose schedules have usually called for 3-hour infusions repeated every 12 hours. Reports are now available describing similar high doses infused over longer periods. Jones et al treated relapsed childhood acute leukemia and non-Hodgkin's lymphoma with 6–12 g/m^2 of ara-C infused over 10 to 48 hours.[65,66] Myelosuppression was the major toxicity, along with hepatotoxicity. In 13 patients treated, cerebellar ataxia and hypersensitivity to the drug were seen once each. Responses were seen, with 1 CR among the 5 ALL patients and 2 CR among the 3 non-Hodgkin's lymphoma patients treated. Unfortunately, in this small series the duration of remission was poor. Ochs et al treated 10 patients with refractory pediatric leukemia using high-dose infusion ara-C.[67] The dose schedules were 3.5 g/m^2/day for 4 days, 3.5 g/m^2/4 days plus 5 g/m^2/day for an additional 4 days, and 5 g/m^2/day for 4 days. Gastrointestinal toxicity was significant at the higher doses, along with pancytopenia. Again, neurotoxicity was not seen. The plasma levels of ara-C varied widely from 10–225 M/L. The CSF levels were 2–5 M/L. Of 10 patients treated, 2 achieved PR. Iacoboni et al also reported on continuous infusion therapy using high-dose ara-C in refractory leukemias and in blast crisis following chronic myelogenous leukemia.[68] Their study was designed to maintain high intracellular levels of ara-CTP, the phosphorylated active metabolite of ara-C. The doses were individualized to maintain 75 M/L of ara-CTP in the blasts. In order to accomplish this, the doses ranged from 300–3,000 mg/m^2/24 hours. Using this approach, they obtained a remarkable 42% (8/19) CR rate, including 40% (4/10) CR in patients with blast crisis. Marrow suppression was again the major complication, with 90% (18/20) having marrow aplasia. Five patients died during the induction. Again, it was remarkable that no patients had cerebellar toxicity.

The conclusions reached from these preliminary high-dose infusion reports indicate that cerebellar toxicity, a devastating effect for those patients receiving the previously reported 3 g/m^2/12 hours given up to 12 doses, has been reduced.

Thymidine

A unique use of thymidine for antineoplastic effect was described by Blumenreich et al.[69] It was appreciated that very high plasma levels of thymidine were cytotoxic. Thus, the authors investigated giving 90–240 g/m^2/day for 14–29 days. Six patients with leukemias and lymphomas were treated. Nausea and vomiting and CNS toxicity were common complications. Hepatotoxicity, diarrhea, and electrolyte imbalances appeared occasionally. Spinal fluid levels reached 2–23.5% of the plasma levels. All patients acquired marrow aplasia. Of 6 patients treated, 1 attained a CR from ANLL and 1 attained a PR from lymphoma lasting 16 and 4 weeks, respectively. This therapeutic effort was problematic because of the large quantity of drug delivered as well as the toxicities encountered. Nevertheless, with caution, other novel approaches such as this are available for investigation.

Thymidine has been investigated as a means to sensitize leukemic cells to the effects of ara-C.[70] Thymidine was given at 30 g/m² by continuous infusion for 24 hours on days 1 and 4, followed by 48-hour infusions of ara-C (days 2 and 3 and days 5 and 6). Among the responders, thymidine recruited cells into the S phase and was associated with higher levels of intracellular ara-C. This altering of pyrimidine metabolism is intriguing and offers areas for further study.

Hydroxyurea

Hydroxyurea (HYD), with a short half-life of about 2 hours, is a reasonable drug to test by infusion. Currently, it is not available in parenteral form other than for investigations. In the murine L1210 system, low-dose infusions of HYD arrested cells in the S phase, whereas higher doses infused for 24 hours killed the leukemic cells.[71] Another report suggested that ara-C, when administered immediately after completion of HYD infusion, was synergistic, whereas ADR and MTX were not.[72] Belt et al gave HYD by continuous infusion for 72 hours and compared its efficacy to HYD given orally every 4 hours.[73] The doses tested by infusion ranged from 2.0–3.5 mg/m²/min. The maximum tolerated infused dose was 3.0 mg/m²/min. and 800 mg/m² every 4 hours when given by mouth. Granulocytopenia was the limiting toxicity in all patients who developed blood levels greater than 2×10^{-3} M/L. It was concluded that the I.V. route produced a modest amount of cell synchronization. One of 15 patients treated responded, that patient having a nonhematologic disease. Because of the significant variation of the rate of absorption of the oral HYD, the authors concluded that I.V. infusion therapy was appropriate for further investigation.

Metals

Cisplatin

Cisplatin (DDP), a drug with major antineoplastic activity, is extensively bound to protein, and has a long terminal half-life but a short beta half-life.[1] The pharmacology of the drug given at 25 mg/m²/day for 5 days has been established by Posner et al.[74] When given by infusion for 5 days, DDP creates less intestinal distress than when given by bolus.[75] When infused to treat murine L1210 leukemia, there was no improvement of response rate over that seen following bolus injections.[76] The drug has not been systematically investigated in the treatment of hematologic neoplasms.

Gallium

Nephrotoxicity limits the use of gallium by I.V. bolus injection.[77] Kelson et al reported the pharmacokinetics of gallium nitrate when given by 7–day infusion at 200 mg/m^2.[78] In 2 patients, the serum levels were 0.9 ± 0.2 mcg/ml and 1.9 ± 0.4 mcg/ml, with 68–107% of the drug recovered in the urine. Warrell et al treated 64 patients with 7-day infusions of 200, 250, 300, and 400 mg/m^2 of gallium nitrate.[79] In this phase 1 study, 300 mg/m^2 was selected as the best dose. Responses were seen following all 4 doses tested, with 34% having "major responses," including 2 CR in heavily pretreated patients with diffuse histiocytic lymphomas. Proteinuria was less of a problem, but hypocalcemia occurred in two-thirds of the patients, along with increased pulmonary complications.

New Drugs

Anthracycline Derivatives

Pharmacologic data are available for continuous infusion of the anthracycline analogue aclacinomycin.[80] This drug has not yet been applied to phase 2 or 3 studies in humans by infusion. Another derivative, mitoxantrone, has been studied in man.[81] It appears to have better efficacy based upon peak drug levels rather than total drug exposure in experiments in which 5 mg/m^2 I.V. bolus per day was compared to 15 mg/m^2 bolus, each given every 3 weeks.[82] Results with infusion of mitoxantrone have not yet been reported for hematologic neoplasms.

Spirogermanium

Spirogermanium, a recently added antineoplastic drug, has neurotoxicity as its dose-limiting side effect.[83] The drug has activity in lymphomas, among other tumors, and has been studied when given by continuous infusion to 18 patients for 4–6 weeks.[83] In this program, 250 mg/m^2/day was well tolerated. Woolley et al[84] demonstrated that the drug used in vitro to treat lymphoma cells was more effective with prolonged exposure. They then tested doses of 100–500 mg/m^2/day for 5 days by infusion in patients. All doses caused phlebitis. Again, neurotoxicity was a primary side effect, including tremors, vesiculations, and confusion, all of which were observed at the higher doses. They, too, determined that 250 mg/m^2/day was tolerated by most patients. This drug will be expected to progress through clinical investigations using similar infusional programs.

Homoharringtonine

Homoharringtonine, a drug that inhibits macrotubule synthesis, has been administered by continuous 5-day infusions in a phase 1–2 study using 0.2 to 3.75 mg/m^2/day for 5 days.[85] Myelosuppression was the dose-limiting toxicity. Coonley et al concluded that most patients could tolerate 3.25 mg/m^2/day for

5 days, although leukemic patients could probably receive more.[85] Neidhart et al infused the drug for 30 days at 1 mg/m²/day.[86] One patient with refractory acute myeloblastic leukemia responded to this dose. An interesting report by Boyd and Sullivan suggested that a maturing effect of the drug on pro-granulocytic leukemia was such that the arrest of cell growth and proliferation parallel the differentiation effect induced.[87] This is another drug worthy of further investigation using infusion systems.

Aziridinylbenzoquinone (AZQ)

Lee et al gave AZQ, an alkylating agent, by continuous infusion at 16–32 mg/m²/day for 7 days to 22 patients with refractory leukemias.[88] The drug was found to have a short monoexponential plasma half-life of 10 to 40 minutes. Marrow toxicity was a strong limiting factor in these heavily pretreated patients with acute nonlymphoblastic leukemia. There were 3 responders out of 17 patients treated, with 7 of the 17 dying with aplastic marrows but without leukemia present. Whitacre et al treated 13 patients with solid tumors, each having had prior chemotherapy and some prior radiation therapy.[89] The infusion doses tested were from 4–8 mg/m²/day for 5 days given every 3–4 weeks. Again, myelosuppression was the dose-limiting toxicity, although it was not very profound. Thus, diaziquone should be studied further using a variety of routes.

Deoxycoformycin

Sinkule et al studied the pharmacokinetics of continuous infusion 2'-deoxycoformycin (dCF), an inhibitor of adenosine deaminase, in patients with refractory acute lymphoblastic leukemia.[90] The doses studied ranged from 20–30 mg/m²/day by infusion given 24, 48, and 72 hours. At 30 mg/m²/day, a steady-state of drug level was obtained at 0.5–1.2 M/L. As a biological marker of activity, the authors measured the adenosine deaminase (ADA). The pre-treatment levels of the deaminase varied from patient to patient. However, there was a greater than 75% inhibition in 14/17 patients following treatment with 25 mg/m² or more per day. They astutely observed that the ADA inhibition was reversible with red cell transfusion. Based on this data, additional investigation is warranted.

Ifosfamide

Ifosfamide is a derivative of cyclophosphamide, with a long serum half-life of 15.2 hours, beta phase.[91] It has been given for 5 days at 60–85 mg/kg/day by infusion. The maximum tolerated dose was 85 mg/kg/day. Dose-limiting toxicities included CNS defects, cardiac dysrrhythmias, and hematuria. Lymphomas were responsive, as were squamous cell carcinoma of skin, fibrosarcoma, and head and neck tumors. Pharmacokinetic data are presented by Klein et al.[91]

5-aza-2'-Deoxycytidine (5 aza/CdR) and 5-Azacytidine

Aza/CdR and its parent compound 5-azacytidine have been shown to pro-mote differentation of leukemia cells in vitro.[92,93] In fashions similar to that seen with ara-C, 5 aza/CdR induces terminal maturation of human monoblasts and myeloblast leukemia cells when nontoxic concentrations are added.[94] They are available for study using low-dose infusion schedules.

Combination Chemotherapy

As would be predicted from the results of investigations using single-agent infusion chemotherapy, investigations have begun using combinations of drugs, with 1 or 2 of the component drugs delivered by infusion. Most studies reported to date have not been designed to compare the efficacy of the added infusion system with that of the more standard noninfusion programs. How-ever, systematic investigations of these issues are required before endorsing one or the other as being the more advantageous. Each investigator has estab-lished a drug schedule predicated upon concepts that are yet to be proven as truly valid. The drug(s) chosen, the doses given, the durations of therapy, and the integration of the infused drug(s) with other drugs given by routine routes are issues to be systematically investigated.

Vincristine Plus Bleomycin

Vincristine has been infused on a variety of schedules in combination with other drugs. Coleman et al reported COPBLAM-III combination chemotherapy for diffuse large-cell lymphoma.[95] In this program, VCR at 1 mg/m²/day was infused on days 1 and 2. In addition, BLM was infused at 7.5 mg/m² on days 1–5 after having initiated therapy with 7.5 mg/m² I.V. bolus. The additional drugs given by a standard bolus were prednisone, procarbazine, ADR, and CTX. The therapy was repeated every 6 weeks inpatient for 6 cycles. Between the inpatient programs, on the alternate third week as outpatients, the patients received bolus VCR plus prednisone, procarbazine, ADR, and CTX. The doses of the last 2 drugs were escalated by 5 and 50 mg/m² per cycle to a maximum of 50 and 500 mg/m² per cycle, respectively. Forty-three of the 54 entered patients were evaluable. Eighty-six percent (37/43) patients achieved CR, with those in the poor prognostic categories having the same response rate as the group as a whole. There were 4 toxic deaths. Notably, BLM-induced lung toxicity occurred in 18 patients, 2 of whom died. The median time to BLM toxicity was 4 cycles. In the previously treated patients with large-cell lymphoma, CR occurred in 3/4 patients, with a PR in the fourth. The conclusion that this program is better than other therapeutic programs rests upon historical experience with large-cell lymphoma. However, a critical appraisal must await appropriately struc-tured, stratified, and randomized studies comparing these drugs in bolus form to the infusion schedules. Moreover, since infusion by design was given only every other cycle, there is concern about the presumed advantage of infusions of VCR and BLM. Moreover, there was a large complication rate from BLM following the doses selected.

Hollister et al reported the use of infusion VCR and BLM followed by high-dose MTX for resistant non-Hodgkin's lymphoma.[96] In this drug program, VCR at 1–2 mg/m²/day was infused for 2 days. BLM was given as 0.25 mg/kg by bolus followed by 0.25 mg/kg/day for 5 days. Responders thereafter received 1,500 mg/m² of MTX with leucovorin rescue on days 15, 22, 29, and 36. The entire program was repeated every 36 weeks. Of the 16 cases treated, 50% responded, including 3 CR and 5 PR, having a median duration of response of 29 weeks. Stomatitis, dermatitis, and leukopenia were the major side effects. Toxicity was recorded as severe in 4, but the significant BLM-induced toxicity seen in the previously described study was not observed. Again, the notion that this is a preferable program to other standard approaches needs to be justified based upon comparative studies.

Vincristine and Etoposide

Kaplon reported the combinations of VCR and VP-16 by infusions in the treatment of refractory non-Hodgkin's lymphoma.[97] This complex study was divided into 3 arms. One arm included VP-16 at 50 mg I.V. followed by continuous infusion of 60 mg/m²/day for 5 days every 3 weeks. The second arm was as above on days 10–15 but preceded by VCR infusion at 0.25 mg/m²/day for 5 days on days 1–5. The third arm was VP-16 at 120 mg/m²/day by bolus on days 6 and 7 preceded by VCR infusion as in the second arm of the study. The response rates in these studies were poor. It was believed that VP-16 in the doses infused produced substantial toxicity. It did not appear, however, that the addition of VCR added substantially to the toxicity.

Vincristine and Doxorubicin

These 2 agents were infused simultaneously for treatment of refractory multiple myeloma.[98] VCR was infused at 0.4 mg/day for 4 days along with ADR at 9 mg/m²/day for 4 days. Dexamethasone was given orally at 40 mg daily for 4 days beginning days 1, 9, and 17. All patients studied were resistant to prior treatments, including alkylating agents and/or ADR. There were 14/23 responders, according to reduction of tumor masses, and 2/6 responders if only Bense-Jones proteins were available for monitoring. Thus 16/29 responded, with improved survival. Response rates were higher for those who had previously responded and subsequently failed, as compared to those who had failed to respond to all previous treatment. Infections, thought due to the steroids, were significant problems.

Daunorubicin and Cytosine Arabinoside

Lewis et al used daunorubicin by infusion for 3 days at 135 mg/m²/day beginning on day 3, along with infused ara-C at 100 mg/m²/day for 10 days in the treatment of ANLL.[99] 6-thioguanine was also given. The authors concluded from this uncontrolled study that this approach using infused daunorubicin created less toxicity with the same response rate as observed following bolus daunorubicin in previously treated patients.

Etoposide and Cytosine Arabinoside

Kalwinsky et al studied use of continuous infusion VP-16 along with ara-C to treat childhood acute myelogenous leukemia.[100] In this study, VP-16 was given at 150 mg/m²/day for 3 days by infusion followed by ara-C given at 200 mg/m²/day subcutaneously every 5 days before beginning conventional daunorubicin, ara-C, and 6-thioguanine. The pharmacology of this program was discussed. However, the clinical outcome was not discussed in the abstract. Price et al performed a feasibility study using VP-16 alone and in combination in the treatment of Hodgkin's and non-Hodgkin's lymphoma.[101] They reported that the duration of the nadir was less with the infusion program, even after 3,200 mg of VP-16. Neutropenia was the dose-limiting toxicity.

Bleomycin

Continuous BLM infusion therapy has been integrated into the combination drug therapy programs. (See *Vincristine and Bleomycin*, above). Ginsberg et al gave BLM at 2 units/day for 5 days by infusion along with CTX, daunorubicin and VCR, given by standard routes and in standard doses to treat non-Hodgkin's lymphoma.[102] There were 58 evaluable patients in this study. No changes were detected in the lung function, suggesting a protection from BLM-induced lung toxicity by infusing the drug. (*Note*: The toxic effects described in paragraphs above occurred with much higher doses.) However, response rates were similar to standard therapies using I.V. bolus BLM. Of note, however, was that 18/21 previously treated patients responded, 6 of whom had received these same agents before.

This approach was modified in a subsequent protocol wherein bleomycin was given (CAVPB) or not given (CAVP), with MTX added in standard or high doses.[103] Here again, the BLM was infused at 2 units/day for 5 days. Again, there were no response benefits from having infused the BLM, since there were no significant differences in response rates between the CAVP and the CAVPB. There was no toxicity from the infused BLM. Moreover, in this study the additional MTX created no change in the complete remission rate or in the duration of remissions. The plasma levels of BLM reached steady-state when the drug was given this way, and the levels fell rapidly, in less than 2 hours, after the infusion was stopped.

Williams et al integrated BLM infusion into a multidrug combination chemotherapy including DDP, VP-16, CCNU, BCNU, and MTX with leucovorin rescue.[104] The BLM was given at 10 mg/m²/day on days 1 through 4. The protocol was extremely toxic and had to be revised. Therefore, to date it is not clear whether there is a therapeutic advantage to infusing bleomycin in drug combinations. The infusion system does not appear to protect from bleomycin toxicity when the high daily doses described are given.

Cyclophosphamide

Guthrie has reported using infusions of CTX in combination with ara-C given by bolus plus VCR and prednisone.[105] CTX was given at 350 mg/m^2 by infusion for 24 hours on days 5, 6, and 7 after the patients had received VCR on day 1, plus prednisone and ara-C on days 5, 6 and 7. Sixty-four percent of the patients with refractory adult acute leukemia attained CR lasting 3–21 + weeks. No cardiac, bladder, ocular, or pulmonary problems developed. Gastrointestinal and neurotoxicity were minimal. Again, however, the true implications of CTX given by infusion versus bolus were not examined in these studies, since comparative studies using CTX by bolus were not investigated.

Cytosine Arabinoside

Several protocols have integrated infusions of ara-C into their structure. Indeed, it is generally accepted as the standard approach for nonlymphoblastic leukemias. Fiere et al added high-dose ara-C infusion to daunorubicin given in a routine way to treat 51 patients with ANLL.[106] Ara-C was infused at 45 mg/kg on days 1–3 and days 8–10. Daunorubicin was given at 1 mg/kg on days 1, 2, and 3. Sixty percent (31/51) patients attained CR, with median duration of remission 7 months. Twelve remained in remission (3–30 months) at the time of the report. Six deaths occurred: 3 early deaths and 3 aplastic deaths. The authors concluded that this combination failed to offer unique advantages, and that longer exposure to ara-C using lower doses was preferable.

Gisselbrecht et al integrated ara-C at 100 mg/m^2 by infusion per day on days 1, 2, and 3 into a protocol using I.V. boluses of daunorubicin, VCR, CTX, and oral prednisone in the treatment of previously untreated patients with diffuse non-Hodgkin's lymphoma.[107] These authors concluded that no detectable difference occurred from using ara-C in this schema. Hainsworth et al used ara-C in a similar fashion in combination with CTX, VCR, MTX, and prednisone.[108] The CTX was given in high doses of 1,500 mg/m^2 on days 1 and 2. MTX was integrated at 200 mg/m^2 on days 8 and 22 with leucovorin rescue. This induction program was conducted twice on days 1 and 28. It was followed thereafter by CHOP for 4–6 cycles. Significant toxicity limited therapy to only 1 course in 7 of the 25 patients. Of the 23 evaluable patients, 17 (68%) attained CR. Six additional patients achieved PR. Of the 17 patients with CR, 12 had been in CR at the time of report from 8–28 months. The conclusion in this uncontrolled study of previously untreated patients was that although the toxicity was great, it was nevertheless manageable, and that the CR rate in an otherwise poor prognostic category was interesting.

Methotrexate

Amadori used MTX at 500 mg/m^2 beginning on hour 60 for 6 hours of infusion in a protocol that also contained VCR and CTX, 5-FU, ara-C, ADR, and prednisone.[109] This intensive chemotherapy program was delivered to 46 patients with diffuse lymphoma. Complete remissions were attained in 81% (37/46) of the patients, with an additional PR rate of 4% (2/46). There was a projected disease-free survival of 4 years in 78% of the patients. Again, this is a very interesting and provocative protocol with exciting results. However, the combinations of drugs delivered, and the use of MTX by infusion, while very interesting, did not have an identifiable role in the construct of this noncomparative study.

Table 1. Hematologic Neoplasms Seen To Be Clinically Responsive* to Single Drug Infusion Chemotherapy

Disease	Drug/reference
Leukemia	Vincristine[10]
Lymphoblastic	Vindesine[20]
	Cyclophosphamide[46,47]
	Ara-C: high-dose[68,69,70]
	Deoxycoformycin[90]
Nonlymphoblastic	Vincristine[9,10]
	Ara-C: low-dose[59,60,61,62,63]
	high-dose[71]
	Thymidine[72]
	Homoharringtonine[85,86]
	AZQ[88]
Progranulocytic	Homoharringtonine[87]
Blast crisis	Vincristine[9]
	Vindesine[20]
	Ara-C: high-dose[71]
Chronic myelomonocytic	Ara-C: low-dose[60]
Myelodysplasia	
R.A.E.B.	Ara-C: low-dose[59,60,61]
Preleukemia	Ara-C: low-dose[54,59]
Lymphoma**	Vincristine[9,10,12,13]
	Vinblastine[13]
	Vindesine[20]
	VP-16[21]
	Streptozoticin[45]
	Ara-C: high-dose[67,68,69]
	Thymidine[72]
	Gallium[82]
	Spirogermanium[84]
	Ifosfamide[91]
	Bleomycin[97]
Multiple Myeloma	Vincristine[11]

*Response is defined to include any evidence of response, including any evidence of tumor lysis to complete response.
**Lymphomas include all types of non-Hodgkin's lymphoma, including previously treated and untreated patients.

Conclusions

The table lists the diseases against which single-drug infusions have shown activity. Negative results are not included in the table because many of the negative studies contained too few patients to be significant. Entries onto the table vary greatly for status of the patients and the disease; primary, resistant, or relapsing diseases; and the definitions of response. However, the tentative results thus far are exciting enough to justify comparative studies of infusion versus noninfusion schema. It is critical that these future investigations be structured to allow for comparative conclusions to be drawn. Likewise, the integration of infusion programs into standard protocols is an issue to be dealt with by comparative studies. These efforts should be made despite the difficulties of acquiring adequate numbers of patients in each of these rare disease groups. This approach to intensification of therapy is a format worthy of definitive study in a cooperative group setting.

26

LUNG CANCER

*Lucien Israel, Jean-Luc Breau, M.D., and
Jean François Morere, M.D.*

THE WELL-KNOWN RESISTANCE OF nonoat cell lung carcinomas to conventional forms of chemotherapy has led us, since 1979, to use continuous, prolonged infusions of cytostatic drugs in order to try to overcome the kinetic resistance and to prolong the inhibition of DNA repair without increasing the toxicity. This chapter reports several consecutive phase 2 trials conducted in collaboration with members of the French Thoracic Oncology club.* All were based on a combination of cisplatin and bleomycin.

Theory and Background

In a pharmacokinetic study,[1] the authors have shown that the administration of cisplatin (DDP) at a dose of $20 \, mg/m^2/day$ over 1 hour for 5 consecutive days results in satisfactory plasma levels of free platinum, which are prolonged for several days after cessation of treatment without producing a toxic peak. This method of administration was first used by Einhorn[2] in testicular cancer. It has been found to be effective in all of the protocols in which it has been used, and it is associated with decreased G.I. and renal toxicity.

Apart from its specific effects, especially against squamous cell carcinomas,[3] bleomycin (BLM) is a DNA polymerase type 2 inhibitor,[4] which means that it inhibits the repair of damage caused to DNA by intercalating agents. The

*G. Akoun (Hôpital Tenon, Paris), J. P. Battesti, J. L. Breau, L. Israel, J. F. Morere, D. Valeyre (Centre Hospitalier Universitaire Avicenne, Bobigny), F. Blanchon, B. Milleron (Centre Hospitalier Général de Meaux), J. Clavier, C. Zabbe (Centre Hospitalier Régional de Brest), J. Corroller, G. Dabouis (Centre Hospitalier Régional de Nantes), A. Depierre, G. Garnier (Centre Hospitalier Régional de Besançon), B. Hamel (Centre Hospitalier Régional Orléans), M. Lavandier, E. Lemarie (Centre Hospitalier Régional de Tours), P. Morere, G. Nouvet (Centre Hospitalier Régional de Rouen), F. Tcherakian (Centre Hospitalier Général d' Auxerre).

combination of DDP and BLM has transformed the prognosis of testicular cancer.[5] Findings in various nonpulmonary cancers[6] suggest that this combination has a synergistic action in all tumors in which DDP is effective and that it may also be active in certain cases in which neither of the 2 agents, used alone, is effective.

Certain studies have shown that the administration of BLM continuous infusion may reduce its toxicity, especially its pulmonary toxicity, without decreasing its therapeutic effects.[7,8,9] It should be added that, in the context of inhibition of DNA repair, BLM must be administered continuously, as the repair processes may continue for several days after the appearance of the damage. The bolus administration of BLM dose not satisfy the pharmacokinetic conditions required for effective inhibition of DNA repair.

In addition to its synergistic action, which is believed to be essentially due to the inhibition of DNA polymerase type 2, the combination of DDP and BLM does not induce any hematologic toxicity because neither of the 2 components causes such toxicity. Marrow toxicity has never been observed, even in patients with reduced marrow reserves due to previous treatments or to diffuse bone involvement. This feature led to the introduction of a third hematotoxic drug in a number of trials in order to evaluate any possible additive effect.

Modalities of Administration of DDP-BLM and Associated Drugs

The combination of DDP and BLM was administered according to the following modalities:

DDP — 20 mg/m²/day for 5 consecutive days, by I.V. infusion at a rate of 1 mg/min. in 250 ml of normal saline, with a light-protected bottle and tubing, after hydration of the patient.

BLM — 5 mg/m²/day for 5 consecutive days, by continuous I.V. infusion, 24 hours/day. The total daily dose was divided into 2 infusions of 250 ml of 5% glucose-saline, each lasting 12 hours.

The daily intravenous fluids consisted of 1 L of 5% glucose with saline, with 3 g of KCl, 2 g of NaCl, 10 mg of 10% calcium, 10 mg of 15% magnesium sulfate, and 500 cc of 10% mannitol infused over 4 hours. In the absence of tumor progression and renal, pulmonary, or neurological toxicity, the 5-day cycles were repeated every 21 days. A daily oral supplement of 1 g of elemental calcium and 250 mg of magnesium was prescribed between each cycle. In cases in which a peripheral venous line suitable for continuous infusion over 5 days was not available, a Port-a-Cath or Infusa-Port was used. The catheter was placed in the superior vena cava via the subclavian vein or the internal jugular vein. A bolus heparinization was performed at the start of the infusion on the 1st day and on the 5th day prior to removing the needle.

With the use of Cormed infusion pumps or Travenol infusers, DDP has been infused continuously over 24 hours, in parallel with the BLM. However, the 2 drugs were never mixed, as the patients were fitted with either 2 Cormed infusion pumps of 1 Cormed and 1 Travenol infuser. In this case, hydration was ensured orally with a minimum of 2 L of fluid per 24 hours and an oral supplement of calcium, magnesium, and potassium.

Since January 1982, in order to prevent the nausea and vomiting associated with DDP, 80 mg of methylprednisolone has been administered at 6 p.m. on the day before each cycle by direct I.V. injection and 120 mg of methylprednisolone has been administered daily from day 1 to day 5, except when there was a contraindication to steroid therapy (past history of gastroduodenal ulcer, poorly controlled diabetes, severe uncontrolled hypertension).[10] When this steroid treatment was inadequate (20% of cases), it was associated with an I.V. injection of 40 mg/24 hours of metoclopramide or an I.M. injection of perimetazine (20 mg/24 hours).

Excluded from this treatment were patients with decompensated heart failure preventing the hydration necessary for the administration of platinum; patients with renal failure, with a creatinine clearance of less than 70 ml/min.; patients with respiratory failure, with flow rates and volumes decreased by more than 50% in relation to normal values or responsible for alveolar hypoventilation as reflected by the arterial blood gases; and patients with preexisting pulmonary interstitial disease.

Prior to each cycle, the patients were examined clinically and the tumor markers were evaluated by chest X ray. The serum electrolytes and the 24-hour urinary creatinine clearance (minimal diuresis required: 1 L) were measured, and respiratory function tests and volumes together with arterial blood gases and evaluation of the carbon monoxide diffusion (CMD).

This treatment was suspended in the absence of tumor progression:

- Because of BLM toxicity, when clinical and/or radiological signs of interstitial lung disease were observed, or when the carbon monoxide diffusion was reduced by 25% or more in relation to the initial pretreatment evaluation when not related to any other cause (bronchial infection, anemia).
- Because of DDP toxicity, when the creatinine clearance fell below 70 ml/min. or when signs of peripheral neurotoxicity or 8th cranial nerve impairment were detected clinically.

Modalities of Administration
of 1 or 2 Complementary Drugs

Mitomycin-C — Mitomycin-C (MIT) was administered on day 1 of each cycle in a bolus dose of 6 mg/m^2.

Vindesine — Vindesine (VDS) was administered by continuous 24-hour infusion for 5 consecutive days at a dose of 1 mg/m^2/day in 1 L of 5% glucose with protection of the veins by flushing with 15 mg of heparin and 25 mg of hydrocortisone hemisuccinate every 8 hours. This drug is now infused by means of infusion pumps.

Etoposide — Etoposide (VP-16) was administered by continuous 24-hour infusion for 5 consecutive days at a dose of 50 mg/m^2/day. Because of its instability in glucose or saline and its solubility (which decreases with time in saline solutions), the daily dose of VP-16 was divided into 3 infusions in 250 ml of normal saline, each over 8 hours. For this reason, this drug cannot be administered by infusion pumps.

Vincristine — Vincristine (VCR) was administered by continuous 24-hour infusion at a dose of 0.2 mg/m^2/day in 500 ml of 5% glucose-saline for 5 consecutive days.

During the administration of VDS and VCR, a daily oral supplement of 1 g of vitamins B$_1$ and B$_6$ is now administered during each cycle and between each cycle in order to delay and minimize the neurological toxicity.

5-fluorouracil — 5-fluorouracil (5-FU) was initially administered for 5 consecutive days by bolus injections of 400 mg/m^2/day. It is now administered by means of Cormed pumps or Travenol infusers over 8–24 hours.

These various combinations were administered to patients with primary bronchial carcinoma. The distribution of these patients in terms of therapeutic protocol and the anatomicoclinical situation is shown in table 1.

A total of 764 patients were treated with these combinations, consisting of 624 squamous cell carcinomas, 53 adenocarcinomas, 81 small-cell anaplastic carcinomas, and only 6 large-cell anaplastic carcinomas.

The evaluation of the response of small-cell anaplastic carcinomas to the DDP-BLM combination was based on a series of 30 consecutive patients. The responses were evaluated on the 14th day in terms of the X rays. These patients were all treated with cycles of the following combination every 2 weeks: cyclophosphamide (CTX) 800 mg/m^2, doxorubicin (ADR) 60 mg/m^2 on day 1, CCNU 60 mg/m^2 divided between day 1 and day 2, and VP-16 100 mg/m^2 on day 1, day 2, and day 3.

In another group of 51 small-cell anaplastic carcinomas, the rotation series started with this conventional combination. The responses were evaluated after 4 cycles of DDP-BLM and the myelotoxic combination. For this reason, this group was not taken into account in the study of toxicity, which was therefore based on 713 patients.

Secondary Therapy Protocols in Relation to Clinical Situations

For patients with squamous carcinoma, adenocarcinoma, and large-cell anaplastic carcinoma, the following protocols were observed:

- In patients treated preoperatively, radiotherapy was administered after surgery to the mediastinum and to the homolateral supraclavicular fossa (mediastinum 5,500 rad, supraclavicular fossa 4,500 rad), in the case of lymph node involvement, followed by treatment with the DDP-VDS combination until toxicity or progression. In the event of cerebral progression, radiotherapy was administered to the whole of the encephalon (3,000 rad in 2 series of 3 days). In the event of progression to another site, relay treatment consisted of various combinations of CTX, ADR, methotrexate (MTX) and thio-tepa.

- Postoperatively, in the absence of preoperative treatment, N+ patients were initially treated with 3 or 4 cycles of the DDP-BLM combination, followed by radiotherapy according to the modalities described above, with postradiotherapy relay with DDP-VDS.
- In the operable localized forms, the initial treatment was replaced, either because of nonresponse or routinely after 5 cycles in the absence of toxicity, by radiotherapy (5,000 rad to the tumor and mediastinum and 4,500 rad to the supraclavicular fossa), followed by the DDP-VDS combination until toxicity or progression.

Table 1. Chemotherapeutic Combinations and Anatomicoclinical Situations

Diagnosis	No. patients	Combination	No. patients
Squamous : preoperative neoadjuvants	30	DDP-BLM	17
		DDP-BLM-MIT	11
		DDP-BLM-VDS	2
Squamous : postoperative adjuvants N+	37	DDP-BLM-radiotherapy-DDP-VDS	
Squamous : localized inoperable	344	DDP-BLM	188
		DDP-BLM-MIT	111
		DDP-BLM-VDS	32
		DDP-BLM-VP-16	10
		DDP-BLM-VP-16-VCR	3
Squamous : metastatic	213	DDP-BLM	107
		DDP-BLM-MIT	79
		DDP-BLM-VDS	19
		DDP-BLM-VP-16	4
		DDP-BLM-VP-16-VCR	4
Adenocarcinoma : postoperative adjuvants N+	11	DDP-BLM-radiotherapy-DDP-VDS	
Adenocarcinoma: localized inoperable	20	DDP-BLM	12
		DDP-BLM-5-FU	6
		DDP-BLM-VP-16	2
Adenocarcinoma : metastatic	22	DDP-BLM	10
		DDP-BLM-5-FU	9
		DP-BLM-VP-16	3
Small-cell anaplastic 1st treatment with a rotation series (radiological evaluation on 14th day)	30	DDP-BLM	30
Small-cell anaplastic Treatment with a rotation series	51	DDP-BLM rotation with CTX-ADR-VP-16-CCNU every 2 weeks	51
Large-cell anaplastic	6		
Preoperative neoadjuvant	1	DDP-BLM	1
Inoperable localized	4	DDP-BLM	4
Metastatic	1	DDP-BLM	1

- In the forms that were initially metastatic, DDP-BLM was followed by DDP-VDS and then by other forms of chemotherapy in the event of toxicity or progression.
- A randomized study is currently in progress in postoperative N+ patients consisting of 3 arms: (1) DDP-BLM — DDP-VDS; (2) DDP-BLM — radiotherapy-DDP-VDS; and (3) radiotherapy alone.

In the cases of small-cell anaplastic carcinoma, the DDP-BLM/CTX-ADR-VP-16-CCNU rotation every 2 weeks was replaced, after the total dose of BLM had been administered (5 cycles), by a rotation of the following 2 combinations every 4 weeks: (A) CTX-ADR-MTX-CCNU (until the total dose of ADR is reached); (B) VP-16 for 3 consecutive days, HXLM 300 mg/day for 14 consecutive days. Thoracic radiotherapy and routine prophylactic cerebral radiotherapy are no longer performed.

Toxicity

The toxicity was evaluated according to the ECOG grades (see table 2). The 51 patients with small-cell anaplastic carcinoma treated by a rotation starting with the myelotoxic combination CTX, ADR, VP-16, and CCNU were excluded from this toxicity study, which therefore concerns 713 patients.

HEMATOLOGICAL TOXICITY

Table 2 shows the number of patients who presented at least 1 episode of grade 2, 3, or 4 leukocyte or platelet toxicity with the various combinations used. This toxicity was minimal with the DDP-BLM combination, but was observed more frequently with the combinations containing myelotoxic drugs. The incidence of hematological toxicity was moderate with the combinations containing MIT or VP-16. One combination (DDP-BLM-5-FU) caused severe platelet toxicity, and the parallel administration of DDP and 5-FU was subsequently abandoned.

It should be stressed that in the rotation protocol for the small-cell tumors, the DDP-BLM combination was resumed as soon as the platelet count rose to 100,000/mm^3, frequently in the presence of persistent leukopenia of between

Table 2. Hematological Toxicity for the Various Combinations

Combination	No. patients	Leukocytes 10^3			Platelets 10^3			L	Plat.
		Grade 2 2.0 < 3.0	Grade 3 1.0 < 2.0	Grade 4 < 1.0	Grade 2 50 < 90	Grade 3 25 < 50	Grade 4 < 25		
DDP-BLM	418	24	1		14	1		5	3
DDP-BLM-MIT	201	25	18		40	27	15	21	40
DDP-BLM-VDS	53	18	21	5	3	3	1	83	13
DDP-BLM-VP-16	19	4	1		2			26	10.5
DDP-BLM-5-FU	15	6	4	3	4	3	2	86	60
DDP-BLM-VP-16-VCR	7	1	2		2			43	28.5
	713								

2,000 and 4,000 leukocytes/mm³, without any infectious complications. There were no cases of death due to hematological toxicity with these combinations.

RENAL TOXICITY

A decrease in the creatinine clearance to less than 70 ml/min. was observed in 32 patients (5.8%) during the induction cycles (an average of 4 cycles). Except for 5 patients, this toxicity was reversible when the DDP was stopped. A decrease in the creatinine clearance to below 70 ml/min. was always observed in the maintenance treatments after a cumulative dose of 1 g of DDP.

NEUROLOGICAL TOXICITY

In this series of 713 patients, there were 26 cases (3.6% of patients) of grade 1 toxicity (moderate paresthesia), 18 cases of grade 2 toxicity (severe paresthesia), and 4 cases of grade 3 toxicity with motor disturbances. This toxicity was most marked with combinations that included VDS (6 cases of grade 1, 5 cases of grades 2 and 3); toxicity was observed in 20% of patients treated with the DDP-BLM-VDS combination. The toxicity of DDP to the 8th cranial nerve was not evaluated by routine audiogram, but only 2 patients presented clinical hypoacusis.

PULMONARY TOXICITY

Clinical and radiological signs of interstitial lung disease were observed in 51 of the 713 patients, i.e., 7.1%, including 20 cases from the DDP-BLM-MIT group (9.6%). Four deaths were directly related to respiratory failure due to pulmonary fibrosis. The carbon monoxide diffusion decreased after each cycle in the majority of patients. BLM was suspended as soon as the CO diffusion was found to be decreased by 25% or more in relation to the values recorded prior to treatment.

Febrile or allergic reactions to BLM were observed in only 12 cases, and grade 2 and 3 stomatitis, which interfered with eating, developed in 9 patients and 2 patients, respectively, treated with DDP-BLM-5-FU (73% of the patients treated with this combination). In 4 cases, diarrhea requiring parenteral hydration occurred in these same cases from the group of 15 patients treated with this combination.

The nausea and vomiting have improved, in terms of their frequency and their severity, since the routine administration of methylprednisolone. Twenty-five percent of the patients suffered from vomiting that interfered with their nutrition, especially during the first 2 days of each cycle. However, these gastrointestinal disturbances were never a reason for refusal of treatment. Four cases of gastrointestinal hemorrhage from gastroduodenal ulcer observed can possibly be attributed to the steroid treatment.

Platelet transfusions were administered in cases with a thrombocytopenia of less than 50,000/mm³ associated with a hemorrhagic syndrome. Patients who developed infection as a result of neutropenia were treated with a combination of Amikacin 7.5 mg/kg every 12 hours by I.M. injection, or by infusion over 30 minutes in the case of thrombocytopenia, and Amoxicillin 1 g twice a day orally or by I.V. injection.

In patients who developed interstitial lung disease, the BLM was stopped and steroid therapy was instituted, at a dose equivalent to 2 mg/kg of prednisolone for 10 consecutive days, followed by a dose of 1 mg/kg for at least 1 month, with very gradual reduction of the doses over 3 months. In the majority of cases, this steroid treatment was able to prevent or at least stabilize the progression toward pulmonary fibrosis.

It is difficult to evaluate the exact role of the steroid therapy administered at the same time as the BLM infusions. Its routine administration to prevent vomiting did not decrease the incidence of interstitial lung disease or the fall in TLCO. Nevertheless, the administration of high-dose steroids at the first sign of interstitial disease appeared to be beneficial.

Based on the hypothesis of the deposition of immune complexes, BLM and antibleomycin antibodies in the pulmonary parenchyma in addition to the direct toxicity of BLM, patients who presented a fall in the TLCO (42 cases) were treated by plasma exchange with a mean volume of 2.700 L (range: 1.800 to 4.300 L) and replacement by 4% albumin.[11] A total of 76 plasma exchanges were performed in this way, with 71 evaluations of the TLCO before and after the exchange (1 patient had 3 plasmaphereses and another had 2 plasmaphereses prior to evaluation of the TLCO). No improvement was observed after 44 exchanges. After the other 27 exchanges (38%), the TLCO was improved by 11% to 30% in relation to the preplasmapheresis values.

In 27 patients, the BLM treatment could be continued after plasmapheresis — for as many as 7 cycles in one case. Although plasma exchange appeared to have a real but insufficient effect, it cannot yet be proposed as routine treatment.

Results

The response to treatment was evaluated for the squamous cell carcinomas, the adenocarcinomas, and the large-cell anaplastic carcinomas after a minimum of 2 cycles. In the group of 30 small-cell anaplastic carcinomas, the results were evaluated on chest X rays taken 14 days after day 1 of the *first* cycle of DDP-BLM. In the other group of 51 patients initially treated with the CTX-ADR-CCNU-VP-16 combination, the responses were evaluated after 4 cycles of A and 4 cycles of B (DDP-BLM), which were administered in rotation every 2 weeks. The criteria of evaluation were those of the ECOG. The cases of stable disease (no improvement or improvement of less than 50%) and progression of disease were grouped under the heading of failures. The responses were described as being complete only when the bronchoscopy was macroscopically normal and the bronchial biopsy was also normal.

Squamous Cell Carcinomas

PREOPERATIVE SITUATION

The number of complete responses (CR), partial responses (PR), and failures for each combination after 3 or 4 preoperative cycles are shown in table 3. The median survival of these patients was not attained at 12 months (4+ to 35+), and 15 patients are still alive. It should be stressed that these patients were intitially considered to be inoperable because of the locoregional extension of the disease.

POSTOPERATIVE ADJUVANT N+ SITUATION

Thirty-seven patients were treated with 4 cycles of DDP-BLM followed by mediastinal and supraclavicular radiotherapy and then DDP-VDS. The median survival was greater than 24 months for stage 1, greater than 16 months for stage 2, and 12 months for stage 3. Ten of the 21 patients with stage 3 disease survived for more than 1 year, and 7 were still alive after 16–30 months.

INOPERABLE LOCALIZED TUMORS

The responses at the end of the induction treatment for the various combinations are shown in table 4. The overall objective response rate for the 344 patients was 73.3%, without any significant difference among the 3 combinations containing a sufficient number of patients: DDP-BLM, DDP-BLM-MIT, and DDP-BLM-VDS. The actuarial survival of these patients (all protocols combined) was 30% at 12 months and 11% at 24 months for the whole group (36.8% at 12 months and 16.5% at 24 months for the responders and 18.6% at 12 months for the nonresponders).

TUMORS WITH DISTANT METASTASES

The response rates for tumors with distant metastases were inferior to those obtained in the localized forms (see table 5). The overall response for the

Table 3. Responses Obtained in 30 Patients with Squamous Cell Carcinoma Who Became Operable After Chemotherapy

Combination	No. patients	CR	PR	Failures	Objective response (%)
DDP-BLM	17	2	11	4	
DDP-BLM-MIT	11	2	7	2	80
DDP-BLM-VDS	2		2		
	30				

Table 4. Response Rate of Inoperable Localized Squamous Cell Carcinomas of the Bronchus in Relation to Combinations Used

Combination	No. patients	CR	PR	Failures	Obj. resp. (%)
DDP-BLM	188	30	107	51	72.8
DDP-BLM-MIT	111	13	70	28	74.7
DDP-BLM-VDS	32	5	15	12	62.5
DDP-BLM-VP-16	10	1	8	1	
DDP-BLM-VP-16-VCR	3		3		
	344				

group of 213 patients was 46%. The overall actuarial survival was 12.5% at 12 months (responders 27.6%, nonresponders 4.7%).

Adenocarcinomas

POSTOPERATIVE ADJUVANT SITUATION WITH POSITIVE NODES

Eleven patients are evaluable at the present time with a schema identical to that of the squamous cell carcinomas. The survivals were as follows: stage 1 (1 patient) 27 months; stage 2 (1 patient) 5 months; stage 3 (9 patients) median survival 13 months. Three patients with stage 3 disease were still alive after 17+, 24+, and 39+ months, respectively.

INOPERABLE LOCALIZED TUMORS

The results are presented in table 6. An overall objective response rate for the 3 combinations of only 45% is lower than that in disseminated squamous cell carcinomas. The median survival time was 10 months (2 to 34+).

TUMORS WITH DISTANT METASTASES

The results are shown in table 7. The overall response rate for the 3 combinations in 22 patients was 40.9%, less than that obtained with the metastatic squamous cell carcinomas. The median survival was 6 months (2 to 36+).

Table 5. Response Rates of Metastatic Squamous Carcinomas in Relation to Various Combinations

Combination	No. patients	CR	PR	Failures	Obj. resp. (%)
DDP-BLM	107	2	39	66	58
DDP-BLM-MIT	79	4	40	35	55.6
DDP-BLM-VDS	19	1	7	11	42
DDP-BLM-VP-16	4		3	1	
DDP-BLM-VP-16-VCR	4		3	1	
	213				

Table 6. Response Rate of Inoperable Localized Adenocarcinomas in Relation to Various Combinations

Combination	No. patients	CR	PR	Failures	Obj. resp. (%)
DDP-BLM	12	1	4	7	45
DDP-BLM-5-FU	6		3	3	
DDP-BLM-VP-16	2	1		1	
	20				

Small-Cell Anaplastic Carcinomas

RESPONSES OBTAINED AFTER THE FIRST CYCLE OF DDP—BLM

Thirty patients were treated by this protocol and were evaluated by simple x-ray examination on the 14th day—the day before administration of the conventional combination, which was administered in rotation. Four apparently complete responses and 19 responses of greater than 50% were observed, for an overall objective response rate of 75%. The other 7 patients each achieved response of less than 50%.

RESPONSES OBTAINED AFTER ROTATION OF
DDP-BLM AND CTX-ADR-VP-16-CCNU

Response and survival could be evaluated in 51 patients. This evaluation was performed after 4 cycles of each combination administered in rotation. The following results were observed:

- In the localized forms, of 26 patients, 92% achieved objective responses (16 CR and 8 PR).
- In the diffuse forms, of 25 patients, 84% achieved objective responses (8 CR and 13 PR). No changes were observed in 4 others.

The limited follow-up in this study prevents evaluation of the survival in relation to the extent of the disease and the response to treatment. It should be noted that the CR rate was higher in the localized forms.

Large-Cell Anaplastic Carcinomas

The responses were evaluated after 4 cycles of DDP-BLM. This combination, in a small number of patients, resulted in only 2 partial responses, with survivals of 14+, 10, 6, 5, 4+, and 4 months.

Discussion

Experience with the various protocols proposed is now sufficiently extensive to permit confirmation of their feasibility. In hospitalized patients, these protocols do not present any particular problems for experienced nurses. The extension of the protocols to outpatients with implanted pumps raises a number of problems. Rather than mixing the various drugs in the reservoir, it is

Table 7. Responses of Metastatic Adenocarcinomas in 22 Patients

Combination	No. patients	CR	PR	Failures	Obj. resp. (%)
DDP-BLM	10		6	4	
DDP-BLM-5-FU	9		2	7	40.9
DDP-BLM-VP-16	3		1	2	
	22				

preferable to connect 2 or even 3 portable pumps to the implanted subcutaneous reservoir (Port-a-Cath or Infusaport), but this greatly increases the total cost. Further technical progress is required, either in the form of 2 or 3 reservoirs included in the 1 portable pump or in the form of adjustable pumps in relation to the emptying time of the reservoir, so that 2 or 3 drugs could be administered successively each day via the same pump.

It should also be emphasized that certain drugs such as VP-16 are unsuitable for this type of administration because their poor solubility requires at least 200 ml of solution per 50 mg of drug in order to avoid deposition on the walls of the catheter during very slow infusions.

Further studies need to be performed on the modalities of administration. For example, if 8 hourly subcutaneous injections of BLM retained the effectiveness of this agent, 1 less reservoir would be required for outpatient chemotherapy. Despite these reservations, these protocols are sufficiently feasible to be administered not only in medical oncology units but in specialized pneumology units as well.

The toxicity of the proposed protocols has been shown to be moderate and totally acceptable, which is probably due to the fact that the plasma levels remain moderate and regular. The major problem is the pulmonary toxicity of BLM. Because this toxicity is aggravated by MIT, it is recommended that this combination be avoided. This toxicity is also aggravated by supplementary radiotherapy and by the use of pure oxygen, including during anethesia following the preoperative administration of BLM. Most important, nearly all of these chronic smoker and bronchitic patients present a chronic obstructive airways syndrome. Some patients also have a constrictive syndrome in the case of a previous pulmonary operation. It is therefore essential to know when to stop the BLM in time. In practice, although we can administer an average of 10 cycles of DDP before inducing renal or neurological toxicity, pulmonary toxicity appears after a mean of only 5 cycles of BLM. BLM should then be replaced by either VDS, according to the current protocol described, or by VP-16, as has been proposed.[12,13] The limitations to the duration of the treatments presented in this chapter constitute a major drawback that will need to be overcome by the development of precise successive protocols using various therapeutic agents. The replacement of BLM by an analogue with less pulmonary toxicity but with equivalent effectiveness would be an important contribution.

The results presented are superior to those of conventional treatments reported in the literature, some of which are presented in table 8, together with their references. These results were found to be reproducible in time and from one center to another. It is believed that one of the reasons for these differences is that the reports in the literature usually group squamous cell carcinomas and adenocarcinomas together, although these 2 types of cancer do not respond in the same way to the DDP-BLM combination. It is essential for articles on this subject to distinguish between these 2 groups. It is possible that one of the principal causes of resistance in squamous cell cancers is the importance of DNA repair, a plausible process, considering that the skin is continually repairing damage due to ultraviolet radiation. Adenocarcinomas probably possess additional mechanisms of resistance that have not yet been elucidated and that cannot be overcome by presently available forms of chemotherapy.

It should also be noted that the highest response rate was observed in small, operable primary tumors. It was lower in inoperable localized tumors and lower still in metastatic cancers. These results reflect the importance of the tumor burden in the response rates, but they also reflect the fact that populations of metastatic cells possess additional mechanisms of resistance. This observation should lead to the earlier use of chemotherapy as part of neoadjuvant protocols. It also suggests that T3N- tumors, which have a much lower metastatic potential,[21] should be more easily controlled than N+ tumors.

The DDP-BLM combination was found to have remarkable short-term effectiveness in the case of small-cell cancers. This means that in the event of failure of primary chemotherapy, more active infusion treatments can be proposed instead of the conventional protocols. This finding has also led to an investigation of the rapid rotation of myelotoxic chemotherapy protocols and a continuous combination of DDP-BLM as initial treatment. The possible superiority of this approach will need to be evaluated by randomized trials.

A rational strategy for current clinical research would be to evaluate, by means of randomized trials, the benefit of continuous chemotherapy compared with the same doses of the same agents administered by bolus. Certain centers should undertake these studies. However, the authors have chosen to pursue continuous chemotherapy and to study, either by successive phase 2 trials or by randomization in relation to the double platinum-bleomycin com-

Table 8. Results of Conventional Treatments as Reported in 7 Studies

Treatment		No. patients/ disease class.	Extent of disease	CR/PR	Obj. resp. (%)	Study/ reference
VDS 3 mg/m^2/week DDP 120 mg/m^2 or 60 mg/m^2 } 4 weeks		81 patients Squamous 30% Adeno 70%	Metastatic 100%	7 CR 27 PR	43	Gralla[14]
VDS 3 mg/m^2/week DDP 100 mg/m^2/4 weeks		43 patients Squamous 70%	Limited 69%	14 PR	33	Elliot[15]
VDS 5 mg/m^2/week or 1.5 mg/m^2/j × 3 j/3 weeks DDP 100 mg/m^2/4 weeks		30 patients Large-cell	Limited 17 Metastatic 13	2 CR 3 PR	53 23	Niederle[16]
VDS 3 mg/m^2/week DDP 120 mg/m^2/4 weeks		19 patients Squamous 86%	Metastatic 88%	2 CR 11 PR	68.4	Briancon[17]
DDP 60 mg/m^2/3 weeks VP-16 120 mg/m^2/3 weeks		94 patients Squamous 72	Not given	{ 3 CR 26 PR } 40		Longeval[18]
		Adeno 22		{ 1 CR 6 PR } 32		
DDP 60 mg/m^2 VP-16 120 mg/m^2 × 3 j } 3 weeks VDS 1.5 mg/m^2 J1-J7)		62 patients Squamous 61% Adeno 27%	Metastatic 60%	5 CR 20 PR	40.3	Klastersky[19]
DDP 60 mg/m^2 VDS 3 mg/m^2 } 3 weeks MIT 10 mg/m^2 } 6 weeks		87 patients Histology not given	Metastatic 100%	8 CR 25 PR	37	Miller[20]

bination, the combination capable of inducing a greater number of complete responses.

In lung cancers, as in most solid tumors, a partial response to treatment results in only a minor increase in the total survival, which is quite obvious in terms of cellular kinetics. The reduction of a cell population by 2 logs offers only a temporary benefit, although this may be useful in the case of slow-growing tumors. A reduction by 4 or 5 logs may eradicate a large number of occult metastases and can induce a very significant improvement in survival. From this point of view, the control of the kinetic resistance by means of continuous chemotherapy, for the same degree of metabolic resistance, may prove to be the determinant.

At present, there are 2 theoretical approaches to the search for increased CR rates. The first approach consists of increasing the number of drugs associated with the DDP-BLM combination, within the limits of tolerance, and the 2nd consists of increasing the duration of administration by means of protocols containing continuous infusions for 7 days, 10 days, and 14 days every 3–4 weeks. The 2 approaches obviously can be combined, and this is currently under study. When the optimal combinations and optimal durations have been determined for the available drugs in terms of the CR rate and the tolerance, it would be legitimate to exactly evaluate, by randomization, the benefit of continuous administration over bolus administration.

Other Trials of Infusion Chemotherapy

This review has focused on the experience of the French Thoracic Oncology Club and on combinations involving DDP and BLM. Relatively few studies have been performed using the infusion schedule in bronchogenic carcinoma with other drugs. 5-FU is an agent traditionally administered as an intermittent bolus and is associated with minimal activity in advanced lung cancer.[22] Recent trials in head and neck cancer, however, have demonstrated substantial activity for the infusion schedule for 5-FU administered in conjunction with DDP.[23] In a study involving 34 patients with advanced nonsmall-cell lung cancer, a combination of 5-FU administered as a 5-day infusion at 1.0 gm/m^2/day in conjunction with bolus DDP was evaluated. Ten patients responded to therapy, including 37% of previously untreated patients and 20% of patients previously receiving chemotherapy.[24] An extension of that study involved combining infusional 5-FU and DDP with primary radiation delivered concomitantly preoperatively for stage 3 nonsmall-cell lung cancer. In a study of 27 patients treated, 18 came to thoracotomy, and in 4 patients (22%) there was no histologic evidence of tumor, and the total response rate preoperatively was 78%.[25]

The contribution of DDP to the regimen is unclear, although in a study in which 5-FU and radiation were delivered together with the 5-FU administered as a continuous infusion, a CR was observed in 10/28 patients.[26] This may be compared to the 3/22 observed in the trial in which DDP was added to the regimen of 5-FU continuous infusion and radiation cited above.

In small-cell carcinoma of the lung, there have been virtually no trials of continuous infusion. Etoposide (VP-16) is an agent with substantial activity in this tumor and one that has demonstrated a greater responsiveness when the drug is delivered more frequently.[27] It is also an agent that could rationally be delivered as a continuous infusion based upon schedule dependency demonstrated in experimental tumor systems and upon the pharmacokinetic behavior of the agent, which has a variably short half-life.[28] A continuous infusion schedule was evaluated for VP-16 in small-cell carcinoma of the lung administered in conjunction with 2 other agents (CTX and ADR).[29] Toxicity was substantial in this group of patients, and the response rate and median survival were only comparable to those reported for bolus delivery of VP-16, suggesting no advantage to the infusion schedule.

Another agent commonly delivered by continuous infusion is cytosine arabinoside (ara-C), which has a singular role in the treatment of acute leukemia. A trial of ara-C in small-cell lung cancer has reported no responses in 10 patients who received extensive prior therapy. The ara-C was then integrated into a 4-drug regimen with CTX, ADR, and VCR. In 25 patients without prior therapy, the response rate and median survival were only comparable to the experience with the 3-drug regimen delivered as a bolus excluding ara-C.[30]

Vinblastine (VLB) combined with DDP has been evaluated in nonsmall-cell lung cancer in a series of reports.[31-37] In half of these reports, the VLB was delivered as a 5-day continuous infusion in conjunction with bolus DDP. Response rates varied, with a general response level of about 25%. Responses were related to performance status, prior therapy, and stage of disease, but the infusion schedule had no definite advantage.

Summary

There is no standard regimen for the treatment of lung cancer, although for the histologic subtype designated as small-cell carcinoma the usual regimen involves CTX, ADR, and VCR, with VP-16 added by some groups. At least 3 of these agents can be practically administered as a continuous infusion, and reports of short-term infusion for all 4 agents have demonstrated clinical activity.

For nonsmall-cell lung cancer, the common regimens today include CTX, ADR, and DDP (CAP), BLM plus DDP, and VLB plus DDP. All regimens obviously involve drugs that may be delivered as a continuous infusion schedule, but the trials reported to date have been relatively few. Newer trials involving 5-FU delivered as a continuous infusion, again with a DDP combination, will expand the experience with this schedule for this tumor. The use of multiple drugs — delivered as admixtures if the compatibility of multiple drugs can be established, delivered sequentially at 8, 12, or more hours per agent, or delivered by continuous infusion of 1 agent interspersed with bolus delivery of additional agents — represents a fruitful area for exploration in treatment for this tumor.

27

TESTICULAR CANCER AND OTHER TUMORS OF THE MALE GENITOURINARY TRACT

Christopher J. Logothetis, M.D.

MALIGNANT TUMORS OF THE genitourinary tract represent a wide spectrum of disease. Included among those diseases are the highly curable primary germ cell tumors of the testis, the most frequent tumor of males between the ages of 20–30 years. The cure for testicular germ cell tumors is dependent on the widely applied chemotherapy regimens developed over the past decade. Also included is prostatic carcinoma, the most frequent tumor of males in the 7th and 8th decades of life. Chemotherapy has a much less important role at present in treating prostatic carcinoma, but it is a hormonally responsive tumor. Urothelial tumors, for which the most rapid advancement in the introduction of chemotherapy has been seen in the past 3 years, have the potential for most dramatic improvement in therapy. Primary clear cell carcinomas of the kidney remain refractory to systemic chemotherapy.

This chapter will necessarily be confined predominantly to a review of infusional chemotherapy for the treatment of germ cell tumors and the development of infusional therapy at the M. D. Anderson Hospital. Reference will be made to the recent introduction of vinblastine (VLB) continuous infusion chemotherapy in the treatment of prostatic carcinoma, and a brief discussion of the potential role of infusional therapy in the management of urothelial tumors will be included.

Vinblastine and Bleomycin Combination in the Management of Germ Cell Tumors

The combination of vinblastine sulfate and bleomycin (VB) is the first chemotherapy regimen to consistently achieve durable complete remissions (CR) and apparent cures in the management of metastatic germ cell tumors. This combination, introduced by Samuels et al, was delivered in a schedule of I.V. bolus VLB and intermittent I.M. bleomycin (BLM) (VB$_1$).[1] The schedule was selected because of the then available information. Since that time, there has been progress in the management of germ cell tumors, with more appropriate integration of chemotherapy with surgery, the introduction of new agents, and with the use of newer dosage schedules resulting in increased therapeutic index. This chapter will briefly discuss the evolution of VLB and BLM chemotherapy in the management of germ cell tumors and the results of a recent study completed with the combination of continuous infusion VLB with continuous simultaneous infusion BLM.

The original VLB-BLM combination (VB$_1$) resulted in frequent CR among patients with germ cell tumors of the testis. Complete remissions were most frequently seen among those patients with modest-volume or minimal-volume disease, whereas those patients with truly advanced disease remained with a very poor prognosis.[2] The original results were improved upon with the introduction of higher doses continuous infusion BLM while also escalating the dose of bolus VLB (VB$_3$) (see table 1).

Although the populations were not comparable in the original VB$_1$ study when compared to the VB$_3$ patients, the impression of the investigators was that there was a higher and more durable CR rate with the VB$_3$ combination.

The toxicity of the bolus VLB combinations with continuous infusion or intermittent BLM were significant and have previously been reported. The constellation of mucocutaneous toxicity and severe myelosuppression in the presence of ileus resulted in a high infectious complication rate. The expertise that developed as experience accumulated with the use of these combinations allowed for the escalation of the dose of VLB. These combinations were very hazardous, but in the appropriate clinical setting, with the liberal use of prophylactic antibiotics and aggressive supportive care, the mortality rate remained remarkably low.[3] The toxicity of this combination included the development of severe mucosal toxicity and modest cutaneous toxicity, with hyperpigmentation and the development of very tender hyperkeratosis over pressure points. Headache and high spiking fevers were frequent during BLM infusion. With the introduction of BLM as a continuous infusion, a reduction in the frequency and severity of the cutaneous toxicity was noted. The previous

Table 1. Comparison of Response by Protocol[1]

Tumor volume	VB$_1$ ± BLM COMF. No. patients (% CR[2])	VB$_3$ No. patients (% CR)
Minimal lung	10 (60)	11 (81)
Advanced lung	21 (23)	12 (52)
Advanced abdomen	12 (33)	17 (17)
Nodal presentation only[3]	3 (0)	7 (57)

[1]Includes patients with embryonal + teratocarcinoma only.
[2]Complete remission.
[3]Mediastinal + supraclavicular ± abdominal nodes.

frequently occurring tender areas of hyperkeratosis and ulceration over the pressure points and hyperpigmentation with pruritis no longer occurred in clinically relevant severity or frequency.

Bleomycin-induced hyperpyrexia is common. When associated with the acute toxicity of bolus or continuous infusion VLB, the clinical picture may mimic sepsis. In the presence of a presumed bleomycin-induced fever associated with clinical toxicity, the practice in the Genitourinary Oncology Section of the M. D. Anderson Hospital is to perform appropriate cultures (blood, urine, mucosal membranes) and to introduce antibiotics early (see table 2). The broad-spectrum antibiotics used must be tailored to the needs of the patient as determined by the gram stains of the mucosal secretions or other inflamed sites. Bleomycin infusion, if associated with an incremental toxicity over 48 hours, should be discontinued because of the likelihood that this may be related to an infectious episode. The classic BLM-induced fever reaches its peak 24–36 hours following the infusion and is decremental in the final day of the infusion. Even in the absence of severe toxicity, an incremental febrile curve at 48–72 hours should lead the clinician to the introduction of broad-spectrum antibiotics. Discontinuation of the chemotherapy is a clinical decision that should be determined by the tumor status.

BLM pulmonary toxicity, manifested either in an idiosyncratic pulmonary interstitial pneumonia or a progressive pulmonary fibrosis, is the most feared complication of BLM therapy.[4] With the introduction of BLM as an infusion and with the appropriate monitoring of its pulmonary toxicity, there has been an almost total absence of clinically significant pulmonary toxicity among patients treated at the M. D. Anderson Hospital. In the most recently treated 100 patients with continuous infusion BLM, not a single BLM-induced respiratory failure has occurred. Many recommendations have been made in monitoring patients with BLM as a continuous infusion. These have included the use of carbon monoxide diffusion, forced vital capacity (FVC), spirometry, arterial blood gases, and exertional arterial blood gases. Although the diffusion capacity total lung volumes are sensitive tests in measuring early evidence of BLM pulmonary toxicity, they also have disadvantages. It must be recognized that a negative effect of very sensitive tests is that BLM would be removed from the therapeutic regimen prematurely. It also must be noted that carbon monoxide

Table 2. Bleomycin Hyperpyrexia

Characteristics

1. Peak bleomycin fever occurs in 24 – 36%.
2. Fever may be associated with chills.
3. Low-grade temperature (< 101) may persist for duration of infusion; fever is decremental after 48 hours of infusion.

Management

1. In presence of clinical toxicity and fever, broad-spectrum antibiotics should be introduced after appropriate cultures.
2. Incremental fever after 48 hours must be considered as infectious in origin and managed with antibiotics. Cessation of bleomycin therapy should follow if tumor status allows.

diffusion requires expertise in its use and has a wide fluctuation depending on the patient's preparation for this test.

At the M. D. Anderson Hospital, the monitoring of BLM is performed with the simple FVC and gallium scan (see table 3). The FVC is a reproducibly reliable test in measuring lung capacity, although it is relatively crude when compared to diffusion capacity. At our institution, a > 10% drop from the initial FVC is indicative of a significant change in pulmonary function. Whether this drop can be attributed to the primary pulmonary lesions or other factors (chest wall, generalized asthenia, lack of cooperation, etc.) may require further evaluation. In our experience, not a single instance of BLM pulmonary toxicity occurred without the presence of a positive gallium scan. A 48-hour gallium scan of the lung is routinely performed with the FVC. The combination of these 2 parameters results in an early detection of BLM pulmonary toxicity. Upon development of a > 10% drop in FVC and a positive gallium scan, BLM therapy is discontinued.

We have recently reported the results of 100 patients treated with the combination of CISCA$_2$/VB$_4$ cyclic chemotherapy.[5] These patients received continuous infusion bleomycin with simultaneous continuous infusion vinblastine. This Velban/BLM combination (VB$_4$) is delivered in a cyclic fashion with CISCA$_2$ (Cytoxan, Adriamycin [ADR], cisplatin) (see table 4). Of the 100 patients treated, 7 have developed a conversion of their baseline gallium scan from negative to positive (see table 5). The diffuse uptake in the gallium scan was associated with a drop in the FVC of > 10% in 1 patient. That patient had open lung biopsy performed and was found to have findings compatible with early

Table 3. Monitoring Bleomycin for Pulmonary Toxicity

1. Gallium scan of lung (48 hours)*
2. Spirometry with forced vital capacity (FVC)

Interpretation

A > 10% drop in FVC must be viewed as a bleomycin-induced lung toxicity if associated with a positive lung gallium scan (lung biopsy should be performed for confirmation).

A > 10% drop in FVC with a normal gallium lung scan should initially search for the causes of decreased FVC (asthenia, progressive tumor).

*Gallium scan performed on patients with > 1,000 granulocytes.

Table 4. CISCA$_2$ and VB$_4$: Schedules and Administration

CISCA$_2$

Cytoxan, 500 mg/m^2 B.S.A. I.V. day 1 and 2
Adriamycin, 40 to 45 mg/m^2 B.S.A. day 1 and 2
Cisplatin, 100 to 120 mg/m^2 B.S.A. diluted 1 mg/ml normal saline given over 2 hours

VB$_4$

Vinblastine, 3 mg/m^2 B.S.A. continuous for 24 hours × 5 consecutive days via a centrally placed line
Bleomycin, 30 u. I.V. continuous for 5 consecutive days simultaneously with vinblastine

BLM-induced pulmonary fibrosis. In 5/7 patients, the gallium scan reverted to normal. All patients had a return to normal of their pulmonary function tests. Only 1 patient developed radiographic evidence of BLM pulmonary toxicity, and all remained clinically asymptomatic. The combination of gallium scan and FVC is a reliable, simple, and reproducible manner of monitoring for BLM pulmonary toxicity. This very sensitive screening procedure for bleomycin pulmonary toxicity did not result in its premature deletion. By employing continuous infusion BLM, we have been able to deliver high doses at 3-week intervals. This schedule is convenient and allows for adequate pulmonary testing prior to each dose. A significant drawback of intermittent I.M. bleomycin schedules commonly used is that they do not allow for frequent testing prior to each dose. During the acute phase of chemotherapy toxicity, patients are unable to perform reliably the pulmonary tests required.

The reduced frequency of BLM pulmonary toxicity when the drug is delivered as a continuous infusion is in keeping with the laboratory data supporting the increased therapeutic index of this agent when delivered in this manner.[6] In the experiments performed by Sikic et al, animals exposed to continuous infusion BLM had a marked reduction in pulmonary fibrosis when compared to those receiving the drug by bolus.

Although we have not regularly introduced other agents with BLM therapy in an attempt to reduce the pulmonary fibrosis, some experimental evidence indicates that the use of nonsteroidal anti-inflammatory agents, when introduced early in BLM therapy, may reduce the frequency of pulmonary fibrosis.

Goldinger et al first observed a postoperative adult respiratory distress syndrome among patients overhydrated or exposed to oxygen intraoperatively with a preoperative exposure to relative high doses of bleomycin.[7] This complication, which is fatal, has been attributed to underlying BLM therapy resulting in a reduced threshold to oxygen toxicity. In our experience with 70 patients submitted to surgery following VLB-BLM therapy and our most recent experience with 32 additional patients, not a single patient has suffered postoperative BLM pulmonary toxicity.[8] The initial 70 patients were treated prior to the reports on postoperative pulmonary toxicity, and no effort was made to avoid higher oxygen concentrations or hydration status. We believe that the absence of this postoperative adult respiratory distress syndrome is attributable to the use of continuous infusion BLM and the manner with which we monitor BLM

Table 5. VB$_4$: Long-Term Toxicity in 100 Patients

Type	No. patients (%)
Bleomycin lung toxicity[1]	
Positive gallium scan	7 (7)
Positive gallium scan + drop in FVC[2] > 10%	1 (1)
Peripheral neuropathy	10 (10)
Raynaud's phenomenon	1 (1)

[1]Only 1 patient had radiographic findings of interstitial pneumonitis with a drop in forced vital capacity.
[2]FVC = forced vital capacity

therapy. At the M. D. Anderson Hospital, BLM is discontinued prior to the development of clinically significant pulmonary toxicity.

Samuels et al have reported on the increased frequency of pulmonary toxicity for patients who had received prior radiation therapy involving portions of the lung followed by BLM.[9] Added caution needs to be exercised when using the drug in such patients.

The experience we have accumulated with BLM therapy supports the evidence produced by Sikic et al that this drug, when delivered as a continuous infusion, results in an increased therapeutic index. We believe that BLM pulmonary toxicity is a totally avoidable complication with the use of continuous infusion and appropriate monitoring of the pulmonary status.

Available pharmacologic data suggest that most tumor cell killing with BLM therapy occurs during G_2 of the cell cycle. Some evidence suggests that cell death with BLM also occurs during the G_1 phase. The reported cell cycle specificity of bleomycin suggests that continuous exposure would result in an increasing cell kill, and the superiority of VB_3 over VB_1 strongly suggests that the therapeutic index is also improved by increased cell kill.

BLM is an active cytotoxic agent with an integral role in the successful therapy of advanced germ cell tumors. It is an ideal agent for combination therapy with myelosuppressive cytotoxic agents because of its minimal bone marrow toxicity. When used as a continuous infusion, the therapeutic index is improved primarily because of a marked reduction in pulmonary and cutaneous toxicity. Intermittent BLM therapy is associated with a high fatal respiratory toxicity (3–5%) and an even higher frequency of clinically restrictive lung disease. The use of intermittent I.M. bleomycin therapy is hazardous and is no longer indicated in cancer chemotherapy.

Vinblastine as a single agent has been demonstrated to be active in the management of germ cell tumors. Complete remissions were encountered in the initial report by Samuels and Howe, but long-term durable CR were rarely encountered. The addition of melphalan (MEL) to VLB did not increase the overall response rate.[10] Experiences with the combination VLB-BLM therapy demonstrated that the total VLB dose, when delivered as a bolus, was directly related to the ultimate response rate. Such differences in dosage and outcome were most frequently seen when the dose of VLB was escalated to a high dose of 0.6 mg/kg.[11] In a prospective randomized trial performed by Einhorn et al, 0.4 mg/kg of VLB with intermittent BLM and cisplatin (DDP) was compared to 0.3 mg/kg of VLB with intermittent BLM-DDP and 0.2 mg/kg of VLB with ADR-BLM-DDP.[12] In that randomized prospective trial, no significant difference in the outcome of each of these 3 protocols was documented. A significant increased infectious complication rate was noted for those patients receiving 0.4 mg/kg of VLB when compared to the lower dose VLB combinations. Although these data have been interpreted as indicating that higher dose VLB does not achieve a more durable or higher CR rate than lower dose VLB, this conclusion appears erroneous. The data presented by Einhorn et al failed to achieve adequate numbers of patients to securely make the statement that 0.4 mg/kg of VLB is not superior to 0.3 mg/kg.

The toxicity of high-dose VLB is unique to this agent. The toxic manifestations include severe myalgias, myelosuppression, hypertension, a rare rhabdomyolysis and myositis associated with patients who are muscular, and G.I. toxicity manifested either by obstipation or frank ileus. These side effects, both in the experience from the University of Indiana and the experience published from the M. D. Anderson Hospital, were found to be directly related to the total dose of VLB. Of greatest concern was the documented infectious complication rate. Such infectious complications were directly associated with the total dose of VLB infused. Although the fatal complication rate of the combination chemotherapy employed at the M. D. Anderson Hospital despite the high dose of vinblastine sulfate used (VB$_3$) was low, it did require intensive therapy and great expertise in its management and has not become widely applicable.

DDP-Velban-BLM (PVB) combinations have been accepted as standard therapy, and many investigators have published their experiences. Recent reports tabulating long-term survival document an improvement in survival for the 3 drugs when compared to Velban-BLM delivered in high doses.[13] The single comparative trial published by Peckman et al also fails to demonstrate a difference between PVB and Velban-BLM (VB$_3$) alone.[14] We attribute this lack of an improvement to (1) the reduction in the total dose of VLB in order to accommodate DDP and (2) the use of intermittent BLM therapy. Cisplatin is clearly a very active agent in the management of germ cell tumors, and its addition to relatively low-dose VLB and intermittent BLM has allowed maintenance of the CR rate at a level equivalent to that with the high-dose VLB combination.

The initial M. D. Anderson Hospital experience of germ cell tumor chemotherapy indicates that the optimal combination chemotherapy would maintain high-dose VLB and continuous-infusion BLM while adding DDP combination chemotherapy to this. The initial efforts were directed toward maintaining high-dose VLB therapy with supportive care and sequential DDP following recovery from the Velban-BLM toxicity. Following that experience, an independently effective regimen (CISCA$_2$) was developed.[15] We now deliver in cyclic fashion the 2 independently curative regimens. The recent results reveal an encouraging 92% long-term CR among 100 patients with advanced germ cell cancer. Most of these patients are in the advanced disease category as initially proposed by Samuels et al (see tables 6 and 7).

Recent improvements have been reported in combination chemotherapy in the management of germ cell tumors. These improvements have included the introduction of a complex multidrug regimen reported by Newlands et al from the Charing Cross Hospital in London (POMB-ACE).[16] POMB-ACE appears to be an effective regimen, but the data derived from that study are very difficult to interpret. Patients with very high beta HCG or HCG levels at presentation remain a poor prognostic category as difficult to treat as those in the CISCA$_2$/VB$_4$ regimen. In addition, patients with AFP at very high levels remain with a relatively poor prognosis when treated with POMB-ACE. The influence of high AFP levels has been effaced with CISCA$_2$/VB$_4$ chemotherapy. Although POMB-ACE appears to be an improvement, the relative effectiveness of POMB-ACE when compared to CISCA$_2$/VB$_4$ is difficult to evaluate. The continued negative influence of the high AFP levels is disturbing. Etoposide (VP-16), first introduced in Europe in the management of patients with germ cell tumors, appears to be a highly effective agent.[17] VP-16 and DDP is an active combination, but is associated with a high relapse rate. The recent development of the combination of BLM-VP-16-DDP (BEP) by Peckham et al is an improvement.[18] In a prospective randomized trial, BEP was found to be equally effective as PVB.[19] Continued mortality from BLM pulmonary toxicity was associated in both arms of that study. Long-term results from PVB have now been reported, and a 56% long-term disease-free survival has been achieved.[20] It can be anticipated that BEP will have equal results. A recent review of experience tabulating results of VAB$_4$, VAB$_5$, and VAB$_6$ also confirms the suspicion that the major cause of the recent improvement in survival of patients with germ cell tumors is improvement in overall prognostic variables over the past 5 years; only secondarily is the improved survival rate due to modest improvements in chemotherapy.[21]

Except for the use of continuous infusion VLB and BLM at our institution and the use of continuous infusion BLM in the various protocols developed at the Memorial Sloan-Kettering Hospital, infusional therapy has not been regularly employed in the management of germ cell tumors. Agents that have a

Table 6. Samuels Staging for Testicular Cancer

3-A	Disease confined to supraclavicular nodes.
3-B$_1$	Either one or more biomarkers elevated or gynecomastia, unilateral or bilateral. Both may be present together. No demonstrable mass.
3-B$_2$	Minimal pulmonary disease: up to 5 nodules in each lung field, and the largest diameter of any single lesion < 2.0 cm. (Total tumor volume does not exceed 40 cm^3.)[1]
3-B$_3$	Advanced pulmonary disease: presence of any mediastinal or hilar mass, neoplastic pleural effusion, or intrapulmonary mass > 40 cm^3.
3-B$_4$	Advanced abdominal disease, defined as abdominal mass > 10 cm.[2]
3-B$_5$	Visceral disease (excluding lung), most often liver but also gastrointestinal tract and brain.

[1]Based on each nodule being spherical. Volume of sphere is 1/6 D^3.
[2]Abdominal mass measured by computerized tomography; hydronephrosis is no longer included in the staging system.

Table 7. CISCA$_2$ and VB$_4$: Disease-Free Survival (DFS) by Stage

Stage	Total patients	DFS No. patients (%)
Clinical 2	22	21 (95)
3-B$_1$	3	3 (100)
3-B$_2$	12	12 (100)
3-B$_3$	16	16 (100)
3-B$_4$	23	21 (91)
3-B$_5$	15	11 (73)
Extragonadal	9	5 (56)
TOTAL	100	89 (89)

potential role in increasing the therapeutic index by infusion and are commonly used in the treatment of germ cell tumors are DDP, ADR, and VLB.

The VLB-BLM combination currently used is a further modification of the initial VB combinations developed at our institution. We continue to employ continuous-infusion BLM and see a near total absence of pulmonary toxicity.

In an attempt to maintain full-dose VLB, we have also adopted continuous infusion therapy for this agent. A recent publication supports the use of continuous infusion VLB, reporting an increased therapeutic index in patients with breast carcinoma. VB_4 consists of the continuous simultaneous infusion of VLB with BLM.

Pharmacological data in an initial pilot study was collected. A radioimmunoassay using an antibody furnished by the Eli Lilly Co. indicated that bolus achieved marked intitial elevations of VLB that rapidly reduced (see figure 1). Continuous infusion VLB reached a steady state at approximately 12 hours. At 0.5 mg/kg and 0.6 mg/kg, the peak level of VLB achieved is 50 and 70 ng/ml. We theorize that the very high peak levels of VLB achieved with bolus may be responsible for the toxicity. Maintaining continuous exposure to the tumor cell with VLB may sustain the high response rate without increasing toxicity.

We have subsequently performed a study with continuous infusion VLB at 3 mg/m². In a pharmacologic study presented at the American Association for Cancer Research (AACR) meetings in 1985, we observed a direct correlation between the peak VLB level achieved at 24 hours and the toxicity.[22] Eleven patients who had VLB levels >6 ng/ml within the first 24 hours developed more profound toxicity compared to those patients maintaining a lower level (see figure 2).

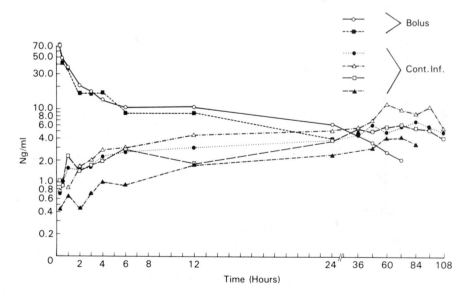

Figure 1. Velban levels, bolus vs. continuous infusion.

Eleven patients were studied through a 5-day infusion of vinblastine sulfate. The dose of vinblastine sulfate was 3 mg/m² daily. The patients' toxicity scores (tables 8 and 9) were performed for the purpose of the study. The toxicity included nonhematological toxicity and infectious complications of myelosuppression. Two groups of patients were identified: group A (5 patients) and group B (6 patients) (see table 9). VLB level was >6 ng/ml in group B and <6 ng/ml in group A. Marked nonhematologic toxicity was noted in group B, whereas patients in group A had very little. The severe complications (pericarditis, rhabdomyolisis, inappropriate secretion of ADH, and severe myalgias requiring analgesics) were all in group B patients. The early peak of VLB level directly correlated with the area under the moment curve in a simple lineographic relationship. Nonhematologic toxicity was present most frequently in those patients with high peak VLB levels, and all patients developed severe myelosuppression. This was common to both groups of patients. The toxicity could also not be related to the clinical presentations of the patients as determined by their nutritional status or tumor volume. Our initial results suggest that there is a direct correlation between the peak VLB level achieved within 24 hours of initiation of infusion and nonhematologic toxicity. Should this be verified in a larger number of patients, pharmacologically directed VLB ther-

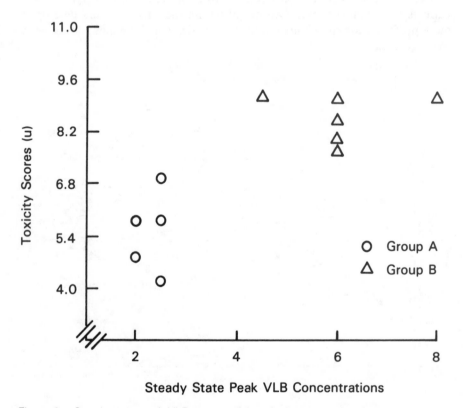

Figure 2.   Steady-state peak VLB concentrations in 2 groups of patients.

apy to achieve the maximum safe dose will be feasible. The study is being expanded.

We believe that pharmacologically directed therapy for patients with germ cell tumors and other malignancies is necessary to achieve safe, yet effective delivery of VLB.

There has been some suggestion in the literature that VLB by continuous infusion may actually be superior to VLB as a bolus in increasing the overall

Table 8. Toxicity Scale for Vinblastine Pharmacology

Nausea/vomiting	1
Ileus	1
Ileus requiring decompression	2
Urine retention	1
Paresthesia	1
Stomatitis	
Grade 1	1
Grade 2	2
Grade 3	3
Myalgia	1
Raynaud's phenomenon	1
Syndrome of inappropriate antidiuretic hormone secretion	1
Orthostatic hypotension	1
Fever of unknown origin with neutropenia	1
Sepsis	1
Pericarditis	1
Rhabdomyolysis	1

Note: Sum of accumulated points equals toxicity score.

Table 9. Nonhematologic Toxicity During Vinblastine Infusion

Toxic manifestation	Group A (5 patients)	Group B (6 patients)
Nausea/vomiting	2	5
Ileus	0	5
Ileus requiring decompression	0	0
Urine retention	0	2
Neuropathy (paresthesia)	0	1
Stomatitis	5	6
Grade 1	5	2
Grade 2	0	2
Grade 3	0	2
Myalgia	0	2
Raynaud's phenomenon	0	0
SIADH*	0	1
Orthostatic hypotension	0	2
Fever of unknown origin with neutropenia	4	5
Sepsis	1	1
Pericarditis	0	1
Rhabdomyolysis	0	1

*Syndrome of inappropriate antidiuretic hormone secretion

response rate. This laboratory information was studied in the treatment of breast carcinoma, and Yap et al initially reported their results suggesting an increased therapeutic index when VLB was delivered in this manner.[23] The data of VB_4 when compared to VB_3 were not comparable. VB_4 is currently used in the context of cyclic chemotherapy; therefore, a comparison of the therapeutic effects of these 2 regimens is impossible. The overall high CR rate and the lack of any initial failure to VB_4 does suggest that patients have a higher therapeutic index with continuous infusion VLB.

A change in the spectrum of toxicity has occurred with the introduction of VB_4. VB_3 toxicity was associated with acute, relatively short-term toxicity, frequently allowing the clinician to rapidly introduce the combination at 2-3-week intervals. Myelosuppression, although severe, was of relatively short duration, and there was rapid rebound. The toxicity was acute and severe, but again of short duration. VB_4 has changed the spectrum of toxicity in that now myelosuppression is now of much longer duration but not as severe. The frequency of ileus and other clinical side effects of VLB-BLM in 100 patients treated are outlined in table 10. Occasional idiosyncratic reactions (pericarditis, urinary retention) do occur. Overall, these appear to be reduced when

Table 10. Toxicity of VB_4 (100 Patients)[1]

	VB_4 Courses[2]	
	Number	Percent
Stomatitis		
Grade 1	98	45.0
Grade 2	39	18.0
Grade 3	6	3.0
Intestinal toxicity		
Obstipation	62	29.0
Paralytic ileus	7	3.0
Pericarditis	7	3.0
Hypertension	9	4.0
Culture-negative leukopenic fever	95	44.0
Culture-positive leukopenic fever	17	8.0
Soft tissue infection	5	2.0
Urinary tract infection	9	4.0
Pneumonia	2	0.9
Drug-induced hepatitis	4	2.0
Pancreatitis		
Rectal abscess		
SIADH[3]		
Anaphylactic reaction		
Clinical systemic candidiasis	1	0.5
Rhabdomyolysis	1	0.5
Viral myocarditis		
Granulomatous disease of unknown		
origin	1	0.5

[1]219 VB_4 courses
[2]Requiring nasogastric tube
[3]Syndrome of inappropriate secretion of antidiuretic hormone

compared to bolus VLB. The degree of myalgias, previously a very significant side effect of bolus VLB, now also is significantly reduced, along with the requirement for I.V. narcotics. Culture-negative leukopenic fevers remain a frequent observation in the VB_4 combinations, occurring in 44% of the courses, whereas only 8% of the courses were associated with culture-positive leukopenic fevers. Soft tissue infections and urinary tract infections occurred, but pneumonia was very rare, and a previously very frequent drug-induced hepatitis was reduced to 2%. Only a single patient suffered rhabdomyolysis. That patient was a very muscular athletic male who experienced muscular pain early in the infusion; he had a very high peak level of VLB and had a rise in CPK with development of myoglobinuria. Among patients with a very muscular habitus, meticulous care with adequate hydration and alkalization of the urine is a necessary precaution. Of interest is that serum-inappropriate ADH secretion, a previously unrecognized occurrence with bolus VLB, now has occurred in a single patient. This is perhaps related to the prolonged serum level exposure of VLB. Pericarditis, which was previously reported to occur with bolus VLB, has occurred more rarely with continuous infusion of the drug; it was present in 7 of the courses, documented by EKG changes in a typical clinical syndrome with a pericardial rub. These EKG changes totally resolved with time and no residual cardiac effect was observed. The frequency and grades of stomatitis are tabulated in table 10. Forty-five percent of the courses were associated with grade 1 stomatitis. The frequency and severity of stomatitis is ameliorated as compared to high-dose bolus VLB.

Our experience with continuous infusion VLB with simultaneous continuous infusion BLM suggests that there is an altered spectrum of toxicity. The idiosyncratic reactions (drug-induced hepatitis, pericarditis) appeared to be reduced. New side effects have occurred (SIADH), but the incidence has been small. Rhabdomyolysis in the very muscular persists as a rare occurrence. Infectious complications frequently occur, but the frequency of paralytic ileus and obstipation appear to be markedly reduced.

Our data indicate also that early peak levels of VLB in the serum are predictors of toxicity.

Prostatic Carcinoma

Agents that are effective in the management of prostatic carcinoma include ADR, mitomycin-C (MIT), and VLB. Other agents of doubtful effectiveness include DDP, methotrexate (MTX), and vincristine (VCR). At the M. D. Anderson Hospital, we have performed a series of sequential trials, the first of which consisted of ADR, MIT, and 5-FU (DMF), a combination that results in a consistent objective response rate.[24] ADR in that study was delivered as an intermittent bolus regimen. Since the studies by Benjamin et al, and with the introduction of new chemotherapy regimens, ADR is used as a continuous infusion. A 24- 96-hour infusion is employed. In view of the increase in stomatitis among patients with a prolonged infusion, 24-hour infusional ADR is delivered in the Genitourinary Oncology Service for patients with prostatic carcinoma. Only those patients with severe heart disease and marked reduction in the ejection fractions at presentation have more prolonged infusions of ADR.

VLB is also an effective agent in the management of prostatic carcinoma. A recent report from our institution documents a 22% objective response rate.[25] Most important, these responses were achieved among patients who had received prior chemotherapy including ADR, MIT, and 5-FU (see table 11). Vinblastine may therefore be a highly effective drug. Vinblastine in that study was used as a continuous infusion at 1.5 mg/m^2 daily for 5 consecutive days. Myelosuppression was a significant but moderate side effect. Most important, an unexpected significant side effect of this regimen was the development of accelerated angina and arrhythmias among patients with established heart disease. Our initial intent was to incorporate an agent in the management of prostatic carcinoma in part due to its lack of cardiac toxicity. It appears that the sympathomimetic effects of VLB can sometimes result in accelerating angina and progression of a previously underlying cardiac disease. Patients receiving continuous infusion should have a prior thorough evaluation for arrhythmias, and these should be managed aggressively prior to the introduction of VLB continuous infusion in the advanced age group of prostatic carcinoma patients (see table 12). Angina must also be adequately controlled prior to the introduction of this agent among patients in this advanced age category. At this dose of VLB chemotherapy, leukopenia frequently occurred, but this could in part be related to poor prognosis and advanced stage with heavy pretreatment of the patients used in that trial. Diffuse marrow involvement and prior radiation therapy or chemotherapy was a frequent occurrence in that study population.

Other potentially effective agents that could lend themselves to continuous infusion in the management of prostatic carcinoma include MIT. The experience at our institution suggests that MIT may be one of the more effective agents in the management of prostatic carcinoma. Laboratory data have been

Table 11. Study Population (Total of 39 Patients)

Characteristic	No. Patients (%)
Performance status[1]	
0 – 1	17 (44)
2	10 (26)
3	6 (15)
4	6 (15)
Predominant site of metastasis	
Axial skeletal or nodal disease	17 (43)
Axial and extremity skeletal involvement	16 (41)
Pulmonary	3 (8)
Liver	3 (8)
Prior therapy[2]	
Radiotherapy	24 (62)
Chemotherapy	25 (64)

[1]Eastern Cooperative Oncology Group criteria
[2]All patients failed hormonal therapy.

presented suggesting that MIT as a continuous infusion increases the therapeutic index and reduces the myelosuppressive effect of this agent. These data have not been reproduced in the single clinical trial performed to evaluate this hypothesis. Therefore, it appears that further trials to ascertain the validity of this concept are justified.

Table 12. Vinblastine Toxicity: Prostatic Cancer

Toxicity	No. of courses
Neutropenic infections	10
Cardiotoxicity	4
Arrhythmias	3
Angina	1
Ileus	1
Myalgias	1

Total: 133 courses

Urothelial Tumors

Urothelial tumors are clearly very responsive to chemotherapy. Although patients treated with advanced disseminated and high-volume disease frequently respond, long-term responses are rare.[26] By the introduction of chemotherapy in lower volume disease, frequent excellent responses are currently seen.[27] Most encouraging are the recently reported complete remissions of long duration either with the earlier introduction of the same chemotherapy regimens that had only modest effectiveness in visceral disease or with the introduction of MTX-DDP combinations.[28,29] The integration of chemotherapy and local therapy (surgery or radiation therapy) appears to hold promise for significant improvements in survival among patients with urothelial tumors. The systematic stages of disease from long local-regional phases to final dissemination lend themselves well to the incorporation of chemotherapy early in the management of urothelial tumors.

Infusion chemotherapy has not been employed in the management of urothelial tumors. Agents that have established use with potential effectiveness as continuous infusion include ADR, VLB, MIT, and DDP. The mean age of the study populations with urothelial tumors at our institution is 62 years. With some frequency, this population includes heavy smokers with COPD. A reduction in the nauseating effects of ADR and reduction in the cardiac side effects of this agent are both desirable in this population; both of these can be achieved by continuous infusion. DDP, perhaps the single most effective agent in the management of urothelial tumors, lends itself to continuous infusion, although the related therapeutic benefit of such an experience remains untested. Intra-arterial infusion and prolonged infusions via hypogastric catheters appear to be another reasonable approach.

28

GYNECOLOGIC MALIGNANCY

Hyman B. Muss, M.D.

GYNECOLOGIC MALIGNANCIES ARE AMONG the most frequent cancers seen in women. In 1985, it is estimated that pelvic malignancy will account for 15% of all new female cancer, including 37,000 new patients with cancer of the endometrium, 18,500 new patients with cancer of the ovary, 15,000 new patients with cancer of the cervix, and almost 4,500 patients with vulvar and vaginal carcinoma, germ cell tumors, and gynecologic sarcomas. Pelvic malignancy will be responsible for 10% of all female cancer deaths.[1] In addition, ovarian cancer remains the third most common cause of female cancer death, followed by cervical and endometrial malignancy.

This review of infusion therapy for gynecologic malignancy will discuss both I.V. and intra-arterial (I.A.) approaches. Intravenous infusion therapy of solid tumors is undergoing renewed interest, due largely to the development of new techniques involving reliable, portable external infusion pumps and implantable delivery devices, which make such therapy more feasible in the outpatient setting. On the other hand, I.A. therapy enjoyed popularity in 1950s and 1960s, but enthusiasm has currently waned due to its technical complexity, need for hospitalization, and the variable and occasionally conflicting treatment results. The explosive development of new chemotherapeutic agents, coupled with new knowledge of the biology of malignant tumors, is likely to renew interest in I.A. approaches for gynecologic malignancy.

Treatment of carcinoma of the cervix, ovary, endometrium, and other gynecologic sites will be discussed in separate sections. To facilitate tabulation of data, a list of abbreviations is presented as table 1. In most publications reviewed, response criteria were similar or identical to those suggested for use by the World Health Organization.[2] Some reports, however, especially in the older literature, used criteria of response that were not precisely defined; when possible, an attempt was made to categorize response in such studies using

The author would like to thank Linda H. Brown of the Medicine Satellite Center for her help in the preparation of this manuscript.

standard criteria. An effort has been made to review all relevant literature. Studies involving only a few patients also have been included because such reports might serve as a basis of further investigation. Because of the small size of many of the trials reviewed, the 95% confidence interval (CI) has been calculated for the reported complete response (CR) plus partial response (PR) rate. Such a calculation is more likely to put small trials with high response rates in proper perspective.

Cancer of the Cervix

Although patients with stages 1 and 2 of cancer of the cervix are generally curable by either surgical or radiation techniques, patients with stages 3 and 4 disease have a poor prognosis, with 5-year survival of 30% and 5%, respectively.[3] Patients who present with advanced local disease, although they may respond initially to radiation therapy, generally recur in the pelvis, with ominous clinical consequences. Such patients with advanced localized disease have in the past been ideal candidates for I.A. therapy, but more recently have been included in I.V. and combined modality therapy programs.

There is good rationale for continuous infusion therapy for carcinoma of the cervix. Most patients have squamous cell histology, and like other squamous cancers, the doubling time would be expected to be long. Shackney and colleagues, in their review of growth patterns of solid tumors, noted a mean doubling time of 87 days for primary squamous carcinoma of the lung,[4] while the doubling time of squamous pulmonary metastases was noted to be 58 days by others.[5] Although one cannot directly extrapolate the growth rate of primary cervix carcinoma from these data, it is likely to be similar. Averette and co-workers labeled normal and neoplastic squamous carcinomas of the female genital tract with tritiated thymidine and measured cytokinetic parameters.[6] These investigators found little difference in the duration of the S and G_2 phases of normal and neoplastic tissues, which were 9 and 5.4 hours, respectively. The labeling index of 27.2% was higher, however, for neoplastic lesions than the index of 16.6% observed for dysplasia. Also, the cycle time for

Table 1. Abbreviations

ACT	— actinomycin		MEL	— melphalan
ADR	— doxorubicin (Adriamycin)		MIT	— mitomycin
Ara-C	— cytarabine (cytosine arabinoside)		MTX	— methotrexate
BLM	— bleomycin		RT	— radiation therapy
CF	— citrovorum factor (leucovorin)		SPI	— spirogermanium[1]
CTX	— cyclophosphamide		VCR	— vincristine
DDP	— cisplatin (cis-platinum)		VLB	— vinblastine
ETO	— etoposide (VP-16)			
5-FU	— 5-fluorouracil		CR	— complete response
GAL	— galactitol[1]		PR	— partial response
HN_2	— nitrogen mustard		95% CI	— 95% confidence interval
HYD	— hydroxyurea			for response

[1]Investigational use only

invasive cancer of 1.4 days was about half as long as that for normal tissue (2.6 days). These data indicate that malignant tissues, even though they have a larger growth fraction, have a cycle time similar to that of normal tissue. Continuous exposure to cytotoxic agents in such tumors is more likely to lead to higher cell kill than with bolus therapy, especially with agents that have short plasma half-lives.

Intravenous Infusion

A variety of I.V. infusion programs have been used in the treatment of advanced cervical cancer. Experience with single-agent therapy, however, has been limited (see table 2). Cisplatin (DDP), the most effective single agent in cervical cancer,[7] with a response rate of 25–30%, has been given by infusion by several investigators. Salem et al treated patients with a variety of malignancies with 20 mg/m^2 of DDP daily for 5 days by continuous infusion. Only 20 patients in this large phase 2 study received DDP alone, with the remainder receiving various other agents in addition.[8] In 4 patients with cervical cancer, no complete or partial responses were recorded; however, it is likely that many of these patients had prior treatment with other agents. Preliminary data from a trial by the Gynecologic Oncology Group comparing DDP 50 mg/m^2 by bolus versus the same dose administered via a 24-hour I.V. infusion indicates a similar response rate for these regimens.[9] Further follow-up in these patients, who have not received prior chemotherapy, should clarify the role of 1-day infusion of this agent. In a phase 1 study, 3 patients with cervical carcinoma were treated with carboplatinum, a DDP analogue, without response.[10] Except for bleomycin (BLM) (see below), the only other single agent adequately studied using prolonged infusion has been vincristine (VCR). Jobson and colleagues treated patients with a 0.25 mg I.V. bolus followed by 0.25 mg/m^2/day for 5 consecutive days.[11] In 11 patients, all of whom had received extensive prior chemotherapy, no responses were noted.

A variety of studies using combination chemotherapy, as well as several using chemotherapy in addition to radiation therapy, have also been completed (see table 2). Three studies[12,13,14] utilized methotrexate (MTX) infusions of low to intermediate dosage for periods of 2–24 hours in combination with other agents. Response rates ranged from 17–45% for these programs. The study of O'Quinn is of special interest.[14] Five of 11 patients treated with his regimen responded, and 6 had their chemotherapy scheduled on the basis of flow cytometry studies from biopsied tumor tissue. It is not possible in this small series to determine if such selectively scheduled chemotherapy is of greater benefit than that given on a fixed timetable, but further studies in this area are warranted. Studies using DDP, doxorubicin (ADR), and fluorouracil (5-FU) infusions in combination with other therapy have also shown substantial response rates in patients with advanced disease.[15,16,17] Yordan and colleagues have treated 11 patients with advanced gynecologic cancer with 5-FU 600 mg/m^2/day using a 4-day continuous infusion along with 50 mg/m^2 of DDP given by bolus on day 1.[18] There have been 8 responses among the first 11 patients treated, including 8 with cervical cancer. Unfortunately, the number of patients studied in most of these trials was small, preventing firm conclusions.

Two groups have combined chemotherapy and radiation therapy as first-line treatment for patients with advanced localized disease. Fluorouracil has been the agent infused in both studies and is attractive when given concurrently with radiation therapy because of its radiation-sensitizing properties.[21] The data from these trials, although preliminary, appear superior to results for radiation alone; however, small numbers of patients and short follow-up times make it difficult to tell whether such combined modality regimens are truly superior to less aggressive treatment.

Table 2. Cervical Cancer: Intravenous Infusion

Author/ref.	Drug	Dose & schedule[1]	Prior chemo Rx	No. patients	CR + PR/(%)	95% CI
Salem[8]	DDP	20/d × 5 d[2]	NS[6]	4	0	0 – 89
Jobson[11]	VCR	0.25/d × 5 d	Yes	11	0	0 – 24
Hakes[12]	MTX VCR	250 – 500/2 h (CF) 1.0 (B)[3]	Some	29	0 + 5 (17)	6 – 36
Forney[13]	MTX CTX ACT 5-FU VCR Ara-C BLM	100/24 h (CF) 600 (B) 0.25 (B) 500 (B) 1.0 (B) 100 Q 6 h × 4 (B) 30 (B)	None	23	0 + 9 (39)	20 – 61
O'Quinn[14]	MTX GAL VCR	1 g/6 h (CF) 100 (B) 1.0 (B)	None	11	2 + 3 (45)	17 – 77
Wade[15]	5-FU DDP	1 g/d × 3 – 5 d 100 (B)	1/7	7	1 + 2 (43)	10 – 82
Sorbe[16]	ADR BLM DDP	40/10 h 10/10 h[4] 50 (B)	None	21	4 + 4 (38)	18 – 62
Lele[17]	DDP ADR CTX	40/6 h 40 (B) 40 (B)	None	20	1 + 3 (20)	6 – 44
Thomas[19]	5-FU MIT RT	1 g/d × 4 d 6 (B) 4,560 rad[5]	None	27	20 + 0 (74)	54 – 89
Kalra[20]	5-FU MIT RT	1 g/d × 5 d 10 (B) 3,000 rad[5]	None	10	6 + 2 (80)	44 – 97

[1]All doses mg/m² unless specified
[2]Most received other drugs concurrently
[3](B)—bolus administration
[4]Total dose
[5]Concurrent with chemotherapy
[6]Not specified

In table 3, infusion chemotherapy programs employing BLM alone and in combination are presented. Because of the initial high response rate reported for BLM when administered as a single-agent bolus,[7] infusion studies were performed to further explore its role in cervical cancer. In a phase 1-2 trial, Ochoa et al[22] noted a 38% CR and PR rate in 32 patients. It is not specified in their report whether these patients had previous chemotherapy. Krakoff et al also used continuous BLM infusion given for a period of 7-11 days.[23] Thirty-two patients who had prior chemotherapy were treated in this fashion, with a 31% response rate. In both of these studies, pulmonary toxicity was substantial, and in each trial, 5 deaths resulted from BLM-induced pulmonary fibrosis.

Table 3. Cervical Cancer: Intravenous Infusion Using Bleomycin

Author/ref.	Drug	Dose & schedule	Prior chemo Rx	No. patients	CR + PR/(%)	95% CI
Ochoa[22]	BLM	0.06 – 0.5/kg/d × 10 d[1]	NS	32	2 + 10 (38)	21 – 56
Krakoff[23]	BLM	0.25/kg/d × 7 – 11 d	Yes	32	2 + 8 (31)	15 – 50
Baker[24]	BLM VCR MIT	30[2]/d × 4 d 0.5 day 1, 4 (B) 20/day 2 (B)	No[3]	41	6 + 10 (39)	24 – 55
Hannigan[25]	BLM VCR	60[2]/d × 2.5 d 1.5 (B)	No	14	0 + 2 (14)	2 – 43
Alberts[26]	BLM VCR MIT DDP	30[2]/d × 4 d 0.5/day 1, 4 10 (B) 50 (B)	No	14	4 + 2 (43)	18 – 71
Surwit[27]	4 4	No RT Concurrent RT	No No	17 7	4 + 4 (47) 1 + 4 (71)	23 – 72 29 – 96
Rosenthal[28]	BLM DDP VCR MTX	10/7 h × 5 d 20/7 h × 5 d 1.0 (B) 40 (B)	No	15	3 + 7 (67)	38 – 88
Israel[29]	BLM DDP	6/d × 5 d 20/d × 5 d (B)	No	5	2 + 1 (60)	15 – 95
Daghestani[30]	BLM DDP	10/d × 3 d[5] 120 (B) day 1	No	24	0 + 13 (54)	33 – 74
Hakes[31]	BLM DDP RT[6]	20/d × 3 d 75 (B) 4,200 rad	No	30	25 + 0 (83)	65 – 94
Bauer[32]	BLM DDP MTX RT[6]	20/d × 3 – 7 d 20/d × 5 d (B) 200 day 15, 22 (CF) "high dose"	No	9	0 + 7 (78)	40 – 97

[1]Until toxicity
[2]Total dose
[3]No prior Rx with study drugs
[4]Same as Alberts[26]
[5]Day 5 to 7
[6]Following chemotherapy

Subsequent to these trials, numerous studies have included BLM infusion as part of a combination chemotherapy regimen.[24-30] A variety of other agents have been used in these studies, with response rates of 14-67%. It is noteworthy that in several of these trials, a substantial number of patients have achieved CR. In this regard, the results of Alberts[26] and Surwit[27] are notable, with CR rates of 28% and 23%, respectively, some patients sustaining remissions of long duration. Unfortunately, in all of these reports, only small numbers of patients have been studied, and none has been randomized against single agents or other regimens. Toxicity for these combination regimens has ranged from moderate to severe, and median survival has generally been less than 1 year in spite of high remission rates. Two recent studies in patients with advanced localized disease have used infusion chemotherapy prior to radiation therapy with impressive preliminary results.[31,32] Hakes et al reported an 83% response rate in 30 patients who had not had prior therapy using 2 cycles of a chemotherapy program combining BLM infusion and DDP followed by radiation therapy.[31] A similar response rate of 78% in 9 patients was noted by Bauer.[32]

The role of I.V. infusion therapy in cervical cancer cannot be ascertained from these studies. There have been very few single-agent infusion therapy studies in untreated patients, and combination regimens using infusion have generally been limited to small numbers of patients, with variable results. Although combination chemotherapy programs appear to be superior to single-agent regimens,[7] phase 3 studies confirming such superiority are lacking. Most responses to chemotherapy are partial and of short duration, with the median survival of patients with advanced disease generally being less than 1 year. The CR rate of 15-29% reported by several investigators[24,26-28] is worthy of note, as only such patients are likely to derive long-term benefit from chemotherapy with the potential for cure. Unfortunately, none of the infusion studies reported contains enough patients to accurately assess the durability of CR. These data indicate a need for large randomized trials in cervical cancer to determine the relative merits of combination chemotherapy versus single-agent treatment and the possible benefits of infusion.

Intra-Arterial Infusion

Intra-arterial chemotherapy for cervical cancer was first tried more than 4 decades ago, with the initial trials using nitrogen mustard.[33-35] Numerous investigations have been carried out since that time, both with single-agent and combination regimens (see table 4). Patients selected for such treatment generally have had advanced localized disease not amenable to cure with surgery or radiation therapy or have had recurrent disease in the pelvis after initial therapy. Methods for arterial access have varied, with both percutaneous and operative procedures used for catheter placement. In addition, several trials have used isolated perfusion techniques.[36,37] Percutaneous approaches generally have used the femoral route, with catheter placement in the descending aorta just above the bifurcation. Intraoperative placement has included unilateral or bilateral catheterization of iliac, gluteal, or hypogastric arteries. The distribution of arterial blood flow in such patients has been estimated by

Table 4. Cervical Cancer: Intra-Arterial Therapy

Author/ref.	Drug	Dose & schedule	Prior chemo Rx	No. patients	CR + PR/(%)	95% CI
Cromer[33]	HN$_2$	6/d × 6–13 d	No	14	0 + 9 (64)[1]	35–87
Boiman[34]	HN$_2$	0.89/kg/d × 16 d	No	8	0	0–31
Krakoff[35]	HN$_2$	0.4/kg (single dose)	No	6	0 + 2 (33)[1]	4–78
Trussell[38]	MTX	50/d × 7–14 d (CF)[3]	No	14	1 + 7 (57)[1]	29–82
Bateman[41]	MTX	5/d × 6–7 d	No	12	0 + 7 (58)[1]	28–85
Laufe[39]	MTX	50/d × 5–6 d (CF)	No[5]	4	0 + 2 (59)[1]	7–93
Calvo[46]	DDP	75–150/4 h	No	2	0 + 2 (100)	16–100
Carlson[40]	DDP	120/2 h	No	9	0 + 3 (33)	7–70
Morrow[48]	BLM	20/7 d 59 10 wk	No	9	0 + 3 (33)	7–70
Kraybill[49]	ADR	0.4/kg/d × 5	NS	1	0	0–95
Lifshitz[50]	MTX VCR	60–200/2 d[4] 1–2 (B)	Some	12	0 + 1 (8)	0–38
Boutselis[36]	5-FU MTX MEL	20/kg/h 5/kg/h 1.5/kg/h	NS	7	0 + 5 (71)[2]	29–96
Averette[6]	MTX HYD VCR	50 d × 4 d (CF) 4 g (PO) 2[3] (B)	No	36	0 + 8 (22)	10–39
Swenerton[51]	BLM VCR MIT	45/d × 2 2[3] (B) × 2 20/6 h	No[5]	20	0 + 3 (15)	3–38
Kim[44]	VCR MIT BLM	2[3] (B)-I.V. 10 (B) 20–40/24 h	No	19	0 + 7 (37)	16–62
Smith[52]	5-FU RT[7] MTX RT[7]	10/kg/d × 15 5,000 rad 10/kg/d × 15 5,000 rad	No No	11 9	4 + 0 (36) 3 + 0 (33)	11–69 7–70
Falappa[42]	MTX ADR RT[8]	10/12 h[6] 10/12 h 5,000 rad	No	25	10 + 10 (80)	59–93
Kavanagh[53]	VCR MIT BLM DDP RT[8]	2[3] (B) 10/4 h × 3 25/30/24 h 100/24 hr Not specified	No	10	0 + 6 (60)	26–88

[1]No standard response criteria
[2]Includes 25–50% response
[3]Total dose
[4]Patients received either single-agent MTX or combination
[5]Three had single agent chemotherapy
[6]Drugs repeated in succession
[7]Concurrent with chemotherapy
[8]Following chemotherapy

several techniques, including the use of radiopaque contrast agents,[33,38,39,40] the administration of fluoroscein with the examination of either tumor or skin with ultraviolet light,[38,41-43] or the administration of isotopes for radionuclide scanning.[44] These studies have indicated that although pelvic tumors are usually amenable to infusion therapy, the distribution of drug may vary. In a recent trial, Kim et al used technetium 99[m]-labeled macroaggregated albumin particles to measure drug distribution in patients given therapy by internal iliac infusions.[44] Increased activity in the tumor bed was seen in 11/19 patients; however, in almost half the trials, significant asymmetry of drug distribution (75:25) was noted. Such data indicate that even with meticulous technique, drug distribution to the tumor may vary substantially.

Initial single-agent therapy with nitrogen mustard[33-35] or MTX [38,39,41,45] resulted in response rates of 0–64%. Oberfield treated 52 patients with a variety of primary pelvic sites with either MTX (50 mg/day for 7 days with leucovorin rescue), 5-FU (5–7.5 mg/kg/day) or fluorodeoxyuridine (0.1–0.3 mg/kg/day), and noted objective responses in 16 patients.[43] In addition, 2 small studies have used I.A. infusion of DDP,[40,46] with several PR noted. The small numbers of patients and variable response criteria make these trials hard to interpret, and almost all responses have tended to be brief, with total median survivals of less than 1 year. Of importance, however, was the frequent and dramatic improvement in disabling pelvic pain that occurred shortly after infusion in many patients. In several trials, more than half of those treated experienced such pain relief, which was attributed to a direct effect of the chemotherapeutic agent on afferent pain fibers in the area of the malignancy.[47] Single-agent BLM infusion was studied by Morrow et al in 16 patients.[48] In this trial, 4 patients developed renal failure thought to be due to BLM, a rarely reported side effect of this drug. The experience with I.A. ADR is too small to determine if this agent has any role in pelvic infusion therapy; however, Kraybill and colleagues have defined a phase 2 schedule for future trials.[49] Combination I.A. chemotherapy has been used by several investigators, with response similar to single-agent treatment.[6,36,44,50,51] Averette et al treated 36 patients with a combination of MTX, hydroxyurea, and VCR.[6] The schedule of drug administration was based on cell kinetic studies in the patients treated, and although only 8 developed a PR (22%), 2 of these patients remain alive and in remission at 7 and 8 years, respectively. These authors also noted a marked decrease in pain in almost two-thirds of the patients.

There have been 3 trials using I.A. chemotherapy with radiation therapy. Smith and co-workers administered radiation therapy concurrently with either 5-FU or MTX.[52] With each agent, approximately one-third of the patients responded to treatment; however, one cannot determine whether such combined modality therapy was superior to either modality when used alone. In 2 other reports, I.A. chemotherapy infusion was followed by irradiation. Falappa et al noted 10 CR in 25 patients using an alternating infusion schedule of MTX and ADR given over a 12-hour period for 8–12 consecutive courses; such responses were noted prior to radiation therapy.[42] Kavanagh et al noted 6 PR in 10 patients utilizing VCR, mitomycin (MIT), BLM, and DDP, the latter 2 agents given by 24-hour infusion.[51] Severe toxicity was noted; however, following 3 courses of chemotherapy, 4 patients had no evidence of malignancy upon repeat biopsy.

The role of I.A. chemotherapy in cervical cancer is unclear. In patients with advanced localized disease, responses usually have been partial and brief; however, a small percent of patients may do well for long periods. Improvement in pain can be dramatic, and I.A. therapy should be considered in patients with intractable pelvic pain due to recurrent gynecologic cancer. The use of I.A. chemotherapy as an adjunct to surgery or irradiation in patients with early-stage disease deserves further trial. Agents with radiosensitizing properties, such as 5-FU,[21] DDP,[54] and others that can infused locally and in high concentrations, would have the advantage of enhancing radiation effects in addition to cytotoxicity. Collins has reviewed the pharmacologic rationale of regional drug delivery[55] and has defined the most favorable circumstances as being the use of drugs with high total body clearances to sites of delivery with low regional exchange rates. Obviously, drugs that require activation in other sites (cyclophosphamide) have no regional delivery advantage unless infused into the site of activation. For I.A. infusion through either low-flow (100 ml/min.) or high-flow (1,000 ml/min.) arteries, several antimetabolites have the maximum theoretical advantage for regional infusion, including thymidine, 5-FU, fluorodeoxyuridine, and cytosine arabinoside (ara-C). Carmustine (BCNU), ADR, and DDP have moderate theoretical advantage when given by such route. MTX, because of its low total body clearance and high regional exchange rate in the liver, theoretically is of little benefit when given by I.A. infusion. Future trials using drugs that theoretically have greatest advantage when given by regional infusion should be considered. DDP and 5-FU, which display such advantage and which might be used concurrently with irradiation, are ideal candidates.

Ovarian Cancer

There have been only a limited number of infusion therapy trials in ovarian cancer; a summary of these reports is presented in table 5. These studies must be measured against the current standard of care — DDP-containing combination regimens. Such combination programs have led to complete clinical responses in about half of those treated.[56] However, the value of such response is tempered by the observation that such clinical remissions have led to modest, if any, improvement in long-term survival, with less than half of those with clinical complete response found to be disease-free at "second look" surgery. DDP[8,57] and vinblastine (VLB)[58,59] have been used as single agents in phase 1 and 2 trials without benefit. In these studies, however, patients had extensive prior chemotherapy, diminishing the likelihood for response. FUDR[60] and VCR[11] have also been used in small number of patients without benefit. Spirogermanium,[61], mitomycin,[62] and carboplatinum[10] have been evaluated in phase 1 trials, but the number of patients treated was small and no conclusions regarding the benefit of these drugs when given by infusion can be drawn. It is unlikely that any agent studied in such heavily treated patients is likely to be beneficial, and further trials are warranted.

Combination chemotherapy using infusion has been used by several investigators. Izbicki et al treated 29 patients, none of whom had received prior chemotherapy, with cyclophosphamide (CTX) and 5-FU.[63] They noted 9 CR and 11 PR in this group, with a median duration of response of 18 months. The dose-limiting toxicity was stomatitis, but life-threatening toxicity was seen in only 1 patient. This combination is intriguing, since it might be used as an alternating noncross-resistant regimen with DDP in a first-line treatment program. Vriesendorp et al administered high-dose chemotherapy with CTX and etoposide (VP-16) to 2 heavily treated patients with ovarian cancer who had failed prior treatment with DDP-containing regimens.[64] Both patients were given autologous marrow for rescue and attained CR of 10+ months' duration. Such an approach deserves further trial in the research setting. Drapkin et al delivered infusions of MTX, VLB, and DDP sequentially over a 72– 96-hour period.[65] Six patients had failed prior combination therapy with DDP. Five responses were seen, but 3 patients experienced severe toxicity.

Table 5. Ovarian Cancer: Infusion Therapy Trials

Author/ref.	Drug	Regimen Dose (M) schedule	Prior chemo Rx	No. patients	CR + PR/(%)	95% CI
Boiman[34]	HN$_2$	0.89 mg/kg/d × 7−8 d (I.A.)[1]	No	8	0	0−45
Krakoff[35]	HN$_2$	0.4 mg/kg × 1 d (I.A.)	No	6	0 + 2 (33)	4−78
Salem[8]	DDP	20/d × 5 d[2]	Yes	22	0[3]	0−13
Kavanagh[58]	VLB	1.0−1.4/d × 5 d	Yes	16	0	0−17
Shah[59]	VLB	20/d × 5 d	Yes	16	0	0−17
Papac[60]	FUDR	1 mg/kg/d × 3−16 d	NS	1	0	0−95
Jobson[11]	VCR	0.25/d × 5 d	Yes	3	0	0−63
Legha[61]	SPI	100−375/d × 5 d 100−200/d × 30 d[4]				
Izbicki[63]	CTX 5-FU	400/d × 3−4 d (B) 1 g/d × 4 d	No	29	9 + 11 (69)	49−85
Vriesendorp[64]	CTX ETO AM[6]	7 g[5]/d × 3 d 900/d × 3 d d 7	Yes	2	2 + 0 (100)	23−100
Drapkin[65]	MTX VLB DDP	1 g/24 h, d 1 (CF) 12−16/24 h, d 2 75−100/24 h, d 3	Yes	10	0 + 5[7] (50)	19−81

[1]I.A.—Intra-arterial
[2]Alone or in combination with other agents
[3]No response mentioned in manuscript but not clearly specified
[4]Median duration for continuous infusion
[5]Total dose
[6]AM—autologous marrow
[7]Standard response criteria not used

Intra-arterial therapy of ovarian cancer has been limited to only a few trials. Two studies of nitrogen mustard disclosed no response in 1 series of 8 patients,[34] and 2/6 PR in another.[35] Using a complicated closed perfusion technique,[37] 1 response lasting 21+ months was seen in 1 of 3 ovarian cancer patients treated. Intra-arterial infusion of ovarian cancer is unlikely to be an effective approach. Patients with ovarian cancer generally present with stage 3 disease, with multiple metastatic sites within the abdomen including peritoneal surfaces, diaphragm, and para-aortic nodes. The vascular supply to such a wide distribution of metastases makes it unlikely that arterial infusion would have any role in such patients; patients with limited disease (stages 1 and 2) are more likely to be adequately treated with surgery.

Except for the study of Izbicki, there have been no adequate trials of I.V. infusion therapy in untreated patients. Further studies of continuous I.V. infusion appear warranted in this malignancy.

Other Sites

Endometrium

Deppe et al treated 13 patients with endometrial cancer with DDP 3 mg/kg as a 2–4 hour I.V. infusion.[66] All patients had received prior chemotherapy, and 2 CR and 2 PR were noted. Toxicity was moderate. Jobson and co-workers treated 2 patients with VCR infusion, but neither responded.[11] Aisner et al treated 2 patients with a continuous infusion of VP-16 in a phase 1 trial, but no benefit was reported.[67] Boiman[34] and Krakoff et al[35] used I.A. nitrogen mustard in 3 patients, with 1 response. Chemotherapy for patients with advanced or metastatic endometrial carcinoma is not yet of substantial benefit. The most effective single agents in metastatic endometrial cancer include ADR and DDP; however, only 9–33% of treated patients achieve response, which is usually partial and brief.[68] Combination regimens have demonstrated better response rates than single agents in small trials, with response as high as 72%; these results are not convincingly superior to single-agent treatment, and in several small randomized trials, no benefit for combination therapy has been shown when compared to single-agent therapy. Infusion therapy for this site is worth further consideration in the research setting.

Vulva and Vagina

As with endometrial carcinoma, only few patients with vulvar and vaginal carcinoma have been treated with infusion chemotherapy. Krakoff et al noted no responses in 6 patients treated with I.V. BLM infusion.[23] Kalra treated 3 patients with 5-FU 1 g/day for 5 days by infusion, MIT 10 mg/m^2 by bolus, and concurrent radiation.[24] Three CR were noted, 2 in the vulva and 1 in the vagina. Cromer treated 2 patients with I.A. nitrogen mustard without benefit.[33] Using MTX, Lifshitz saw no response in 2 patients with vulvar cancer,[50] and Kraybill[49] noted no response in 1 patient treated with ADR. Vulvar and vaginal carcinomas are uncommon, and obtaining adequate numbers of patients for trial is difficult. Like other squamous cell carcinomas, infusion therapy using 5-FU, DDP, MIT, and other agents with or without irradiation is worthy of investigation, and should be considered by large institutions and cooperative groups that have the ability to accrue adequate numbers of patients for study.

Germ Cell Malignancies

Ovarian germ cell tumors are uncommon, potentially curable malignancies that generally appear in young women. Recent programs using treatment similar to that of metastatic testicular carcinoma have demonstrated substantial CR rates in such patients, many of whom are probably cured.[69] Carlson et al treated 7 patients with ovarian germ cell tumors with a combination of VLB, BLM, and DDP.[70] DDP 100 mg/m^2 was infused over a 24-hour period. VLB was given on days 1 and 2, and BLM was given weekly. One patient had received prior chemotherapy. Seven CR were noted, and most of these patients continue to do well. Whether this method of using VLB-BLM-DDP is superior to other schedules is not clear. The briefer treatment duration, however, is probably more cost-effective than the commonly used 5-day regimens, and further trials with Carlson's schedule are warranted.

Conclusion

Intravenous infusion therapy has not had adequate study in gynecologic malignancies. Except for cervical cancer, where a large number of trials have used bleomycin infusion generally in combination with other agents, only sparse data are available. It is unlikely, however, from the information available that single-agent infusion therapy is likely to be superior to bolus therapy with currently available agents. Nevertheless, continuous infusions, especially when given over protracted periods, are attractive for study because of the slower growth rate and doubling time of gynecologic malignancies. The availability of new technology that makes it possible to use protracted continuous infusion in the outpatient setting should lead to further investigation in these areas. The use of infusion chemotherapy concurrent with irradiation, especially with agents that are radiosensitizing as well as cytotoxic, is especially attractive for further study.

Intra-arterial therapy trials, which appear to have fallen out of favor a decade ago, are worthy of reconsideration. Such trials should be considered for untreated patients who have disease limited to the pelvis and whose likelihood of cure with conventional methods is small. In such patients, treatment with I.A. chemotherapy prior to or concurrent with radiation therapy or surgery may hold promise. Chemotherapy prior to irradiation or surgery has resulted in impressive preliminary results in carcinomas of the head and neck,[71] esophagus,[72] and anus.[73] Squamous cell tumors of the cervix, vulva, and vagina should be considered for similar approaches in selected patients.

29

SOFT TISSUE AND OSTEOGENIC

SARCOMAS

Jacob J. Lokich, M.D., Richard Lackman, M.D., and
Arthur J. Weiss, M.D.

TUMORS OF THE SOFT tissue and bone, classified as mesenchymal tumors, are relatively rare; the annual incidence in the United States is fewer than 5,000 cases. A major proportion of these tumors occur in the pediatric age group in the form of osteogenic or other bone sarcomas and rhabdomyo sarcomas. The adult types of sarcomas are the soft tissue variants, dominated by the malignant fibrohistiocytoma. The natural history and clinical behavior of the various categories of soft tissue sarcomas are related to the stage and histologic grade of the tumor, site of the primary tumor and, to some extent, the pathologic subtype.

In reviewing the chemotherapeutic approach to the mesenchymal tumors, it is important to separate the clinical trials for soft tissue sarcoma and those for osteogenic sarcoma as well as distinguish childhood from adult sarcomas. In addition, it should be recognized that the evaluation of response in the sarcomas, particularly osteosarcoma, is distinctive in that the parameters employed often relate to a pathologic quantitation of tumor necrosis and survival related to the fact that chemotherapy is often a part of the multimodality approach to primary tumors.

This selective review of the chemotherapy of soft tissue and osteosarcoma will focus on the relatively sparse clinical trials in which systemic or regional infusion of chemotherapeutic agents has been applied for the 2 classes of sarcomas. Experience in adult tumors will be emphasized.

Standard Bolus Chemotherapy

The chemotherapy of mesenchymal tumors has been dominated by the use of doxorubicin (ADR), most commonly in combination with other drugs, although newer agents such as cisplatin and ifosfamide have more recently been explored, predominantly in previously treated patients.

Soft Tissue Tumors

The 4 major drugs evaluated in soft tissue tumors are ADR, methotrexate (MTX), cisplatin (DDP), and ifosfamide (see table 1). Although other drugs such as dacarbazine (DTIC), vincristine (VCR), actinomycin D, and cyclophosphamide (CTX) have also been employed in multidrug regimens, the individual activities of these agents in soft tissue tumors have been difficult to glean from the literature, and the contribution of each of these agents to the anthracycline component is as yet unclear.

ADR single-agent therapy at a dose of 75 mg/m^2 at 3-week intervals continues to be evaluated in clinical trials. The drug is presently being studied as a single agent in prospective trials compared to the newer anthracycline analogues, and in the study by Bramwell et al, in 38 evaluable patients a 32% response rate was observed, with 1 complete response (CR).[1] Although phase 2 studies of anthracycline-based combinations suggest an augmentation of the response rates—particularly the CR rate—for combination chemotherapy, comparative trials do not show an advantage for multidrug regimens. In the original series of combined CTX, VCR, ADR, and DTIC, the response rate was similar to that achieved with single-agent anthracycline.[2]

MTX as a single agent has been employed in both standard-dose[3] and in high-dose regimens with leucovorin rescue.[4] In a report on 3 regimens by Subramanian and Wiltshaw, MTX was administered at a dose rate of 2.5–10 mg orally daily for 15 days or by infusion for up to 36 hours both systemically and intra-arterially. In this study, it is difficult to dissect the various treatment schedules in terms of the contribution to the 39% response rate observed in 41 patients, but the activity for MTX is clear. High-dose MTX combined with leucovorin as revealed in collected series does not appear to have substantive activity in soft tissue sarcoma, in contrast to the experience in osteogenic sarcoma.

Table 1. Antineoplastic Agents Evaluated with Treatment of Soft Tissue Tumors (Bolus Schedules)

Agent/reference	Response rate	
	Single agent	Combination
Doxorubicin[1,2]	11/38 (29%)	28/95 (30%)
Methotrexate[3,4]	15/41 (39%)	12/57 (21%)[1]
Cisplatin[4]	6/73 (8%)[1]	
Ifosfamide[5,6]	15/40 (38%)	6/12 (50%)

[1]Collected series

DDP has similarly been evaluated sporadically, but in a collected series of 3 reports totaling 73 patients, only an 8% response rate was achieved.[4] It is perplexing that DDP and high-dose MTX, which have apparent activity in osteo-genic sarcoma, appear to have no meaningful activity in soft tissue sarcomas. This apparent paradox may be related to the lack of a rigorous evaluation of these agents in previously untreated patients.

Ifosfamide is the newest agent with activity to be identified in soft tissue sarcoma. In a large series of 40 patients, one-third of whom had received prior therapy, a 38% response rate was observed, with 6 patients achieving CR.[5] In addition, multidrug regimens with ifosfamide combined with etoposide (VP-16) or with DDP in smaller series have achieved response rates of 50% or greater.[6]

Osteogenic Sarcoma

Chemotherapy trials in osteogenic sarcoma are distinctive in that drug activ-ity in metastatic disease is different from the activity as defined by tumor necrosis in primary tumors. Adjuvant trials, particularly in the context of limb-sparing surgery, emphasize tumor necrosis as a criterion of response. Table 2 indicates a collection of selected trials in which, for the most part, standard criteria of objective tumor response have been employed. The 3 most prominent agents employed in advanced osteogenic sarcomas have been ADR, DDP, and MTX.

The initial trial of ADR was reported by Cortes et al in a series of 87 patients evaluated in a phase 1 trial followed by a phase 2 study in advanced disease and, finally, in an adjuvant trial.[7] In the phase 2 trial, 7/17 patients responded, and in this trial ADR was administered as a bolus on 4 consecutive days at a dose of 20 mg/m^2/day. Trials of combination chemotherapy with ADR as a primary agent had been variably reported. In the small study by Pratt et al, 5/19 patients responded to ADR combined with DDP.[8]

DDP appears to have activity in osteogenic sarcoma, in contrast to its lack of activity in soft tissue sarcoma. Ochs et al observed responses in 5/8 patients with advanced osteogenic sarcoma, all of whom had received prior adjuvant ADR therapy and 6 had received high-dose MTX as well.[9] The bolus schedule for DDP included some patients who received 20 mg/m^2/day for 5 consecutive days

Table 2. Antineoplastic Agents Evaluated in Treatment of Osteogenic Sarcoma (Bolus Schedules)

Agent/reference	Response rate	
	Single agent	Combination
Doxorubicin[7,8]	7/17 (41%)	5/19 (26%)
Cisplatin[8,9]	5/8 (62%)	5/19 (26%)
Methotrexate[10,11]	38/44 (88%)	22/57 (38%)
Cyclophosphamide		
CYVADIC[2]		7/29 (24%)
BCD[11]		17/21 (77%)

and some who received a bolus of 120 mg on a single day. Combination chemotherapy reports with DDP are sparse. The report of DDP-ADR combination chemotherapy indicated above was in previously untreated patients with one exception, and the response rate of 26% is not different from that in a single-agent experience.

MTX has been active in osteogenic sarcoma only in the context of high-dose delivery systems with leucovorin rescue, and as a generality the dose of delivery has been upward of 12 g/m^2.[10] The response rate of 88% was by primary tumor evaluation, and this is complemented by responses in pulmonary metastasis in 4/5 patients so evaluated. Combination chemotherapy regimens in which high-dose MTX is added are difficult to evaluate in terms of response rate because the majority of such trials have been performed in the context of adjuvent therapy. In fact, in the study by Rosen et al of 57 patients, only 22 (38%) responded to the high-dose MTX alone based on analysis of the histologic effect on the primary tumor. However, within this subgroup, only 1 of 22 patients has subsequently relapsed, indicating that the tumor effect may predict for prognosis.

Although CTX has become a part of the primary adjuvant treatment of osteosarcoma for some groups, the effectiveness of this drug as a single agent has not been defined. The original CYVADIC program reported a response rate of 24%, and the more recent program of Rosen et al, in which CTX is combined with a bleomycin (BLM) and actinomycin-D, achieved a response rate of 77%.[11]

Regional Infusion Chemotherapy

Intra-arterial (I.A.) delivery of antineoplastic agents has been employed exceptionally and predominantly in osteogenic sarcoma of the extremities. The most common agents applied have been ADR and, more recently, DDP (see table 3).

Following the initial pilot study demonstrating the feasibility of I.A. delivery of ADR, Eilber et al employed regional infusion in a combined modality treatment program for osteogenic sarcoma. Sequentially, ADR infusion for 3 days with preoperative radiation was combined with limb-sparing surgery.[12] The series was subsequently expanded from the initial 17 patients to a total of 83 patients and an additional 100 patients with soft tissue sarcoma.[13] In the collected experience at this single institution, the median survival for osteogenic sarcoma was greater than 48 months, and in the patients with soft tissue sarcoma, a 76% survival at 2 years was achieved. Inasmuch as the thrust of these studies involved adjuvant or multidisciplinary therapy, there are no specific data on tumor response except as measured by local control and survival.

Extended ADR infusion over 8 days without concomitant radiation but with surgery performed on day 12 was studied by Azzarelli et al.[14] All patients had extremity soft tissue sarcomas; 6/13 demonstrated tumor reduction, and 8 remained without evidence of disease. The systemic effect of the drug was demonstrated by a nadir for leukopenia of 1,900 WBC per cc and alopecia in all patients. Jaffe et al used ADR infusion for much shorter periods in a small series of patients in which tumor necrosis up to 90% was observed in more than half the patients.[15]

The clinical activity of DDP in osteogenic sarcoma has been established and extended to I.A. delivery, although the pharmacologic advantage for I.A. infusion or for this agent is unclear.[16] Two studies have employed related short-term infusion of DDP for 2 hours in pediatric and adult osteogenic sarcoma.[17,18] The dose of delivery has been 120 to 150 mg/m², and in both groups adjunctive chemotherapy in the form of systemic infusion ADR[18] or high-dose MTX[17] has been added. The measurement of response was on the basis of tumor necrosis that correlated precisely with survival in that greater than 90% tumor necrosis was associated with an 85% disease-free survival compared to 24% disease-free survival in patients with less than 90% tumor necrosis.

The experience with the antimetabolites MTX and 5-FU has been meager. MTX had a remarkable response rate, as indicated earlier in the study by Subramanian and Wiltshaw in which an unstated proportion of patients received regional MTX.[3] Jaffe et al employed high-dose MTX delivered over a 6-hour period in 9 patients, 4 of whom demonstrated tumor necrosis.[19] The experience with 5-FU has been reported by Akahoshi et al in a large series of patients with soft tissue sarcoma.[20] However, patients received only a weekly bolus of this drug in spite of the extended period up to 48 days of treatment. They also received bolus MIT and MTX on a weekly basis, with some patients also receiving radiation.

In a multiagent program at Thomas Jefferson University, the fluoropyrimidine floxuridine (FUDR) is administered intra-arterially along with ADR and DDP, employing the regimen described in figure 1. Sequentially, ADR is administered at a dose of 8 mg/m²/day as a continuous I.A. infusion until toxicity is shown. Cisplatin is administered as a bolus infusion just prior to and after

Table 3. Regional Delivery of Antineoplastic Agents for Extremity Soft Tissue (STS) or Osteogenic Sarcoma (OS)

Agent/study	Reference	Dose Rate	Infusion duration	Tumor	Comment
Doxorubicin					
Eilber et al	12	30 mg/d	72 h	OS	86% TN*; 14/17 survive
Eilber et al	13	30 mg/d	72 h	STS	76% survival; 100 pts.
Eilber et al	13	30 mg/d	72 h	OS	Med. survival > 48 mo
Azarelli et al	14	100 mg/m²	8 d	STS	13/13 TN
Jaffe et al	15	45 – 75 mg/m²	6 – 24 h	OS	3/5 TN 90%
Cisplatin					
Jaffe et al	17	150 mg/m²	2 h	OS	6/11 TN
Benjamin	18	120 mg/m²	2 h	OS	58% 2 g survival 40 pts.
Methotrexate					
Jaffe et al	19	12.5 mg/m²	6 h	OS	4/9 TN
5-fluorouracil					
Akahoshi et al	20	1 – 1.5 g	weekly	STS	56 pts., TN present

*TN = Tumor necrosis

completion of the intra-arterial course of ADR. FUDR at 18 mg/m²/day is administered for a 4- 8-day period. The regimen has been associated with the usual spectrum of toxicity, including ADR-associated stomatitis and FUDR-associated local cutaneous erythema. In 18 patients, objective tumor regression was observed in all patients measured clinically or by computerized tomography. The program is ongoing.

Systemic Infusional Chemotherapy

The major agents administered systemically on an infusion schedule have been ADR and DDP (see table 4). From a single institution in a combined modality program for osteogenic or soft tissue sarcoma, 4-day continuous infusion ADR was administered predominantly in conjunction with additional agents. In the osteogenic sarcoma program, adjunctive I.A. DDP was administered in patients with primary tumors. In the soft tissue sarcoma program, ADR was administered for a similar interval admixed with DTIC. The latter study in patients with advanced disease achieved a response rate of 53% in patients with metastatic disease, comparable to the previous experience in soft tissue sarcoma employing a bolus rate for ADR. In a much smaller trial of patients

Drug	Dose rate	Duration
Adriamycin	8 mg/m²/d	Daily to toxicity or cumulative dose of 120 mg/m² (15 days)
5 FUDR	0.5 mg/kg/d	Daily admixed with Adriamycin to development of cutaneous reaction
Cisplatin	120 mg/m²	6-hour infusion, day 4 and day 13

Figure 1. Three-drug intra-arterial infusion schema for extremity soft tissue and osseous sarcoma administered preoperatively.

Table 4. Systemic Infusion Chemotherapy for Soft Tissue or Osteogenic Sarcoma

Agent/study	Reference	Tumor	Dose rate	Comment
Doxorubicin				
Benjamin et al	18	OS	22.5 mg/m²/d × 4 d	58% 2 yr survival
Legha et al	21	STS	15 to 22.5 mg/m²/d × 4 d	15/28 (53%) response
Lokich et al	22	STS	3 mg/m²/d × 30 d	1/14 response
Cisplatin				
Gasparini et al	21	OS	100 mg/m²/24 h × 1 d	7/37 (19%) response
Gasparini et al	24	OS	40 mg/m²/24 h × 3 d	5/5 response Combined with MTX and VCR
Periwinkle alkaloids				
Vinblastine	25	STS	1.5 mg/m²/24 h × 5 d	0/15 response

receiving protracted infusion ADR at a dose of 3 mg/m²/day, only 1/14 patients, most of them extensively treated previously, responded.[22]

Systemic infusion of DDP has been reported in sequential trials by Gasparini et al[23,24] in osteogenic sarcoma. The initial study administered the agent at a dose of 120 mg/m²/24 hours for a single day in patients extensively treated previously with high-dose MTX, ADR, and VCR. Seven of 37 patients responded, for a response rate of 19%. In an earlier report, a 3-day infusion of DDP administered at a dose of 40 mg/m²/24 hours in conjunction with MTX and VCR achieved responses in 5/5 patients.

The only other agents evaluated on the infusion schedule have been vinblastine (VLB) and vindesine (VDS).[25] In this study in soft tissue sarcoma, VLB was administered at a dose of 1.5 mg/m²/24 hours for 5 days and VDS at a dose of 1.2 mg/m²/day for 5 days. No responses were observed in the entire series in heavily pretreated patients.

Combined Modality Therapy

The adjuvant applications of chemotherapy in osteogenic and soft tissue sarcoma are complicated by a relative paucity of prospective randomized trials in these rare tumors and by the diversity of approaches employing a variety of chemotherapy regimens, regional delivery systems, and limb-sparing surgery. Nonetheless, the randomized[26] as well as nonrandomized studies[27] strongly support a role for chemotherapy in primary management of these diseases.

Infusional delivery systems, both regional and systemic, have had relatively limited clinical trials for the known active agents in these tumors in spite of pharmacologic and toxicologic advantages for the major active agents, including DDP, ADR, and ifosfamide.[28]

Just as systemic infusional ADR has been the major program at M. D. Anderson Hospital, regional infusion of this agent also has been the major program at UCLA used in conjunction with radiation therapy to provide an opportunity for limb-sparing surgery. Infusional ADR and concomitant radiation has been tentatively explored in the management of recurrent soft tissue sarcomas by Rosenthal et al.[29] In a small study of 8 patients, ADR was administered at a dose of 12 mg/m²/day as a continuous infusion for 5 days, with concomitant radiation therapy at a dose of 150 rad/day. Most patients had either prior radiation or prior ADR by bolus schedule. Seven of 8 patients responded to this therapy, and 5 were CR. In spite of the extensive prior therapy, radiation sensitization appears to have been achieved in this combined modality approach to recurrent tumors. A potential role for the interdigitation of infusional ADR and radiation in primary therapy is therefore suggested.

Summary and Conclusions

The number of chemotherapeutic agents active against the mesenchymal tumors is relatively limited. Furthermore, in prospective comparative trials, the use of multiagent regimens has not meaningfully increased response rates over those achieved with single agents when the single agent is anthracycline.[30] In the absence of the identification of new agents or multidrug regimens — the major efforts directed at improving chemotherapy — alternative methods can be explored.

Another potential direction for improving the effectiveness of chemotherapy for soft tissue and bone sarcomas may be by developing regional delivery systems of improving the therapeutic index by optimizing the schedule of drug administration. Of the known or presumed active drugs in mesenchymal tumors, infusional schedules and regional delivery have been employed relatively infrequently (see table 5). The established stability for most of these agents does permit an infusion schedule for delivery in an outpatient setting, with substantial improvement in the therapeutic index by virtue of minimization of toxicity. The potential improvement in cytotoxic effects on tumor cells has not been identified, however, and will require prospective comparative trials. Other than the 3 standard agents in the treatment of mesenchymal tumors (ADR, DDP, and MTX), regional and systemic infusion schedules are virtually unknown and are potentially important and fruitful areas for future investigation.

Table 5. Antineoplastic Agents Optimal for Infusion Delivery and Status

Agent	Infusion route	
	Systemic	Regional
Adriamycin	+ +	+ +
Cisplatin	+ +	+
Methotrexate	o	+
Ifosfamide	o	o
Bleomycin	o	o
Vinblastine	—	o
5-fluorouracil	o	o
Cyclophosphamide	o	o

o   Not evaluated
—   No activity
+   Incompletely evaluated
+ + Active

30

UNCOMMON TUMORS

Jacob J. Lokich, M.D.

THE EXTENSIVENESS OF THE spectrum of rare or uncommon tumors makes a selective review of infusion chemotherapy for these tumors appropriate. A common characteristic of the uncommon tumors is the variable natural history across the range of tumor categories. For example, islet cell tumors characteristically have a long natural history even in the presence of metastases, whereas at the other end of the spectrum, tumors such as hepatocellular carcinoma may be associated with an extraordinarily short survival related to rapid tumor growth. Another common feature of the more rare tumors is the fact that many are often treated with a drug or combination of drugs that has become standard for that tumor (see table 1). Because the tumor categories are rare, the ability to perform prospective comparative trials to analyze the impact of variations on the chemotherapy schedule of delivery such as bolus versus infusion has not been possible. This chapter will review selected rare tumors in which infusional chemotherapy has been employed in anecdotal or abbreviated phase 2 trials as well as consider the potential for infusion delivery for

Table 1. Rare or Uncommon Solid Tumors and the Chemotherapeutic Drug of Choice

Tumor	Incidence*	"Standard" Drug Therapy
Sarcoma	4,500	Doxorubicin, cisplatin
Melanoma	9,000	Dacarbazine (DTIC)
Hepatoma	4,000	Doxorubicin
Islet cell tumors	250	Streptozotocin, DTIC
Carcinoid tumors	†	Streptozotocin, doxorubicin, cisplatin
Thymoma	‡	Cisplatin

*Number of cases reported annually
†No reliable data; primary sites include G.I. tract, lung, thymus, etc.
‡No reliable data

those tumors in which a specific drug is recognized to be effective but has not yet been studied within that tumor category.

To the uncommon tumors listed in table 1 would be added the collective group of childhood tumors; tumors of the endocrine glands including the pituitary, thyroid, and adrenal gland; ocular tumors; adnexal tumors (eccrine or appocrine tumors), and a multitide of others. However, for many of these tumors, with the exception of childhood tumors, chemotherapy experience has been too limited to permit even speculation about the application of the infusion schedule to clinical trials. The focus of the chapter, therefore, will be on malignant melanoma, hepatocellular carcinoma, and islet cell tumors and other tumors of the apudoma class.

Malignant Melanoma

Malignant melanoma is a relatively uncommon tumor, with only 9,000 new patients annually, but it represents a tumor with a consistent lack of responsiveness to chemotherapy. Dacarbazine (DTIC) and the nitrosoureas are considered the standard agents in the treatment of advanced malignant melanoma (see table 2),[1-8] but it is evident that the modest response rates to these agents make them suboptimal. With a single exception, these agents have not been administered as a continuous infusion, although the pharmacology of DTIC is such that this agent more ideally would be administered on an infusion schedule if drug stability were established.

Streptozotocin has been employed as a 5-day infusion in the treatment of melanoma in a single report.[8] The rationale for this phase 2 trial in melanoma was based upon the fact that streptozotocin is in fact a nitrosourea, a group of compounds that are effective in melanoma; it is also an agent that, like DTIC, is effective in islet cell tumors; and finally, melanoma is akin to tumors with neurosecretory capability in that intracellular granules are identifiable. Two transient responses were observed in 14 patients with advanced measurable melanoma receiving continuous infusion streptozotocin.

Table 2. DTIC or Nitrosourea Single-Agent Regimens for Advanced Melanoma

Agent/study	Reference	No. patients	CR + PR	(%)
DTIC				
Costanzi et al	1	127	9	(15)
Costanzi et al	2	110	21	(19)
Einhorn et al	3	113	19	(17)
Nathanson et al	4	115	32	(28)
Luce et al	5	125	20	(16)
Nitrosourea				
BCNU	6	99	19	(19)
CCNU	7	48	2	(4)
Methyl CCNU	1	119	18	(15)
Streptozotocin	8	13	0	

A host of other agents have been employed in the treatment of advanced melanoma, always employing a bolus schedule (see table 3). There is some modest activity for most of the agents indicated, and 3 in particular— thio-tepa, actinomycin D, and cisplatin (DDP)—lend themselves to an infusion schedule based on pharmacologic considerations. The other agents also have pharmacologic advantage with the infusion schedule, including the antimetabolites (5-fluorouracil [5-FU], 6-mecaptopurine, methotrexate [MTX]), the antibiotics (mitomycin-C [MIT]), and the periwinkle alkaloids (vincristine [VCR] and vinblastine [VLB]). It would seem reasonable, therefore, to consider these agents on infusion schedules and reexamine their activity with this tumor. The relative feasibility of infusion capability is based on pharmacologic studies only (+) or phase 2 or 3 clinical trials demonstrating a superiority of infusion (+ + + +).

A single study of a 5-drug regimen for advanced malignant melanoma employed 3 agents by bolus delivery (DDP, Adriamycin, and VP-16) and 2 agents by continuous infusion for 3 days (bleomycin [BLM] and 5-FU). Of 27 patients, 23 of whom had received prior therapy, 7 complete remissions (25%) and 4 partial remissions were observed for a total response rate of 41%. It is obviously not possible to determine what contribution infusion 5-FU and BLM may have provided in this group of patients; however, each of the component agents has modest to no activity in the treatment of malignant melanoma delivered as a bolus.

Interferon as a treatment for melanoma has been proposed based upon the fact that this agent represents a biologic response modifier, and malignant melanoma in particular is characterized by immunologic peculiarities such as spontaneous regression and regression in response to intralesional injections of BCG. Occasional responses to systemic bolus interferon administered on a daily or 3-times-a-week schedule have been observed. However, the short half-life of interferon again provides a pharmacologic rationale for delivering this agent as a continuous infusion. To date, although phase 1 studies for continuous

Table 3. Potential Agents Suitable for Clinical Trials of Infusion Therapy in Melanoma

Agent	Reference	Bolus activity	Infusional feasibility
Thio-tepa*		5/24 (21%)	+ + +
5-Fluorouracil*		1/20 (5%)	+ + + +
6-Mercaptopurine*		2/29 (7%)	+
Methotrexate*		3/41 (7%)	+ +
Actinomycin D*	9	8/23 (35%)	+ + +
Mitomycin C*		9/65 (14%)	+ +
Vincristine*		3/26 (12%)	+ +
Vinblastine*		7/58 (12%)	+ + +
Cisplatin	10	3/11 (27%)	+ + + +

*Represent collected series of small studies reported in Mastrangelo et al. 'Cutaneous Melanoma.' In: Principles and practice of cancer treatment. Rosenberg, Hellman, DeVita, eds.

infusion have been completed, there are no clinical studies directed at establishing the antitumor effects of this schedule for this drug.

Regional Delivery

Malignant melanoma represents one of the first tumors to be studied employing regional infusion. First introduced by Creech et al in 1957, the concept was based upon the capability of isolating the limb by vascular occlusion and infusing an agent permitting a high dose to be delivered "topically" to the tumor and minimizing host effects. Melanoma lends itself to this technologic application because of the clinical and biologic behavior of the tumor.

The agent most commonly employed in limb perfusions is melphalan (MEL), an alkylating agent with modest activity when administered systemically. The regional delivery of this agent is generally over 1 hour or less using regional perfusion system, related to the limitations of vascular occlusion. Another component to regional delivery in the perfusion system has been the introduction of hyperthermia pioneered by Stehlin et al. Regional perfusion for melanoma has been comprehensively reviewed by Cumberlin et al.[12]

Regional drug delivery has also been employed in melanoma metastases to the brain using either carmustine (BCNU) or DDP delivered as a bolus as opposed to an infusion.[13,14] The responses observed in small series have been impressive and warrant further exploration of regional delivery, possibly using an infusion schedule. The complication rate from both regional extremity perfusion as well as carotid arterial bolus delivery for brain metastases and the technologic considerations and complexities dictate the absolute need to determine whether an advantage exists for a regional delivery in this as well as other tumors.

The infusion chemotherapy experience in melanoma is obviously sparse. New drugs have been the focus for developing effective treatment, but the opportunity to reexamine old drugs on infusion schedules may be fruitful, particularly because some of the old drugs have demonstrated modest activity. The regional delivery systems have not truly involved an infusion, and continuous infusions are, in fact, not practical for the sites for which regional delivery have been employed, i.e., the extremities and the CNS. Nonetheless, the bolus delivery system using regional access has demonstrated some remarkable effects. As such, prospective clinical trials would be worthwhile in selected groups of patients using regional delivery.

Hepatocellular Carcinoma

Hepatocellular carcinoma shares an annual frequency comparable to that of soft tissue sarcoma, with 4,000 new patients annually in the United States. This tumor is, however, the most common tumor in the world at large. It demonstrates a number of unique clinical and biological features, including the secretion of a tumor-associated substance, alphafetoprotein; and a number of epidemiologic clues to the etiology of the tumor exist, including the predisposing condition of cirrhosis and the common association with hepatitis B antigenemia implicating this virus in the etiology.

The mortality for hepatoma is virtually 100%, with the rare exception being surgical excision of isolated solitary nodules. Systemic chemotherapy for hepatoma has predominantly involved 2 agents, 5-FU and doxorubicin (ADR) (see table 4). Both agents have been delivered as a bolus in these trials, and responses have been observed only exceptionally. For ADR, a substantial response rate was observed in earlier trials, but subsequently as a single agent and in combination with other drugs, the anthracyclines as a group have been generally ineffective.

Both 5-FU and ADR may be delivered as a continuous infusion, but short-term infusion of either agent has not been reported in hepatoma. Protracted infusion for each agent identified responses in 2/4 patients with 5-FU and 3/4 patients with ADR alone or ADR admixed with cyclophosphamide (CTX).[15,16]

For hepatocellular carcinoma, clinical trials employing infusional ADR or the antipyrimidines, as well as possibly other agents including the alkylating agents, would be of potential interest. The alkylating agents in particular have not been extensively evaluated in hepatoma. Drugs within this class that lend themselves to infusion because of their relatively short half-life include thio-tepa, MEL, and MIT. Other agents that could be applied on an infusion schedule systemically for hepatoma include MTX and VP-16.

Regional infusion trials in hepatoma have employed the same 2 major agents: antipyrimidines (5-FUDR) and ADR. Although the anatomic distribution of hepatocellular carcinoma provides a substantial rationale for regional infusion of chemotherapy, there are no compelling data to indicate the superiority of regional delivery for these agents.

Table 4. Chemotherapy of Hepatocellular Carcinoma and Biliary Tract Tumors

Drug/study	No. patients	Response rate	Median survival
5-Fluorouracil			
Falkson et al	43	0	6 weeks
Kennedy et al	12	6/12	45 weeks
Link et al	21	0/21	9 weeks
Combinations[1]	112	19/112	8 – 23 weeks
Doxorubicin			
Olweny et al	53	23/50	—
Johnson et al	44	14/44	—
Vogel et al	41	7/41	—
Chlebowski et al	52	6/52	—
Combinations[2]	59	8/59	—

[1]5-Fluorouracil plus MeCCNU (44 patients); streptozotocin (23 patients); BCNU (19 patients) or cytosine arabinoside (16 patients).
[2]Doxorubicin plus MeCCNU (21 patients) or 5-fluorouracil (38 patients).
Adapted from Lokich J. Chemotherapy of hepatobiliary tumors. Bottino et al, eds.

Apudomas

The apudoma class of tumors includes a spectrum of malignancies related to the endocrine system that are widely distributed in the body. The tumors include islet cell tumors of the pancreas, carcinoid tumors and, at the other end of the rare spectrum, chemodectoma and paraganglioma, as well as tumors of the thymus and adrenal glands. Of the various classes of tumors, islet cell tumors perhaps are the most common, with an annual incidence of 250 cases.

Islet cell tumors of the pancreas are treated typically with streptozotocin, an agent that is particularly specific for such tumors. In a prospective randomized trial reported by Moertel et al, streptozotocin administered weekly as a standard bolus was compared to streptozotocin combined with 5-FU, and the 2-drug combination was superior.[17] Continuous infusion of streptozotocin employing short-term durations of up to 5 days has been studied by Lokich et al in malignant melanoma and has been applied to islet cell tumors. It is evident that in a tumor generally characterized by an indolent course, the tumor cell kinetics must be such that a relatively small proportion of cells are in cycle. In that sense, and in particular with a short half-life chemotherapeutic agent such as streptozotocin, the protracted tumor cell exposure over time would presumably have a more optimal effect on the tumor. Thus, future clinical trials might consider employing streptozotocin on an infusion schedule. Therapeutic activity has been established for the infusion schedule (see figure 1), and 5 of 6 patients treated to date have responded to short-term streptozotocin infusion.

The second agent employed for islet cell tumors is DTIC. This agent has been discussed previously as the "standard" drug in the treatment of metastatic melanoma. In islet cell tumors, DTIC appears to be a highly effective agent,

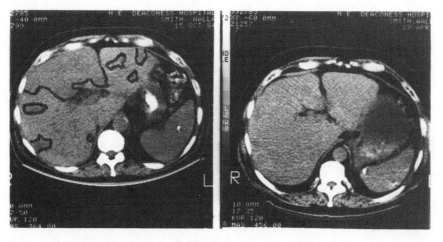

Figure 1. Computerized tomographic scan of the liver involved with metastatic islet cell tumor before and following 6 courses of streptozotocin administered as a 5-day continuous infusion by the systemic route.

with a response rate that was greater than 50% in a small group of patients,[18] but no trials of continuous infusion scheduling have been reported. ADR is the agent currently being evaluated in islet cell tumors. As indicated previously, ADR is an agent with an established capability of delivery as an infusion of either short-term or protracted duration. If ADR is active on a bolus schedule in islet cell tumors, an expanded application employing an infusion schedule would be reasonable.

Carcinoid tumors are histologically and biologically related to islet cell tumors, and the chemotherapy of carcinoid tumors has been similar. Table 5 lists the results of a number of trials of chemotherapy for carcinoid tumors updated by Harris[20] and by Moertel.[21] Streptozotocin has had a controversial application for carcinoid tumors, with major differences in antitumor effect reported by different investigators. ADR is active, based on a retrospective analysis of patients treated with a variety of multidrug regimens.[22] ADR in combination with DDP administered on a bolus schedule has been reported in a small series of 12 patients with advanced apudomas.[23] In 6 patients with carcinoid tumors, 3 demonstrated an objective tumor regression, and an additional patient had clinical and/or biochemical improvement, suggesting a drug effect. Thus, in this small series, two-thirds of the patients demonstrated a response to this 2-drug regimen. More recent programs are exploring interferon in the treatment of carcinoid tumors based upon a report that interferon improved the clinical symptoms and reduced the secretion of 5 HIAA in 4 patients with the syndrome in conjunction with the carcinoid tumor.[24]

The experience with infusion chemotherapy in this class of rare tumors is limited, as is the reported experience with standard "bolus" chemotherapy. Nonetheless, in spite of this sparse experience it is evident that some agents such as streptozotocin, DTIC, ADR combined with DDP, and even interferon have some drug effect, and for most of the agents an infusion schedule has been identified to be feasible, with some improvement in the therapeutic index by virtue of reduced toxicity.

Table 5. Chemotherapy of Islet Cell Tumors and Carcinoid Tumors

Class tumor/drug	Reference	Response rate (%)
Islet cell tumors		
Streptozotocin	17	36
5-fluorouracil	19	25
DTIC	18	
STZ + 5-FU	17	63
Carcinoid tumors		
STZ	21	50
5-FU	21	40
5-FU + STZ	21	32
Doxorubicin*	22	62
DOX + Cisplatin	23	50

*All patients received Adriamycin-containing multidrug regimens.

Thymoma

Tumors of the thymus gland are especially uncommon and are biologically and clinically interesting because of the association with paraneoplastic syndromes. Histologically, there exists a spectrum of tumor categories ranging from sarcoma or spindle tumors to epithelial tumors and apudoma type tumors (carcinoid tumors).

The chemotherapy trials with this tumor have been limited, but recent reports have suggested that DDP is an important agent to be considered.[25,26] In one trial, 10/11 patients responded to a 4-drug regimen that included bolus delivery of DDP, ADR, VCR, and CTX; 4/10 were complete responses. Infusion schedules have not been applied for these agents with this tumor, but the potential role for such a schedule is clear.

Summary and Commentary

A number of rare and uncommon tumors have not been included in the discussion. For example, mesothelioma is a tumor often treated in the category of other mesenchymal tumors, such as soft tissue sarcoma, and the experience with infusion chemotherapy is virtually nil, although Lokich et al identified 1 major response to infusion ADR of 6 patients treated. Another class of tumors not discussed includes the endocrine tumors, accessory organ tumors (sweat glands, etc.); pediatric tumors collectively; unusual nervous system tumors, such as chordoma; and many others. The literature for any chemotherapy employed for these tumors is too limited or, as in the case of pediatric tumors, too specialized to review in this chapter.

It is evident that in the uncommon tumors selected for discussion for infusional chemotherapy, the agents considered to be the standard drugs for a specific tumor have not been evaluated in infusional trials. Furthermore, the single agents that have been found to be inactive in bolus schedules could potentially be reexamined in these uncommon tumors employing an infusion schedule.

SECTION IV

Regional Infusion

31

HEAD AND NECK CANCER

Richard H. Wheeler, M.D., and Shan R. Baker, M.D.

REGIONAL THERAPY IS NOT applicable to all malignancies or patients. The important factors that must be considered when planning a regional approach for drug delivery include (1) a tumor natural history that demonstrates primarily local aggressiveness rather than widespread metastatic dissemination, (2) a definable and accessible arterial supply that provides selective access to tumor blood supply with minimal normal tissue distribution, and (3) the availability of antineoplastic agents with favorable pharmacokinetic properties and demonstrable antitumor activity against the tumor being treated. The clinical course and anatomic tumor distribution of the majority of patients with primary head and neck cancer fulfill these criteria. Although the clinical incidence of distant metastases is increased in advanced stage patients who achieve loco-regional control, the majority of patients still develop and die of loco-regional disease.[1,2] This is a group of patients who could benefit from improved local control rates through new therapeutic approaches. Ultimately, the proper place of regional chemotherapy in the overall management of patients with head and neck cancer must be defined by randomized trials documenting improved tumor regression rates, with prolonged patient survival or cure compared to systemic therapy. However, considerable improvement in efficacy over historical experience must be accomplished before a randomized study can be realistically expected to show a therapeutic benefit for intra-arterial (I.A.) drug delivery.

Regional Infusion: Background and Experience

The concept of regional drug delivery is not of recent origin. The rationale for I.A. injection of antiseptic substances was elaborated by Parlavecchio at the end of the 19th century.[3] Over the next 25 years, the I.A. route was used in anesthesia and in the treatment of neurosyphilis.[4,5] Intra-arterial chemotherapy of head and neck cancer was first reported by Klopp, who administered nitrogen mustard by this route and reported tumor regression not obtainable by I.V. administration of therapeutic amounts of the same drug.[6]

Until the late 1950s, the administration of I.A. chemotherapy agents was largely confined to alkylating agents. Although improved tumor response was reported, use was limited by the severe normal tissue toxicity. Antimetabolites were given by the I.A. route in early clinical studies.[7] However, single daily arterial administration of these agents produced toxic and therapeutic effects similar to those seen with the systemic route of administration. Recognition that antimetabolites may require a more prolonged duration of drug exposure to achieve maximum antitumor effects directed attention toward prolonging the duration of I.A. administration.

Methotrexate (MTX), the most active single agent for squamous cell cancer of the head and neck for more than 3 decades, has been the drug most commonly used intra-arterially. In an early evaluation of the pharmacologic advantage of regional therapy, Clarkson and Lawrence Jr. demonstrated that a 3- to 4-fold higher concentration of MTX was present in the distribution of the external carotid artery compared to the concentration in the systemic circulation.[8] In the majority of studies, concomitant systemic leucovorin was also administered. Sullivan et al treated head and neck cancer with continuous I.A. infusion of MTX and gave leucovorin I.M. every 6 hours. Partial responses (PR) or complete responses (CR) were observed in 10/18 patients treated.[9] These results were compared in a nonrandomized fashion with another series of patients who received comparable courses of therapy with continuous I.V. methotrexate and intermittent leucovorin. Based on clinical observation, the authors concluded that continuous 24-hour administration of MTX increased toxicity and antitumor effect of a given dose 10-fold or more compared to I.V. administration. As summarized by Carter, multiple other investigators have used a similar treatment regimen (see table 1).[10-22] The duration of therapy and daily doses administered have varied considerably. The criteria used to judge response were far from uniform, and the regression rates reported have varied from 27 to 76%. The cumulative overall response rate in the series cited is 53% which, as noted by other reviewers, is the same as that reported for systemic MTX.[22,23]

Other systemically active single agents have been administered intra-arterially for head and neck cancer, including the fluoropyrimidines bleomycin (BLM) and cisplatin (DDP). Johnson et al treated 70 patients with head and neck cancer using 5-fluorouracil (5-FU).[24] Most patients received 15 mg/kg/day for 4–5 days followed by 7.5 mg/kg/day for several more days. Objective response of greater than 50% reduction of tumor size occurred in 25 (36%) of the patients. Freckman treated 36 head and neck cancer patients with intra-arterial 5-FU (500 mg/24 hours for 10–14 days), with 12 (33%) patients responding.[25] The toxicities observed included mucositis and skin erythema within the infused area.

Intra-arterial BLM, used as a single agent or in combination with MTX, has produced response rates of 18–70%.[26-31] Burkhardt and Holtje used 9–12 units daily for a median of 32 days and noted 5 of 7 complete remissions.[27] However, Richard and Sancho gave 30 units over 10–12 hours daily for 6–10 days to 27 patients and obtained responses in only 5 patients.[28] The major toxicities observed have been stomatitis and skin rash in the perfused region. Pulmonary toxicity has been observed with high cumulative doses. Bitter, using cobalt-57-tagged BLM, has demonstrated higher tumor concentrations of the drug following I.A. administration compared to the same dose given I.V.[32]

DDP is a highly active systemic agent in squamous cell carcinoma of the head and neck, producing response rates of 27–31% in single-agent trials.[33,34] The dose-limiting toxicity is renal impairment, with stomatitis and myelosuppression occurring infrequently. Organ distribution studies in the dog following systemic or intracarotid drug administration have demonstrated 5-fold lower renal levels following I.A. injection.[35] Lehane et al have treated 26 patients with head and neck cancer (19 had not prior therapy) with 100 mg/m² of I.A. DDP infused over 1 hour and observed responses in 25 patients.[36] No loco-regional toxicity was observed. All patients had mild to moderate nausea and vomiting.

Intra-arterial combination drug therapy has been used by multiple investigators. Representative results are shown in table 2. Response rates ranging from 62 to 87% have been reported. Although the response rates reported are generally higher than those reported for single-agent MTX trials, randomized comparisons have not been conducted.

Intra-arterial chemotherapy has also been used to treat previously untreated patients with stage 1, 2, or 3 head and neck cancer without the addition of the standard treatment of radiotherapy or surgery.[42] BLM (total dose 180 mg) and MTX (240 mg/m²) with leucovorin factor were used. Clinically, CR was achieved in 2/2 T1 tumors, 7/8 T2 tumors, and 4/8 T3 tumors. CR was achieved in 8/10

Table 1. Intra-Arterial Methotrexate

Reference	Dose schedule	No. patients	No. responses (%)
10	50 mg/day with concomitant leucovorin	13	3 (23)
11	50 mg/day; leucovorin 30 mg/day	30	8 (27)
12	40 – 50 mg/day; leucovorin 0.085 – 0.125 mg/kg/day	13	7 (54)
13	50 mg/day; leucovorin 20 mg/day	16	5 (31)
14	50 mg/day; leucovorin 18 mg/day I.M.	74	56 (76)
15	340 – 610 mg total dose over 10 – 14 days with intermittent leucovorin	7	0 (0)
16	50 mg/day with concomitant leucovorin	21	7 (33)
17	50 mg/day; leucovorin 24 mg/day	45	25 (56)
18	Up to 25 mg/day; leucovorin 12 mg/day	11	7 (64)
19	25 – 50 mg/day; leucovorin 27 mg/day	14	4 (29)
20	50 mg/day + leucovorin	28	17 (61)
21	50 mg/day with leucovorin 24 mg/day	68	42 (62)
TOTALS		340	181 (53)

patients with necks classified as N0, 3/5 with N1 necks, and 2/2 patients with N2 disease. Despite the high CR rate, the 5-year survival of 27% was not impressive, and the author concluded that radiation or surgery should be combined with I.A. chemotherapy.

The introduction of I.A. chemotherapy led quite early to its combination with other modalities in cancer therapy. Reese et al administered I.A. triethylenemelamine in combination with radiation therapy to treat 3 patients with retinoblastomas.[43] Bolman et al used I.A. nitrogen mustard combined with irradiation to treat various gynecologic malignancies.[44] In a nonrandomized study, Jesse compared intra-arterial MTX to 5-FU in 38 previously untreated patients with head and neck cancer. Both drugs were used in combination with irradiation.[45] Local control of disease for greater than 15 months was obtained in 14% of patients receiving MTX and radiotherapy and 46% of those receiving 5-FU and radiotherapy.

Most investigators have reported single-arm studies with I.A. chemotherapy preceding irradiation with or without surgery. Response rates of 67–100% have been published, with CR in up to one-third of patients.[31,40,46–49] A nonrandomized comparison of the efficacy of combined I.A. chemotherapy preceding standard treatment was performed by Auersperg et al.[50] Of 74 patients with locally advanced carcinoma of the oral cavity and oropharynx, 38 were given radiotherapy and 36 received I.A. chemotherapy followed by radiotherapy. Intra-arterial chemotherapy consisted of MTX with leucovorin (7/36), BLM (5/36), MTX and BLM (7/36), MTX and podophyllic acid ethyl hydrazine (4/36), or vinblastine (VLB) with BLM and MTX (13/36). Intra-arterial chemotherapy was continued to CR or maximum objective response. Radiotherapy was commenced 10–14 days after completion of I.A. chemotherapy. Surgical resection was performed when possible. Intra-arterial chemotherapy produced an objective response in 28/36 patients and a CR in 13/28 responders. One of 38 radiotherapy-treated and 6/36 I.A. chemotherapy-treated patients were free of disease at 3 years. Median survival times were approximately 6 months with radiotherapy and 11 1/2 months for the chemotherapy group. The chemotherapy group had significantly higher survival rates than the radiotherapy group at 5–14 months, but not at greater than 14 months.

Only 2 studies have used concurrent randomized controls to evaluate the efficacy of I.A. chemotherapy combined with radiotherapy. Nervi and colleagues studied 140 patients with advanced squamous cell carcinoma of the

Table 2. Intra-Arterial Combination Chemotherapy

Reference	Agents*	No. patients	No. responses (%)
37	MTX/5-FU/BLM	15	13 (87)
38	VCR/MTX/BLM/ADR or MIT	47	29 (62)
39	VCR/BLM/MTX/MIT	72	57 (80)
40	VCR/BLM/ADR	97	66 (68)
41	MIT/BLM	30	26 (87)

*Abbreviations: MTX, methotrexate; 5-FU, 5-fluorouracil; BLM, bleomycin; VCR, vincristine; ADR, Adriamycin; MIT, mitomycin-C.

oral cavity, oropharynx, or maxillary antrum.[51] Seventy-two patients were randomized to receive I.A. MTX (90–120 mg in 25–40 days according to tolerance) followed by radiotherapy (7,000–7,500 rad). Both interstitial and external radiotherapy was given to 38 of the MTX-treated patients; the other 68 patients were treated with radiotherapy only. All patients were followed for at least 4 years. In the MTX group, the 4-year survival rates in patients with stage 1, 2, 3, and 4 disease were 93%, 66%, 40% and 10%, respectively. In the radiotherapy only group, 4-year survival rates were 50% in stage 2, 41% in stage 3, and 10% in stage 4. There was no advantage overall with the addition of chemotherapy. MTX infusion followed by a combination of external and interstitial radiotherapy gave significantly better local tumor control and survival rates as compared with radiotherapy alone in patients with cancer of the oral cavity (82 patients). These improved results were attributed to the increased use of interstitial radiotherapy in this group of patients rather than to a synergism between MTX and radiotherapy.

Bagshaw and Doggett reported on a controlled study of I.A. chemotherapy plus irradiation versus irradiation alone.[52] Local control of disease was achieved in 32% (7/22) of patients receiving MTX plus radiation therapy versus 38% (6/16) of patients treated with radiotherapy alone.

In the final analysis, most studies utilizing I.A. chemotherapy followed by irradiation or surgery may have yielded some improvement in short-term control, but randomized studies have not demonstrated a significant increase in long-term survival. The high response rates reported in previously untreated patients are matched by recent reports using systemic drug combinations in a similar patient population.[53]

Limitations and Complications of Regional Infusion

Despite more than 3 decades of experience, the use of I.A. chemotherapy for the treatment of head and neck cancer remains controversial. As illustrated above, the overall reported response rates are not substantially different from the therapeutic results obtained with systemic therapy. The additional complications associated with establishing and maintaining arterial access have further dampened enthusiasm for this approach. It is clear that considerable improvement in regional therapy technique and efficacy will be necessary before widespread clinical acceptance of I.A. infusion is attained. This improvement must be based on knowledge of the anatomic and pharmacologic factors that determine the success of regional therapy and the development of safe and reliable delivery systems.

The 2 major anatomic considerations are the extent and location of the malignancy and the vascular supply of the involved region. The therapeutic advantage of regional therapy, high local drug concentration with a low systemic exposure, becomes a major disadvantage when the tumor extends or metastasizes beyond the infused volume. Most I.A. chemotherapy conducted to date has been delivered through catheters placed in the external carotid artery (ECA) by way of the superficial temporal artery, the superior thyroid artery, or other accessible branches. Lesions that cross the midline require the insertion of two catheters.

The ECA arises from the common carotid artery near the upper border of the thyroid cartilage and passes upward to supply the vast majority of the integument, musculature, skeleton, and mucosal lining of the face and upper aerodigestive tract. Unilateral india ink injections of the ECA in fresh cadaver specimens demonstrate ink staining of the mucosal surfaces of the nasal passage, oral cavity, oral pharynx, and hypopharynx, as well as the skin of the face, forehead, anterior scalp, and upper neck to the level of the thyrohyoid membrane inferiorly.[54] Ink staining extends to the midline of the head and neck. This anatomic study is confirmed clinically in patients receiving ECA I.A. chemotherapy by observing ipsilateral stomatitis and alopecia extending only to the midline.

In general, long-term I.A. therapy has been applicable only to lesions supplied by the ECA. The regional lymph nodes in the mid- and lower neck, along with tumors confined to or extending into the neck beyond the nutrient field of the external carotid artery, are excluded from the infused volume. Implantation of a catheter into the thyrocervical trunk (TCT) can allow infusion of the cervical region and can be used in conjunction with the standard craniofacial infusion through the ECA.[54]

The TCT is a short, thick vessel arising from the first portion of the subclavian artery close to the medial border of the scalenus anterior. It divides almost immediately into 2 constant branches, the inferior thyroid and the suprascapular arteries, and a variable third branch, the transverse cervical artery. The inferior thyroid artery divides into 2 branches that supply the posterior-inferior part of the gland, portions of the trachea, and the upper cervical esophagus. The inferior thyroid artery also supplies the muscles and mucous membrane of the hypopharynx and lower portion of the larynx and the deep muscles of the neck. The suprascapular artery distributes branches to the sternocleidomastoideus, subclavius, and neighboring muscles. The transverse cervical artery arises from the TCT in 80% of cases. It divides into a superficial and a deep branch supplying much of the trapezius, levator scapulae, and neighboring deep cervical muscles.

India ink injections of the TCT trunk in fresh cadaver specimens demonstrate excellent staining of the integument and deep structures of the lower neck.[54] Dissection of the deep structures of the neck in these cadavers demonstrate ink staining of a fine network of vessels surrounding the lymph nodes of the lower jugular chain. Ink extends superiorly to the level of the mid-neck. Staining of the mucosa of the hypopharynx, pyriform sinus, and upper cervical esophagus is also apparent. Dye extends well beyond the midline in the hypopharyngeal and postcricoid mucosa.

For the vast majority of anticancer drugs, the dose/response curve is steep.[55] In other words, relatively small changes in dose rate have a major impact on the percentage of cells killed. The implication for cancer chemotherapy, in general, is that maximum tumor regression will be obtained by using the highest dose possible, i.e., the maximum tolerated dose (MTD). Because normal tissue cell kill follows a similar steep curve, the clinical MTD is defined as the highest dose rate that produces an "acceptable" level of toxicity. The therapeutic advantage of regional therapy is defined by the increase in tumor drug exposure compared to that achieved by systemic therapy at the MTD.

With in vitro and animal tumor models, a 2-fold increase in dose can result in a 3- to 10-fold increase in tumor cell kill.[55] The few clinical trials that examine the effect of dose rate on objective tumor response have been hampered by the paucity of highly active agents in many solid tumors and by the relatively small dose rate differences employed. In addition, many studies have compared low-dose, nontoxic therapy with full-dose therapy and do not answer the question of extension of the dose/response curve beyond the MTD of systemic therapy. To the extent that regional therapy can achieve a greater than 2- to 3-fold increase in the dose delivered to the tumor, it will provide a mechanism to further evaluate the dose/response curve.

The duration of drug exposure is also an important determinant of cytotoxicity. For many agents, particularly drugs that are cytotoxic only during 1 phase of the cell cycle, the duration of exposure above a critical concentration is more important than the concentration achieved.[56-59] However, agents capable of killing resting or cycling cells are primarily concentration-dependent and are best administered by intermittant bolus with sufficient time between doses to allow normal tissue recovery.[57,60-63] Effective chemotherapy, systemic or regional, must take into consideration these important variables of dose and duration. Properly designed infusion treatment regimens should be based on the mechanism of action and the cycle specificity of the drugs used and on the anticipated growth kinetics of the tumor being treated.[57,64]

The major factors determining drug concentration are the dose rate and the regional blood flow. The higher the dose rate (quantity/unit time) and the lower the regional blood flow (volume/unit time) the greater the drug concentration in the local tumor blood supply.[65] Tumor drug exposure will then be determined by the rate of diffusion or transport of drug across capillary endothelium into the extracellular fluid.[66] Tumor drug exposure can be maximized by increasing the dose rate, infusing into regions of low blood flow (or decreasing the blood flow) and by using rapidly diffusing antineoplastic agents.[67]

The pharmacokinetic principles affecting regional therapy have been extensively reviewed.[66,69] The therapeutic advantage (R_d) of an I.A. infusion (assuming the same dose rate is used I.A. and I.V.) is defined by the equation:

$$R_d = \frac{(AUC_T)/(AUC_S) \text{ I.A.}}{(AUC_T/AUC_S) \text{ I.V.}} + 1$$

where AUC is the area under the concentration $\times$ time curve of drug exposure, T refers to the tumor and S to the systemic circulation.[65] For infusion into a body region that does not metabolize drugs (such as the head and neck), equation (1) reduces to:

$$R_d = \frac{Cl_{TB}}{Q_i} + 1$$

where Cl_{TB} is the total body drug clearance and Q_i is the regional blood flow. The regional advantage can be increased by using agents with a high total body clearance and by infusion into regions with a low regional blood flow.

Ultimately, the tumor drug exposure attained is limited by the toxicity produced, either local or systemic. The amount of systemic toxicity depends upon the systemic drug level and varies with the total body clearance of active drug, the first-pass extraction of drug as it goes through the regional capillary bed, and the degree of A-V major vessel shunting around the capillary bed. Local toxicity is primarily determined by the drug sensitivity of normal tissues within the infused volume.

Even given a high first-pass extraction in the capillary bed, substantial systemic toxicity may occur if a high percentage of the drug is shunted from the arterial to the venous circulation via precapillary shunts. The A-V shunting that occurs during head and neck infusion has been determined in patients receiving I.V. therapy and is shown in table 3. The shunt varied from less than 10% to more than 40%.[70]

Although systemic toxicity can occur with I.A. therapy, in the majority of instances the dose-limiting side effects are local.[71] The major determinant of local toxicity is the drug sensitivity of the normal tissue within the regional area. Avoidance of agents that characteristically produce toxicity in the infused area would be appropriate. For regional therapy of head and neck

Table 3. Systemic Shunting of Intra-Arterial Tc-MAA

0.5 mCi Tc-MAA was injected intravenously (A[I.V.]) and lung field was acquired on computer for 5 min. (C[I.V.]). 2.0 mCi Tc-MAA was then injected intra-arterially (A[I.A.]) and lung field was again acquired (C[I.A.]). Syringes were then assayed for residual counts, corrected for decay, and actual injected dose determined. Shunt index (SI) was calculated as

$$SI = \frac{C(I.V.)}{A(I.V.)} \times A(I.A.) \times 100$$

Patient no.	Artery	% Shunt*
1	L. ECA	11
2	R. ECA	43
3	L. ECA	29 (35)
4	L. ECA	8
5	L. ECA	25
	R. ECA	41
6	L. ECA	11
	R. ECA	38
7	L. ECA	19 (9)
	R. ECA	15
8	L. ECA	10
	R. ECA	28 (24)
9	L. ECA	20
Mean ± S.D.		23 ± 11

*Numbers in parentheses represent separate determinations.

cancer, this is impractical because the majority of efficacious drugs (MTX, BLM, fluoropyrimidines) frequently produce mucositis.

Because toxicity follows a steep dose/response curve similar to tumor cytotoxicity, physiologic conditions that increase drug delivery to the tumor relative to normal time would be advantageous. A low total regional blood flow improves the regional advantage of I.A. therapy by increasing the drug concentration at a given dose rate. However, once drug/blood mixing has occurred, drug delivery becomes proportional to the blood flow rate, with greater blood flow providing higher drug delivery.[67]

Radionuclide techniques have been used to quantitate blood flow to the tumor and to reference normal tissue in patients undergoing I.A. chemotherapy for head and neck cancer.[70] The results of this evaluation are shown in table 4. Quantitative blood flow was determined from the slope of the washout curve of I.A. injected [133]Xenon. The mean tumor blood flow was 13.6 ± 6.7 ml/100 g/min., while the mean blood flow to the scalp was 4.2 ± 2.1 mg/100 g/min., providing a mean tumor/normal tissue ratio of 3.9 ± 2.7. These studies show that at least part of the therapeutic advantage of regional chemotherapy in patients with head and neck cancer is due to a tumor/normal tissue blood flow ratio that favors drug delivery to the tumor contained within the infused volume.

Appreciation of the physiologic conditions that determine drug distribution within the infused volume also suggest pharmacologic manipulations that

Table 4. Quantitative and Qualitative Tumor and Normal Tissue Blood Flow

10 mCi [133]Xenon was rapidly injected intra-arterially. The t½ for [133]Xenon clearance was determined by semi-automated computer generated exponential fit of the second portion of the downslope of the time activity curve. Blood flow calculated as

$$\frac{\ln 2}{t\tfrac{1}{2}} \times \lambda \times 100$$

Partition coefficient (λ) was 0.7 for scalp and 1.0 for tumor.

Patient no.	Artery	Blood Flow (ml/100 g of tissue/min.)		
		Tumor	Scalp	Ratio
1	L. ECA	12.3	3.1	4.0
3	L. ECA	22.3	3.4	6.6
4	L. ECA	11.5	6.2	1.9
5	L. ECA	10.9	5.2	2.1
6	L. ECA	6	3.1	1.9
	R. ECA	10.5	4.6	2.3
7	L. ECA	15.6	1.5	10.6
	R. ECA	5.9	1.8	3.2
9	L. ECA	27	8.6	2.8
Mean ± S.D.		13.6 ± 6.7	4.2 ± 2.1	3.9 ± 2.7

could improve selective drug delivery. The smooth muscle of the precapillary arteriole is sensitive to a variety of vasoconstrictors.[72] Brief infusions of these agents will constrict the arterioles in normal tissues and decrease overall blood flow. Tumor neovascularity lacks the smooth muscle layer sensitive to these vasoconstrictors.[73,74] Thus, vasoconstrictors have the additional potential to produce a relative shunting of blood toward tumor vessels to increase the tumor/normal blood flow ratio. The effects of norepinephrine infusion on blood flow T/NT using intra-arterially infused ^{99m}Tc macroaggregated albumin and single photon emission computed tomography have been explored.[75] Improvements in the T/NT blood flow ratio were observed, although effective vasoconstrictor dose rates varied widely. The use of vasoconstrictors thus has the potential to improve the therapeutic response of various forms of I.A. chemotherapy. Further studies are needed to determine the optimum vasoconstrictor agent and dose rate and to pharmacologically quantitate the improvement in regional advantage.

In addition to the variable evidence for improved therapeutic results, clinical application of regional chemotherapy in head and neck cancer patients has been retarded by reports of the many complications associated with I.A. treatment. Most complications and disadvantages were related to the use of an indwelling catheter. Keeping the catheter in place requires accurate surgical technique, good nursing care, and a cooperative patient. Clotting of catheters is an ever-present complication. When injections are made, considerable care must be exercised to prevent air embolism and to avoid dislodging small terminal clots formed in the lumen and around the catheter.[76]

Arteritis and infection of the skin around the catheter at the skin level eventually develops in all external catheter systems. Arteritis may lead to hemorrhage, leaking of infusate around the catheter, and septic embolus. Likewise, unless meticulous care is taken, the lumen of the catheter may become infected and lead to sepsis.

Neurologic sequelae may also occur from air embolism or inadvertent dislodgment of an atherosclerotic plaque into the internal carotid system. Migration of the infusion catheter from the external carotid artery into the common or internal carotid artery may expose the brain to direct infusion of antineoplastics, resulting in seizures or neurological impairment.[77]

When the side effects of the antineoplastic agents administered are added to the physical complications of catheter insertion and maintenance, complication rates of up to 40% have been reported.[78,79] In 1 study, fibrin coating along the catheter was found in 20 patients studied by pull-out arteriography and was associated with clinical symptoms.[76] Major thrombus formation occurred around the catheter tip in 28% of the infused vessels. Systemic heparinization did not reduce the incidence of thrombus formation.

The newer soft and flexible silicone elastomer catheters with extremely small lumens (OD 2.5 mm, ID 1.2 mm) have proved to be effective conduits for administering long-term I.A. chemotherapy. The small lumen does not readily allow retrograde blood flow into the catheter. The softness and flexibility of the catheter prevents migration or penetration of the catheter through the vessel wall. The extreme flexibility of the catheter requires that it be implanted surgically via an arterotomy since it cannot be easily advanced within an artery. By selecting a branch of the external carotid artery for access, an arterotomy is performed near the origin of the vessel from the external carotid artery. The catheter tip is advanced until the tip is just flush with the lumen of the external carotid artery. This technique allows drug to be delivered directly into the bloodstream of the external carotid artery without the need for the catheter to occupy any of the lumen of the vessel.

Use of External and Implantable Pumps

Refinements of the infusion apparatus used to maintain I.A. infusions have paralleled improvements in the techniques of arterial cannulation. Early investigators used bulky external pressure pumps or systems driven by air pressure.[80-86] The technique of continuous I.A. infusion was simplified by a chronometric infusion pump described by Watkins.[87-89] This spring-activated pump was used to dispense 3–5 ml of infusate per 24 hours. A disposable plastic reservoir within the apparatus contained 25 ml of the infusate, a supply sufficient for several days of treatment. The apparatus, harnessed to the chest, enabled prolonged I.A. infusion chemotherapy on an outpatient basis. The pump, named the Chemofusor, was powered by a miniature mercury battery. A single roller fixed to a drive plate rotated against the infusion tubing to create the pumping action. The Chemofusor, worn by the patient in a carrying holder, afforded continuous I.A. infusion chemotherapy in ambulatory patients.

Despite these improvements in infusion technology, the need for prolonged hospitalization and/or the complications accompanying the use of externalized catheters and pumping devices continued to hamper wide application of I.A. treatment. The recent development of a totally implantable infusion system circumvents many of these technical limitations. The design, animal trials, and initial experience with this device as a delivery vehicle for heparin for patients with refractory thromboembolic disease, have been described in detail[90-94] and are reviewed in a separate section of this book. To deliver I.A. chemotherapy to head and neck cancer patients, implantation of the pump and delivery catheter are accomplished under general anesthesia.[95] Neoplasms confined to the head and upper neck are perfused through the external carotid artery. A branch of the external carotid artery that does not perfuse a region of the neoplasm is selected to receive the catheter. An arterotomy is performed and the catheter is threaded into the vessel. The catheter tip is advanced until it is flush with the lumen of the external carotid artery. After the catheter has been inserted, the distal vessel can be ligated and the catheter securely tied in place within the vessel with several separate ligatures. Additional branches of the external carotid artery that are not directly perfusing the area of the cancer are ligated.

Implantation of the infusion pump requires an incision parallel to and 2 cm below the clavicle. A subcutaneous pocket is made superficial to the fascia of the pectoralis major muscle. The sterile pump is introduced into the pocket and secured to the deep fascia by nonabsorbable sutures placed through loops attached to the sides of the pump. The arterial catheter is directed toward the subcutaneous pocket created in the subclavicular fossa. The catheter is tunneled through the subcutaneous tissues of the neck and upper chest wall and is connected to the outlet catheter from the pump. The incisions in the neck and chest are closed in layers without drains.

At the University of Michigan, 25 pumps have been implanted in 20 patients.[96] Two patients had 2 pumps implanted to provide bilateral head infusion; 3 pumps have been replaced. Eight of these patients have received dual-catheter infusion systems. There have been no episodes of bleeding. An abrupt decrease in flow rate has occurred in 3 patients receiving dichloromethotrexate (DCMTX) infusions for head and neck cancer. The pump was replaced in 2 patients, and DCMTX crystals were noted in the arterial catheter or resistance element. DCMTX has subsequently been dissolved in 0.5% sodium bicarbonate to increase drug solubility, and no further infusion malfunctions have occurred. Two patients have developed infections of the pump pocket. One infection occurred while the catheters were externalized for 3 weeks awaiting pump delivery. The second infection occurred following skin breakdown over the catheter in a patient who had undergone a previous radical neck dissection and neck irradiation. The patient characteristics and pump performance are detailed in tables 5 and 6.

Accurate identification of an artery for cannulation is essential when administering I.A. chemotherapy to ensure complete infusion of the tumor vasculature. A number of methods have been developed for this purpose, including radiographic visualization and the use of injectable fluorescein or methylene blue dyes.[26,97-99] Radionuclide techniques also have been employed

Table 5. Patient Population Treated with Infusaid Pump

No. treated	20
Male/female	13/7
Median age (range: 18 – 72)	55
Prior radiation	16
Prior chemotherapy	6
No prior therapy	4
Cell type	
Squamous	13
Basal cell	2
Undifferentiated	2
Salivary gland	2
Sarcoma	1
Primary site	
Tongue/tonsil	9
Palate	2
Ethmoid sinus	2
Parotid	2
Skin	2
Larynx	1
Floor of mouth	1
Max. sinus	1

to assess the infused volume. Rapoport et al injected I^{131} labeled albumin macroaggregate followed by scanning of the head and neck to determine infusion patterns and to provide a method of selective catheterization of appropriate branches of the external carotid artery for direct infusion of tumors.[100] Kaplan et al infused radionuclides at low flow rates, approximating those used for drug delivery, to define patterns of intrahepatic infusion.[101] The presence or absence of radiolabeled albumin flow to focal tumor defects was compared to a prior [99m]technetium-sulfur colloid liver/spleen scan to assess adequacy of the infusion.

A similar technique has been utilized to assess infusion patterns in head and neck cancer patients treated with I.A. chemotherapy.[102] Following a slow injection of ^{99m}Tc-tagged macroaggregated albumin through the pump sideport, computerized tomographic and static postinjection scanning is performed. This allows determination of the infused area and permits detection of CNS infusion that could result from improper catheter placement or collateral circulation.

The therapeutic results obtained in patients treated through the implanted system are summarized in tables 7–9.[96] Patients eligible for I.A. therapy were defined by (1) histologically demonstrated primary malignancy of the head and neck, (2) tumor confined to the distribution of the external carotid artery and/or the thyrocervical trunk, (3) performance status ≥ 50 Karnofsky, (4) creatinine clearance ≥ 50 ml/min., WBC $\geq 4,000$/ul, platelet count $\geq 150,000$/ul, bilirubin < 1.5 mg/ul, and (5) no prior radical neck dissection on the side of the tumor unless an accessible vascular supply could be

Table 6. Infusaid Pump Performance

No. Implanted	25
Single catheter	17
Dual catheter	8
No. infusion days	7,500+
Median duration of therapy (range: 3 + −31 +)	7 + months
Infections	2
Bleeding	0
Emboli	2
System failure	3

Table 7. Intra-Arterial Single Agents

Agent	No. patients	Median MTD	Spectrum of toxicity	Response
DCMTX	6	4 mg/m²d × 14 d (3.4 – 6.0)	local—5 patients systemic—1 patient	2/5
FUDR	6	0.02 mg/kg/d × 14 d (0.015 – 0.04)	local—6 patients systemic—0 patients	1/3
BLM	5	>4 u/d × 7 d (1 – >4)	local—1 patient systemic—0 patients	0/3

demonstrated by angiography. Patients who had received prior MTX or DDP were not excluded; however, patients who had received systemic BLM did not receive this agent intra-arterially.

FUDR, DCMTX, and BLM were instilled into the pump chamber for continuous infusion. FUDR and BLM were dissolved in normal saline containing 200 units/ml sodium heparin. DCMTX was dissolved in 0.5% sodium bicarbonate without heparin. DDP (1 mg/ml) and mitomycin-C (MIT) (total dose in 30 ml of normal saline) were given by short-term infusion through the side port of the pump using a Harvard pump connected with polyetheline tubing to a bent

Table 8. Intra-Arterial Cisplatin + FUDR

Patient no.	Arteries	No courses	DDP (mg/m²)	FUDR (mg/kg/14 d)	Syst.	Local	Response
			MTD		Toxicity		
1	ECA	1	50	0.1	N/V	Skin	PR
2	ECA	4	50	0.015	N/V	Muc	PR
3	ECA	3	50	0.02	N/V	Muc	PR
4	ECA	2	50	0.025	N/V	Muc Skin	PR
5	ECA	4	50	>0.03	N/V	None	PR
6	ECA	6	70	0.02	N/V	Muc	PR
7	ECA × 2	2	70	0.02	N/V	Muc	PR
8	ECA	4	100	0.02	N/V	Muc	PR
9	ECA	1	100	>0.02	N/V	None	NR
10	ECA + TCT	2	100	0.01	N/V	Muc	NR

Abbreviations: MTD, maximum tolerated dose; DDP, cisplatin; ECA, external carotid artery; TCT, thyrocervical trunk; N/V, nausea/vomiting; MUC, mucositis; PR, partial response; NR, no response.

Table 9. Intra-Arterial Bleomycin + Mitomycin-C ± Dichloromethotrexate

Patient no.	Arteries	No. courses	MIT (mg/m²)	BLM (u/d) × 7 d	DCMTX (mg/m²/d) × 14 d	Syst.	Local	Response
			MTD			Toxicity		
1	ECA	1	4 × 1	4	—	None	None	NE
2	ECA	2	4 × 1	4	—	None	None	PR
3	ECA	4	4 × 2	4	—	Pul Myelo	None Extr	PR
4	ECA	1	3 × 1	4	3	None	None	NR
5	ECA	4	3 × 2	4	3	Liver	Muc	PR
6	ECA, TCT	2	3 × 2	4	3	None	Muc	NR
7	ECA, TCT	1	4 × 2	4	4	None	None	NE
8	ECA × 2	4	4 × 2	4	5	None	Muc	SD
9	ECA × 2	4	4 × 2	4	4	None	Muc	SD
10	ECA × 2	3	4 × 2	4	3	None	Muc	PR

Abbreviations: MTD, maximum tolerated dose; ECA, external carotid artery; TCT, thyrocervical trunk; MUC, mucositis; PR, partial response; NR, no response; NE, not evaluable.

Huber needle inserted into the side port. Cisplatin was infused over 90 minutes and MIT over 30 minutes.

The 20 patients have received 39 different treatment regimens using the implantable pump. Seventeen single-agent treatment regimens and 20 combination drug programs have been evaluated. The versatility of the Infusaid system has allowed multiple therapeutic trials in individual patients. Five patients have received 3 separate treatment regimens, and 8 have received 2 programs. Ten patients have responded to at least 1 regimen, and 3 additional patients have had minor responses (>25 to <50% tumor regression) of at least 5 months' duration. Seven of 14 patients who had the pump implanted more than 1 year ago have received therapy for at least 1 year, and 4 patients have had functioning systems for more than 2 years.

A total of 16 objective responses were attained during these drug trials. In 7 patients, disease progression has occurred within the infused volume after a median of 7 months (range 4–14+ months). Five patients progressed outside the infused area after a median of 4 months of therapy (range 2–7 months).

DCMTX was used as a single agent in 6 patients. Therapy was initiated at a dose rate of 1 mg/m²/day × 14 days and escalated with each subsequent course to toxicity. The MTD was limited by local toxicity (mucositis) in 5 patients. Two of 3 patients who had not received prior chemotherapy (all were previously irradiated) attained a PR lasting 7 and 8 months, respectively. One patient did not have measurable disease at the time DCMTX was administered.

Single-agent FUDR was evaluated in 6 patients. Dose escalation was halted from an initial level of 0.01 mg/kg/day × 14 days by the development of stomatitis in all patients, and no systemic toxicity was observed. One patient had skin toxicity (erythema of the skin overlying the lesion) concommitant with the development of mucositis. Five patients were previously treated with I.A. chemotherapy (DCMTX 3, DDP 2), with 1 patient attaining a PR lasting 4 months.

Five patients received BLM as a continuous 7-day infusion. One patient developed stomatitis at a dose rate of 1 unit/day × 7 days. The other 4 patients had no toxicity at a dose rate of 4 units/day. Dose escalation was halted at this level (about 30 units/course) since the goal for this agent was to find a tolerable dose rate that could be given for multiple courses without exceeding the cumulative dose that produces pulmonary toxicity.

The results obtained with the combination of DDP + FUDR are shown in table 8. The initial patients were treated with 50 mg/m² of DDP, and the dose was escalated to 100 mg/m² in later patients. The dose rates of FUDR delivered in combination and the toxicity observed are identical to the results obtained with single-agent FUDR. DDP, therefore, appears to have little or no regional toxicity at this dose. DDP was given with systemic hydration and mannitol. One patient had a fall in creatinine clearance to 40–45 ml/min. following the 6th course of therapy and the drug was discontinued. All other patients maintained a clearance in excess of 50 ml/min. No clinically evident hearing loss was noted in this population. Objective PR were attained in 8/10 patients. The median duration of response was 4 months, with a range of 4–12 months. Ten patients have been treated with BLM + MIT ± DCMTX (see table 9). Five of the

8 patients evaluable for response have attained partial regressions that have lasted 4–14+ months.

The major aims of this investigation were to evaluate the use of the Infusaid pump for long-term regional therapy in patients with head and neck cancer and to develop single-agent and combination drug regimens to use with this system. This study (1) established the safe initial dose rates for the drug combinations DDP + FUDR and BLM + MIT + DCMTX; (2) delineated the spectrum and magnitude of drug toxicity; (3) showed that the critically active agents can be administered near or at the single agent MTD; and (4) demonstrated that these drug combinations are active in head and neck cancer. Additional experience will be necessary to further define objective response rate and applicability of these regimens. However, the Infusaid pump has proven safe and effective, has high patient acceptance, and permits long-term continuous I.A. infusion in ambulatory head and neck cancer patients.

Summary

The principal objective of regional chemotherapy, as for cancer chemotherapy in general, is tumor cell kill. The rationale for regional delivery is based on the steep dose-response curve exhibited by most antineoplastic agents. Intra-arterial chemotherapy has the potential advantages of (1) increased drug concentration at the tumor site, (2) decreased systemic drug levels and toxicity, and (3) continuous tumor cell exposure to an antineoplastic agent. Despite decades of experience, the place of I.A. therapy in the treatment of head and neck cancer remains undefined. Published series have reported a wide range of response rates and complications. The recent development of a totally implantable pump system for I.A. infusion overcomes the majority of technical impediments to regional therapy and makes long-term I.A. therapy practical in an outpatient population. Further advances in the regional therapy of head and neck cancer will come from the aggressive application of pharmacologically rational drug combinations in primary and recurrent disease. Ultimately, randomized comparisons of systemic and I.A. therapy must be conducted to establish the efficacy of a regional approach.

32

REGIONAL INFUSION FOR

METASTATIC LIVER TUMORS

Yeu-Tsu Margaret Lee, M.D., F.A.C.S.

IN THIS COUNTRY, AMONG autopsy series, nearly half of the patients with malignancies died with liver metastasis.[1] Using a conservative figure, assuming that only 10% of the 200,000 new cases with carcinoma of the digestive tract and 250,000 with cancer of the lung and breast have liver metastasis at initial diagnosis, at least 45,000 patients with liver metastasis would be discovered each year.

For all hepatic tumors limited to the liver, surgical resection is the treatment of choice whenever possible. But the resectability rate is rather low, and there is always a significant associated surgical mortality. For the majority of patients who are not surgical candidates or who have unresectable cancers limited to the liver, regional modalities of treatment have been actively investigated. Such nonsystemic therapeutic approaches have included infusion chemotherapy via the hepatic artery or portal vein (with catheter placed either percutaneously or surgically); hepatic artery ligation or embolization (either alone or in combination with other forms of therapy); radiotherapy (administered either externally or internally with radioactive isotopes); and other more experimental approaches such as hyperthermia and liver transplantation. Indications and results of these different therapeutic approaches have been reviewed elsewhere.[2]

This chapter will emphasize hepatic arterial infusion chemotherapy of metastatic liver tumors and summarize clinical experience to date. Results dealing with the totally implantable pump are covered elsewhere in this book. Some investigators used hepatic artery infusion chemotherapy after permanent or temporary occlusion of the hepatic artery. Some oncologists introduced chemotherapeutic agents into the portal vein system in conjunction with or instead of hepatic artery infusion chemotherapy. In certain institutions, opera-

---

The assertions or opinions contained herein are the private views of the author and are not to be construed as official or as reflecting the views of the Department of the Army or the Department of Defense.

tive ligation of the hepatic artery has been replaced by percutaneous embolization performed by the radiologist. All of these varied and diversified approaches reflect the active ongoing research aimed at improving the management of unresectable liver metastases.

Incidence and Natural History of Metastatic Liver Tumors

The liver is the major organ most commonly involved by metastatic neoplasm. In a large report of 10,736 patients who died of various types of malignancies, about 25% had no metastasis at time of autopsy, 34% had only extrahepatic involvement, and 41% had liver metastasis.[1] For adenocarcinoma of the systemic circulation, the comparable figures were 21%, 34%, and 45%, respectively. For adenocarcinoma, which normally drains into the portal vein system, the figures were 19%, 24%, and 58%, respectively.

In patients with colorectal cancer, hepatic metastases were present in 40–80% at autopsy.[1,3,4] At the time of initial laparotomy, liver metastases are reported to be present in approximately 9–30% of those with colorectal cancer[5,6] and in 50–63% of those with cancer of the pancreas or gallbladder.[7] For patients with breast cancer, 42% had liver metastases diagnosed shortly before death and 71% were found to have metastases postmortem.[8] Younger patients had a higher chance of developing liver metastases than patients older than 50 (80% versus 56%).[9]

In one series of 390 patients with various untreated liver metastases seen 1940–66, the median survival time was 75 days from diagnosis.[10] For patients with metastases from carcinoma of the stomach, the median survival was 60 days, and for those with carcinoma of the pancreas or biliary tract, 42 days. Patients with metastases of colorectal cancer had the longest median survival (146 days), with 20% of the patients surviving over 1 year.

For patients with carcinoma of the colorectum specifically, those whose liver metastasis was diagnosed at initial surgery fared better.[5] One study showed that the median survival of those with solitary liver metastasis was 36 months, as compared to 7 months for those with multiple metastases.[11] Another study of 252 patients with unresected liver metastasis (1943–76) showed that the median survival time of patients who had solitary and multiple unilobar lesions were 21 and 15 months, respectively.[12] The 3-year survival rates for solitary, multiple unilobar, and widespread metastases were 21%, 6%, and 4%, respectively.

In the literature, more than 10 staging systems have been proposed.[2] The mere presence of so many different staging systems implies that the most practical classification scheme remains to be identified. The natural history of patients with liver metastasis is influenced by many factors, such as age and sex, performance status, site and stage of the original lesion, histologic type, degree of differentiation, disease-free interval, symptom duration, number and extent of hepatic metastases, prior therapy of the hepatic metastasis, laboratory tests of enzymes, liver functions, and tumor markers.

Using the multifactorial analysis of 22 prognostic factors in 175 patients with liver metastasis from colorectal carcinoma, Lahr et al[13] found 7 independent factors that influenced survival rate: alkaline phosphatase, bilirubin, albumin, involvement of 1 or 2 lobes, number of metastastic nodules (1–5 versus 5 +), primary tumor resected or not, and chemotherapy given or not. The first 2 factors, when elevated, were most important. In fact, the median survival of patients with bilirubin level greater than 5 mg% was less than 30 days. Other than number and location of metastases, the maximal dimension of any single hepatic metastasis did not correlate with survival. In this study, the relative extent of metastatic liver involvement (% replaced or some type of staging system) was not studied.

Studying patients with liver metastases diagnosed before 1966, Jaffee et al[10] showed that hepatic metastasis exerted an overriding influence upon the natural course of the patient despite concurrent pulmonary, peritoneal, and/or lymph node involvement. Thus, aggressive treatment of secondary cancer of the liver appears to have a rational basis.

Rationale and Methodology of Infusion Chemotherapy via Hepatic Artery

Regional and continuous chemotherapy to the liver has the advantages of achieving higher local concentration of drug in the tumor, prolonging the contact of drug with tumor cells, reducing systemic toxicity, and increasing the therapeutic benefit/risk ratio. Long-term infusion chemotherapy has the theoretical advantage of sequential destruction of tumor cells as they randomly enter their vulnerable metabolic phase. Delivering chemotherapy directly to the tumor through its arterial supply was initiated in 1950[14,15] and repopularized in the 1960s by Sullivan et al[16] and Clarkson and Lawrence.[17]

The infusion catheter can be placed in the hepatic artery either percutaneously or directly at the time of celiotomy. Both techniques are fairly standardized.[18-20] Hepatic arterial anatomy and anomalies are well described and have been classified recently with the wider use of arteriograms.[21] For patients who cannot tolerate general anesthesia or who refuse surgery, a catheter can only be inserted percutaneously. The overall success rate reaching the liver via either the brachial or femoral artery is about 85%. The advantages and disadvantages of percutaneous insertion versus operative placement of catheters and the respective and common complications of the 2 approaches have been described in other chapters of this book and elsewhere.[2]

Some newly reported complications deserve comment. One patient had a Silastic catheter placed into the distal end of a transected hepatic artery. One month later, a hepatic artery and bile duct fistula developed.[22] Patients receiving FUDR intra-arterially (I.A.) via the hepatic artery frequently developed significant increase in alkaline phosphatase, transaminase and/or bilirubin, a condition once called "chemical hepatitis." But Hohn et al[23] documented the pathology as sclerosis of the extrahepatic ± intrahepatic bile ducts. Severe G.I. toxicity could be seen endoscopically in 46% of patients given I.A. infusion chemotherapy: 29% had discrete ulcers and 17% had diffuse gastritis or duodenitis.[24] Peptic ulcer was present in 11% of 82 patients by biopsy.[25] One patient had biopsies of antral and duodenal ulcerations, which showed marked epithelial atypia initially reported as adenocarcinoma. Subsequent partial gastric resection proved the lesion to be benign. On review, 56% of biopsies of peptic ulcer cases also had marked cytological atypia.

Newer radioisotope-labeled macro-albumin can check the position of the hepatic catheter and perfusion pattern either intraoperatively or during follow-up with a portable gamma camera.[26] Macro-aggregated albumin can be given at a slow rate (40 ml/hour) similar to the I.A. chemotherapy infusion rate. Thus, such study reflects more accurately the true pattern of regional perfusion. Even without change in the position of the arterial catheter, there were changes in the arterial flow patterns due to (1) collateral formation, (2) arterial spasm, (3) progressive arteritis ± thrombosis, and (4) laminar flow.[27] In 14–51% of the cases, there was extrahepatic perfusion in the regions of the stomach, pancreas, spleen, and small bowel.[28,29] This correlated with increased incidence of gastritis with infusion chemotherapy. Tumor arteriovenous shunt was present in 38% of the cases, but this incidence decreased as tumors decreased in size.[29] Kaplan et al[30] found that there was significantly greater G.I. toxicity with infusion therapy when more than 20% of the injected tracer appeared in the lung, because a greater amount of drug bypasses the hepatic parenchyma, resulting in decreased hepatic detoxification of chemotherapeutic agents.

Because Sullivan et al[16] demonstrated in 1959 that hepatic I.A. infusion of methotrexate (MTX) gave better response than systemic I.V. therapy, most of the early reports employed MTX. Subsequently, many investigators used 5-fluorouracil (5-FU) or floxuridine (FUDR), while others used mitomycin-C (MIT), cisplatin (DDP), dacarbazine (DTIC), doxorubicin (ADR), etc. Currently, more than 20 different cytotoxic drugs have been used by the I.A. route for malignancies of various types.[31] Ensminger et al[32] demonstrated that there is a higher extraction of FUDR than of 5-FU from blood traversing the liver. At an equivalent molar dose, which was 10 times that used in conventional hepatic I.A. therapy, 94–99% of FUDR and 19–51% of 5-FU were extracted in 1 pass. Stagg et al[33] cited data showing that continuous hepatic arterial infusion of FUDR is the most effective treatment of hepatic metastases of colorectal carcinoma. However, others found that it was impossible to state whether 5-FU or FUDR had any therapeutic advantage.[34]

Satisfactory objective response is usually defined as a decrease in tumor volume by more than 50%, as measured by the sum of products of the 2 largest perpendicular dimensions of each of the tumor masses[35] and the return to normal or nearly normal levels of liver function tests. Other criteria, such as improved hepatic scan, biochemical liver function tests, or improved angiogram, have also been used.[36] But physical examination, blood tests (including carcinoembryonic antigen), and scans are not reliable methods to measure response. With hepatic angiograms, some tumors showed a transient increase in size followed by a decrease; some grew bigger as the liver span became smaller.[37]

Studying patients who had liver resection or transplantation, Mittal et al[38] showed that even computerized tomography missed 47% of primary liver cancers, 31% of metastatic tumors, and 20% of benign lesions. The missed nodules varied in size from 0.1–1.6 cm (79% were greater than 1 cm). A new organ-specific contrast agent selectively concentrated by malignant tumor of the liver can enhance initial detection and subsequent follow-up study of liver tumors.[39] The newer generation of high-resolution computerized tomography scanning, particularly with volumetric analysis, may provide both accurate and reproducible data.[33]

Most clinical reports of response rates do not specify the duration of response. Labelle et al[40] reported that their 82% objective response rate dropped to 47% if the response had to be maintained for at least 3 months.

Although some workers, especially those using short-term I.A. infusion therapy of 21 days or less,[41] reported nearly equivalent responses with hepatic I.A. infusion and systemic I.V. chemotherapy, most clinical studies indicated at least a 2-to-1 superiority of hepatic I.A. infusion over systemic chemotherapy for hepatic metastases. For advanced gastrointestinal cancers, the objective response rate with 5-FU by systemic I.V. administration varied from 13% without prior loading to 33% with an initial loading course, compared to 36% and 71% when the drug was administered directly via the hepatic artery.[2] Although currently there is no controlled and randomized data (vida infra) showing that I.A. chemotherapy is more effective than I.V. chemotherapy, indirect evidence is provided by the fact that among patients who had progression of liver metastases with systemic I.V. 5-FU or FUDR chemotherapy, subsequent hepatic I.A. infusion of the same drug produced response rates in one-third to two-thirds of the patients.[2,33]

Up to now, there also has been no randomized study showing that the survival of patients who had hepatic I.A. infusion chemotherapy as the first-line therapy, even with objective response, was significantly better than that of patients treated by the I.V. route. One report showed that hepatic I.A. infusion as a second line of therapy following the failure of I.V. chemotherapy resulted in significant improvement of survival from 12 to 18 months.[20] Thus, most investigators prefer to give hepatic artery infusion chemotherapy to patients who have failed conventional systemic treatment. Some physicians use stricter criteria for selecting patients for I.A. infusion chemotherapy, such as major symptoms from liver metastasis, hepatomegaly of at least 6 cm below the right costal margin, age less than 65 years, and anticipated survival greater than 1 month.[42]

Ansfield et al[43,44] preferred systemic 5-FU as the initial treatment for patients who have liver metastases, either found at surgery or developed on follow-up examinations. However, I.A. 5-FU was used as the initial therapy in jaundiced patients or those with liver metastases from lung, melanoma, or primary breast cancer because such tumors were relatively unresponsive to systemic 5-FU. They gave continuous I.A. infusion of 5-FU via a percutaneously placed catheter for only 21 days and maintained the response with weekly systemic I.V. therapy under close observation. When it became apparent that there was reactivation of liver metastases, they gave the patient another 21-day I.A. 5-FU infusion. As long as the patient responded, repeated infusions were alternated with 4–6 months of weekly I.V. doses. About 15% of their patients had multiple I.A. infusions. Even in patients with greater than 5 cm hepatic enlargement, 55% had objective response, and I.V. maintenance therapy of 5-FU increased the mean duration of response (6–7 weeks to 4–6 months). Reed et al[45] first gave FUDR infusion chemotherapy via a brachial artery catheter. When the tumor diminished markedly in size after 4–6 weeks of therapy, the peripheral catheter was replaced with a permanent catheter inserted at laparotomy.

Therapeutic Results of Hepatic Arterial Infusion Chemotherapy

Patients with liver metastases of colorectal carcinoma account for the majority of cases treated with hepatic I.A. infusion chemotherapy (see tables 1, 2, and 3). Scattered numbers of metastases from other sites are also candidates for infusion therapy. Some authors give I.A. chemotherapy for short duration (less than 30 days) and continue with systemic treatment (table 2). Most oncologists aim to treat on a long-term basis (table 3).

Because of the heterogeneity of the patient population, different drugs and treatment schedules, and varied methods of reporting data, it is difficult to evaluate and compare the therapeutic results. Reed et al[45] reported that 76% of colorectal cases had objective improvement, with a median survival of 13 months versus 2 months for nonresponders (p = 0.001). Others have shown that the survival time of the responding patients is 3 to 4 times longer than that of nonresponders and no-treatment controls (16 versus 5 months).[56]

For noncolorectal liver metastasis, the response to hepatic I.A. chemotherapy is reported to be good for lesions of the gallbladder, biliary tract,[45] breast, stomach, lung, and esophagus.[66] In patients with liver metastases of carcinoma of the breast, Peetz et al[63] found that the addition of I.A. chemotherapy and endocrine ablation to systemic chemotherapy significantly increased survival (mean survival = 21 versus 11–15 months). For liver metastasis of breast carcinoma that has failed to respond to prior systemic chemotherapy, including combinations with ADR, Wallace et al[31] have used hepatic I.A. infusion of DDP or Velban. The response rates were 25% and 30%, respectively. When they tried a combination of DDP (100 mg/m^2 for 4 hours) followed by a continuous infusion of Velban (1.6 mg/m^2/day × 5), the response rate was increased to 80%.

Some investigators reported that malignant melanoma responds poorly, but Kondi et al[74] reported a patient who had a 14-month objective response to I.A. bleomycin (BLM) and oral hydroxyurea. Some melanoma metastases in the liver had transient response to I.A. infusion of DTIC. Storm et al[73] treated 10 patients with I.A. DTIC plus localized hyperthermia. Three patients had disease regression and 5 had disease stablized for 3–14 months (median 6.5 months) and survived 4–18 months (median 8.5 months).

In general, patients who showed objective response benefited both in quality (improvement in Karnofsky score) and length of survival. In patients with colorectal cancers, Cady and Oberfield[52] noted that those with either no symptom or symptoms of 6 months or longer survived considerably better than those with symptoms lasting 1 to 6 months. Patients over 60 years of age, those with transaminase (SGOT) of more than 80 units, albumin of less than 3.5

Table 1. Hepatic Arterial Infusion Chemotherapy for Liver Metastasis of Colorectal Carcinoma

Investigators/reference	Year	A[1]	No. patients	I.A. infusion chemo Rx drug(s)	Duration	Response rate (%)	Survival Overall	Survival Responder	Survival Non-responder
Brennan et al[46]	1963	B[2]	13	5-FU	1 – 3 M	70	?	?	?
Freckman[47]	1971	F[3]	271	5-FU or combination	1 – 8 M	36 at 6 M	?	12 M	4 M
Cady and Oberfield[36]	1974	S[4]	55	FUDR	6 – 9 M	57	?	16 M	5 M
Fortuny et al[48]	1975	F	25	5-FU* or MIT#	2 – 10 day	?	?	9.5#, 12 M*	?
Oberfield et al[49]	1979	B	66	5-FU, FUDR	1 – 24 M	54 (15% CR)	?	11 M	4 M
Douglass[50]	1979	?[5]	48	5-FU + MIT + VCR + Velban	Q3 M	56	?	17 M	?
Grage et al[51,52]	1979	S,B,F	30	5-FU	21 day	34			
Patt et al[35]	1981	B,F	55	FUDR + MIT	8 M	43 (5% CR)	11 M	?	?
Wallace et al[31]	1984	F	31	FUDR + MIT	Q M	—	8 M	?	?
Bedikian et al[53]	1984	F	27	FUDR ± MIT		43	?	10 M	?
Fortner et al[54]	1984	S	73	5-FU + MTX ± CTX ± Act-D	+ 14 day	?	11.5 M	?	?
			694						

[1] technique of placement of the hepatic artery infusion catheter
[2] via brachial artery
[3] via femoral artery
[4] at time of abdominal surgery
[5] data not given
* 5-fluorouracil
# mitomycin-C

Table 2. Hepatic Arterial Infusion Chemotherapy for Liver Metastasis of Various Primary Malignancies (Short-Term I.A. Chemotherapy of 30 Days or Less)

Investigators/reference	Year	A[1]	No. patients	Colorectum	Pancreas	Stomach	Breast	Melanoma	Liver	Biliary tract	Other	Drug(s)	Response rate (%)	Survival (median) Responder	Survival (median) Nonresponder
Rochlin and Smart[55]	1966	F[2]	51	24	6	—	2	4	4	—	11	5-FU	36	?[5]	?
Ariel and Pack[56]	1967	F	{ 22	12	—	1	—	4	1	—	4	5-FU + MTX	27	?	?
			59	23	5	5	1	6	3	2	14	Same + RT	47	?	?
Massey et al[57]	1971		38	10	6	—	5	—	3	3	11	5-FU	44	?	?
Tandon et al[58]	1973	F	122	67	21	6	16	—	—	3	9	5-FU	64 at 3 M	8 + M	—
Kraybill et al[59]	1977	B[3],F	13	—	—	—	2	—	—	—	11	ADR	2/2 islet cell, 1/2 breast		
Misra et al[60]	1977	S[4]	23	2	—	2	—	—	4	13	2	5-FU + MIT	65	9.4 M	2 M
Petrak and Minton[42]	1979	F	62	28	3	1	8	6	6	3	7	5-FU, others	46	5 – 9 M (overall)	
Robinson[61]	1979	F	134	108	13	2	5	1	6	—	5	5-FU	55		
Helsper et al[62]	1981	F	86	45	7	4	9	2	8	7	4	5-FU, others	64 colon / 77 breast		
Peetz et al[63]	1982	F	48	—	—	—	48	—	—	—	—	5-FU mostly, few ADM	—	19 M (I.V. + I.A. + endocrine) / 6 M (I.V. + I.A.)	
			650												

[1]technique of placement of the hepatic artery infusion catheter
[2]via femoral artery
[3]via brachial artery
[4]at time of abdominal surgery
[5]no data given

Table 3. Hepatic Arterial Infusion Chemotherapy for Liver Metastasis of Various Primary Malignancies (I.A. Infusion Chemotherapy of 30 Days or Longer)

Investigators/ reference	Year	A[1]	No. patients	Colorectum	Pancreas	Stomach	Breast	Melanoma	Liver	Biliary tract	Other	Drug(s)	Response rate (%)	Survival (median) Responder	Non-responder
Burrows et al[64]	1967	B[2]	109	↓	94	↑	—	2	—	—	13	5-FU or FUDR	59, 25	?[5]	?
Labelle et al[40]	1968	B	59	33	9	6	8	—	—	—	3	FUDR	47 (at 3 M)	?	?
Donegan et al[65]	1970	S[3]	13	10	1	—	—	1	—	—	1	5-FU	60 (colon)	?	?
Watkins et al[66]	1970	S	184	108	19	5	6	6	10	11	19	FUDR	54 (colon) / 71	15 M (colon)	4 M
Stehlin et al[67]	1974	S	108	51	3	3	23	9	—	—	19	mainly 5-FU	?	7 M (colon)	3 M
Davis et al[41]	1974	B	26	—	20	6	—	—	—	—	—	5-FU	—	{ 4 M (pancreas) / 11 M (stomach)	—
Ansfield et al[68]	1975	B	419	381	15	12	—	4	9	—	—	5-FU	55	7 M	2 M
Pettavel and Morgenthaler[69]	1978	S	107	57	—	5	9	9	11	—	16	5-FU + FUDR	{ 75 / 85 (colon)	10 M / 18 M	? / ?
Sundqvist et al[70]	1978	B	46	15	7	5	—	—	11	—	8	5-FU	43	12 M	4 M
Patt et al[71]	1978	B,F[4]	30	16	2	1	5	2	2	—	2	{ FUDR (colon) / DTIC (melanoma)	50	?	?
Calvo et al[72]	1980	B,F	20	2	—	—	9	5	—	—	4	DDP	45	?	?
Reed et al[45]	1981	B,S	124	88	4	—	—	—	13	10	—	FUDR	76 (colon)	13 M	2 M
Storm et al[73]	1982	B,F	10	—	—	—	—	10	—	—	—	DTIC+hyperthermia		8.5 M	?
Falk et al[78]	1982	F	157	98	6	7	6	—	21	—	10	5-FU + MIT	?	12 M	3 M
Wallace et al[31]	1984	F	71	31	—	—	40	—	—	—	—	{ DDP + Velban / FUDR + MIT	{ 25 – 80 (breast) / 45 (colon)	9 M / 14 M	3 M / 6 M
			1,483												

[1]technique of placement of the hepatic artery infusion catheter
[2]via brachial artery
[3]at time of abdominal surgery
[4]via femoral artery
[5]data not given

g/100 ml, and hepatic involvement of more than 50% had a shorter expectancy of survival. Surprisingly, a bilirubin level of more than 3 mg% indicated better opportunity for survival (median survival of 5 patients was 21 months versus 9 months for 43 patients without jaundice). The response rate was slightly higher for patients with synchronous liver metastases, and nonresponders received less 5-FU and FUDR compared to responders.[49] Chemical hepatitis and various drug-related toxicities were listed, but no correlation with response rates was noted. Patients who had operative catheterization and infusion chemotherapy without any technical complications had longer median survival than those intolerant of therapy or with complications (21 versus 8 months).[66]

In 1979, Grage et al[51] reported on the only prospective randomized study of short-term hepatic I.A. infusion of 5-FU versus peripheral I.V. 5-FU in patients with colorectal metastasis. The 2 approaches differed only in the initial loading course. The 30 patients given I.A. therapy received continuous infusion of 5-FU over 21 days (20 mg/kg/day × 14 and 10 mg/kg/day ×7). In another 31 patients, I.V. 5-FU was given over 12 days (12 mg/kg/day × 4 and 6 mg/kg/day Q.O.D. × 4). Both groups were maintained on weekly 5-FU (15 mg/kg, maximum = 1 g). Patients completing the initial loading course received 350 mg/kg of 5-FU in the I.A. group versus 72 mg/kg by the I.V. method. Although the response rate in the I.A. group was higher (34% versus 23%), the difference was not statistically significant (nor were duration of response and survival rate). The complications of stomatitis, leukopenia, and thrombocytopenia were similar, but the I.A. group had significantly more nausea and vomiting and diarrhea than the I.V. group (76% versus 25% and 41% versus 12%, respectively). The survival curve of 12 patients who had catheters placed at laparotomy appeared better than that of 18 patients who had catheters placed percutaneously.[52] Some significant morbidity associated with the infusion catheter was noted (2 femoral artery thrombosis, 6 bleeding, 3 catheters needed repositioning). Many detailed aspects of evaluation of response and failures were subject to criticism.[75] Since this was a multi-institutional study (12 institutions each entered 1–18 patients) composed of heterogeneous and relatively few patients with many technical problems, the findings in this study remain to be confirmed.

In 1984, Bedikian et al[53] retrospectively studied 179 patients who had metastatic carcinoma confirmed to the liver treated with at least 1 cycle of chemotherapy and who could be evaluated 4 weeks later. With no prior chemotherapy, 152 patients received 5-FU-containing I.V. therapy and 27 had hepatic I.A. infusion of an FUDR-containing regimen. The overall response rate was significantly higher for the I.A. group (43% versus 12%), but not the median duration of response (8 versus 10 months). The overall survival was similar (10 versus 11 months).

Although the activity of MIT given as a single agent by hepatic I.A. infusion was less than that of 5-FU — 46% versus 83% in one study[48] — Misra et al[60] used both for 2–4 weeks followed by I.V. maintenance therapy and reported a 65% response rate. Patt et al[76] reported a high response rate (83%) with MIT and FUDR by hepatic artery infusion of colorectal metastasis (adding ADR for hepatomas or metastasis of other primaries[77] and using DDP for carcinoma of the breast, melanoma, and sarcoma).[72] In the above 2 series, more than half of patients (13/24) who were refractory to MIT or 5-FU given I.V. as a single drug responded to this combination infusion therapy.

Kano et al[81] from Japan treated 72 patients with hepatic metastases (discovered concomitently with gastric carcinoma) with hepatic I.A. infusion and/or systemic chemotherapy alone (using single or 3 drugs) after resection of the primary tumor. In this nonrandomized study, the mean survival was 9 months for the hepatic I.A. infusion and systemic chemotherapy group, 7 months for the 3-drug systemic group, 4 months for the single drug group, and 3.5 months for those given no chemotherapy. The survival rates at 1 year were 21%, 12%, 6%, and 7%, respectively. Hepatic I.A. infusion with MIT and 5-FU was better than with 5-FU alone. The benefit of any chemotherapy is hard to document, because Koga et al[82] from Japan showed that for patients with metastasis from gastric cancer, noncurative resection of the stomach significantly increased survival for those with limited liver metastasis. (Mean survivals for metastases of one lobe: gastrectomy patients 20.6 months versus 4.2 months without gastrectomy; for those with scatter metastases to both lobes, 12.4 months versus 4.1 months.)

Falk et al[78] believed that high-dose intermittent hepatic I.A. infusion of 5-FU (48% for 3–5 days, Q 6–8 wks) gave better quality of life than weekly chemotherapy. They reported that the addition of MIT did not increase the survival result of I.A. 5-FU alone. Tilchen et al[79] treated 4 patients with unresectable unilobar hepatic metastasis of colorectal cancer with percutaneous I.A. infusion of MIT and FUDR. After 2 months, partial remission was achieved in all, and 3 patients had complete resection of the hepatic tumor. These 3 patients remained disease-free for 13+ to 21+ months without any further treatment. With decreased operative mortality of hepatic surgery, Hodgson et al[80] have debulked multiple liver metastasis (range 1–8) in 16 patients and added postoperative hepatic I.A. chemotherapy via catheter. At a median follow-up of 15 months, the 1-year survival rate was 62%, and 2-year, 33%.

Oily contract medium (Ethiodol) used in lymphangiographic studies can be injected into the liver to delineate liver neoplasms.[83] Using a new anticancer agent (styrene maleic acid conjugated neocarcinostatin) solublized in Lipiodol and administered via the feeding artery (2–4 doses given at intervals of 3–8 weeks), Konno et al[84] treated 24 patients with mostly unresectable malignancy. Serum CEA levels decreased in 11/12 patients and tumor size decreased in 7/13 liver metastases. Preliminary survival data on patients with liver metastasis was better than on comparable but untreated patients (mean survival 8.5 versus 3.7 months).

Several oncologists noted that patients who had inadvertant or intentional occlusion of the hepatic or celiac artery had higher response rates and longer survival times than those without arterial occlusion. With 5-FU and FUDR infusion therapy via a percutaneously placed catheter, the median survival of those with complete or partial occlusion of the artery was 7–11 months versus 4 months for those without occlusion.[49] With infusion of MIT and FUDR, the median survival time for patients with hepatic artery occlusion by embolization was 15 months, compared to 8 months for those without occlusion.[35]

These findings indirectly confirm the rationale for using deliberate ligation of the hepatic artery as a treatment for unresectable liver metastasis.

Hepatic Artery Ligation (HAL) and Arterial Infusion Chemotherapy

It has been estimated that the hepatic artery normally supplies 25% of the blood to the liver and provides 50% of its oxygen. The portal vein provides 75% of the blood and 50% of the oxygen to the liver.[85] The concept of treating liver cancers by interruption of their arterial supply was suggested by Marko-witz in 1952.[86] The premise for this approach is that both primary and meta-static tumors of the liver receive their blood supplies almost exclusively from the hepatic arterial system, whereas nonmalignant liver tissues have a double supply (the hepatic artery and the portal vein).

In 1966, Nilsson et al[87] first reported using hepatic artery ligation (HAL) as the only treatment of liver metastasis in 7 patients. It appears that patients with carcinoid syndrome from metastatic lesions in the liver derived definite benefit from ligation of the hepatic artery alone.[88,89] Metastatic visceral leiomyosarcoma may have prolonged survival, too.[90] For other lesions, the benefit of HAL appeared to be less certain.

Clinical and experimental evidence shows that ligation of the hepatic artery does cause selective necrosis of the center of a large tumor, but there is almost always a margin or shell of viable malignant cells at the periphery of the devascularized nodule.[2] Thus, tumor regression after HAL is short-lived, and there is a definite rationale to add chemotherapy (1) either into the hepatic artery distally or via branches of the portal vein or (2) systemically. Almost all patients who had HAL after 1970 are so treated; their results are summarized in table 4.

The techniques of ligation of the hepatic artery and dearterialization have been well described.[19] Almersjo et al[97] found no correlation between the extent of dearterialization and survival time. These investigators also compared 36 patients who had resection of metastatic liver cancer with 30 patients who had hepatic dearterialization.[97,107] The overall operative mortality for the resection group was 30%, and for HAL, 14%. Berjian et al[90] reported mortality of 13%, which would have been improved if they had excluded patients with portal hypertension.

After ligation of the hepatic artery distal to the gastroduodenal artery, there is an immediate and significant rise of serum lactic dehydrogenase, creatine phosphokinase, transaminase, and a mild elevation of alkaline phosphatase and bilirubin.[108] All abnormal tests tend to return to preoperative levels within a week. It appears that hepatic arterial ligation for metastatic tumors in the liver can be well tolerated unless far-advanced cirrhosis, hepatic decompensa-tion, coagulopathy, renal failure, and/or portal hypertension are present. Even in selected patients with ≥ 50% of liver involved with colorectal metasta-sis, HAL can be performed with 2% mortality and minimal morbidity.[105]

Table 4. Hepatic Artery Ligation and Infusion Chemotherapy for Liver Metastasis

Investigators/reference	Year	No. patients	Colorectum	Pancreas	Liver	Biliary tract	Carcinoid	Sarcoma	Melanoma	Other	Chemotherapy	Response rate (%)	Survival Median	Survival Range
Murray-Lyon et al[91]	1970	11	5	—	—	—	3	—	2	1	I.P.V.* 5-FU	—	12 M	1–20 M
Koudahl and Funding[92]	1972	20	6	4	4	2	2	—	—	2	I.V. 5-FU	—	5 M	—
Zike et al[93]	1974	38	25	—	5	1	—	—	—	7	I.A. 5-FU	—	13 M+	—
Cushieri et al[94]	1975	17	8	—	9	—	—	—	—	—	I.A. 5-FU,MTX	50	12 M (mean)	—
Sparks et al[95]	1975	19	13	—	—	—	1	1	2	2	I.V.	43	—	2–20 M
Ramming et al[96]	1976	16	9	—	7	—	—	—	—	—	I.A. 5-FU	80	11 M	3–14 M
Almersjo et al[97]	1976	40	10	3	10	4	1	3	—	9	I.P.V. 5-FU	—	12 M (colon) 10 M (breast)	—
Nagasue et al[98]	1976	14	2	—	6	—	—	2	—	4	I.P.V. 5-FU ± ADR	71	7 M	—
Lee[99]	1979	9	2	—	4	2	—	1	—	—	I.A. FUDR or ADR	71	—	—
Evans[100]	1979	28	28	—	—	—	—	—	—	—	I.V.	50	12 M	—
Smith[101]	1979	100	?	?	12	21	?	?	?	?	(45 patients)	—	12 % at 2 years	—
Fortner and Papachristou[102]	1979	134	54	—	31	—	9	—	15	25	I.A. ± I.P.V. 3–4 drugs	—	18 % at 2 years	—
Berjian et al[90]	1980	15	2	2	2	1	3	—	4	1	I.P.V.	40	14 M	—
Taylor[103,104]	1981	35	35	—	—	—	—	—	—	—	I.P.V. 5-FU	—	—	—
Wallace et al[11]	1984	24	24	—	—	—	—	—	—	—	I.A. FUDR + MIT	53	15 M	—
Petrelli et al[105]	1984	97	97	—	—	—	—	—	—	—	5-FU + other drugs	—	9.5 M	—
Laufman et al[106]	1984	19	19	—	—	—	—	—	—	—	5-FU + MIT	—	13 M	—
		636												

*infusion into portal vein

Petrelli et al[105] did a comprehensive retrospective review (1975–82) of 97 patients with $\geq 50\%$ of liver involvement with colorectal carcinoma who were treated with HAL. After HAL, patients were also treated with a number of 5-FU-containing combinations, but this did not affect survival. The overall median survival time was 9.5 months. Three factors significantly influencing survival after HAL were: (1) performance status (12.3 months of normal activity versus 2.6 months of 100% bedridden); (2) extent of metastasis (10 months for those with only intrahepatic metastasis, 8.8 months for liver and lung metastasis, and 7 months for synchronous intra-abdominal metastasis); and (3) alkaline phosphatase value (12.4 months for those below 2 times normal, 7 months for those above).

Many investigators emphasized that substantial palliation (improvement of pain and general well-being) can be achieved by HAL plus infusion of various chemotherapeutic agents. To avoid the deleterious effects of sudden ligation of the hepatic artery and to combine the effect of complete arterial interruption (which produces central tumor necrosis) with I.A. infusion chemotherapy (which effects the rapidly proliferating cells at the periphery of the tumor), various techniques of temporary, delayed, or intermittent occlusion of the hepatic artery have been devised.

El Domeiri[109,110] used an arterial balloon catheter inserted surgically. The balloon was inflated twice daily and kept inflated for 45–50 minutes during the 3-week infusion chemotherapy. He compared results among 29 patients with cancer of the colorectum: 13 had systemic chemotherapy, 9 had hepatic I.A. infusion chemotherapy, and 7 had I.V. therapy plus intermittent arterial occlusion. None of the patients who had systemic chemotherapy responded. Patients who received intermittent arterial occlusion and chemotherapy had longer periods of objective response than did those treated by I.A. chemotherapy alone. In experimental animals, Karakousis et al[111] showed that injection of ADR distal to the occluded hepatic artery or portal vein for 30 minutes resulted in higher liver tissue drug levels than those achieved after hepatic I.A. or intraportal vein (I.P.V.) injection without occlusion. Liver drug levels were significantly higher than those reached in systemic I.V. administration.

Bengmark and Fredlund[112] also described a method of transient and delayed occlusion of the hepatic artery. Total dearterialization of the liver is done at initial abdominal exploration, but the hepatic artery is only cannulated and not ligated. Two external polyethylene catheters placed around the hepatic artery are tightened for about 16 hours 2–5 days after the operation (24-hour occlusion resulted in permanent thrombosis). In 23 patients, there was no operative mortality (repeated inhibition of blood supply could be done 2 and 6 months later). 5-FU was infused 2–4 days after tightening of the slings (15–20 mg/kg/day $\times$ 4 days, 10 mg/kg/day $\times$ 21 days, and then systemic I.V. 5-FU every 2 weeks). Tumor regression was seen in more than 50% of the patients.[113] For patients with metastatic colorectal cancer, the median survival was 11 months. Patients with known extrahepatic tumor at operation had much shorter survival times (mean = 5 months versus 21 months of those without).

Lise et al[114] used both delayed temporary occlusion of the hepatic artery and infusion chemotherapy of 5-FU, MIT, and vincristine (VCR) in 14 patients: 54% had objective responses and the median survival time was 12.5 months. They concluded that delayed occlusion by an external tourniquet method appeared safer than intraoperative HAL. However, among 20 patients reported by Tylen et al,[37] 3 had infected necrotic tumor requiring laparotomy, 3 had 5-FU leakage into the abdominal cavity, 3 had thrombosis of the hepatic artery, and 5 developed aneurysms (3 needed operative ligation). They said that hepatic abscesses could be prevented by giving a broad-spectrum antibiotic postoperatively (ampicillin, 6 g/day, 1 g via I.A. catheter).

Aronsen et al[115] designed another method of intermittent blockage of hepatic artery flow using enzymatically degradable microspheres. With continuous infusion of 5-FU (500 mg/day) into a percutaneously placed catheter in the common hepatic artery, they injected polysaccharide microspheres 3 times a day during a 14-day period. The treatment course was repeated 3 months later. Four of 12 patients had regression of over half of the tumor, and 2 of these 4 had thrombosis of the hepatic artery.

Ensminger et al[116] showed that infusion of carmustine (BCNU) into the hepatic artery generates at least a 4-fold greater drug exposure for hepatic tumor without increasing systemic exposure. Dakhil et al[117] injected BCNU (50 mg/m^2) and degradable starch microspheres into the hepatic artery catheter. There was a transient reduction of hepatic blood flow by 80–100% and a reduction of systemic nitrosourea levels by 30–90%. One patient with cholangiocarcinoma had partial response and a few patients had stable metastatic disease.

Portal Vein Infusion Chemotherapy

In animal tumor systems and in patients, it has been shown that after ligation of the hepatic artery, the vascular plexus at the periphery of the tumor is filled by perfusion via the portal vein.[118] Some investigators therefore added infusion chemotherapy into branches of the portal vein immediately following HAL. Almersjo et al[119] compared 29 patients treated with portal infusion of 5-FU only with 18 patients who had a combination of HAL and portal infusion. The survival was better in the latter group (mean 10.8 versus 7.4 months of portal infusion alone). Many of their patients had repeat laparotomy 2–3 months after the 3-month infusion chemotherapy.[97] A portal catheter could be reinserted in 10% of the patients. Some patients had a third catheter. Of interest is the fact that in 4/40 patients who had reexploration, the previously unresectable liver tumor became resectable.

Laufman et al[106] treated 19 patients with liver metastasis from colon cancer with HAL and portal vein infusions of MIT (10 mg/m^2 I.V. Q2M) and 5-FU (1.2 g/m^2/day × 5 monthly). Of 17 evaluable patients, all improved clinically, with marked decrease of CEA levels, and 12 had tumor response (2 complete, both <30% replacement; 10 partial, 7 had 30–60%, and 2 had 60–74% replacement). Median survival of all patients was 13 months after HAL, with 4 patients still alive at 13, 16, 41, and 61 months.

Fortner and Pahnke[7] described the use of a Ramondi Silastic catheter, which has an antireflux valve at its heparin-treated tip that prevents retrograde flow of blood and subsequent clot formation. He has placed this catheter in the hepatic artery as well as in the inferior mesenteric and middle colic veins. Among 134 patients with unresectable hepatic metastasis (1970–78), 102 had HAL and cannulation, 23 arterial or portal catheter only, and 39 had other procedures.[102] The overall operative mortality was 7%. Among the 77 patients adequately treated (2 cycles of chemotherapy during the first 3 postoperative months), the 2-year survival rate was 18%, and 3-year, 3%. These results were better than with those who received therapy through peripheral veins (8% and 0%, respectively). The authors did not separate the results of patients receiving hepatic I.V. infusion from those receiving I.P.V. infusion.

In a recent report, 117 out of 247 patients (1971–82) with unresectable colorectal hepatic metastases had operative exploration and insertion of infusion catheters: 29 hepatic I.A., 24 portal I.V., and 64 both.[54] Fifty-nine patients also had HAL. The 30-day postoperative mortality rate was 1.7%, and morbidity, 37.6%. The majority of patients were treated with 3 or 4 drugs in combination (MTX + 5-FU and ADR, or actinomycin + Cytoxan). The median survival from time of catheter placement of 109 evaluable patients was 11.5 months. The investigators studied the effect of 20 variables in the observed survival time in detail (site of catheter and chemotherapy regimen had no influence). Only 3 variables influenced survival significantly: percent of hepatic replacement by tumor, lymph node metastases, and history of prior chemotherapy. No patient with liver replacement greater than 80% lived more than 8 months. The data indicated little benefit from any therapy after more than 50% of the liver was replaced by tumor. Wagner et al[12] showed that patients with bilobar widespread hepatic metastasis had poor prognoses with or without extrahepatic spread.

Taylor[102] treated 35 patients with colorectal liver metastasis with HAL combined with portal vein cytotoxic perfusion. In patients with tumor of less than 20% of the liver volume, the median survival was 15 months; when 20–70% of the liver was replaced, the median survival fell to 10 months; and when more than 70% of liver was involved, the mean survival was 5.5 months. Fortner et al[54] divided extent of liver replacement into 3 categories: $\leq 50\%$, 50–80%, $> 80\%$. Within each group, patients could be further subdivided into A or B (had nodal metastasis and/or prior chemotherapy). The 1-year survival rates for 1-A and 1-B were 83% and 50%; and for 2-A and 2-B, 41% and 20%.

Taylor[104] reported a nonrandomized clinical trial of different forms of regional infusion chemotherapy in 24 patients who had liver metastasis found during resection of Dukes B/C colorectal cancer. Six had no treatment, 6 had HAL and hepatic I.A. infusion, 5 had umbilical vein infusion (I.P.V.) because HAL and catheterization could not be performed, and 7 had HAL + I.A. + I.P.V. All patients in the treatment groups received 5-FU (1 g/day) continuously for 10 days. Three patients in the HAL + I.A. + I.P.V. group had almost complete regression of liver metastasis by liver scan plus clinical examination 6 months later. This combination improved the survival greatly (mean 9.8 ± 3.4 versus 4.1 ± 3.8 months). Otherwise, no benefit was found with HAL + I.A. or I.P.V. alone as compared with the control group.

In 1975, Taylor et al[103] started a randomized prospective trial to assess the value of adjuvant treatment of patients who had resection of Dukes A, B, C colorectal cancers but without liver metastasis—using only umbilical vein (I.P.V.) 5-FU infusion chemotherapy for the first 7 postoperative days. With a median follow-up of 34 months, 39% of the untreated control group and 21% of the treated group have died. Specifically, 17/38 deceased patients in the control group had liver metastasis, compared to 5/19 I.P.V.-infused patients. It is obvious that the findings of such studies remain to be confirmed, and if adjuvant chemotherapy can prevent or delay the appearance of liver metastasis, it would represent an important breakthrough in cancer management.

Transcatheter Embolization and Arterial Infusion Chemotherapy

Transcatheter arterial infusion chemotherapy and vascular occlusion by embolization has evolved over the past 10 years. Indications, contraindications and many approaches and variations in techniques are still being developed. Many different materials are available for embolization, including autologous clot, tissue, and foreign substances.[31]

Ivalon particles (250–590 μm) were used for peripheral hepatic artery or small collateral embolization (HAE), and the stainless steel coil was used for proximal hepatic artery occlusion. Gelfoam cubes were injected for segmental artery embolization between Ivalon particles and coils when necessary.[120] Gelfoam powder or particles also can be used to thrombose peripheral hepatic arterial branches.[121]

The classical distribution of the hepatic artery originating from the celiac axis occurs in 55% of patients.[122] Because multiple hepatic arteries and variations in anatomy occur in half of the normal population, hepatic artery anomalies make certain patients technically difficult for arterial infusion chemotherapy. Chuang et al[120] randomized their study according to vascular anatomy: Patients with a single hepatic artery received I.A. infusion chemotherapy, while those with multiple hepatic arteries received sequential lobar or segmental embolization. For patients who had arterial collaterals developed after occulusion of the hepatic artery (by surgical ligation, embolization, or secondary to catheter-induced thrombosis), Soo et al[123] tried additional chemotherapy infusion or embolization through the extrahepatic collaterals. Their success rate of selectively catheterizing the hepatic artery is 95%; for left or right gastric artery, 65%; and for pancreaticoduodenal or gastroduodenal artery, only 50%. Superselective embolization to the phrenic, pancreaticoduodenal, or gastroduodenal arteries created no major problems if prophylactic antacid and cimetidine were used. But infusion of chemotherapy to neighboring organs occasionally resulted in gastric ulcer. In 10 patients, the investigators recatheterized the occuluded hepatic artery by placing a guidewire through the thrombus and then inserting the catheter for infusion.[124]

A postembolization syndrome consisting of fever, nausea and vomiting, and right upper quadrant pain was experienced by most of the patients for 2–7 days. Paralytic ileus occurred in one-third of the patients, lasting 3–4 days.[125] Abnormal liver function tests became more abnormal for 5–7 days and sometimes for as long as 3 weeks.[126] Nonspecific gas-forming occurred in all the embolized livers within hours to days. This was due to air introduced during embolization and to gas released by tumor necrosis. No hepatic abscess was observed in the first 200 HAE procedures despite the lack of routine use of prophylactic antibiotics, which were used only when patients needed to have the catheter repositioned or when there was evidence of infection, fever over 5 days, septicemia, etc.[31,124]

Wallace et al[125] have performed over 350 HAE for both primary and metastatic neoplasms; a majority of the patients had failed systemic or hepatic I.A. infusion chemotherapy. Other indications for HAE included (1) to facilitate surgery of resectable neoplasm, (2) to eradicate a tumor that surgery failed to remove completely, and (3) to control pain, hemorrhage, or arteriovenous shunting from the tumor. The median survival for metastatic colorectal carcinomas after I.A. chemotherapy was only 8 months. After embolization following failure of I.A. chemotherapy, the median survival was 15 months.[124] Among the first 100 patients, 7 died within 1 month; 3 died of hepatic failure that might have been related to the procedure.

In 6 patients with liver metastasis from an unknown primary site, Patt et al[77] intentionally occluded the hepatic artery following attainment of maximal benefits from I.A. infusion of multiple drugs (FUDR, ADR, and MIT). The survival from initiation of therapy appeared to improve from 6 to more than 10 months. In another report, Patt et al[127] saw no benefit of adding embolization when patients with colorectal metastasis either responded or failed hepatic I.A. infusion of FUDR and MIT, which were given after failure of systemic I.V. 5-FU.

Allison et al[128] used gelatin sponge embolization of multiple hepatic carcinoid metastases in 2 patients, both of whom had immediate and lasting relief from flushing attacks. The embolization procedure could be repeated. Martensson et al[129] treated 8 patients, and the liver tumor mass reduced in size in 7 patients for at least 6 months. The carcinoid syndrome disappeared in 5, but the symptom relapsed in 2 after 6 months. For endocrine tumors, it is recommended that the patient be treated with pharmacologic antagonists for a day or two before embolization to minimize the effects of hormone release during the procedure and later with tumor necrosis.[125] Carrasco et al[130] treated 18 patients with apudomas metastatic to the liver with HAE (7 carcinoid, 5 nonsecreting, 4 gastrin, and 2 others). Partial remission occurred in 11 patients (some had additional hepatic I.A. chemotherapy). Symptomatic improvement was dramatic in some, but impact on survival could not be demonstrated.

In patients with liver metastases of renal carcinoma, Chuang and Wallace[131] performed hepatic artery embolization first, followed in 4–6 weeks by renal tumor infarction, nephrectomy, and Depo-Provera. One patient treated in this manner had 90% necrosis of the hepatic metastases documented by surgery and histopathology. Shermeta et al[132] described a child with a large, unresectable hepatic tumor whose artery was too small to allow embolization with conventional substances such as Gelfoam, autologous clot, Ivalon, etc. Accordingly, isobutyl 2-cyanoacrylate was used for injection. The tumor mass shrank significantly and allowed resection by a left hepatectomy. Kato et al[133] designed a "chemoembolization" procedure by giving selective I.A. infusion of ethylcellulose-coated microcapsules of MIT. Four patients with hepatic neoplasms had some reduction of tumor size, and 8 of 12 patients with advanced carcinoma of the kidney, bladder, or cervix had successful radical operation after chemoembolization.

Currently, according to the interventional radiologists, contraindications to hepatic arterial embolization are still being formulated.[126] Cirrhosis, portal vein or biliary tract obstruction, and extensive metastatic disease are only relative restrictions. Even for patients with tumor replacing 70% or more of the liver, sequential partial embolization over several months can be done with relatively few untoward effects. They have been reluctant to embolize in patients who have jaundice caused by hepatocellular damage or tumor thrombosis obstructing the portal vein with extensive collateral network. As with HAL, response of hepatic malignancy to embolization is short-lived. Thus, the radiologists concluded that "a search for more effective cytotoxic agents is still of utmost importance."

Summary and Conclusions

With the availability of portable infusion pumps, Silastic central venous catheters (Broviac or Hickman), easy insertion techniques, and a low catheter-related infection rate even in myelosuppressed patients, long-term and ambulatory infusion of 5-FU, FUDR, and other drugs for systemic or regional chemotherapy is gaining popularity with patients and physicians.

Several prospective randomized and controlled studies are now in progress comparing I.A. infusion therapy with systemic treatment. Recent studies have selected patients for hepatic I.A. chemotherapy much more carefully and have studied the extent of disease in more detail. For instance, some authors suggested that before considering treating patients with liver metastasis of colorectal cancer, they should have a Karnofsky performance status of greater than 50; no evidence of extrahepatic tumor as shown by physical examination, chest roentgenogram, abdominal CT scan, and barium enema or colonoscopy; reasonable hepatic function (bilirubin <5 mg/dL; prothrombin time <15 s; albumin >3 g/dL; absence of gross ascites); no evidence of active infection; estimated life expectancy of at least 2 months; and adequate bone marrow and renal function.[33]

Studies using implantable pumps used more stringent criteria of patient selection and paid more attention to ancillary therapy, including preoperative and postoperative supportive care. Balch et al[134] said patients with tumors involving more than 50% of the liver were not good candidates. They used 1 or 2 trials of hepatic infusion with a percutaneously placed catheter to determine if the tumor was responsive. Preoperatively, patients with significant weight loss (5–10% of ideal weight) received 1 week of continuous enteral alimentation of 2,000 to 3,000 kcal/day. All patients had good-to-excellent performance status. Thus, clinical results published recently and in the future should be much better than those reported in the past.

With more effective control of liver metastasis by regional therapy, extrahepatic lesions have become more of a problem. The natural history of patients with liver metastasis is changing. Metastatic cancer of the liver no longer has a dominant influence upon survival as previously reported.[10] Watkins et al[66] reported that extrahepatic metastasis was the cause of death in 17% of their patients treated with infusion therapy and that carcinomatosis with liver involvement was the cause in another 31%. Cady and Oberfield[36] noted that 59% of their responders to hepatic artery infusion died with or from extrahepatic metastases. Reed et al[45] noted that of their 16 responders who died while still in hepatic regression, 31% died from extrahepatic disease. Recent data on patients treated with long-term hepatic I.A. infusion chemotherapy using an implantable pump also showed that extrahepatic metastases developed in 30% of the patients while receiving infusion therapy.[135,136] Thirty-five of 81 patients (43%) relapsed while receiving regional chemotherapy, and only 8 of the 35 (23%) had tumor progression in the liver. Lung was the most common site of metastasis (54% of all); other sites included abdominal nodes (31%), bone (18%), and peritoneum (9%). Because patients tolerate long-term hepatic infusion chemotherapy with minimal toxicity, Lee[99] suggested as early as 1979 that regional therapy for liver metastasis probably should be supplemented by systemic chemotherapy as well.

In conclusion, metastatic carcinoma of the liver is a virulent and fatal disease. Surgical resection is the treatment of choice whenever possible. Many reports show that hepatic arterial infusion of chemotherapeutic agents can give favorable response in 55–80% of the cases and can prolong survival in comparison with untreated patients or patients receiving systemic chemotherapy. Ligation of the hepatic artery or embolization have been used for palliation of symptoms and have produced short-term responses. Several reports showed that unresectable tumors become resectable after hepatic arterial or intraportal infusion chemotherapy, or transcatheter embolization. These reports are encouraging and emphasize the importance of multimodality cancer treatments.

33

HEPATIC ARTERIAL INFUSION CHEMOTHERAPY: CLINICAL TRIALS WITH THE IMPLANTABLE PUMP

Alfred E. Chang, M.D., Philip D. Schneider, M.D., Ph.D., and Paul H. Sugarbaker, M.D.

CONTINUOUS INFUSION OF CHEMOTHERAPY agents into the arterial system of the liver has several theoretical advantages. The continuous administration of chemotherapy to the tumor prolongs drug exposure to the tumor cells undergoing DNA synthesis, thus increasing the cell-kill fraction. Previous anatomical studies in laboratory animals and humans have demonstrated that most hepatic tumors derive a majority of their blood supply from the hepatic artery as opposed to the portal vein.[1,2] This phenomenon, along with the ability of the liver to metabolize certain chemotherapeutic drugs, allows a much higher local concentration of drug to reach the tumor, with reduced systemic effects. The extensive clinical experience with regional hepatic arterial therapy in the treatment of primary and metastatic liver tumors by means of extracorporeal pump devices is reviewed elsewhere in this volume. Suffice it to say that long-term ambulatory therapy with such systems remains inconvenient and has been associated with mechanical and infectious complications.[3]

A totally implanted device for continuous drug infusion, the Infusaid pump, is designed to maintain constant low flow rates, avoid external power sources, provide a reservoir of sufficient size to preclude frequent refilling, and allow percutaneous filling.[4] The first clinical use of the device was to deliver heparin anticoagulation therapy.[5] Its first use in delivering chemotherapy to hepatic tumors was reported in 1980.[6] Since then, a large body of data has accumulated from many centers on use of the implantable pump for regional delivery of chemotherapy for the treatment of liver tumors. The implantable pump has proven to be very reliable without mechanical complications and is rarely subject to the infectious complications and other catheter-related problems seen with external pumping devices.[7-13] The implantable pump preserves patient comfort and convenience through multiple treatments. Multiple hospitalizations with compromise of a patient's life-style can occur if treatments are administered via external pump devices. The following sections will review clinical experience reported in the treatment of colorectal hepatic metastases using regional arterial chemotherapy delivered with the Infusaid pump. The most common application of intra-arterial therapy (I.A.) has been in this group of patients. Prospective randomized clinical trials evaluating the efficacy of hepatic I.A. chemotherapy given by the Infusaid pump will be reviewed. To date, hepatic I.A. therapy has not been established as "standard" therapy for colorectal hepatic metastases as implied by other publications.

Nonrandomized Clinical Trials

A number of phase 2 studies have documented the response rates, survival, and toxicities associated with I.A. therapy using the Infusaid pump for the treatment of colorectal hepatic metastases (see table 1). The drug used in the

Table 1. Results of Intra-Arterial Chemotherapy Using the Infusaid Pump in Patients with Colorectal Liver Metastases

Author/reference	Regimen	No. patients	No. responses (%)	Median duration of response (mo.)	Median duration of survival (mo.)
Barone et al[7]	5-FU 5–10 mg/kg/d or FUDR 0.2 mg/kg/d and RT	18[a]	10 (56)	NP[c]	8
Cohen et al[8]	FUDR 0.3 mg/kg/d for 14 d ± BCNU 150 mg/m² I.V.	39	21 (54)	NP	12
Weiss et al[9]	FUDR 0.2–0.3 mg/kg/d for 14 d, then NS for 14 d	17	5 (29)	6	13
Balch et al[10]	FUDR 0.3 mg/kg/d for 14 d, then NS 14 d	81[b]	71 (88)	7	12
Niederhuber et al[11]	FUDR 0.3 mg/kg/d for 14 d, then NS for 14 d	50	(83)	13	18
Kemeny et al[12]	FUDR 0.3 mg/kg/d for 14 d, then NS for 14 d	41	15 (37)	8	NP
Shepard et al[13]	FUDR 0.3 mg/kg/d for 14 d + mitomycin-C 14 mg/m², then NS for 14 d or FUDR for 14 d, then NS for 14 d, then DCMTX 2 mg/m² for 14 d	53	17 (32)	NP	17

[a]Includes 9 patients treated with 5-FU via external pumps
[b]Includes 15% of patients with extrahepatic disease
[c]Not published

implantable pump in all these studies, 5-fluorodeoxyuridine (FUDR), was associated with response rates of 29–80%. The variability in response rates was related at least in part to the different response criteria defined by each investigator. These criteria included decrease in size of liver by physical examination; decreased liver lesion size by radionuclide scan, ultrasound or computerized tomography (CT) scan; decrease in CEA or other liver function tests; improvement in Cardio-Green liver clearance; or any combination of these parameters. The duration of responses was in the range of 6–13 months. In the collected series of 299 evaluable patients listed in table 1, 2 studies documented a total of 7 complete responses (CR) to I.A. therapy, or 2% of the entire group.[7,13] These CR were documented by operative or autopsy findings or the resolution of all liver lesions by CT scan for at least 3 months. Six of the studies commented on the response rates or survival data in patients who had received prior systemic chemotherapy versus those who had not been previously treated.[7–10,12,13] Five of the 6 studies indicated that the response rates and/or survival were not affected by prior conventional systemic therapy.[7–10,13] Kemeny et al reported that prior chemotherapy did appear to influence responses because 12/23 (52%) previously untreated patients had responses compared to only 3/18 (17%) in previously treated patients.[12] Prior treatment of patients with high doses of multiple drugs, as done at Memorial Sloan-Kettering Institute, may have an effect, but there is no obvious reason for a low response rate in this study in previously treated patients. In addressing this issue, Buroker et al documented responses in 8/21 (35%) patients receiving FUDR I.A. therapy via an external catheter and pump in patients previously given 5-fluorouracil (5-FU) bolus therapy.[14]

Survival from the time of pump implantation in these reports ranges from 8–18 months. Balch et al, in comparing their pump patients to a historical control group from their institution, found a significant survival advantage in the pump-treated group after correction for various prognostic factors.[10] A mathematical model predicting the clinical course of patients with colorectal hepatic metastases has been described by Lahr et al.[15] Using this model, based upon 7 prognostic variables, both Balch et al and Neiderhuber et al reported a survival advantage in pump-treated patients compared to no treatment as predicted by the model.[10,11] Because of possible unforeseen bias in selection of patients, there is a need for randomized studies to address the issue of the efficacy of pump therapy. It is interesting to place the survival data obtained from these studies in context with the natural history of untreated colorectal hepatic metastases. An important study reported by Wagner et al examined the survival of 252 patients with biopsy-proven unresected hepatic metastases when no extrahepatic disease was found at laparotomy.[16] These patients were documented to have bilobar, multiple unilateral, or solitary lesions, with median survivals of 11, 15, and 21 months, respectively. These data demonstrate that these patients live considerably longer than previous reports seemed to indicate. The data reinforce the notion that prospective randomized studies in the development of treatment strategies for colorectal metastases are mandatory, and that a no-treatment control arm is not irrational.

The presence of extrahepatic disease is a significant prognostic factor in the I.A. treatment of patients. Two studies specifically address this issue.

Neiderhuber et al, who treated 43 patients with extrahepatic disease using I.A. therapy, reported a median survival of 9 months from date of pump implantation. The median survival of these patients represents a major decrease compared to patients with disease confined to the liver who were treated within the same institution and had a median survival time of 18 months. Shepard et al reported no tumor response in 9 patients treated when extrahepatic tumor was present; median survival in these patients was only 4.9 months. Until the efficacy of I.A. therapy can be established in patients with disease confined to the liver, it would appear that patients with extrahepatic disease should not undergo this costly experimental therapy outside the context of a study protocol.

The anatomic sites of relapse in patients who have responded or remain with stable disease has been documented in 3 studies. Of 28 patients who responded or had stable disease, Shepard et al reported that 14/28 (50%) relapsed in extrahepatic sites only, 9/28 relapsed in liver and extrahepatic sites, and 5/28 relapsed in liver only. Of 13 responders who died or progressed, Kemeny et al reported that 5 developed extrahepatic disease, 2 progressed in liver and extrahepatic sites, and 5 had progressive liver disease only. Weiss et al reported 5 responders who all relapsed — 4 in extrahepatic sites and 1 in liver and extrahepatic sites. Combining this information reveals that only about 50% of patients with responding or stable disease will relapse in the liver as a component of I.A. regional therapy. It is likely that this represents a significant alteration in the natural course of this disease and how patients succumb. Neiderhuber et al indicated that of the patients who died when therapy was administered for disease confined to the liver, 73% died of progressive extrahepatic disease. In all reported series, the most common sites of extrahepatic relapse were pulmonary and intra-abdominal.

The toxicity of hepatic I.A. therapy has been well documented. Significant potential complications associated with hepatic I.A. therapy require experience and careful attention in order to minimize adverse side effects. A foremost consideration for the patient is the major abdominal surgery required for placement of a catheter. Also, arteriography is needed for arterial cannulation. About 60% of patients have standard arterial anatomy, with the right and left hepatic arteries arising from the common hepatic distal to the gastroduodenal artery; however, the remaining patients may require customized approaches to obtain total hepatic perfusion.[17] Careful attention must be given to ligating run-off branches to the duodenum, stomach, and pancreas in order to avoid chemical-induced injury to the stomach and duodenum, and a cholecystectomy should be performed prophylactically. Cohen et al have described a technique involving the percutaneous transaxillary catheterization of the hepatic arterial tree with subsequent attachment of the catheter to an implanted pump.[18] This procedure avoids a laparotomy and can be performed under local anesthesia. The gastroduodenal artery is occluded by percutaneous transarterial techniques. Problems associated with this technique are inability to accurately stage the extent of the patient's intra-abdominal disease, catheter dislodgement, and inability to completely devascularize run-off vessels to adjacent organs.

The major problems seen with I.A. FUDR infusions are G.I. and hepatic toxicities. The G.I. problems are manifested as duodenitis, gastritis, and peptic ulceration. A true estimate of this problem is difficult to establish unless it is documented endoscopically. Kemeny et al found severe G.I. toxicity in 19/41 (46%) of patients by endoscopy.[12] Twelve (29%) of their patients had discrete ulcers and the rest were found to have diffuse gastritis or duodenitis. Significant liver enzyme elevations have been documented in 20–100% of patients in reported series. Drug-related jaundice has been noted in these same series in 15–33% of patients. These serum abnormalities, which commonly revert to normal over a period of several weeks, indicate the need to obtain liver function tests every 2 weeks for purposes of dose modification. Kemeny et al recommend the careful monitoring of SGOT as a sensitive indicator of I.A. FUDR hepatopathy. This form of hepatopathy has been described occasionally as "chemical hepatitis."

Hohn et al reported a unique feature of I.A. FUDR toxicity that eventuates in biliary sclerosis.[19] This entity presents itself as an elevation in serum alkaline phosphatase in the absence of any significant hepatocellular injury or inflammation in liver biopsies; however, periportal inflammation and round cell infiltration are common. This complication, which can result in permanent intrahepatic and extrahepatic bile duct narrowing not associated with recurrent or progressive tumor (see figure 1), mandates cessation of therapy. In 3 reported series, the problem of biliary sclerosis was documented in 11/121 (9%) of patients.[12,19,20] It appears that any patient receiving I.A. FUDR who sustains persistent elevations in alkaline phosphatase should undergo cholangiography. Other toxicities reported with I.A. FUDR are anorexia, fatigue, nausea and vomiting, and diarrhea; however, these are usually not severe. Myelosuppression is not a problem.

The significant responses seen with continuous infusion I.A. FUDR via the implantable pump have been confirmed by many investigators. This therapy is associated with major toxicities. The costs of the treatment and the potential complications underscore the need for controlled studies to establish the extent to which treatment improves survival and whether the benefit outweighs the treatment toxicity. The question must also be asked whether this treatment improves the quality of life of these patients, as suggested by some investigators.[11] Only carefully run prospective, randomized trials will be able to address these questions.

Prospective Randomized Controlled Trials

The literature yields only 1 completed randomized controlled trial that addresses the issue of infusional I.A. therapy of colorectal hepatic metastases.[21] On the basis of significant response rates with I.A. 5-FU using external pumping devices, the Central Oncology Group in 1971 initiated a controlled clinical trial of I.A. 5-FU therapy compared to systemic 5-FU. Response rates, duration of response, and survival in patients with colorectal liver metastases were documented in 2 groups of patients. Patients had to have disease confined to the liver and were randomized to receive I.A. or systemic (I.V.) therapy. No crossover in the treatment arms was allowed. Patients selected for I.A.-therapy had catheters placed percutaneously or operatively. I.A. therapy consisted of 5-FU administered continuously for a period of 14 days at 20 mg/kg/day, followed by an additional 7 days at a reduced dose of 10 mg/kg/day. I.V. therapy consisted of 5-FU at 12 mg/kg/day given daily by I.V. push for 4 days, followed by half this dose every other day for an additional 4 treatment days. Patients completing the full loading course received 350 mg/kg of 5-FU on the I.A. arm versus 72 mg/kg of 5-FU by the I.V. route. All patients were subsequently

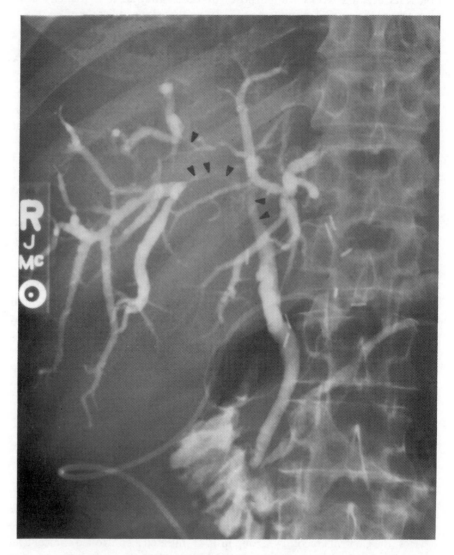

Figure 1.   Periportal inflammation and round cell infiltration can result in permanent intrahepatic and extrahepatic bile duct narrowing not associated with recurrent or progressive tumor. This complication mandates cessation of therapy.

placed on maintenance 5-FU consisting of weekly I.V. injections at a dose of 15 mg/kg.

Sixty-one patients were entered into the study—30 I.A. and 31 I.V. There were no significant differences in response rates, duration of response, or survival between the 2 groups. More G.I. toxicity was seen in the I.A. group than in the I.V. group. The major drawback in this study was the limited nature of I.A. therapy used and the subsequent switch to maintenance systemic therapy in the I.A. arm. A true test of the efficacy of I.A. therapy in prolonging survival would require protracted therapy. Patient inclusion did not require exploratory laparotomy, nor was CT available at the time to more accurately assess the presence or absence of extrahepatic disease. Also, catheter placement was not standardized to ensure total liver perfusion. Thus, the results of this study cannot accurately predict the efficacy of contemporary technical advances represented by the implantable pump and modern diagnostic tests.

At present, there are 6 ongoing National Cancer Institute-supported trials of I.A. regional versus I.V. systemic therapy for colorectal hepatic metastases. Table 2-A lists the groups, the methods of staging, and the eligibility. Table 2-B gives the treatment arms, the provision for crossing over the systemic failure to intrahepatic therapy, and the end points of each trial. Critical differences between the various trials include: (1) whether to perform surgical staging on all patients; (2) whether to include patients with limited extrahepatic disease; (3) whether patients who fail systemic drug therapy should be crossed over to receive intrahepatic therapy; and (4) whether response rate or survival is used as the end point. All the trials compare I.A. infusion to variations of

Table 2-A. Prospective Randomized Trials of Regional (I.A.) Versus Systemic (I.V.) Chemotherapy for Colorectal Liver Metastases

Group*	Laparotomy for staging	Eligibility
Hepatic Tumor Study Group	All patients	1. Liver mets only—laparotomy only 2. Measurable disease
North Central Cancer Treatment Group	I.A. patients only	1. Liver mets only—preop radiologic exam 2. Measurable or nonmeasurable disease in liver
Northern California Oncology Group	I.A. patients only	1. Liver mets only—preop radiologic exam 2. Measurable disease
Memorial Sloan-Kettering Cancer Center	All patients	1. Liver mets only—laparotomy 2. Measurable disease
Piedmont Oncology Group	I.A. patients only	1. Liver mets predominate; no extrahepatic mass >3 cm—radiol exam or laparot
National Cancer Institute	I.A. patients only	1. Liver mets only—radiologic exam 2. Measurable or nonmeasurable disease in liver 3. No peritoneal carcinomatosis

*All groups pursue extensive radiological evaluation.

"standard" chemotherapy treatment. It should be noted that none of these studies includes a no-treatment control group. There are theoretical and practical reasons for the differences in the various studies. With the completion of these trials, it is hoped that a rational decision concerning the continued use of I.A. FUDR chemotherapy for colorectal hepatic metastases can be made.

A central problem in the approach to entering patients into the pump trials concerns the issue of the staging laparotomy. As discussed earlier, there is evidence that patients with extrahepatic disease do significantly worse with I.A. FUDR therapy compared to patients with disease confined to the liver.[11,13] There is also some suggestion from the data by Kemeny et al that the extent of liver involvement by tumor is a significant prognostic indicator in patients receiving I.A. FUDR.[12] A staging laparotomy provides accurate information about response rates and survival in patients stratified for comparable disease. However, the advantages of a staging laparotomy to obtain extent of disease information can have a costly impact on the patient. Patients randomized to I.V. therapy may have a laparotomy for staging purposes only. If a trial included only patients with disease confined to the liver, there would be a substantial

Table 2-B. Prospective Randomized Trials of Regional (I.A.) Versus Systemic (I.V.) Chemotherapy for Colorectal Liver Metastases

Group	Treatment arms[a]	Systemic failure crossover?	End points	Patient accrual[b]
Hepatic Tumor Study Group	A. I.A. FUDR B. I.A. FUDR + syst 5-FU, MIT C. Syst 5-FU: 5-day infusion q 4 wk	No	1. Tumor response 2. Survival	42
North Central Cancer Treatment Group	A. I.A. FUDR B. Syst 5-FU: 5-day infusion q 5 wk	No	1. Survival 2. Time to progression 3. Tumor response	27
Northern California Oncology Group	A. I.A. FUDR B. Syst FUDR: cont. inf.	Yes	1. Tumor response 2. Time to progression 3. Survival	103
Memorial Sloan-Kettering Cancer Center	A. I.A. FUDR B. Syst FUDR: cont. inf.	Yes	1. Tumor response 2. Survival	93
Piedmont Oncology Group	A. I.A. FUDR B. Syst 5-FU: weekly bolus	Yes	1. Tumor response 2. Survival	15
National Cancer Institute	A. I.A. FUDR B. Syst FUDR: cont. inf.	No	1. Survival 2. Time to progression 3. Tumor response	28

[a]I.A. = Intra-arterial infusion—alternate 2 weeks on/off
Syst = Systemic continuous infusion—alternate 2 weeks on/off.
FUDR = 5-fluoro-2-deoxyuridine.
MIT = mitomycin-C.
[b]Number of randomized patients reported at Third Saddlebrook Conference (Feb. 1985)

number of patients excluded from that trial if radiological criteria alone had been used for staging. An alternative approach is to operatively stage only patients randomized to I.A. therapy who require a laparotomy for pump placement. This latter strategy uses the available radiologic screening modalities to assess the patient's extent of disease and to begin systemic therapy for patients randomized to systemic treatment without subjecting them to the potential morbidity of a laparotomy. However, this alternative approach may lead to underestimation of the extent of intra-abdominal disease in patients receiving systemic treatment.

There presently is no "standard" therapy for prolonging survival in patients with metastatic colorectal liver cancer. Systemic 5-FU has been associated with a low response rate of 20% and has not been proven to prolong survival in these patients. Ideally, the optimal study evaluating the efficacy of I.A. therapy should utilize a no-treatment control arm. As can be noted, none of the current trials has adopted this strategy. The major reason has been the fear that patients would be reluctant to participate in such trials if no treatment was to be a potential option. Therefore, all the trials have incorporated some form of systemic chemotherapy. The form of these systemic treatments has been either 5-FU or continuous infusion FUDR. The latter approach evaluates the issue addressed by Lokich, who suggested that the continuous infusion of FUDR may be the major determinant of the utility of this therapy rather than the route by which it is given.[22]

A final issue introduced by some of these trials is the "crossover" design, which allows failures of 1 arm to receive the alternative treatment. In such studies, the primary end points become response rates and time to progression. If response rates do in fact correlate with survival, "crossing over" is not an important problem. This information, however, is not yet available for I.A. FUDR therapy, and the major question is still whether the therapy prolongs survival. Trials by 3 groups directly address this question by using a noncrossover design: the North Central Cancer Treatment Group, the National Cancer Institute, and the Hepatic Tumor Study Group. It is probable that all 3 trials will, in fact, provide an indication of survival, and additional information can be gained from crossover trials aside from tumor response and time to progression.

The conduct of all these trials has been plagued by poor patient accrual (see table 2-B). At an update of all these trials at the Third Saddlebrook Conference (February 1985), there was a consensus among all principal investigators in the clinical trials that patient referral for the studies has been poor.[23] The reason for this appears to be the false perception among many practicing clinicians that I.A. FUDR therapy has already been established as a standard approach to treating patients with colorectal hepatic metastases. This problem has worsened with the establishment of cost reimbursement for pump implantation by third-party insurance groups. Because of patient accrual problems, the Hepatic Tumor Study Group has closed its trial. The Northern California Oncology Group has accrued 103 patients. This trial randomizes patients to I.A. or I.V. continuous FUDR via the implantable pump. Patients who fail in 1 arm of the study are crossed over to the other arm. Preliminary results from this trial are not available because the principal investigators believe that early dissemination of the data may jeopardize patient accrual. Patient entry will continue until a total of 150 patients is reached. The trial at Memorial Sloan-Kettering Cancer Center also randomizes patients to I.A. or I.V. continuous FUDR. Similarly, patients who fail are crossed over to the alternate treatment arm. This trial has randomized 93 patients, of whom 59 have received pump treatment; 34 were excluded due to resectable disease, extrahepatic disease, or findings of no tumor.[23] There were 26 evaluable patients in the I.A. group, with 10 partial responses; 8/24 patients in the I.V. group had partial responses. At present, there are no differences in response rates or survival between the 2 groups. Of interest is the fact that 13/26 I.A.-treated patients developed extrahepatic disease, compared to only 4/24 in the I.V. group. This study is still accruing patients. None of the studies has reached any final conclusion at this early date. The preliminary findings of the National Cancer Institute trial are discussed in greater detail in the next section.

National Cancer Institute Trial

Since May 1982, a prospective randomized study evaluating the efficacy of I.A. versus I.V. FUDR via the Infusaid implantable pump for treatment of colorectal hepatic metastases has been performed by the Surgery Branch, NCI. Only patients with unresectable hepatic metastases confined to the liver as documented by noninvasive studies (full lung tomograms, EOE enhanced liver and abdominal CT scan, radionuclide liver and bone scans) were eligible. Patients randomized to I.A. therapy received monthly FUDR at 0.3 mg/kg/day for 2 weeks. I.V. FUDR was administered at a monthly dose of 0.125 mg/kg/day for 2 weeks through catheters placed in the superior vena cava. After every 3 cycles of chemotherapy, tumor response was determined by CT or radionuclide liver scans. A response was defined as a $\geq 50\%$ decrease in size or disappearance of evaluable tumor. If any lesion was found to increase 25% or if new metastases developed, that patient was considered to have progressed. Patients continued with treatment if they were documented to have stable or responding lesions. If progression of any lesion was noted, therapy was discontinued. No crossover between I.V. or I.A. therapy was performed.

A total of 28 patients (15 I.V., 13 I.A.) have been randomized on study. Three additional nonrandomized I.A. pilot patients who fulfilled the eligibility criteria have been treated. The median duration of follow-up was 15 months. The Mantel-Haenzel test was used to analyze results, and all p values were 2-sided. For all randomized patients, the 2-year actuarial survival times for the I.V. and I.A. patients were 37% and 57%, respectively; they were not significantly different ($p = 0.44$) (see figure 2). Four randomized I.A. patients did not receive FUDR treatment because of extrahepatic disease found at abdominal exploration. Three I.V. patients did not receive treatment because of a postoperative death (1) and documented extrahepatic disease (2). If these patients are excluded from the analysis and the 3 additional I.A. pilot patients are included, a total of 24 evaluable patients (12 I.V. and 12 I.A.) who received appropriate FUDR chemotherapy can be analyzed (see figure 3). The 2-year actuarial sur-

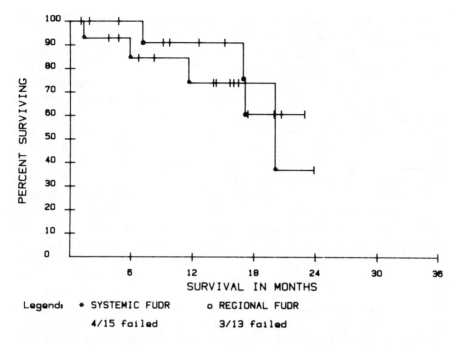

Figure 2.   Comparison of randomized patients: Hepatic mets colorectal protocol.

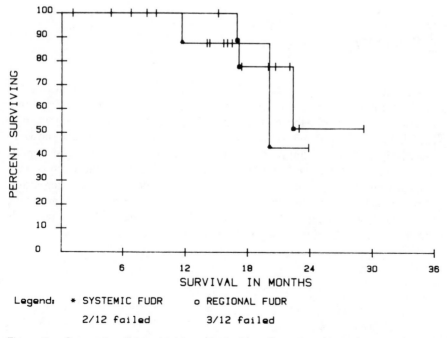

Figure 3.   Comparison of evaluable patients: Hepatic mets colorectal protocol.

vival times for the evaluable I.V. and I.A. patients were 44% and 51%, respectively; they were not significantly different (p = 0.51).

After 3 cycles of chemotherapy, all patients were examined for tumor responses. Of the 12 evaluable I.V. patients, 3 responded, 4 had stable disease, 4 progressed, and 1 was too early to assess. The 12 evaluable I.A. patients had 7 responders, 4 with stable disease, and 1 who progressed. Subsequent follow-up showed that all 7 I.V. patients who responded or had stable disease went on to progress initially in the liver. Seven of the 11 I.A. patients who achieved a response or had stable disease went on to progress initially in the liver (5) or lung (2). The median time to progression for the I.V. and I.A. patients was 13 and 14 months, respectively (p = 0.16).

Significant toxicity has been associated with I.A. FUDR. Hepatopathy in 11/12 I.A. patients was detected by abnormal liver function studies. This chemical hepatitis required FUDR dose reduction, usually with resolution of the hepatopathy; however, 1 patient went on to develop biliary sclerosis documented by liver biopsy and ERCP. Five of 12 I.A. patients developed peptic ulcers or gastritis documented by U.G.I. studies or autopsy findings. Two of these patients presented with perforated duodenal ulcers. Four of 12 I.A. patients had thromboses of a portion of the hepatic arterial system detected by technetium-macroaggregated albumin scans. The I.V. patients had less toxicity. Only 1/12 patients developed chemical hepatitis. The most common toxicity seen in this group was severe diarrhea, noted in 6/12 patients. One I.V. patient developed a subclavian vein thrombosis.

To date, preliminary results from this trial reveal no differences in overall survival or time to progression between I.A. or I.V. FUDR therapy. This protocol is still actively accruing patients for study.

Summary

Current trials must be completed. However, there is evidence that this will not be simple. Dissemination of this new technology has slowed accrual into several of the trials previously mentioned. The use of I.A. FUDR therapy can be associated with significant toxicity. Until this form of therapy can be shown to effectively palliate or improve survival in patients with colorectal hepatic metastases, the treatment should be administered only in the context of a clinical trial. The implantable pump has proven to be reliable and acceptable to patients. However, the pump is not an answer to the problem of metastatic liver cancer; it is merely a device for the delivery of agents that are presently limited in their effectiveness against colorectal cancer.

34

REGIONAL INFUSION FOR PRIMARY
HEPATIC CARCINOMAS

Charles M. Balch, M.D., and Marshall M. Urist, M.D.

CONTINUOUS REGIONAL CHEMOTHERAPY FOR treating hepatic tumors is a rational pharmacological approach as palliative treatment in selected patients such as those with locally advanced hepatocellular carcinoma. Virtually all of these patients have a short life expectancy (average of 2 months).[26,22] They die from progressive hepatic failure and only occasionally have metastases to other visceral organs, such as lung, bone, or brain.

Continuous regional chemotherapy has the following advantages: (1) it delivers a higher concentration of drug directly to the liver tumor, since it avoids the dilutional effect that otherwise occurs with a systemic (I.V.) injection; (2) many antimetabolites have a more effective antineoplastic effect when administered by continuous infusion rather than by pulse injection; (3) there is significant hepatic extraction of many drugs when injected directly into the hepatic circulation, particularly floxuridine (FUDR) and, to a lesser extent, 5-fluorouracil (5-FU), mitomycin-C (MIT) and Adriamycin (ADR); this further increases the concentration of the drug at the site of the liver neoplasm; and (4) continuous infusion (either intra-arterially or intravenously) has a lower peak serum concentration, thus decreasing toxicity such as cardiotoxicity with ADR or marrow depression with FUDR and 5-FU. There are some disadvantages to this approach as well. First, there is less systemic exposure of the drug so that metastases at extrahepatic sites are not treated to the same degree. Second, there can be significant local toxicity, especially chemical hepatitis, cholecystitis, and gastritis.

In the past, fluoropyrimidines (5-FU or FUDR) have been used either systemically or intra-arterially (I.A.) to the liver in patients with hepatomas. However, the response rates have generally been low and of relatively short duration; only a few patients lived more than 12–18 months.[6,10,16] This is especially true for systemic administration of fluoropyrimidines, with some reports of patients doing better with I.A. infusions in nonrandomized comparisons.[1,6,7,23] In one randomized study conducted by the Eastern Oncology Group involving 168 patients from North America and South Africa, systemic ADR was the most active agent compared to oral 5-FU (alone or in combination with methyl CCNU or streptozotocin), accounting for 9 of the 15 responses.[11]

At present, ADR, either alone or in combination with other drugs, is the agent of choice in the treatment of hepatomas. Using standard I.V. dose schedules, response rates range from 9–44%.[2,8,11,14,18,19,25] Higher response rates of 56–70% have been reported with drug combinations using ADR on an I.A. basis to the liver.[20-22,24] When ADR is given on an infusional basis, there is a 2-fold extraction in the tissues to which it is first exposed, and its incidence of cardiotoxicity is diminished because the peak serum concentration of the drug is substantially lower.[13,17] For these reasons, ADR is an appropriate drug to use on a regional infusional dose schedule in patients at risk of dying from their liver tumor. One study, however, did not show any advantage of I.A. ADR over the I.V. route in a selected series of 8 patients.[5] A randomized prospective study comparing these 2 routes of administration would be important to resolve this issue.

It is important to distinguish the different subtypes of hepatomas that may be amenable to this form of treatment. The most common subtype is the diffuse hepatocellular carcinoma that often arises in a cirrhotic liver of patients with underlying viral or parasitic liver disease. These patients generally have minimal hepatic reserves, and the tumor is usually refractory to all forms of chemotherapy, including ADR. The survival rate is short (about 75 days), and they are usually *not* candidates for regional ADR chemotherapy. The second subtype is fibrolamellar hepatoma.[12,15] These are generally nodular forms of tumors that occur in younger individuals with an average age of 25–30 years. They are more often resectable, and even unresectable patients have a more indolent clinical course than those with diffuse tumors. The third subtype is nodular hepatomas arising in a normal liver of older individuals with little or no cirrhosis. The histologic pattern is different from fibrolamellar carcinomas. These patients also have sufficient hepatic reserves, and the tumors are amenable to a regional chemotherapy approach if the primary tumor is not resectable.

There are several methods of delivering regional ADR chemotherapy to the liver. The simplest method is the Seldinger technique of catheter placement in the hepatic artery via the left axillary artery or one of the femoral arteries. If the patient has a dual hepatic blood supply, at the University of Alabama at Birmingham we prefer to embolize the replaced right hepatic artery and redirect the hepatic flow through the left hepatic artery arising from the celiac axis. This approach avoids the risk of thrombosing the superior mesenteric artery, a possible result from placement of an indwelling catheter in this vessel. The second approach is the placement of a permanent catheter in the hepatic artery (or one of its side branches). This requires a laparotomy for implantation, but has the advantages that all downstream vessels can be ligated; there is little or no risk of catheter migration; and all subsequent regional chemotherapy can be given on an oupatient basis rather than requiring repeated hospitalization for percutaneous I.A. drug infusions. Cohen and colleagues[9] have described a method for a permanent transaxillary placement of a hepatic artery catheter that avoids the necessity for a laparotomy. It is our preference to give an induction regimen of I.A. ADR chemotherapy using the Seldinger technique and then implant a permanent catheter in those patients with a documented objective response after 1 or 2 courses of the drugs.

An implanted hepatic artery catheter can be connected to a subcutaneous port such as an Infusaport or Port-a-Cath. This is preferable to the external catheter because of its increased risk of infection. The chemotherapy can then be administered by the implanted port using an external pump or hand injection. There is some risk of arterial thrombosis when these catheters are flushed only intermittently. For this reason, we have used an Infusaid drug infusion pump (model 400) for constant flushing with heparin-saline solution in order to maintain catheter patency. The ADR is then infused directly into the catheter via the side port. The surgical technique of pump implantation and catheter placement has been described previously.[3-4] It is not possible to deliver a therapeutic dose of ADR by placing the drug directly into the Infusaid pump itself because of its low flow rate (3 cc/day). Recently, we have used a modified Infusaid implantable drug infusion pump with a high flow rate (10–22 cc/day) so that ADR can be placed into the pump and delivered over a 4- to 5-day period. The pump is refilled with a saline-glycerol solution, which increases the viscosity and slows the flow to a rate of 2–3 cc/day to permit less frequent refills. The pump flow rate can be adjusted by raising the viscosity with glycerol-saline solution. Using this approach, all chemotherapy can be administered on an outpatient basis. It should be emphasized that this ADR infusion pump is still being evaluated on an investigational basis.

The UAB Experience with Regional Adriamycin Chemotherapy for Hepatoma Patients

An ongoing phase 2 trial is being conducted at The University of Alabama at Birmingham for selected patients with surgically unresectable hepatocellular carcinoma. Patients with evidence of diffuse disease arising in a cirrhotic liver are excluded. Adriamycin chemotherapy is administered as a 72-hour I.A. infusion to the liver in 3-week cycles. In some cases, ADR was first given for 1 or 2 cycles using a percutaneously placed catheter in the hepatic artery. Patients later underwent a laparotomy and placement of a permanent catheter. In our initial experience, an Infusaid pump was attached to the hepatic artery catheter to maintain catheter patency, and the ADR infusions were given through the side port of the pump directly into the catheter. Alternatively, an implanted port was attached to the hepatic artery and then flushed at regular intervals to maintain catheter patency. The former approach was preferred because there was some risk of thrombosis when the implanted ports were used rather than constant infusion of saline. One patient developed thrombosis of the hepatic artery that was relieved by flushing the catheter with a streptokinase solution. Patients were monitored for marrow suppression (with hematological profiles) and for cardiac toxicity using exercise-gaited radionu-clide injection scans (MUGA).

A consecutive series of 13 patients with histologically confirmed unresect-able hepatomas were treated according to the above protocol with regional ADR chemotherapy through a hepatic artery catheter. Three of 13 patients had chronic active hepatitis, 4/13 had hepatomas arising in a mildly cirrhotic liver, and only 4/13 had elevated alpha-feto protein levels.

Six of 13 patients (46%) showed a 50% or greater decrease in the dimen-sions of their tumor by CT scan or ultrasound, while an additional 6 patients (46%) had either stable disease or a reduction in tumor size less than 50%. Only 1 patient continued to have progressive disease while receiving the ADR chemotherapy. Sixty-five percent of patients were alive at 1 year, and the median survival was 20 months (see figure 1). These results compare to an expected median survival of only 10 months in most published series.

Five of 13 developed cardiotoxicity as evidenced by a decrease in their ejection fraction below 50%. None of the patients had irreversible cardiac failure after appropriate treatment with inotropic drugs and cessation of ADR chemotherapy. Only 3 patients developed total alopecia, and 1 patient required delay in treatment because of transient bone marrow toxicity. When ADR was stopped, other drugs were used, either alone or in combination with 5-FU, FUDR, cisplatin (DDP), and MIT. None of the patients had a significant objec-tive tumor response to second-line chemotherapy.

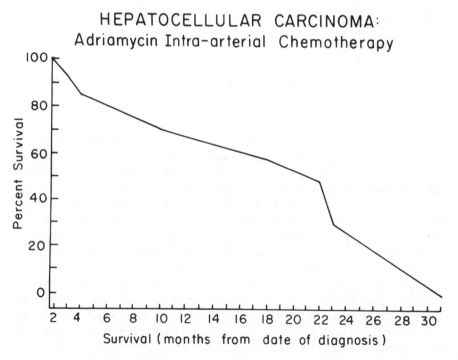

Figure 1.   Overall survival (percent) of patients with hepatomas treated by intra-arterial Adriamycin.

The following case histories illustrate the management approaches used in these patients, their treatment responses, and complications.

Case History 1

MM was a 77-year-old male who presented with a massive hepatocellular carcinoma involving the central portion of the liver. He underwent exploratory laparotomy in August 1981 and was found to have surgically unresectable lesion. The remaining left lobe of the liver was normal to inspection and palpation, and there was no evidence of cirrhosis. A Silastic hepatic artery catheter was placed in the gastroduodenal artery and an Infusaid pump was implanted for maintaining catheter patency. He then received ADR at 60 mg/m^2 at 72-hour infusions in 3- to 4-week cycles. He had an excellent response to chemotherapy, with his measurable lesion being more than 8 cm in diameter and then regressing to a point where it was no longer detectable. The patient received a total of 1,135 mg of ADR. His only toxicity was alopecia.

Because the patient had reached his limit of ADR and had a 54% ejection fraction by exercise MUGA scan, the ADR was discontinued and he never developed clinical evidence of cardiac failure. He then received sequentially FUDR, DDP, bleomycin (BLM), and MIT over a 1-year period. Despite these interventions, his tumor began to grow, and he developed jaundice due to diffuse hepatic disease. He died 3½ years after initiation of his treatment.

Case History 2

JD was a 41-year-old female who presented with a massively enlarged liver that extended to the pelvic brim. She had no jaundice but was easily fatigued, had weight loss, and right upper quadrant pain. CT scan showed a massively enlarged liver (see figure 2). A needle biopsy showed hepatocellular carcinoma. The patient underwent 2 courses of ADR chemotherapy at 60 mg/m^2 through a percutaneous catheter in the hepatic artery using the Seldinger technique. After 3 months, she had a dramatic response with marked diminution of her tumor. She began to work full time and was asymptomatic. The patient then underwent exploratory laparotomy and implantation of a hepatic artery catheter and an Infusaid drug infusion pump to maintain catheter patency. There was massive involvement of the liver with hepatoma. A biopsy showed clear cell variant of hepatocellular carcinoma. The uninvolved liver showed only mild fibrosis in the portal areas and no evidence of cirrhosis.

The patient subsequently underwent 72-hour infusions of ADR through the side port of the pump. Her cardiac performance was stable, she had no marrow depression, and there was only temporary alopecia. Her pump had a flow rate of 3 cc/day, which did not enable administration of ADR through this drug delivery device. This pump later was replaced under local anesthesia with a modified high-flow Infusaid pump having a calculated flow rate of 10 cc/day. Four-day infusions of ADR (100 mg) were administered by the implanted pump on an outpatient basis. A 25% solution of saline and glycerol was used in the pump between courses of chemotherapy to slow the flow rate to 3 cc/day and decrease the number of physician visits for pump refills. She received 4 courses of ADR chemotherapy with this device and had no toxicity whatsoever. She subsequently developed transient episodes of hypoglycemia and liver enlargement that appeared to be due to regenerating liver nodules. An extensive metabolic and endocrine workup failed to reveal the cause of the hypoglycemia. The patient had now received 1 1/2 years of ADR chemotherapy with a total dose of 1,045 mg (745 mg/m²).

Because of her age and overall good clinical status, the patient underwent orthotopic hepatic transplantation. At the time of this surgery, the patient had a liver weighing 5,000 g, with both nodules of well-differentiated hepatocellular carcinoma and regenerating liver. There was no evidence of extrahepatic disease. There was marked fibrosis around the hepatic artery. The patient's postoperative course was complicated by periods of cholestasis without evidence of allograft rejection, osteoporosis, and pneumonia. She is now 2 years after hepatic transplantation and 43 months after initiation of her therapy. There has been no evidence of recurrent or metastatic tumor, chronic graft rejection, or ADR cardiotoxicity.

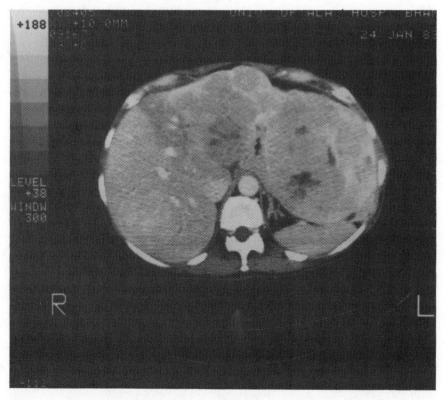

Figure 2.   CT scan of the liver of a 41-year-old female showing massive hepatomegaly and replacement of parenchyma by hepatoma before intra-arterial Adriamycin chemotherapy.

Case History 3

BM is a 60-year-old male who presented in August 1981 with a large, solitary hepatoma. He underwent laparotomy, which showed a 10–12 cm mass in the superior central portion of the liver near the confluence of the hepatic veins. The lesion was judged to be unresectable. A biopsy showed a hepatocellular carcinoma, and the remaining hepatic parenchyma did not show any evidence of cirrhosis. A Silastic catheter was placed in the gastroduodenal artery and connected to an Infusaid model 400 pump in the abdominal wall to maintain catheter patency. The patient then received ADR over the next year, for a total dose of 173 mg (450 mg/m²). He had alopecia and nausea but no other complications. The tumor decreased to 4 cm in diameter and had changes by ultrasound indicative of tumor necrosis and scarring within the remaining tumor. The patient's cardiac ejection fraction declined over 12 months to 50% by MUGA scan, but the patient was clinically asymptomatic. Because of these changes in subclinical cardiac performance, the ADR was stopped, and the patient was given two courses of FUDR chemotherapy at 0.3 mg/kg/day in a 5-day cycle. He had moderate symptoms of chemical hepatitis with upper abdominal pain. The patient then refused all further chemotherapy but continued with regular follow-up examinations. Surprisingly, he was completely asymptomatic and had a normal level of physical activity over the next 2 years. He then developed multiple pulmonary metastases, although the lesion in his liver remained unchanged at 4 cm in transverse diameter. A percutaneous needle biopsy of the lung confirmed the diagnosis of metastatic hepatocellular carcinoma. The patient's clinical course has been declining slowly, but he remains alive 4 years from the time of initial diagnosis.

Case History 4

BS is a 48-year-old male with a diffuse hepatocellular carcinoma in a cirrhotic liver that was discovered at the time of exploratory laparotomy for symptomatic cholelithiasis. The patient had placement of a hepatic artery catheter and implantation of an Infusaid pump. He received only 2 courses of ADR chemotherapy and had no response. Two months later, he became jaundiced and died within a few weeks of rapidly progressing disease and hepatic failure. This relatively young and asymptomatic patient was treated early in our series and exemplifies the lack of response even to intensive treatment in patients with diffuse hepatocellular carcinomas arising in a cirrhotic liver.

Experience at M.D. Anderson Hospital and Tumor Institute

Patt and colleagues at the M. D. Anderson Hospital have also obtained excellent results using regional arterial chemotherapy in the treatment of patients with primary hepatic neoplasms.[20,21] Thirty patients with primary hepatocellular carcinoma were treated with intra-arterial chemotherapy every 4–5 weeks. The chemotherapy consisted of ADR (40 mg/m² infused over 2 hours), MIT (10 mg/m² infused over 2 hours), and FUDR (75 mg/m² as a continuous infusion over 5 days). There were 3 complete remissions and 18 partial remissions (>50% reduction in tumor diameter), for a response rate of 70%. Two additional patients (6.6%) experienced a partial response that was less than 50%. Only 3 patients had no changes observed in their disease (10%), while 4 others had definite progression of their tumor (13.3%). The responding hepatoma patients had a median survival of 10 months from beginning of treatment, as opposed to only 4 months among the nonresponders (p = 0.03). Five patients survived 35 +, 32 +, 11 +, 11 +, and 30 months from the initiation of arterial therapy. Marrow depression occurred in 24% of patients, and alopecia was observed in all patients. Twelve of 30 patients died of liver failure, 4 succumbed to extrahepatic disease, and 6 died from a combination of hepatic and extrahepatic disease. Three patients died from unrelated causes, 2 due to heart failure and 1 due to a myocardial infarction. The 2 patients with congestive heart failure had ADR doses not exceeding 200 mg/m^2. The authors concluded that arterial infusion of ADR, MIT, and FUDR could offer significant palliation in these patients, prolongation of survival, and in some cases, long-term survival in patients with hepatomas that could achieve a chemotherapy-induced or a surgically-achieved complete remission.

Summary

The results of regional ADR chemotherapy (either alone or in combination with MIT and FUDR) showed significant prolongation of life in a selected series of hepatoma patients treated at 2 institutions. The median survival of 20 months at UAB and 10 months at the M.D. Anderson Hospital offers some encouragement that this approach is justified in selected hepatoma patients. It is likely that the better survival rates in UAB patients were due to more stringent selection criteria, since we excluded patients with jaundice and those with diffuse hepatocellular carcinoma arising in a cirrhotic liver (with one exception, as noted in the case histories). It is significant that 20–30% of patients in both series achieved a survival exceeding 2 years, since such durable responses have not been noted previously using other drug regimens or routes of administration. In fact, the success of this form of treatment enabled subsequent surgical treatment, including a successful liver transplantation in 1 patient and resection of the hepatoma in 4 others that were previously judged to be unresectable.

These results will need to be confirmed with further clinical trials, both at our 2 institutions and by other investigators. Randomized clinical trials should be established comparing intra-arterial versus intravenous routes of administration, as well as comparisons of ADR alone versus ADR combined with other drugs.

35

HEPATIC ARTERY LIGATION AND
PORTAL VEIN INFUSION

A. Gerard, M.D., and J. C. Pector, M.D.

BECAUSE OF THE POOR results obtained with systemic chemotherapy for secondary liver tumors, therapeutic locoregional approaches have been used, and the vascular pattern of these tumors has been studied.

By injecting metastasized human liver, we have known for a long time that the vascularization of these tumors is mainly of arterial origin.[1,2] Later, arteriographical studies confirmed this observation while showing the existence of a great variation in vascularity when comparing one tumor to another.[3,4] Liver tumors have been studied in the animal, either induced by hepatocarcinogenic material or obtained by transplanting tumor fragments or tumor cells in suspension. In any case, arterial blood is prevalent in tumor circulation.[5-8] The histological type of the tumor seems to influence its type of vascularity.

Nilsson and Zettergren showed that the vascular system of experimental liver carcinomas is more important when the tumor is well differentiated than when it is not.[5] The contrary was observed in cholangiocarcinoma.[5] The same authors showed, by portography, a portal vascularization of the tumor in well differentiated liver carcinomas, the portal system remaining at the periphery in poorly differentiated liver carcinoma. The portal system does not seem to irrigate the tumor in cholangiocarcinoma.

The tumor size also strongly influences its vascular pattern. This point has been demonstrated by Ackerman[9] using injections of silicone rubber and by Kido[10] studying the injection of marked albumin or of microspheres with angiographic techniques as well as by Honjo and Matsumura,[8] who used injections of coloring matters.

The conclusion from these experimental studies is that small liver tumors are surrounded with both arterial and venous vessels. When the tumor grows, its vascular pattern becomes mainly arterial. However, if the tumor is still increasing, its center becomes progressively avascular and necrotic, the tumor periphery being then much more vascularized than its center, with a portal system remaining at the tumor's periphery.

There is no consensus in published studies concerning the relative proportion of blood flow to tumor and liver. For some authors,[11,12] the vascularity of experimental tumors is more important than in the normal hepatic parenchyma; several investigators[13] observed an equal blood flow, while for some others,[14] the tumor blood flow is not as important as in the hepatic parenchyma. In man, it seems that the metastases are perfused to a lesser extent than the normal hepatic parenchyma when measured with [133]xenon.[11,16]

Effects of Hepatic Artery Ligation on Liver Parenchyma

Hepatic artery ligation (HAL) in man formerly was considered lethal because the hepatic arteries were thought to be terminal arteries.[17] Indeed, HAL in the dog causes death, but this can be avoided if antibiotics are administered.[18] Later, intrahepatic anastomoses were performed. The relative innocuousness of HAL in man was clinically demonstrated.[19] An increase in the hepatic extraction of oxygen from portal blood can be observed after HAL.[20] On the other hand, Lindell demonstrated that in the rat, if marked microspheres are injected intra-arterially, (I.A.) a fraction of arterialized blood remains in the portal blood.[21] His hypothesis is that there is an arteriovenous shunting in the splanchnic organs.

The effect of HAL on the total hepatic blood flow is controversial. Some investigators think that the portal blood flow decreases temporarily as a response to HAL.[22,23] Others disagree.[24,25] The temporary occlusion of the hepatic artery seems to decrease the total hepatic blood flow. However, recovery follows quickly after normalization of the arterial blood flow.[23,26] If the total hepatic blood flow is estimated 15 days after definitive HAL, no effect can be observed.[27] The differences in the hepatic flow probably are due, at least in part, to the various methods used to estimate the flow.

Effects of Hepatic Artery Ligation on Liver Metastases

The injection of silicone rubber has evidenced, after HAL in the animal with hepatic tumors, a rim of portal vessels in the periphery of the tumor.[11,28] Blood flow measures, performed with [133]xenon, confirmed this experimental observation in man.[16]

The first HAL was performed by Rienhoff and Woods in the hope that cutting down the oxygen saturation of the blood reaching the metastases would retard growth.[29] Later (1967), Nilsson et al observed the efficacy of HAL in rats with experimental liver tumors and then performed the same procedure on patients, reporting encouraging results.[30] HAL resulted in subtotal or total necrosis of liver tumors, both in men and in animals. In order to test the therapeutic value of HAL on experimental tumor in rats, Nilsson et al compared the efficacy of HAL to explorative laparotomy only.[30] In a series of 116 rats with Rous sarcoma, they observed a double survival time in rats where HAL was performed. Furthermore, the phenomena seen after hepatic dearterialization were studied by Bengmark and Rosengren, who showed that after HAL, regeneration of arterial vascularization is extremely rapid, revascularization being observed by arteriogram after 3–4 days.[31] Moreover, HAL can be performed with good survival rate and few complications while inducing considerable tumor regression. Nevertheless, the optimistic influence of these procedures has not been confirmed in subsequent clinical trials, and it is generally accepted today that HAL alone does not significantly prolong survival time in comparison to the natural history of untreated patients.[32] The main advantage found with this procedure has been the relief of pain in patients with hepatomegaly.

Effects of Portal Infusion on Liver Metastases

Bengmark et al showed the efficacy of cytotoxic drug infusion through the portal vein.[33] They reported a case with metastases in the two lobes originating from the colon, judged at laparotomy to be impossible to resect completely. A metastasis of 3 cm was resected in the left lobe and a catheter was threaded cephalad into the portal vein. A total dose of 31 g 5-fluorouracil (5-FU) was given over a period of 6 weeks. Ten weeks later, a new laparotomy was performed. No recurrence was seen in the left lobe, which had apparently grown and regenerated. In the right lobe, the tumors were found to be smaller and with histologic signs of degeneration. It was possible to resect the right lobe. The anatomical and experimental observations mentioned above show that growth and development of liver metastases are dependent upon their blood supply. A rational approach for their treatment should lead to a combined procedure including infusion through the portal vein and HAL.

Effect of HAL and Portal Infusion on Liver Metastases

The combined procedure of an occlusion of the hepatic artery and an infusion of the liver with a cytotoxic drug via the portal vein was initiated by Fortner et al.[34] They treated 11 patients without complications using a neurosurgical catheter that has an entire reflux slit valve at its tip and is closed simply with a reservoir of the single inlet type at the outer end. This method was satisfactory for the administration of chemotherapeutic agents intrahepatically. Moreover, the procedure of HAL was found especially attractive because it induces considerable necrosis of the tumor, leaving a rim of viable tumor that is nourished predominantly by the portal vein system. A chemotherapeutic agent is then directed toward these residual neoplastic cells. However, this method allows cyclic administration through the systemic route and excludes continuous infusion.

Nagasue et al[35] reported 17 patients with primary or secondary liver tumors treated by dearterialization of the liver and intraportal infusion of mitomycin-C (MIT), Adriamycin (ADR), and 5-FU. If their results were not always satisfactory in terms of increase in survival, these authors pointed out the efficient palliative effects of this treatment. Recently, Laufman et al observed clinical improvement and a marked decrease in carcinoembryonic antigen levels after HAL and portal vein infusion of MIT and 5-FU for liver metastases from colon cancer.[36] They concluded, on a series of 19 patients, that locoregional treatments administered for these conditions yielded better results than systemic chemotherapy.

In order to achieve a higher concentration of drug delivered to the metastases, helping to destroy a larger volume of tumor cells, Taylor reproduced HAL and infusion of a cytotoxic agent with 2 catheters, one in the hepatic artery and one in the portal vein.[37] This interesting prospective study was carried out as a clinical trial comprising 3 therapeutic arms. The first group was treated by HAL and I.A. infusion of 5-FU. The second group was treated by HAL with I.A. and portal infusion of 5-FU. The third group was a control group. All patients for whom HAL was not possible were treated with portal infusion of 5-FU alone. The survival of the group treated by HAL and I.A. and portal infusion of 5-FU was clearly better in a statistically significant manner than that of the other groups. These results are particularly promising. Nevertheless, the number of patients in each group is very small: Only 24 patients were included in the whole study.

In 1980, the authors of this review started a pilot study on the efficacy of HAL and portal infusion in patients with liver metastases from colorectal origin. The choice for an occlusion of the hepatic artery with temporary ischemia must be made among temporary occlusion by tourniquet,[38] an intravascular balloon catheter,[39] or embolization with enzymatically degradable microspheres.[21] Up to now, no reports have evidenced their efficacy; we found that the first step for a regional approach in this study had to be limited to a HAL such as arterial occlusion.

The criteria for eligibility of patients to be included in this pilot study are summarized in figure 1. Figure 2 shows the surgical procedure. During laparotomy, the hepatic artery and its left and right branches are dissected, double-ligated with 00 silk sutures, then cut off as close to the liver as possible, along with any accessory hepatic arteries that may have been located by preoperative angiography. The lesser omentum, triangular ligaments, and falciform ligaments are transected in an attempt to retard the development of collateral arterial circulation to the liver. The middle colic vein is identified and tied distally. A catheter is threaded cephalad until its tip lies in the portal vein. The efficacy of the perfusion is checked by fluorescin peroperatively. Initially, a Raimondi catheter, usually used by neurosurgeons, was placed. The catheter was tied in place and its distal end was passed through the abdominal wall, using a small stab wound. It was then sutured in place at the skin level, flushed with a solution of 1,000 units of heparin and connected immediately to the perfusion with an Ivac pump for long-term infusion. The disadvantage of this procedure is the duration of hospitalization. Patients receive 5-FU 600 mg/m²/day during a 20-day session for the first course of chemotherapy.

To avoid prolonged hospitalization, infection, and displacement of the catheter, and to provide repeated access to the vascular system without trauma or complications, we replaced the percutaneous catheter by a port system. This device is totally implantable; patients are not subject to frequent heparin flushes or dressing changes, nor are their normal activities restricted. Moreover, the portable pump used allows treatment on an outpatient basis.

The patients were followed up by clinical examination, liver enzyme tests, and CEA serum level tests every 6 weeks, and a computerized tomography (CT) scan of the liver was performed every 3 months. Six of the 8 patients showed a partial response (PR) judged by measurable disease and by the CEA serum level. A measurable tumor was defined as a known mass measured by means of a liver CT scan to evaluate tumor invasion and as a primary indicator of tumor response. The same method of measurement must be used to evaluate response to therapy. A reduction of at least 50% in the sum of the products of the longest perpendicular diameters of the clearly measurable lesion mass is evaluated as a PR.

If the above criteria are not met, if there is a less than 25% increase in any measurable lesion, and if no new areas of malignant disease are found, the lesion can be qualified as being objectively stable. When the increase is more than 25% and when new areas of malignant disease appear, the lesion is classified as an objective progression, which is the end point for determining the duration of response. In our pilot study, 6/8 patients showed a PR, with an average duration of 4–11 months and a median time to progression of 8 months (see figure 3). There were 5 patients with a hepatic involvement between 25–75% and 3 patients with less than 25% hepatic involvement. Survival duration is parallel to the duration of progression. For patients obtaining PR, the survival average is between 11 and 24 months, with a median survival time of 11 months (figure 4).

Figure 5 shows, as an example, the evolution of the CEA serum level of a patient treated by a anterior resection for rectal carcinoma. He was asymptomatic and was evaluated to have 30% liver involvement during laparotomy. When the hepatic artery was ligated, the CEA serum level was 67 ng/ml. During

---

— Histologically confirmed malignancy in the liver (synchronous or metachronous)

— Resection of a primary colorectal carcinoma

— Preoperative evaluation indicating disease confined to the liver

— Unresectable and diffuse liver tumor

— No portal hypertension (less than 16 cm H_2O)

— Karnofsky of 60 or more

— Age less than 70 years old

— No contraindication for surgery

— Preoperative selective hepatic angiography

---

*HAL = hepatic artery ligation; PI = portal infusion

Figure 1.   HAL + PI* for liver metastases: criteria for eligibility.

the postoperative period, the patient received a first course of 5-FU consisting of 1 g/day for 20 days and 3 other courses of 10 g 5-FU administered 3 times every 6 weeks. CEA serum level decreased to 3 ng/ml. But 3 months later, the CEA serum level reached 28 ng/ml and increased continuously. The portal infusion of cytotoxic drug had to be interrupted. It should be noted that 7 months after HAL and portal infusion, the liver CT scan showed a remarkable regression of the main metastases (figures 6 and 7), although the CEA level was higher than at the time of the surgical procedure. This increase suggests the

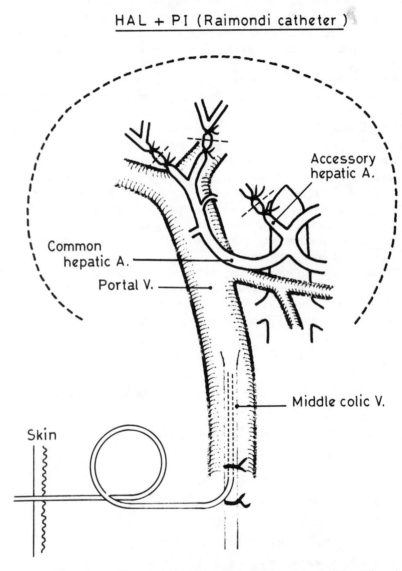

Figure 2.   Surgical procedure for HAL and catheterization of the middle colic vein. The dotted line represents the transection of triangular and falciform ligaments.

spread, out of the liver, of the neoplastic disease and does not reflect the lack of efficacy in the local control of liver metastases.

After these encouraging results, in 1981 the European Organization for Research on Treatment of Cancer (Gastrointestinal Group) activated a randomized comparative study to evaluate the effectiveness of HAL and portal infusion of 5-FU versus a surgical procedure that apparently will not have an influence on survival and will be only symptomatic as HAL alone. Patients with a resected colorectal primary tumor and unresectable liver metastases are stratified according to the measurability of the lesions and the presence or absence of symptoms at the time of entry in the trial. The same criteria as used in our pilot study with regard to the evaluation of progression, the stability of the disease, and remission are applied.

Patients are randomized in 2 groups. In the first group, they are treated by HAL and portal infusion of 5-FU for at least 10 days. Courses lasting 10 days are repeated every 6 weeks until progression of the disease. In the second group, patients undergo HAL alone. During laparotomy, the same procedure as described above is performed. An evaluation of the volume and the number of the metastases must be reported as accurately as possible. Neoplastic tissue involvement of the liver must be classified into two groups: less than 25% involvement and 25–75% involvement.

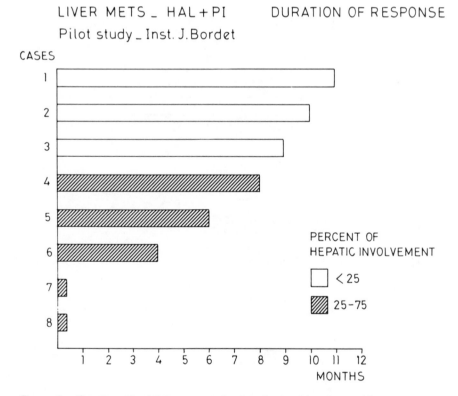

Figure 3.   Duration of partial response for 8 patients with colorectal liver metastases treated in pilot study with HAL and portal infusion of 5-FU.

5-FU is given as a continuous infusion in 5% dextrose, 600 mg/m²/day for 10 days per course, repeated every 6 weeks. Portograms are performed by injecting contrast medium into the catheter before the first day of infusion. The regularity of the infusion can be checked by the administration of Tc radioisotope through the catheter at the same flow rate as that used for portal infusion.

Forty patients are currently registered for the study. A formal comparison of the 2 treatments cannot be carried out with respect to response rate, time to progression, or duration of survival because of the small number of patients registered. Moreover, half of the patients cannot be evaluated yet because they have only recently been entered on the study. Median time to progression in the whole group of patients registered for whom follow-up is available is approximately 5½ months. Median duration of survival in the same group of patients is 11 months. Nevertheless, data on toxicities and side effects of the treatments administered are available. No postoperative mortality has been experienced with HAL. A few local and general complications have been observed, but were never life-threatening. Toxicity due to chemotherapy has been very low, and no chemical hepatitis has been reported. No sclerosing cholangitis has been noted (it was observed after cytotoxic drug infusion by arterial route).

At the beginning of the clinical trial, we used an external catheter without beads. This technique presented complications in 4 patients due to catheter

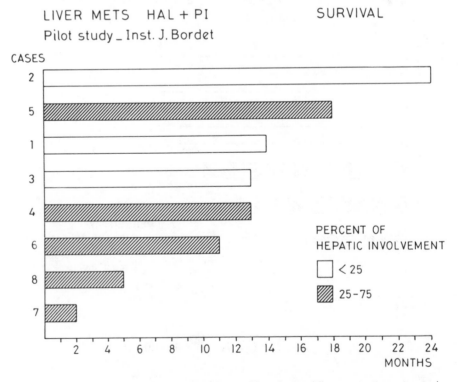

Figure 4.   Duration of survival for 8 patients with colorectal liver metastases treated in pilot study with HAL and portal infusion of 5-FU.

displacement. Since then, we have performed the liver infusion through a port system and a catheter fixed to the vein with ligature around the beads, and no more displacements were observed. Two partial portal thromboses were shown

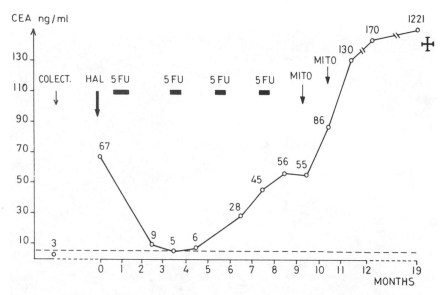

Figure 5.   CEA serum level at the time of anterior resection for primary rectal carcinoma and 1 year later, before and after HAL and portal infusion of 5-FU for diffuse unresectable liver metastases. This patient received 4 courses of 5-FU, 20 g during the first course and 10 g during the other courses.

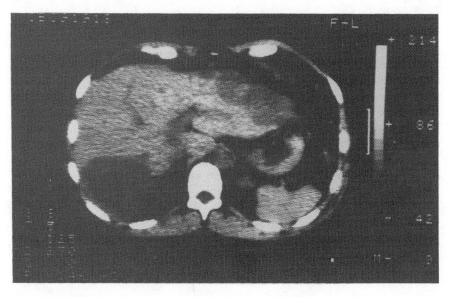

Figure 6.   Liver CT scan before treatment for liver metastases.

by angiography and resulted in stopping the liver infusion after the 3rd and 5th courses of 5-FU, respectively. When compared to the quality of survival of patients who presented immediate progression, the quality of life of the patients was definitely improved.

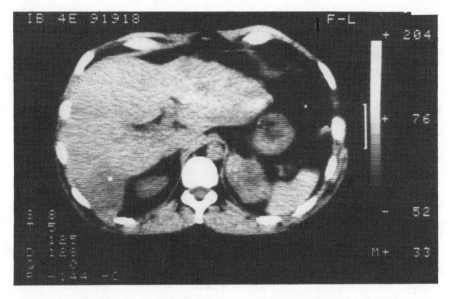

Figure 7.   Liver CT scan 6 months after HAL and portal infusion of a cytotoxic drug. The comparison between figures 6 and 7 shows a remarkable regression of the main metastases.

Conclusion

Among the various treatment possibilities for liver metastases of colorectal cancer, an occlusion of the hepatic artery, combined with portal infusion of a cytotoxic drug, seems to be a rational approach. Experimental data show that HAL increases the necrosis of the tumor and that most of the remaining viable neoplastic cells receive their blood supply from the portal system. The preliminary results of this trial are promising. HAL and 5-FU portal infusion have very low toxicity, without clinical hepatitis and without G.I. bleeding. More clinical trials with new drugs and other procedures assuming longer obstruction of the hepatic artery blood flow are needed to improve this approach in the treatment of liver metastases. In fact, HAL is followed by revascularization. Moreover, we need to study other cytotoxic drug schedules. Finally, cytotoxic drugs now available have not been found to be substantively effective, and new agents need to be identified.

SECTION V

Special Categories of Infusion Chemotherapy

36

REGIONAL INFUSION FOR
BRAIN TUMORS

Fred H. Hochberg, M.D., and Deborah O. Heros, M.D.

Introduction

EACH YEAR, 8,000 INDIVIDUALS in the United States develop and succumb to primary intracranial malignancies. An additional 70,000 have metastatic invasion of the CNS and spinal cord by systemic cancer. For the neurologic oncologist, patients with these neurologic tumors represent uniquely difficult problems of management. The uniform morbidity and mortality associated with these malignancies account for one-fifth of the entire cost for the care of cancer patients in this country.

The most common primary malignant tumor of brain is the glioblastoma multiforme. This malignant growth of supporting brain cells, or glia, is most common among men in the 5th and 6th decade. It may represent the malignant degeneration of benign glial tumors and appears more likely among individuals with long-term histories of seizures and psychiatric abnormalities. Delineation of glioblastoma by computerized tomography (CT) or magnetic resonance (MR) scans has revealed it to be a unifocal, localized, often circumscribed tumor occurring in the subcortical white matter. Approximately 75% of the tumors fall within the distribution of the carotid arteries. Half of these malignancies occur within a single division of the carotid artery (the anterior cerebral artery or middle cerebral artery). Less common are tumors occurring in branches of the basilar or vertebral arteries.

Despite intensive efforts to improve the radiation and chemotherapy of glioblastoma, the median survival remains under 1 year. Fewer than 20% survive 2 years. The Brain Tumor Study Group (BTSG), a consortium of 10 separate teaching institutions, evaluated survival associated with a variety of treatments of this tumor.[50] Postoperative patients with no further therapy survived 14 weeks. The addition of carmustine (BCNU) improved this to 18.5

weeks. Radiation therapy to 6,000 rad median tumor dose (provided to whole brain) was associated with a 35-week survival, which did not change significantly with the addition of BCNU therapy to patients who had received previous radiation. Further reports by the BTSG[49] reemphasized the relative lack of benefit from chemotherapy administered to previously irradiated patients; however, a 20% improvement in survival attends the current I.V. use of BCNU in irradiated patients.

It is expected that newer radiation therapy approaches including high-dose radiation (to 7,000–8,000 rad median tumor dose) being explored by the Radiation Therapy Oncology Group, along with the use of interstitial radiation implants, may further improve the survivals.[45] At this writing, it appears that the maximum benefit from surgical and radiation intervention has been reached. Only the addition of new approaches to the administration of chemotherapy will change these dismal statistics.

The Rationale for Intra-Arterial Chemotherapy

Clinical studies involving the administration of chemotherapy to animals with intracerebral glial malignancies (induced by viral or carcinogen injection) reveal that there are no significant barriers to the transport of drug molecules into the bulk of a malignant rumor. Ninety percent of the bulk of a primary malignant brain tumor has no significant functional barrier to the entry of molecules the size of most chemotherapeutic agents. The remaining 5–10% of the tumor exists as infiltrating cells occupying an area of brain adjacent to the main bulk of tumor. These tumor cells receive their nutrients from blood vessels across which most chemotherapeutic agents cannot pass. They must, therefore, be reached by diffusion of drug from the main bulk of the tumor. The most effective agents known for glioma treatment, the nitrosoureas, readily cross the blood/brain barrier and thus have access to both the major bulk of the tumor and to those cells or cell clusters in the surrounding brain.

That glioblastoma is a localized malignancy is an assumption of recent years. Recurrences of tumor are local; 80% of malignant gliomas fail attempts at control within the original margins. The remainder of tumor recurrences are within 1 cm of the original CT scan margin of the tumor.[25] Thus, the infiltrating portion of the tumor, although theoretically of great concern, has less to do with the demise of patients than does the failure to treat the tumor within its original confines.

BCNU, parenterally administered, is the most commonly used chemotherapeutic agent for the treatment of glioblastoma. It represents one of the group of lipid-soluble nitrosoureas capable of crossing the blood/brain barrier. In animal and tissue culture model systems, these agents have steep dose/response curves.[33] Although they are of minimal benefit, these agents show efficacy in randomized human clinical studies. Additionally, several factors make BCNU an ideal choice for intra-arterial (I.A.) infusion: (1) a short half-life (8–15 min.) and (2) high brain extraction fraction.

These features, combined with the ease of angiographic catheter placement techniques, make arterial infusion methods well within the grasp of most neurologic centers. Retrofemoral catheterizations of the carotid and vertebro-basilar circulation are routinely performed in all neurologic and neurosurgical centers. The procedures require no more than 1 hour and carry a less than 2% risk of hemorrhage into the femoral triangle, infection, or stroke.

The Cytokinetic Rationale for Arterial Infusions

Ensminger has underscored the cytokinetic rationale for arterial infusion therapy.[12] He notes that malignant tumors of brain often have short doubling times and are in a replicative state. Secondly, the normal brain neuronal and supporting tissue are not replicating. The vast majority of chemotherapeutic agents used for brain tumors (methotrexate [MTX], cytosine-arabinoside [ara-C], BCNU) are cytotoxic to replicating tissues primarily. Ensminger and Collins have systematically explored the potential value of I.A. therapies. The high arterial flow rates (200 ml/min.) to brain tissue make BCNU, diaziquone (AZQ), and cisplatin (DDP) ideal drugs for I.A. administration. For these agents, the drug clearance in the body provides a relative advantage for I.A. infusions that is 5–10 times that for equidose I.V. infusions. The computerized modeling of drugs administered in this fashion for the treatment of brain tumors was systematically explored by Fenstermacher and Cowles in 1977.[14] At infusion rates of 25 mg/min. for 4 minutes, they predicted a 10-fold multiplication of drug entering brain tissue 1 minute after the end of infusion. Concentration × time benefits are 3-fold those of I.V. administration. These advantages do not carry concomitant increases in systemic exposure. Systemic arterial and bone marrow exposures are equivalent for I.A. and I.V. infusion routes.

These initial experiences led Crafts to evaluate I.A. BCNU administration (1–20 mg/kg/week) to monkeys without implanted brain tumors.[6] In this study, doses to 15 mg/kg did not produce CNS damage. Extending these initial observations, Levin et al measured activity of ^{14}C-BCNU administered by I.A. (carotid) and I.V. routes.[33] Arterial administration produced 190–280% higher brain nucleic acid-bound drug levels than did the use of I.V. administration. These levels were measured from the infused hemisphere. A similar advantage existed when comparing the effect of arterial infusion of radiolabeled drug concentrations in the infused versus noninfused hemisphere. The authors indicated that these approaches would allow for BCNU dose reduction, with concomitant reduction in BCNU-induced myelotoxicity.[6]

Direct measurement of BCNU concentrations has been performed using ion monitoring mass spectroscopy and high-pressure liquid chromatography (HPLC).[43,33] Levin found that BCNU disappeared in vitro with first order kinetics and a half-life of 11.6 minutes. Using HPLC, the author found a plasma half-life of BCNU approaching 15 min. In red blood cells, the half-life may be twice this value. Evaluating the relative benefits of I.A. administration (10–60 min. infusion) at a single dose of BCNU (10 mg/kg), ipsilateral brain levels are 2- to 4-fold greater than could be achieved with equivalent BCNU doses administered by vein.

Other Agents

Other agents including ACNU, DDP, and AZQ have been recently evaluated as potential I.A. drugs (see table 1). Yumitori[57] demonstrated that ACNU could be delivered safely by continuous intracarotid infusion in 13 patients with malignant brain tumors.[51] Egorin[19] evaluated AZQ and found no significant advantage to intracarotid infusion when compared to I.V. infusion. Early experience using vincristine (VCR) intra-arterially suggested that safe delivery is possible. Because VCR is one of the most effective agents in vitro against malignant gliomas, a reappraisal of I.A. VCR is indicated.[39]

BLOOD/BRAIN BARRIER MODIFICATION

Fenstermacher[15] and Neuwelt[38] have evaluated the benefits of transient disruption of the blood/brain barrier by the use of I.A. mannitol prior to the I.A. injection of chemotherapeutic agents. This approach might be expected to further increase the benefit of I.A. infusion therapy by an additional factor of at least 2-fold, although drug exposure of ipsilateral normal brain may increase neurotoxicity proportionately.[3]

Table 1. Agents Used for Intra-Arterial Infusion of Primary Brain Tumor

Agent	Reference	Rationale
MTX	Perese et al 1962	In vitro sensitivity
VCR	Owens et al 1965	In vitro sensitivity
Nitrogen mustard	Klopp et al 1950 French et al 1952 Hatiboglu and Owens 1961	Possible sensitivity
Thio-tepa	Aronson et al 1963	Possible sensitivity
BCNU	Greenberg et al 1984 Hochberg et al 1985	Penetrated blood/brain barrier Demonstrated antitumor activity
DDP	Feun et al 1983 Feun et al 1984 Stewart et al 1983	Demonstrated antitumor sensitivity
AZQ	Egorin et al 1984	Penetrated blood/brain barrier Demonstrated antitumor activity
BCNU + DDP	Kapp and Vance 1984	Potential synergism
ACNU	Muroaka 1983 Yameshita et al 1983 Yumitori et al 1984	Potential antitumor activity in vitro
VLB	Mealey 1962 Wilson 1962 Wilson 1964	In vitro sensitivity
BCNU + DDP + VM-26	Stewart et al 1984	Potential synergism

Clinical Experience

Methods

Decisions regarding I.A. chemotherapy invariably involve information that is obtained by careful evaluation of the CT scan. The planning of the arterial site for infusion depends in large part on the major arterial blood supply to tumor tissue. Not uncommonly, the physician is asked to identify the major growth area of tumor, which may lie in a different distribution from that of the larger mass of tumor tissue, thus necessitating split doses delivered into both the internal carotid and vertebral arteries. Similarly, at the time of recurrence, a tumor initially in the middle cerebral distribution may be found to be well within the range of the posterior cerebral artery.

Arterial infusions are most often accomplished by retrofemoral catheterizations. These catheterizations, making use of a 5-French catheter, can be done within 40 min. The drugs to be used are administered in final volumes of 100–150 cc of 5% dextrose in water or normal saline over 1 hour. Drugs such as BCNU that require careful attention to solubility, either in reduced alcohol solvents or in alternative solvent systems, may require continuous agitation during infusion. Easily solublized drugs, such as ACNU and DDP, may require little agitation. Pain associated with these infusions may be treated by premedication with morphine sulfate (5 mg), application of ice packs, or local anesthetic retro-orbital blockade performed by a skilled ophthamologist or anesthesiologist. Intermittent external positive pressure to the orbit by an inflatable cuff during the infusion may diminish the pain in some patients.

Experience at the Massachusetts General Hospital

Between 1982 and 1985, 130 patients received a total of 387 infusions at the Massachusetts General Hospital (see table 2). Patients were treated according to 4 protocols (see table 3).

PROTOCOL 1. RECURRENT GLIOBLASTOMA

Thirty-six patients were treated through 70 BCNU infusions given below the origin of the ophthalmic artery. Nine additional infusions were carried out above the ophthalmic artery using flotation balloon techniques. An initial group of 12 patients received 37 infraophthalmic infusions at varying doses: Three patients each were treated at 5-week intervals with 4 separate doses of BCNU (250, 350, 450, 600/mg/m^2).

The toxicities associated with this approach have included neurotoxicity and toxicity to the orbit and its contents. Major toxicity in 90% of patients is due to leakage of BCNU into the ophthalmic artery. This is associated with significant ipsilateral pain lasting the duration of the infusion. Visual abnormalities and retinal arterial obliteration have been well described in the literature.[27,28] Seizure activity occurs at all dose levels up to 600 mg/m^2. Hematologic suppression (WBC < 2000, plts < 50,000) occurs in less than 5% of patients. Systemic toxicity (hepatic, renal, pulmonary) has not been noted in any patients receiving cumulative doses of 1,500 mg/m^2. For these patients, whose glioblastoma was treated at least 5 months from the date of initial operation, the median survival was 58 weeks from the date of recurrence. From initial operation, these patients lived a median of 94 weeks. Ninety percent of patients survived 1 year, and approximately 40% survived 2 years.

PROTOCOL 1-B

Nine patients have received 16 infusions into the vertebrobasilar circulation for treatment of malignant gliomas supplied by the basilar or posterior cerebral circulation. Although these infusions are accomplished with ease and result in only mild retrooccipital or neck discomfort, the prognosis for this

Table 2. Infusion Results at Massachusetts General Hospital

Population	No. patients	Infusions		Survival	
		Infra	Supra	Operation to death	Recurrence to death
Recurrent GLBM[1]	36	70	9		
				84 wk	58 wk
					40 wk
Post-XRT GLBM[1]	26	94		64 wk	
(Supraop)[1]	18	5	57	49.5 wk	
Pre-XRT GLBM[2]	20	59		52+ wk (70% PR or CR)	
Recurrent GLBM[3] (DDP)	31	77		NA	
	130	321	66		

[1]BCNU 240 mg per m^2 over 1 hour q 5–6 wk
[2]BCNU 240 mg per m^2 every 4 wk pre XRT
[3]DDP dose escalation 60–105 mg per m^2 q 5 wk
  GLBM-glioblastoma

Table 3. Protocols Used at Massachusetts General Hospital

Protocol	Patient group	Drug/dose
1	Recurrent glioblastoma	BCNU Escalation 250 mg/m^2, 350 mg/m^2, 450 mg/m^2, 600 mg/m^2
1-B	Glioblastoma within distribution of vertebrobasilar circulation	BCNU 240 mg/m^2
2	Infraophthalmic postradiation glioblastoma	BCNU 240 mg/m^2
2-B	Supraophthalmic postradiation glioblastoma	BCNU 240 mg/m^2
3	Infraophthalmic preradiation glioblastoma	BCNU 240 mg/m^2
4	Recurrent glioblastoma	Cisplatin dose esclation 60, 75, 90, 105 mg/m^2

patient group appears pessimistic in comparison to that of individuals with supratentorial glioblastoma. Patients treated from the time of recurrence (5 months from initial diagnosis) lived an additional 40 weeks.

PROTOCOL 2

Following the initial experience with dose escalation treatment of patients with recurrent glioblastoma, a fixed dose of 240 mg/m^2 (400 mg total dose) in 4 cc of alcohol and 125 cc of normal saline was provided to patients who had completed postoperative whole brain or localized radiation therapy (5,000–6,000 rad median tumor dose). Twenty-six patients were treated at 5-week intervals with 5 separate infusions for a total of 94 infusions. These carotid infusions were provided below the origin of the ophthalmic artery. With one exception, the complication rate was similar to that associated with the treatment of recurrent glioblastoma. It is apparent that the addition of chemotherapy to recently irradiated brain tissue produces profound cerebral edema in up to 15% of patients. For this patient population, the median life expectancy is 46 + weeks from the date of biopsy, with 65% of patients exhibiting partial (PR) or complete response (CR).

PROTOCOL 2-B. SUPRAOPHTHALMIC CHEMOTHERAPY
OF IRRADIATED GLIOBLASTOMA

Eighteen patients received 57 infusions of chemotherapy into the supraophthalmic carotid artery. Methodology for this approach has been described elsewhere.[7] This supraophthalmic approach reduces the incidence of eye pain and toxicity to less than 10%. When present, the pain is attributable to back-flow along the carotid artery. However, the life expectancy for this population is not improved by this technique. Patients survived a median of 49.5 weeks from the date of initial operation, a life expectancy less than that associated with infraophthalmic infusions. This experience suggests that dose-related white matter toxicity resulting from the combined effects of irradiation and drug may be a limiting condition for this patient population. However, dose adjustment for catheter placement was not considered.

PROTOCOL 3. PREIRRADIATION I.A. CHEMOTHERAPY OF GLIOBLASTOMA

Several factors suggest that preirradiation chemotherapy might be preferable to postirradiation approaches.[2] It is commonly assumed that radiation therapy continues to offer profound improvements in the quality of life. However, patients receiving current radiation therapy approaches do no better than patients irradiated 15 years ago. There is reason to believe that drug passage from the artery into irradiated tissue may be less than similar passage into nonirradiated tissue. Blood vessel hyalinization, necrosis, and edema may reduce drug transport and indeed may increase the toxicity. Preradiation chemotherapy is used preferentially in the treatment of lymphoma, colon cancer, and a variety of lung and hematologic malignancies. Because drugs currently available for the treatment of glioblastoma have proven to be efficacious when tested against model systems, the lack of apparent clinical efficacy may be the result of the scheduling of these drugs (i.e., after radiation).

Twenty patients have received 59 infraophthalmic infusions of BCNU (240 mg/m²). These patients received BCNU every 4 weeks in separate infusions. Careful evaluation of preinfusion CT scans allowed patients to be irradiated in the event of tumor resistance to chemotherapeutic agents. The side effects associated with this approach were indistinguishable from those receiving treatment of recurrent glioblastoma. At present, patient survival is 52+ weeks, with 70% of patients achieving either PR or CR with this approach. However, the experience with this approach is too recent to adequately determine its general applicability.

PROTOCOL 4. CISPLATIN INFUSION OF RECURRENT GLIOBLASTOMA

Cisplatin (DDP) arterial infusion techniques have been explored by 2 groups.[46,47,16,17] We have treated 31 patients through 77 infraophthalmic infusions in this fashion. Patients were treated on a dose escalation protocol, receiving chemotherapy every 5 weeks at 1 of 4 different chemotherapy doses (DDP 60, 75, 90, 105 mg/m²). This approach appears better tolerated than does BCNU and is not associated with pain or significant white matter toxicity. However, two patients treated at 105 mg/m² have developed profound white matter damage.

Clinical Experience at the New England Medical Center Hospitals

The experience at the New England Medical Center Hospitals using I.A. BCNU in the therapy of malignant gliomas has included the use of BCNU 150 mg/m² in 5% dextrose in water I.A. at intervals of 6–8 weeks for a maximum of 5 courses following the diagnosis of tumor progression after radiotherapy. Twenty patients received a total of 52 infusions of BCNU between July 1983 and September 1985. Response to treatment was analyzed by CT scan volume reconstruction. A reduction in the enhancing portion of the tumor volume was noted in 8 patients. One patient is still alive without evidence of tumor growth, 4 patients developed tumor progression within 6–26 weeks, and 3 died despite the failure to document regrowth in CT scan. Tumor volume remained stable in these patients for 6, 42, and 84+ weeks, respectively. In the 4 patients who experienced an increase in tumor volume, the doubling time, as calculated by CT scan volume reconstruction, was longer than the expected average tumor doubling time. Four patients had tumors within the watershed areas between the distribution of 2 arterial systems. As predicted, tumor growth was directed into the nonperfused area despite arrest of tumor growth within the perfused region. Toxicity included ipsilateral visual loss in 1 patient following the 5th infusion, despite avoiding the use of alcohol as a diluent. Seventeen patients had low absorption lesions with mass effect during the course of therapy. Although consistent with edema, leukoencephalopathy could not be excluded.[27]

Currently, the patients are receiving a course of combined radiation including external irradiation (6,000 rad) and interstitial [192]iridium brachytherapy (8,000–10,000 rad) delivered in the midcourse of external irradiation. Intra-arterial BCNU is then administered as adjuvant therapy 3 weeks after the completion of radiotherapy. The number of patients undergoing this combined therapy approach is small, but this approach appears to be well tolerated. Efficacy has not been established.

Review of the Literature

Three neuro-oncology departments have provided much of the available data concerning the role of I.A. chemotherapy in patient populations: Roswell Park Memorial Institute, the University of Michigan, and the M. D. Anderson Hospital. Although the earliest data concerning the use of I.A. chemotherapy emerged from the work of Levin et al at the University of California at San Francisco[33] and Sweet et al at the Massachusetts General Hospital (unpublished data), it was not until the report by West[51] that the possibility of using I.A. BCNU became a realistic consideration. West provided I.A. infraophthalmic carotid BCNU between 80–100 mg/m² every 4 weeks to 20 patients with metastatic cancer to the nervous system. Complications included focal eye pain (70%) and seizure activities (11.6%). Myelosuppression was not significant. Although these data were preliminary, response rates of 36% (melanoma) and 44% (lung cancer) suggested that this approach was efficacious. The data were extended by Madajewicz, who failed to find response in any metastatic brain melanoma, but reported a 50% response rate in patients with metastatic lung cancer to brain.[34,35] Responses endured up to 14 months. Extending these observations, West et al now infuse mitomycin (MIT) through infraophthalmic carotid artery routes in doses of 5–20 mg/m² every 6 weeks. This drug was chosen for its efficacy against lung cancer of adenocarinomatous origin (personal communication). BCNU, however, is reserved for patients with small-cell carcinoma of the lung and squamous cell cancers that have remained sensitive to this agent. Investigations currently under way in the treatment of metastatic brain tumor include those of Casino[5] and Yamada.[54]

Neuro-oncology groups (West at Roswell Park and Greenberg at the University of Michigan) provided much of the early data concerning the use of BCNU in the treatment of glioblastoma. In 1983, West treated 25 patients with postoperative postirradiation glioblastoma through 72 courses of BCNU with the addition of systemic VCR and procarbazine.[52] BCNU complications included those noted above. Seven of 10 patients, previously without irradiation, responded to this approach, with survivals of 9–22 months. Two of 3 patients with recurrent gliomas responded and survived to 37+ and 45+ months; 15 patients (60%) responded to combined therapy after radiation, with a median survival of 12.7 months.

Greenberg et al[20,21] have treated 65 patients with glioblastoma. Nineteen of these have received chemotherapy with BCNU in alcohol solvent and have survived 54 weeks after radiation therapy. Twelve patients treated prior to radiation therapy survived 56 weeks. The alternative BCNU solvents used by Greenberg and others[43] have reduced toxicity, but have not been associated with improved survival or quality of life.

Alternative Agents

Feun has treated 35 patients, 23 with primary malignant brain tumors and 12 with brain metastases, with DDP (60–120 mg/m²) into the carotid artery below the ophthalmic artery.[16] Six of 20 patients with primary brain malignancies responded, with a median response duration of 33 weeks (13 weeks for all patients, responders and nonresponders). Half of the patients with brain metastases responded with a 30 + week response; responses for patients with stable disease without clear evidence of response were 12 + weeks. It appears that doses of DDP up to 75 mg/m² are tolerated without significant associated toxicity. Similar data emerge from the previous studies of Stewart (1982), who noted that CNS toxicities occurring in 5% of patients included visual and auditory abnormalities but without significant evidence of renal or hematologic toxicity.[46]

Sakai treated 17 patients with a variety of intracranial malignancies with Adriamycin (ADR) in varying doses (up to 20 mg) every 2 weeks.[44] He measured drug levels of ADR that appeared at higher concentrations in tumor tissue than in surrounding brain. Responses were noted in 4/6 glioblastoma and in 2/4 metastatic brain tumors treated.

Combination drug I.A. chemotherapies have been used by Yung and Stewart. Yung (personal communication) currently provides combinations of BCNU (100 mg/m²) and DDP (60 mg/m²) into the infraophthalmic carotid artery. He has treated 40 patients with glioblastoma in this fashion and 20 patients with metastatic cancer to the nervous system. Partial responses occur in 40% of patients, with median time to tumor progression being 30 weeks.

Stewart treated 37 patients with a combination of I.A. BCNU, DDP, and VM-26.[48] Responses were noted in 68% of primary brain tumor patients and 56% of brain metastases, with previous cranial irradiation and intravenous chemotherapy reducing the likelihood of drug response. Retinal toxicities occurrred in 56% of patients receiving doses of BCNU equal to or greater than 100 mg/m² and DDP above 60 mg/m².

Supraophthalmic Carotid Artery Infusions of BCNU and Other Agents

As noted previously, at the Massachusetts General Hospital we have treated a total of 27 patients through 66 supraophthalmic infusions of BCNU (9 infusions in patients with recurrent glioblastoma and 57 with previous irradiated glioblastoma). Although offering theoretical appeal, this approach has practical difficulties that have been well explained by a number of authors.[28,7] A variety of catheter tips are used in this fashion. We have used a fixed tube that can be inserted within a 5-French catheter. A fenestrated balloon is used to administer chemotherapy.[7] Kapp et al use a flexible tip catheter with an expanded end to facilitate drag in flowing blood.[30] In either case, infusions may be carried out into the first division of the middle cerebral artery; however, skilled hands are needed for this approach, and dose levels of drug that can be accepted by the CNS when delivered at this level are still uncertain.

Toxicity

Several authors have indicated toxicities associated with infraophthalmic carotid infusions, predominantly of BCNU[26,28] These toxicities have been indicated previously. However, the increasing use of BCNU administered into previously irradiated patients has produced significant white matter toxicity or leukoencephalopathy that may be unique to BCNU and radiation. Calcification may occur. The pathologic basis for this abnormality appears to include a necrotizing white matter abnormality associated with occlusion of small arterioles. This may appear at intervals of 1–10 weeks after infusion. Toxicities resemble the retinal vasculitis reported by ophthamologists studying patients treated in this fashion.[9,19,22,37] Complications included visual loss, vascular toxicity with retinal infarction, and an unusual pigmentary retinopathy associated with DDP infusions.[37]

Systemic toxicity from I.A. administration of various chemotherapeutic drugs is rarely observed and has not been a limiting factor for this application. Mild and temporary thrombocytopenia may be seen with I.A. BCNU. We have not seen any pulmonary or hepatic toxicity, even in patients receiving the largest cumulative doses of BCNU. Renal impairment has not been associated with I.A. DDP. We use systemic mannitol prior to and during the infusion of DDP.

New Approaches

Two studies have explored the disruption of the blood/brain barrier with mannitol prior to the infusion of MTX and other chemotherapeutic agents.[4,38] These approaches would appear to further enhance drug passage by a factor approaching 3 times in comparison to approaches without barrier modifications. With the exception of primary CNS lymphoma, however, the clinical benefits of this approach have yet to be seen.

Modifications of Intra-Arterial Administration

Several laboratories have explored the administration of noncycle-specific materials by continuous infusion into the carotid artery. Phillips made use of implantable pumps with catheters embedded into the carotid artery through a retrotemporal approach.[42] Similar approaches have made use of radiosensitizers such as BUDR and IUDR. Techniques for the removal of these agents from the venous system draining the intracerebral circulation may be developed. Dedrick[8] and Oldfield[40] have explored these approaches as means of removing BCNU that has passed through tumor tissue. The relatively rapid metabolism of BCNU may suggest that this elaborate system is unnecessary. However, this system may have important applications for the use of agents with longer half-lives and for continuous infusion systems.

The availability of human-human and mouse-human monoclonal antibodies may lead to I.A. infusion of these products. Epenelos performed the I.A. infusion of a radiolabeled monoclonal antibody in a patient with a recurrent glioblastoma.[13] The radioactive monoclonal antibody against epidermal growth factor receptor provided a preferential source of radiation, resulting in tumor regression and clinical improvement. As our understanding of the various cell surface markers and tumor antigens becomes more sophisticated, and as monoclonal antibody therapy conjugated to radiolabeled particles or chemotherapeutic agents become more specific in the field of neuro-oncology, I.A. infusion will provide an excellent means of delivery. Liposome-bound chemotherapeutic agents may also be administered by I.A. infusion; this is another potentially exciting method of drug delivery for the future therapy of brain tumors.

In summary, I.A. infusion of various chemotherapeutic agents has been performed safely and effectively in the treatment of primary and metastatic brain tumors. As our understanding of tumor therapy becomes more sophisticated in terms of new chemotherapeutic agents and antibodies directed against tumor specific antigens, I.A. delivery will certainly play an important role.

37

THE CLINICAL USE OF 5-FLUOROURACIL AND OTHER HALOPYRIMIDINES AS RADIOSENSITIZERS IN MAN

John E. Byfield, M.D., Ph.D.

Introduction

THE HALOPYRIMIDINES WERE THE first rationally synthesized anticancer agents. The development of 5-fluorouracil (5-FU) by Duschinsky et al[19] and its application by Heidelberger and his group[23] were the first useful fruit harvested from the work of the preceding decades that had outlined the steps in nucleic acid biosynthesis. The clinical benefits of these applications are probably yet to be fully applied.

The halopyrimidines are a family of analogues of normal cellular compounds absolutely required for RNA and DNA synthesis. They act through competition with or substitution for nucleic acid contituents that are the basis for the transmission of the genetic information. The family divides into 2 basic groups: the first is the 5-FU group, whose members are uracil analogues; the second is the bromouracil/iodouracil group, which are thymidine analogues. All of these compounds were first synthesized in the late 1950s based on analysis of the atoms available for substitution that were closest in size to either the hydrogen present at the 5′ position of uracil (fluorine) or the methyl group at the 5′ position of thymine (bromine or iodine). The reader is referred to the reviews by Heidelberger[23] and Prusoff and Goz[40] for a summary of the original work.

Almost all halopyrimidines have the capacity to radiosensitize (RS) growing cells to radiation. This property has been recognized virtually since their

479

introduction.[4,6,23,33,49] Despite this long history, successful clinical exploitation has been slow. The current clinical status of halopyrimidine RS, particularly that of 5-FU, is the subject of this chapter.

Preclinical Studies

Biology of the Halopyrimidines

The halopyrimidines have been studied intensively and continuously for the past 3 decades. Their literature is vast and, in many aspects, somewhat ambiguous. From a biochemical standpoint (which underlines some important clinical features), it may be noted that each of the 2 halopyrimidine groups have 2 possible subgroups. The first are the free bases (5-FU, 5-iodouracil [5-IU], and 5-bromouracil [5-BU]) in which the 5' group of uracil has been replaced by a halogen. Of these, only 5-FU is important, since the other 2 (5-BU and 5-IU) are not significantly used by human cells in vivo. The second group are the nucleoside derivatives of each base. In these latter compounds, either a pentose or deoxypentose sugar is added to create analogues of uridine and thymidine, respectively (e.g., 5'-fluorouridine and 5'-bromo-2'-deoxyuridine). At the clinical level, only BUDR and IUDR (5'-bromo-2'-deoxyuridine and 5'-iodo-2'-deoxyuridine) are currently under clinical study. Both the free bases and the nucleosides may enter mammalian cells, but all cytotoxic activity (including RS) is mediated by some form of phosphorylated derivative (e.g., 5'-fluoro-2'-uridine monophosphate, 5-FDUMP).

The most important distinction between 5-FU and the 5-bromo and 5-iodo compounds stems from their specific stereochemistry. 5-FU is a uracil analogue, and most, if not all, of its activities are mediated via an effect on uracil and RNA metabolism.[3] Bromine and iodine substitution create thymine/thymidine analogues whose actions, by and large, are mediated through their substitution for thymidine in DNA. However, one derivative of 5-FU, the 5-FDUMP mentioned above, inhibits the enzyme thymidylate synthetase,[23] preventing thymidine formation and thereby blocking DNA synthesis. At this specific biochemical point, the metabolism of RNA and DNA interconnect in a major way. Because of this important interaction, the overall metabolic actions of 5-FU are quite complex. Moreover, its cytotoxic activities probably vary from cell line to cell line and from species to species. To add to the complexity, the closely related compound 5-FUDR, when activated by phosphorylation to 5-FDUMP, again acts at the same point. However, 5-FUDR is not a radiosensitizer, has a quite different toxicity spectrum when infused into patients (compared to infused 5-FU), and has been almost exclusively administered by arterial infusion. A full understanding of the implications of these subtle biochemical and pharmacologic variations will be necessary before full clinical exploitation of these compounds against specific tumor types is possible.

Molecular Bases of Halopyrimidine Radiosensitization

For the purposes of this review, RS will be defined as the effect of making living cells more sensitive to ionizing radiation. There are 2 totally different processes by which this can occur. The commonest current meaning refers to compounds that can substitute for molecular oxygen and thereby make *hypoxic* cells more radiosensitive. Hypoxic cells are about 3 times less sensitive to X rays than oxygenated cells;[48] therefore, molecular oxygen is a radiosensitizer. This RS phenomenon is quite different from the RS effects of the halopyrimidines. For all practical purposes, halopyrimidines (5-FU, BUDR, and IUDR) have no effect on hypoxic cells since they act only on growing cells, i.e., cells that are synthesizing RNA and DNA. The hypoxic component of a tumor is doing neither and will therefore be unaffected by these compounds. This review is devoted solely to *"oxic"* RS. *Hypoxic cells are thought to be a significant source of x-ray treatment failure but, as will be shown, the correct use of oxic RS can eliminate this problem through the process of reoxygenation.*

At the molecular level, RS by BUDR is better understood than is RS by 5-FU. In order for BUDR to radiosensitize cells it must be incorporated into cellular DNA.[23,28,46] Because it is a close analogue of thymidine, BUDR is avidly taken up into most cells and incorporated into cellular DNA via the same enzymatic pathways as thymidine (the "salvage" pathways). Considering the fundamental importance of thymidine and DNA to the correct function of the cellular genes, it is remarkable how well cells tolerate BUDR. However, both genetic expression and cell survival *are* affected in a fundamental fashion, and clinical cell toxicity by BUDR (and IUDR) occurs as shown below. From the standpoint of therapy, the most important effect of the presence of BUDR (and IUDR) in cellular DNA is its interaction with the free radicals formed by X rays in the cellular water. These react with the bromine atom of BUDR (as compared to the relatively nonreactive methyl group of the normally present base thymidine) and lead to DNA damage and cell death.[50,51] The degree of RS achieved by BUDR is a function of the amount of thymidine substituted by BUDR.[46]

Because only actively dividing cells are synthesizing DNA, BUDR can only radiosensitize growing cells. For this reason, the basic rationale for the use of BUDR as a RS is in such regions as the brain or liver where the X ray dose-limiting normal tissues have very low mitotic rates. However, BUDR is rapidly degraded in humans, first to bromouracil followed by dehalogenation.[23] Therefore, programs using *slowly* infused drug are required to achieve RS of human tumors.[28] This is necessary because the BUDR must be constantly available during the 6–12 hours required for the DNA biosynthetic process. Although it differs in some important respects, most notably a reduced capacity for resensitization to fluorescent light, IUDR behaves similarly to BUDR, and the same fundamental scheduling factors prevail.[27,30]

The mechanism by which 5-FU radiosensitizes[4] is poorly understood,[11] but is undoubtedly quite different from that of BUDR and IUDR. For example, 5-FU RS requires that the drug be present *after* rather than before X ray exposure,[11] i.e., the opposite of the case for BUDR and IUDR.[46] 5-FU in vivo is converted into both 5-fluorourdine-monophosphate (5-FUMP) and 5-fluoro-2'-deoxyuridine monophosphate (5-FDUMP). The former leads to 5-FU incorporation into RNA, whereas the latter blocks DNA synthesis. Both of these effects may be cytocidal. However, little 5-FU is incorporated into DNA, and that which does enter probably is rapidly removed.[24] Accordingly, some factor quite different from a BUDR-like action must be involved in 5-FU RS.

Although the fundamental biochemical mechanism of 5-FU RS is not known, tissue culture experiments[11] have clearly shown that there are 3 basic prerequisites that must be met in order for cells to reach a 5-FU RS state: (1) the 5-FU must be present *after* each X ray exposure; (2) enough 5-FU must be available to yield a cytotoxic effect from the drug alone; and (3) the duration of 5-FU exposure must be at least 1 full cell cycle in length (usually 24+ hours). Because of the short half-life of 5-FU in man (10–15 min.),[37] these prerequisites can be met only by continuously infused 5-FU.[11] Thus, quite different reasons lead to the same conclusions for BUDR and 5-FU; only infusional schedules of many hours duration can produce the conditions required for in vivo halopyrimidine RS in man.

Quantitative Aspects of Halopyrimidine Radiosensitization

Figure 1 outlines in schematic form the quantitative cellular aspects of 5-FU RS as demonstrated in tissue culture. The basic assay for such studies are cell survival curves performed using colony counting methods. In each experiment, known numbers of the cells under study are subjected to increasing doses of radiation. Clonogenic survival is then determined by assaying the surviving colonies formed after 10–14 days in culture. This type of assay permits rapid and quantitative examination of the effects of drug concentration, sequencing, etc., on cell clonogenic survival in tissue culture.

If the cells are exposed to radiation alone (upper line), a typical "radiation survival curve" is generated. Such curves usually have a shoulder of various widths followed by a long straight curve of exponential cell killing (when plotted in a semilog plot as is the case here). Curves for 5-FU alone are similar[16] when survival is plotted versus 5-FU concentration (for each fixed 5-FU exposure duration). As shown, a typical clinical X ray dose (200 rad) kills about 30% of the cells, while about 70% *survive* (hence the term X ray survival curve). If sufficient 5-FU is present for 24 hours or more after the radiation exposure, then enhanced cell killing (RS) occurs. A "sufficient" 5-FU concentration is one that will induce demonstrable cell killing alone.[11] Under these combined drug and X ray conditions, additional cells are killed. In figure 1, 5-FU toxicity is shown by point A, where 50% of cells have been killed by the 5-FU alone (since the percent survivors is 50% at *zero* rad X ray dose). When the 2 modalities are combined, more cells are killed (90%) than would be expected if the toxicities were only additive (line B). In this illustration, "additive" killing would be the simple product of the cytotoxic effects of 5-FU (50% killing) and radiation (30% killing). Numerically, additive toxicity is therefore 0.7×0.5, or 35% survivors (and therefore 65% killing). Instead, more cells are killed (90%) and only 10% of the cells have survived. This is termed radiosensitization, which is one form of cytotoxic synergism.

Work in the author's laboratory has shown that the greater the killing by 5-FU, the greater will be RS.[11] This is illustrated in figure 1 by point D, where

90% of the cells are killed by 5-FU alone. With this degree of killing by 5-FU alone (90% tumor cell killing), only 3% of the cells will survive the combination treatment (point C). This aspect has important clinical implications because it shows that: (1) RS is most likely to occur if the tumor is "responsive" to 5-FU alone, and (2) the more 5-FU that can be administered to each patient, the more likely it is that RS can be achieved.

Multiplied over a series of 15–35 x-ray treatments, the effects of RS can be dramatic. For example, one might assume that treatment involves a gastric cancer containing the maximum concentration of 10^9 stem cells per gram of

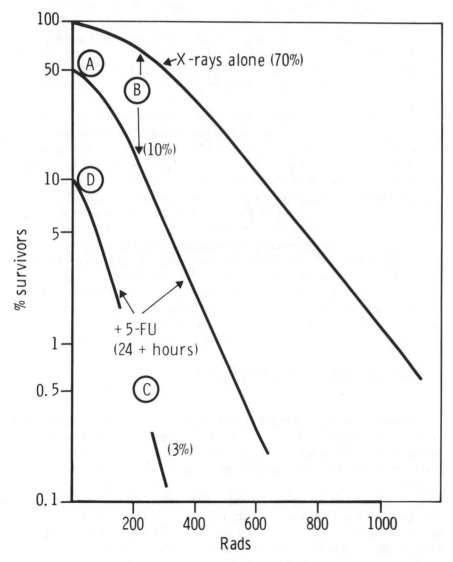

Figure 1. Effect of 5-fluorouracil on the radiation survival of human cells in culture (see text for explanation).

tumor. If the tolerance of the surrounding tissues is such that only 4,000 rad total radiation may be given, then:

- 5-FU alone will reduce the tumor by 50% each treatment cycle; such cycles can be given every other week as, for example, for the 11 weeks used here (5 infusion cycles). Thus $(0.5)^5$ reduces the surviving tumor stem cell fraction to 0.03, or 3 out of each initial 100 cells survive. This would be considered a good clinical partial response. However, tumor stem cells resistant to 5-FU would have been proportionately increased, leading eventually to treatment failure.
- Radiation alone leaves 70% of the tumor stem cells surviving after each 200-rad fraction; as noted, tolerance of nearby organs limits the x-ray treatment dose in this abdominal area to 20 fractions (4,000 rad). Hence $(0.7)^{20}$ reduces the tumor to 7.9×10^{-4} tumor cells surviving after the 4,000-rad dose. This would be scored as a clinical complete response, since the 7.9×10^4 surviving tumor cells would be just below clinical detection by ordinary tests. However, the patient would be subject to early recurrence.
- Consider, then, the *combination* given under minimal RS conditions where 30% of tumor cells survive each treatment. This would be only 5% more killing than an additive effect of 35% surviving. The total treatment (delivered as 4 treatment cycles, each including a 5-day 5-FU infusion combined with 5 X ray fractions of 200 rad each). This therapy would yield a reduction in surviving tumor cells by $(0.35)^{20}$, which yields a final surviving fraction of only 7.6×10^{-10} cells. Because there were only 10^9 stem cells per gram of tumor to begin with, this regimen becomes curative. (Tumor cell repopulation is ignored for simplicity's sake in each, but would affect each process in the same fashion). The reader will then remember that as the degree to which RS is increased (by increasing 5-FU levels or 5-FU sensitivity), so is the dose of radiation required for tumor sterilization reduced. This reinforces the importance of the need to use as much 5-FU as can be tolerated each cycle when used for RS.

Pharmacology of Infused 5-FU

It should be apparent that the clinical challenge is to create the conditions needed to establish RS within the patient. To do this, the pharmacology of 5-FU must quantitatively recreate the RS requisites established in the preclinical work described above. To do this, the pharmacology of infused 5-FU must be fully understood.

The most important aspects of the pharmacology of infused 5-FU are (1) nonlinear clearance;[37] (2) a threshold for change in clearance in the clinical infusion range;[13] (3) the potential for significant drug accumulation at higher infusion rates;[13] and (4) impaired clearance in patients with significant liver function abnormalities, including metastatic disease.[20] A clear understanding of these factors will facilitate the use of 5-FU as an RS in the future.

It has been recognized for several years that the clearance of 5-FU is nonlinear, instead falling steadily as the dose rate of administration of 5-FU increases.[17,37] Radiation of a patient has no discernible effect on 5-FU pharmacology.[12] The effect of nonlinear clearance is to *decrease* the percent 5-FU that can be removed by a single passage through the body as the infusion dose load increases (see figure 2). This observation is of more than academic interest, since it implies that *at very low 5-FU infusion rates, the clearance is effectively the cardiac output*.[13] This means that all drug that enters the body at low infusion doses is, on average, immediately removed. Because the liver, or more accurately, the splanchnic bed,[1] is the only known source of catabolism (degradation) of 5-FU, the obvious conclusion is that other parts of the body are using the drug without immediately degrading it.

Our working hypothesis is that this noncatabolic "use" of the drug is, in fact, its incorporation into RNA. Based on the work of Heidelberger's group,[36] one can calculate that if about 4% of the body's cells were growing exponentially, a 70 kg man could fully use all 5-FU infused at up to 15 mg/kg/24 hours. Thus, the hypothesis of a significant contribution of "anabolic" or biosynthetic "clearance" appears quantitatively tenable. This model has the attraction of directly relating both side effects and tumor response to drug infusion rate.[13] Other interpretations, such as pulmonary catabolism, are possible, but seem to us less likely.[17]

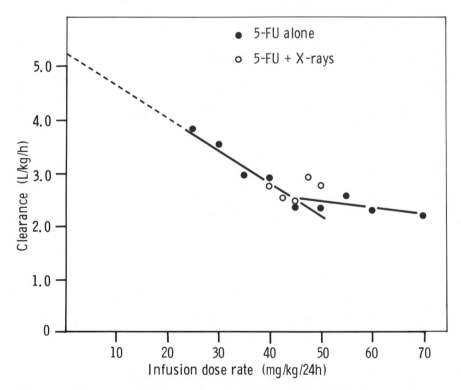

Figure 2.   Clearance of 5-fluorouracil as a function of infused dose rate in man. Reprinted with permission (ref. 12).

The main effect of nonlinear clearance on the plasma 5-FU levels achieved as a function of infusion dose rate is shown in figure 3. It can be seen that there is a linear relationship between the administered dose and the mean plasma 5-FU level. However, the curve extrapolates to a dose of about 15 mg/kg/24 hours for a zero plasma 5-FU level. It is at 15 mg/kg/24 hours that clearance reaches its maximum, namely the cardiac output (figure 2). We interpret this as fol-lows: Above an infusion rate of about 15 mg/kg/24 hours (in the average patient), one component of clearance becomes saturated. No more drug can be removed by this mechanism, and clearance begins to fall. This "extra" 5-FU appears in the bloodstream and can be measured. Clearance continues to fall until it reaches an asymptote equivalent to the splanchnic/hepatic blood flow (figure 2). Thereafter, it is constant ("linear") and equivalent to the hepatic blood flow. The implication of this interpretation is that at low infusion doses, peripheral utilization (a low capacity consumer) dominates 5-FU clearance, whereas at high dose rates (e.g., bolus injections), hepatic blood flow is the

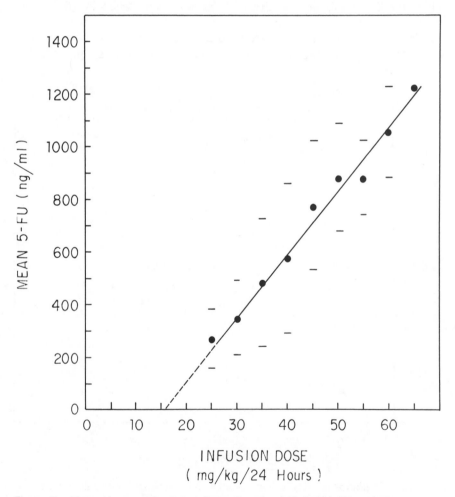

Figure 3.   Mean plasma 5-fluorouracil as a function of infused dose rate in man.

major source of drug removal. The former is important because it is responsible for many side effects and for tumor response (and RS). The latter is purely a catabolic phenomenon.

These aspects of 5-FU pharmacology previously have not been fully appreciated, but are important in understanding the parameters for 5-FU infusions and for RS. We have shown elsewhere that the sensitivity of human tumor cells to 5-FU is a clear function of both the external concentration of the drug (i.e., the measured drug level outside the tumor cell) *and* the duration of 5-FU exposure.[16] By comparing the plasma 5-FU concentration (which is the effective external level in vivo) with the plasma 5-FU levels obtained during infusional therapy in man (see figure 3), one can attempt to determine what 5-FU infusion doses are needed for tumor cell killing and therefore for RS.[11] The correlation between these C × T factors and clinical results are surprisingly close.[13] However, the figure also shows that one must be aware of the translation of serum 5-FU concentration/infusion dose rate curve to the right, which comes from there being 2 disparate sources of drug "clearance" in the infusional dose range. Once this is understood, some of the mysteries of dose/response curves for both clinical toxicity and tumor response disappear.

In summary, while it is widely agreed that the calculated clearance of 5-FU is "nonlinear," the sources for this nonlinearity are controversial. It is the writer's belief that there are 2 basic components of 5-FU clearance: (1) 5-FU incorporation into cellular RNA, which is a saturable phenomenon, is thought to be the basis for almost all drug "cleared" at doses below 15 mg/kg/24 hours; and (2) hepatic catabolism, which is the basis for all other 5-FU clearance. In this model, at high dose rates (including bolus injections), most of the clearance of 5-FU would be in the liver. In the range of "intermittent continuous" infusions (20–65 mg/kg/day), clearance is divided between the 2 sources and is declining rapidly with increasing 5-FU dose (figure 2). The latter is especially important in colon cancer patients because many such patients have liver metastases, which we have shown further reduces 5-FU clearance.[20] According to this concept, all truly continuous infusions[32] must be conducted at rates below 15 mg/kg/24 hours or less (to avoid drug accumulation), and this turns out to be the case.

Therapeutic Implications of 5-FU Pharmacokinetics

There are 2 major implications of the pharmacology of infused 5-FU. First, the existence of clearance values equivalent to the cardiac output is consistent with removal of drug by many growing cells, probably all growing cells. Second is the somewhat complex physiological implications of the presence of 2 clearance mechanisms, 1 of which is directly involved in 5-FU clinical toxicity.

One piece of evidence that drug removal is involved in the toxic (and presumably therapeutic) effects of 5-FU is shown in figure 4. In this analysis, the total amount of 5-FU infused to the point where toxicity developed (dose rate × total time to toxicity) is plotted against the dose rate. The data are drawn from 2 fundamental papers in the clinical literature on 5-FU infusions.[32,43] The 2 studies were performed at different institutions in different time periods. At very low infusion dose rates there is no toxicity (figure 4). Sufficient drug has not been given to induce demonstrable cell death. After a threshold has been passed, all infusion dose rates appear to induce the same limiting toxicity (stomatitis). These data were not adjusted for liver abnormalities (which affect clearance) and were obtained mainly from colon cancer patients. Nevertheless, figure 4 shows that the *total* infused dose needed to reach toxicity is remarkably constant.

We interpret this kind of evidence as suggesting that 5-FU accumulation in cells is steadily occurring. Eventually, the cell has accumulated enough and a toxic event occurs (cell death). This is manifest clinically as stomatitis, i.e., failure of the stem cells of the oral cavity to replace lost cells. We believe that

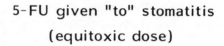

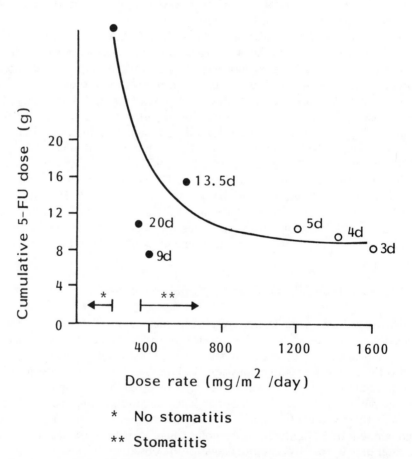

Figure 4.   Cumulative dose of 5-fluorouracil required to induce dose-limiting stomatitis in man. Also shown is the duration of the infusion in days. From refs. 32 (closed circles) and 43 (open circles).

most of the drug infused at doses up to 15 mg/kg/24 hours is involved in this kind of phenomenon, and that this element is a major factor in all clinical infusions of 48 hours or more duration when taken to toxicity. Accordingly, infusions of almost any duration (i.e., infusions lasting at least 24 hours or 1 cell cycle in duration) should have (1) similar toxicity patterns and (2) similar response rates. The exception to this are short-term, high dose-rate infusions, which we have shown to have dose-limiting CNS toxicity that is not a cell renewal phenomenon.[13]

The second major feature of 5-FU clearance that affects its use is its *accumulation in the plasma* during infusions *above* 15 mg/kg/day. (This feature is documented in ref. 13.) It probably occurs because the first element of clearance (anabolism) has been saturated. The 5-FU that emerges from the nonhepatic tissue beds effectively acts as an additional infusion source. Eventually, a new equilibrium plasma 5-FU level should be reached. However, accumulation occurs for longer than would be expected, and it is possible that the tissue compartments are simultaneously being slowed in their anabolic activity by the effects of the 5-FU. So far as we could determine, slow accumulation of the drug is occurring during all 5-FU infusions lasting 72–120 hours when the infusion dose rate is 20–65 mg/kg/24 hours. These dose rates are well above those used in the "continuous" infusions piloted by Lokich et al,[32] and these considerations do not apply in the latter context. The absence of drug accumulation at low dose rates (less than 15 mg/kg/day) undoubtedly makes such infusions safer and more manageable.

For shorter infusions (typically 5 days or less in duration), however, plasma 5-FU accumulation is important for 2 reasons. The most obvious consideration is that the effective drug infusion rate is slowly increasing, and the likelihood of toxicity is also therefore increasing. The most important implication has to do with the clinical variable of the *duration of a therapeutic infusion*. For infusions *to limiting toxicity*, one can reasonably project that the maximum therapeutic amount of drug has been given. On the other hand, in many clinical protocols toxicity is not considered in response analysis, although there is good evidence for a dose/response effect with 5-FU.[2] We have shown that the likelihood of a tumor cell's dying (*or being radiosensitized*) from 5-FU is a strict function of the 5-FU C $\times$ T factors the cell encounters.[11,16] Any reduction of *either* the C *or* T will reduce both toxicity and response. Thus, the response rate from a 96-hour 5-FU infusion at a constant dose rate will not be as great as that from the same amount of drug given for 120 hours. To the degree that almost all drug is "used," this factor is reduced. Thus, for a truly continuous infusion (to toxicity) such as Lokich has used,[32] this factor is minimized. However, for a constant C $\times$ T, as the duration of an infusion is *reduced* the percent drug "used" by tumor cells also falls, and the relative importance of plasma accumulation increases. Because the survival of human tumor cells following 5-FU exposure is of a semilog nature,[16] a reduction of the C $\times$ T factor by 20% means a much greater reduction in cell killing. All of these factors come into play in the planning and execution of 5-FU clinical studies if optimal results are to be obtained.

Pharmacology of BUDR and IUDR

The pharmacology of BUDR is somewhat different from that of 5-FU in the range of clinical doses needed for RS.[41] Over most of the desired range, the clearance of both BUDR and IUDR is linear.[30,41] Slightly more IUDR is needed compared to BUDR to achieve similar plasma concentrations. Both IUDR and BUDR are rapidly degraded into the free halogenated bases, iodouracil and bromouracil. These are analogues of thymine and are, as such, mainly inactive against human cells. Both BUDR and IUDR can be infused safely in man[27,28,29,39] and can produce plasma levels consistent with those thought to be required for RS. However, both agents are toxic to the bone marrow and, in addition, BUDR sensitizes the entire skin because of its photosensitizing properties.[29] The current feeling is that arterial treatment will be required for these agents and that IUDR may be more useful than BUDR. The reader is referred to recent reviews by the National Cancer Institute group for further details of these highly interesting studies.[27-30,41]

Clinical Studies of 5-FU Radiosensitization

Variations in the Clinical Use of Infused 5-FU

There are many combinations possible in a regimen in which "radiation," 1 or more drugs, and surgery are combined. As is to be expected, a form of "evolutionary" mixing has occurred in the development of existing 5-FU RS programs. To simplify these variations, they will be divided into 2 basic "models":

THE DETROIT MODEL (WAYNE STATE UNIVERSITY)

This type of program developed from the initial studies of Nigro et al on squamous cell anal cancer.[38] It includes coincident infused 5-FU and a modest dose of external beam radiation, both used as a preoperative measure. There is no reduction in the extent of surgery employed. The preoperative therapy is used solely to improve survival. Mitomycin-C (MIT) is included, as it was in the initial regimen. The duration of the 5-FU infusion is usually 96 hours. The origins of the program are empiric. Evidence now appears solid that it has improved the prognosis of at least 1 human cancer (anal) when compared to surgery alone.[18]

THE UCSD MODEL (UNIVERSITY OF CALIFORNIA, SAN DIEGO)

This regimen is based on the preclinical studies by the author's group in which the basic requirements needed to achieve 5-FU RS were identified.[11] These are: (1) 5-FU must be continuously infused for at least 24 hours *after* each radiation treatment is used; (2) ideally, enough 5-FU is used to produce adequate[13] toxicity (grade 2 stomatitis) from the 5-FU alone; and (3) treatment is given in *cycles*, with toxicity appearing and disappearing during scheduled rest periods. The biological basis for an improved therapeutic ratio is the use of recruited, dose-limiting normal cell repopulation.[15] The dose-limiting normal tissues (usually the oral mucosa) are purposefully caused to "outgrow" the tumor within the constraints of an acceptable dose of radiation with respect to late effects. This model is shown in figure 5.

The "standard" regimen the author now recommends for squamous, transitional, cloacogenic and breast carcinomas is as follows:

- 25 mg/kg/24 hours continuously infused 5-FU given each day for 5 days (120 hours). This is preferably given on an outpatient basis.
- Five x-ray treatments of 200 rad each given at times 0, 24, 48, 72, and 96 hours into each infusion.
- Following each of these combination treatment periods (i.e., the above treatments together), there is introduced a defined rest period lasting 9 days; this should be extended until toxicity has subsided but *not* significantly longer. Toxicity (stomatitis plus minimal marrow toxicity and occasional skin reactions) appears during the first part of the rest period and then subsides.

    Only the neutrophil plus band count is used for following marrow reactions because of the well-known (and clinically irrelevant) lymphopenia induced by radiation.

    The entire period of treatment, toxicity, and healing is termed a "treatment cycle."

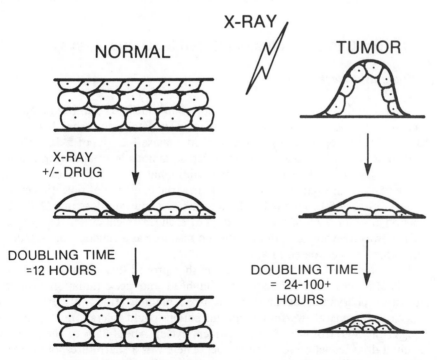

Figure 5.   Biological model of 5-fluorouracil radiosensitization (see text). Reprinted with permission (ref. 15).

- The total cycle time is therefore 14 days (5 days on therapy, 9 days on rest); the total *number* of cycles is defined by the total radiation dose tolerable for the treatment region, which is not different from that used when radiation alone is given.
- The treatment goal is total clearance of tumor within the x-ray treatment field. If the patient has no systemic tumor spread at the time of treatment, the goal is therefore cure. Surgery is reserved for clear-cut treatment failures in all tumor sites, except for biopsy of any suspicious regions.

This "standard" UCSD regimen is not currently considered as definitive, but is believed to be the best thus far developed for squamous and transitional cell cancers (and their variants, such as basaloid, large-cell, etc.). Alternative schedules may be better, particularly in nonsquamous cancers. Without doubt, additional agents such as cisplatin (DDP) can be added to this regimen.[42] The role of any such agents remains to be defined, as described below. The author believes that the biological basis of this regimen is RS by 5-FU coupled to the cyclical recruitment of normal tissue stem cells. There is rarely significant marrow toxicity with this method, even with pelvic radiation.

The most notable modification of the Detroit model has been made at the Princess Margaret Hospital in Toronto, where surgery, except for salvage, has been omitted, and additional radiation doses (usually without drug) have been employed. The Princess Margaret regimen may be regarded as an interesting and certainly useful "hybrid"; it is almost exactly intermediate between the Detroit and San Diego methods. Its specific applications are described below.

Current Clinical Status of Infused 5-FU and X rays

Head and Neck Cancers

Several studies have recently been reported in which 5-FU has been used in a schedule in which RS might be anticipated. To date, only 1 has been published.[15] In that report, our group described a phase 1–2 trial of 5-day infused 5-FU combined with radiation in advanced squamous head and neck cancer. We have also recently published some additional phase 1 data on 72-hour infused 5-FU in this patient group.[12] The first trial consisted of repeating cycles of 5-day infused 5-FU coupled with radiation at a constant dose rate (250 rad/fraction given on each of the first 4 days of each treatment cycle). The goal of the trial was to evaluate both toxicity and response as a function of 5-FU dose rate, which was escalated in a phase 1 format.

The commonest toxicity, and the one that proved dose-limiting, was stomatitis. Because both infused 5-FU and head and neck radiation produce stomatitis/pharyngitis as their major toxic manifestation, this effect was expected. In general, we found that no patient could tolerate more than 25 mg/kg/day 5-FU (for each 5-day treatment cycle). About 25% of the patients required dose reduction to a lower level. There was a sharp threshold for the induction of stomatitis, which was never seen in a dose-limiting or dose-reducing form at the lowest dose tested (20 mg/kg/day). We had found similar results in our first series of patients with esophageal carcinoma.[9] All 20 mg/kg/day patients completed therapy without requiring dose reduction. We believe, therefore, that 20 mg/kg/day is too low a dose for many patients; we suggest 25 mg/kg/24 hours (for 120 hours per cycle) as "standard therapy," even with head and neck radiation.

Much-reduced patient survival was also seen with 20 mg/kg as opposed to a higher dose, suggesting a therapeutic dose/response relationship.[15] This underscores the relationship between toxicity and response that has been suggested for bolus 5-FU.[2] Our study of head and neck cancer patients strongly suggested that toxicity, response, and survival appeared linked as predicted by the theoretical basis of this treatment.[11] The study also clearly showed that therapy can be given in a cyclical fashion in head and neck patients with results at least equivalent to conventional radiation.

Three other studies have recently been reported in which a similar approach has been offered to patients with advanced cancer of the head and neck. These are summarized in table 1. One of these[22] used the Detroit model (preoperative therapy including MIT, 1 used the modified (Detroit) Princess Margaret version with higher radiation doses and surgery reserved for salvage,[25] and the third used full-dose radiation and added DDP to infused 5-FU, also reserving surgery for salvage.[42]

A most promising modification of the UCSD program has recently been presented by Showell et al.[42] They reported their work in which infused 5-FU (800 mg/m^2 for 120 hours) and radiation were combined with DDP for the treatment of advanced head and neck cancer. They found a 56% complete response (CR) rate if defined as total return to a normal-appearing anatomy, but a higher (90%) rate if tumor-free (but anatomically distorted patients) were considered as CR. Survival appeared to relate to the latter and was far better than would ordinarily have been expected. The cyclical therapy used produced considerably reduced toxicity, as predicted by our model.[15]

A modified Detroit program was used by Hahn et al, with infused 5-FU combined with MIT and external beam radiation in 44 patients with advanced head and neck cancer.[22] Their program used a split course treatment with 3,000

Table 1. Results of Treatment With Infused 5-Fluorouracil and Radiation in Advanced Head and Neck Cancer

Institution/ reference	No. patients	CR (%)	Survival	
			Median	2-Year
Northwestern[42] (+ cisplatin)	27	60	2 years	70%
Princess Margaret[25]	57	—	—	66%
UCSD[15]	18	75	2 years	70%
RTOG* historical controls	—	—	13 months	—
RTOG CT — XRT*	—	—	15 months	—

*Unpublished Radiation Therapy Oncology Group data

rad in 3 weeks, with the drugs being given "up front," i.e., a bolus of MIT (10 mg/m^2) on day 1 and a day 1–4 infusion of 5-FU (1.0 g/m^2). In the subsequent surgery, they found a 62% negative primary specimen and a 33% negative neck specimen. The authors regarded their results as promising as compared to their historical experience in this poor-prognosis patient group.

The preliminary results of the Princess Margaret approach[25] are similar (see table 1). These investigators employed a total dose of 4,000 rad with 2 RS cycles and MIT, using surgery only for specific indications. Their CR rate of 50% (defined by the more rigorous recurrence-free status at 1 year or more) was also felt to be somewhat improved over radiation for these bad-risk patients, especially hypopharyngeal cancers.

Although comparison of these regimens in such a complex patient group as advanced squamous head and neck cancer is difficult, there is some suggestion that the more aggressive regimens produce higher CR rates (see table 2). However, to date probably no regimen has produced the best results possible, because no report, including the author's, has attempted to optimize the program in each patient in every treatment cycle.

Squamous Esophageal Cancer

The current available data for infused 5-FU and radiation in esophageal cancer are outlined in table 3. In 1979, we reported the first clinical trial of infused 5-FU and radiation in esophageal cancer.[9] 5-FU was also first used specifically as an RS in that trial. The trial used a dose of 20 mg/kg/24 hours 5-FU and a 5-day infusion duration. It also introduced the use of cyclical therapy for the first time. Although primarily of an exploratory phase 1 nature, the study yielded a CR in 5/6 patients, showing that the approach was both possible and useful in man. Toxicity was minimal, and in some patients the drug dose was undoubtedly inadequate. Noteworthy is the observation that the first patient so treated lived more than 5 years free of disease before being lost to follow-up. Since that time, additional patients have been treated; the survival data in table 3 are taken from the overall curves.

Two patients in that initial series developed second (lethal) carcinomas. One was of the hypopharynx, for which the patient underwent a second series of infusions with X rays without substantial problems. These observations showed that there was no demonstrable cumulative toxicity with the regimen,

Table 2. Radiosensitizing 5-Fluorouracil Cycles Versus Response Rate in Advanced Head and Neck Cancer

No. RS Cycles	CR (%)	Total dose (rad)	Reference
1	57	5,000	22
2	50	4,500	25
7[1]	60	7,000	42
5 – –7[2]	75	7,000	15

[1]5-FU given at 800 mg/m^2 (= 1.36 g in 70 kg patient)
[2]5-FU given at 25 mg/m^2 during majority of treatment cycles (1.75 g in 70 kg patient)

at least outside the x-ray treatment field. Second cancers are a significant source of reduced survival in cured esophageal cancer patients.

In 1981, Steiger et al at Wayne State University reported their larger results of what has been termed here as the Detroit approach, primarily using a combination of a 4-day 5-FU infusion and 3,000 rad radiation (2 RS cycles plus 1,000 rad).[45] A single bolus of MIT was given on day 1. Responding patients subsequently underwent esophagectomy. That series also first reported the substitution of DDP for MIT in their most recent patients. The authors felt this approach gave reasonable palliation in medically unresectable patients and, for resected patients, yielded better results than any thus far reported in the surgical literature. Among the resected patients, 29% had no tumor in the resected specimen. The authors felt that DDP was much better than MIT (see table 4). However, the difference in the tumor-free specimen rate when the MIT group was compared to the DDP group was modest. The 2-year survival in the resected group was 30% compared to an expected (historical) 9%.

Leichman et al have recently updated the DDP portion of the study, with overall similar results.[31] Median survival of the entire group has been 18 months, while those whose response was sufficient to have surgery was 24 months. All long-term survivors were tumor-free at resection (including lymph nodes). Sixty percent of this subgroup of patients have lived at least 2 years. These results clearly relate tumor clearance (that is, a CR) with long-term survival. The authors also concluded that their results were better than those they had previously achieved using a MIT-containing regimen, although comparative data were not given.

Table 3. Results of Conservative Management Versus Preoperative Chemo-Radiotherapy in Esophageal Cancer

Institution/ reference	Pts entered	CR (%)	Survival	
			Median	2-Year (%)
UCSD[9]	6	83[1]	22 mo	30
Princess Margaret[26]	35	48[2]	12 mo	28
Wayne State[31]	21	25[3]	18 mo	24

[1]Clinical and radiographic evaluation
[2]Defined as 2-year clinical relapse-free
[3]Surgically confirmed

Table 4. Comparison of Mitomycin-C to Cisplatin Added to Infused 5-Fluorouracil, Radiation, and Surgery in Esophageal Cancer

Drug	No. patients entered	Surgery	Curative resection possible	Tumor-free	% Patients	
					All	Resected
MIT	30	23	18	6	20	33
DDP	21	19	15	5	25	33

Data from refs. 31 and 45

These results may be compared to a report from Princess Margaret Hospital investigators in which the "hybrid" regimen was used.[26] Their esophagus "hybrid" approach used definitive x-ray doses (5,000 rad or more) but only 2 or 3 RS cycles. MIT is included, and surgery other than posttreatment biopsy is omitted. The results, reported by Keane et al, also employed 2 slightly differing schedules of RS 5-FU, in 1 case giving 1 RS cycle and in the other case, 2 such cycles (in a split-course approach after a 4-week rest). The 5-FU dose was 1.0 g/m². Continuous radiation seemed better than split-course. Survival was 48% at 1 year and 28% at 2 years. The local control rate at 2 years was 48%. The authors concluded that these results were clearly superior to their historical results from radiation alone.

These 3 studies give the major current results available for the use of 5-FU used as an RS in esophageal carcinoma. Several conclusions may be drawn. The first is that partial responses (PR), while offering palliation for this disease, have no significant impact on long-term survival. The Detroit data show clearly that a CR is necessary.[31] However, this observation also leads one to question the role of surgery in this approach. If only tumor-free patients (at surgery) are cured, then perhaps the surgery played little to no part in the cures. The overall results reported by Keane et al would certainly tend to support this hypothesis (see table 3).

The other major question that arises from the same analysis relates to the question of treatment intensity. For example, should all of the radiation be given in the context of RS (as in the San Diego model) or just part, as at the Princess Margaret? Because the author's initial series used a relatively low dose of 5-FU (20 mg/kg/day), there is no way of knowing whether or not higher, more adequate 5-FU doses might not do better. Similarly, there is no firm evidence to support the use of any specific alkylating agent in this approach, and the addition of either MIT or DDP remains a theoretical improvement, perhaps adding only toxicity (see tables 3 and 4). These are important questions that can be answered only in future trials.

The question of 5-FU dose was discussed as a general problem above. However, it must be noted that since RS is clearly 5-FU dose-dependent,[11,16] it seems likely that a higher CR rate can be achieved than has yet been reported. The data of Leichman et al nicely show the relationship of a CR with survival. No such relationship would be apparent if death from metastatic disease was the sole important parameter in esophageal cancer. Future studies in esophageal carcinoma should address this question directly.

Gastric, Biliary Tree, and Pancreatic Carcinoma

To date, there have not been any series with significant patient numbers published describing the effects of RS 5-FU in either gastric or pancreatic cancer. In our own institution, gastric cancer is uncommon; most available patients received some form of systemic chemotherapy (usually FAM) prior to consideration of 5-FU and X rays. Several patients were treated with 5-FU as an RS, and most patients showed response, with 1 CR in the treatment field. Overall, gastric cancer appeared almost as responsive as esophageal cancer. In addition, we have not noted any difference in response between esophageal adenocarcinomas and the squamous variant. Larger studies of gastric cancer would be useful, because the trials of bolus 5-FU and radiation at both the Mayo Clinic[35] and by the Gastro-Intestinal Study Group[21] have showed a positive impact of such treatment, even with bolus 5-FU.

Similarly, only anecdotal responses with prolonged survival have been seen in biliary tree cancers. Again, our own experience is too limited to comment further upon, and significant reports by others have not yet appeared. The effects of the halopyrimidines combined with radiation on the normal biliary tree are discussed below.

In the case of pancreatic carcinoma, there are no major series as yet, and our own experience has not been promising. To date, we have not seen a single CR. In the author's opinion, partial responses are of little significance in this disease.

Metastatic Colorectal Cancer in the Liver

We have recently reported our results[7,8] of treating metastatic colorectal cancer in the liver using continuously infused 5-FUDR and 3,000 rad whole liver radiation. It should be noted that 5-FUDR is not a radiosensitizer per se (author's unpublished data). The preliminary results, including the surgical aspects of subcutaneous pump placement, are available to the interested reader[5] and will not further be reviewed here. Our major observation was that the approach is feasible and can lead to permanent CR. Treatment must be delivered early and before derangement is severe (defined as an elevation to greater than twice normal values of either alkaline phosphatase or bilirubin). No benefit from therapy occurred in patients with the latter levels of liver compromise from metastatic disease.

In our initial series, several patients developed evidence of treatment-induced liver disease, which proved fatal in one case (in a patient with a CR). From a recent analysis of the toxicity of therapy, it seems likely that the most sensitive cell system to the combination is the biliary tree epithelium. The reader is referred to a recent review by the author on these topics, including the current status of possible radioprotectors of hepatic cells.[7] Until further data are available, total liver radiation should be limited to 2,000 rad. A recent series using arterially infused 5-FU produced similar results.[34] We consider this approach as still experimental but useful in selected patients, especially patients who have failed systemic therapy but whose disease is still limited to the liver. However, it should be noted that all of our long-term surviving patients eventually developed disease outside the liver, mainly lung and brain metastases.

Cervix Cancer and Lower Bowel Radiation Tolerance

Thus far, there has been a single trial of this approach in cervix cancer. The Detroit model was used as modified at the Princess Margaret.[47] Surgery was not used because all patients were considered too advanced for resection. Radiation was split-course and combined with two 72–96 hour 5-FU infusions, 1 given at treatment inception and the other at the resumption of radiation treatment after the mid-course break.[47] Thus, 2 cycles of x-ray RS with 5-FU were used along with further nonsensitized x-ray therapy. MIT was also used at the beginning of each infusion.

The authors considered the results to be quite promising.[47] In stage 3-B patients, rapid tumor resolution was found. A CR rate of 74% and 1-year control rate of 70% was obtained, compared with an expected control rate of 43% from historical controls. Patients with recurrent disease also appeared improved over past results. The authors believe a randomized trial was indicated based on these results.

The program is of further importance because the areas receiving radiation are similar to those used for lower G.I. radiation, including bladder and rectal carcinomas. Acute lower bowel radiation toxicity did not appear much different from that expected from radiation alone; some adverse late effects on the bowel were found, but at an incidence level similar to radiation alone (G. Thomas, personal communication). Further studies on this common squamous cancer are in progress.

Squamous Cell Anal Cancer

The results of the various programs used against squamous cell anal cancer are reviewed in this volume and have been summarized elsewhere.[18] Squamous cell anal carcinoma is the first tumor in which it is now clear that 5-FU, used in what is recognized to be a RS regimen, can produce long-term disease-free survival tantamount to cure.[38]

The main series of studies that have reported some variant of this approach are listed in table 5, which is modified from the data summarized by Cummings et al.[18] The studies in anal carcinoma can be divided into 3 groups: group 1—those series in which this approach was added to conventional surgery, usually an abdominal-perineal resection; group 2—a single series in which the chemotherapy preceded the radiation (which is a form of control for the coincident drug and x-ray series); and group 3—the series in which no major surgery was performed. Because the original study of Nigro et al using presurgical radiation and drug was widely copied, the surgical adjuvant data have longer follow-up. However, local failures in the conservative series remain very uncommon, and a large difference in local control rate is clearly unlikely to appear (see table 5).

Two major conclusions can be drawn from the table 5 results: (1) the use of infused 5-FU and radiation produces a very high CR rate in squamous anal cancer that is confirmed pathologically in those patients who have surgery and is long maintained in patients treated conservatively; (2) the use of surgery, and certainly radical surgery, with the elimination of normal bowel continuity, can now be questioned in most patients. It is of interest to note that the single series in which the 5-FU and radiation were *not* given simultaneously (thereby making RS impossible) produced a significantly lower response rate. However, other explanations, such as difference in stage, etc., could also be responsible for the notably better response rates in the "RS" series. Nevertheless, the results suggest that RS may well be occurring and contributing to the results of treatment.

The final observation that may be noted is the overall good results in the author's series in which MIT was omitted.[10] Although the number of patients studied was modest, the stage distribution was typical of such series and included patients with advanced stages who nevertheless achieved durable CR. This suggests that the contribution of a potentially leukemogenic alkylating agent may be modest at best. Future studies undoubtedly will address this question.

Rectal Carcinoma

Experience with infused 5-FU used as an RS is quite limited in rectal carcinoma, even though the tumor is considerably more common than squamous anal cancer. Sischy recently updated his series in which a "Detroit" approach (preoperative therapy including MIT) was applied in marginally operable rectal carcinomas.[44] Using 1.0 g/m^2 5-FU for 96 hours, he found that 31% of the resected specimens contained no carcinoma and only 24% of perirectal nodes contained cancer, compared with 53% of their historical controls. Local control in patients eligible for such 5-year evaluation was 84.9%. The treatment proved much less effective against recurrent disease.

Our own experience is more limited than that of Sischy et al but of a similar trend. We have been able to achieve CR in occasional patients who are inoperable for various reasons, but the tumors are clearly more resistant to this treatment than are squamous cell anal cancers. A rigorous evaluation of treatment parameters has not yet been possible. The author believes that this is a

Table 5. Results of Therapy with Infused 5-Fluorouracil (I5-FU), Radiation, with and without Mitomycin-C or Surgery, in Squamous Cell Anal Cancer.

Reference	Tumor-free		Subsequent local recurrence	Follow-up (months)
	Clinical	Pathology		
Group 1 (coincident I5-FU, mitomycin-C and preoperative radiation)				
A	24/28	21/26	0	6 – 108
Group 2 (I5-FU and mitomycin-C, then X rays, then surgery)				
B	13/27	16/30	2	5 – 74
Group 3 (It-FU, mitomycin-C, and X rays without surgery)				
C	9/10	9/10	0	4 – 24
D	29/30	—	1	6 – 60
E*	11/11	9/10	0	24 – 48

*No mitomycin-C used

Sources: A—Nigro et al (Cancer 1983; 51: 1826); B—Michaelson et al (Cancer 1983; 51: 390); C—Flam et al (Cancer 1983; 51: 1378); D—Cummings & Byfield (ref. 18, this review); E—Byfield et al (Cancer Treat Rep 1983; 67: 709).

major area for useful research at this time, since the 2 tumors derive from closely related tissues and can be easily followed. There is a wide variety of evidence that rectal carcinomas are somewhat radiosensitive. 5-FU remains a prime drug in the treatment of these tumors once they have metastasized. This is obviously an area for concentrated clinical study.

Current Clinical Status of BUDR and IUDR

To date, the available clinical data using BUDR as a clinical radiosensitizer are more limited than for 5-FU. Two groups have reported pilot data on the use of infused BUDR and X rays in the treatment of gliomas.[39,41] The NCI group has reported on phase 1 and pharmacologic studies of BUDR and IUDR.[27-30] When infused into the vein in man, both BUDR and IUDR produce a significant bone marrow toxicity.[28] At tolerable doses, sufficient BUDR enters bone marrow colony-forming cells to produce significant RS when the cells are studied in vitro.[29] Whether more slowly growing tumor cells are equally sensitized is presently unknown. Unfortunately, BUDR also strongly sensitizes the skin, making venous infusions troublesome.[29,41]

Current clinical studies using IUDR and BUDR infused through arterial catheters (where a high likelihood of RS is inherent) as well as systemic IUDR infusions are in progress. Both of these approaches have considerable clinical promise, being firmly based in the well-established phenomenon of halopyrimidine RS.

Conclusions

Clinical applications of halopyrimidine RS are promising, but much work remains to be done. Clinical difficulties with systemic BUDR and IUDR infusions are significant, and arterial infusions for such diseases as glioblastoma are in progress. The original difficulties encountered with such an approach were primarily technical in nature and may now be avoidable.

The current results with infused 5-FU used as a RS are highly promising. In 1 tumor (anal squamous cell cancer), this approach has already accomplished the 2 main goals of cancer therapy, i.e., life prolongations *and* a reduction in the need for radical and deforming surgery. The initial results in other squamous tumors, such as head and neck cancer, suggest that the same may be possible for laryngectomy. Pilot data in transitional cell bladder cancer (M. Rotman, personal communication) have also yielded impressive local control rates obviating (thus far) the need for cystectomy in most patients.

The optimal combination of infused 5-FU and radiation in a given cancer is not simple. Unlike most other anticancer agents, 5-FU is taken up by cells in significant amounts. This contributes to an unusual pharmacokinetic picture that must be understood for optimal application. Radiation fractionation is almost infinitely variable. For best results, each of these components must be controlled in a rational fashion in each patient. Nevertheless, this approach has considerable promise, especially in the squamous-transitional tumors, and can probably be done completely as an outpatient regimen. With appropriate development, it also seems quite plausible that the requisite infusional nature of the regime can be replaced by an absorbable slow-release oral prodrug.[14] Further advances almost certainly can be expected.

38

INTRAPERITONEAL "BELLY BATH"

CHEMOTHERAPY

Maurie Markman, M.D.

INTRACAVITARY CHEMOTHERAPY REPRESENTS AN emerging application of new technology in pharmacokinetic modeling used in an attempt to deliver potentially more effective chemotherapy. The introduction of chemotherapeutic agents into body cavities lined by serosal membranes is certainly not new, but the concepts and practice have evolved substantially. The introduction of antineoplastic agents into the peritoneal space, for example, does not just provide "topical" application directly on the tumor but, perhaps just as important, there is a consequential redistribution of the drug to the tumor via the systemic vasculature following absorption into the systemic circulation. In this sense, at least 1 component of the intracavitary application of the chemotherapy is infusional in nature, with a longer tumor exposure time as compared to the bolus systemic chemotherapy. Thus, as with other infusional techniques, the direct delivery of drugs into the peritoneal cavity attempts to improve the efficacy of therapy by increasing local concentrations of moderately active antineoplastic agents as well as increasing exposure time of slowly dividing tumor to cell cycle phase-specific drugs.

This chapter is divided into 4 sections dealing with (1) the use of intracavitary agents to control malignant effusions by a sclerosing effect; (2) a discussion of the basic pharmacokinetic principles of the administration of chemotherapeutic agents for their cytotoxic, rather than sclerosing properties; (3) a review of both the acute and chronic toxicities of intraperitoneal chemotherapy; (4) and finally, a review of the clinical trials employing single-agent and multidrug chemotherapy utilizing the "belly bath" technique.

Intracavitary Sclerosing Therapy

One of the earliest attempts to apply chemotherapeutic agents in malignant disease was to administer them directly into the body cavity containing the tumor.[1-4] Unfortunately, while ascites and pleural fluid reaccumulation were often successfully controlled following intracavitary treatment, shrinkage of tumor masses was rarely observed. In addition, local side effects (particularly pain) were often quite severe. Thus, the administration of intracavitary chemotherapy became restricted to those situations where *sclerosis* of the body cavity was the desired result.

Today, standard treatment of malignant pleural effusions includes the intrapleural administration of several chemotherapeutic agents, including bleomycin (BLM),[5-8] nitrogen mustard,[9-11] and doxorubicin (ADR).[9] These agents also have been delivered intraperitoneally, but with less success. It should be mentioned that the intracavitary administration of radioactive colloids has also been successfully employed in the management of malignant effusions.[12-14] Finally, as will be discussed in greater detail in the following section, a major difference between standard sclerosing therapy and the use of intraperitoneally (I.P.) delivered chemotherapy to produce cell kill is the treatment volume for the administered drug. With sclerosing therapy, a *small* treatment volume is employed with a high concentration of active drug. With I.P. chemotherapy, a *large* treatment volume (with a lower drug concentration) is used to deliver the antineoplastic agent. It is hoped that this latter technique will minimize normal tissue irritation and reduce the risk of producing sclerosis.

Pharmacokinetic Rationale for Intraperitoneal Chemotherapy

It is not the intent of this review to provide a basic course in pharmacokinetics. However, to fully understand the rationale behind the direct I.P. administration of chemotherapeutic agents, it is important to discuss briefly the general principles upon which this technique is based.[15-16]

One can most easily understand the basis for I.P. therapy by viewing the body of a patient receiving this treatment as consisting of 2 compartments, the first being the peritoneal cavity into which the drugs are instilled and the second being the rest of the body (2-compartment model). Drugs instilled into the peritoneal cavity will diffuse out into the systemic circulation. The rate at which the concentration falls will be a function of the volume (V_{pc}) in the peritoneal cavity, the surface available for diffusion (A), the permeability of this surface (P), and the difference in free drug concentration between the peritoneal cavity (C_{pc}) and the plasma (C_p). Peritoneal cavity clearance is equivalent mathematically to the product of permeability × area (PA). Equation 1 defines this relationship:

Equation 1.
$$\frac{dC_{pc}}{dt} = \frac{PA\ (C_{pc} - C_p)}{V_{pc}}$$

If it is assumed that all the drug leaving the peritoneal cavity enters the systemic compartment, then the concentration of drug in the plasma is determined by several factors, including the volume of this compartment (V_D), the rate at which drug is entering it ($PA\ [C_{pc} - C_p]$), and the rate at which drug is cleared from the plasma (kC_p). This relationship is defined mathematically by equation 2:

Equation 2.
$$\frac{dC_p}{dt} = \frac{PA\ (C_{pc} - C_p) - kC_p}{V_D}$$

Equations 1 and 2 can be integrated to show that if the concentration in the peritoneal cavity can be maintained at a constant level such that the system comes into a steady-state, then the ratio of the concentration in the peritoneal cavity to that in the plasma is inversely related to the clearance from the 2 compartments (equation 3).

Equation 3.
$$\frac{C_{pc}}{C_p} = \frac{Cl_p}{Cl_{pc}} + 1$$

An extremely important principle of I.P. chemotherapy can be derived from an examination of equation 3. The greater difficulty a chemotherapeutic agent has in leaving the peritoneal cavity (low clearance) and the more rapidly the drug is cleared once it reaches the systemic circulation (high plasma clearance), the higher the concentration ratio between the peritoneal cavity and plasma. Differences in the area under the concentration versus time curve (AUC), an indirect measure of drug exposure, will be enhanced by increasing differences in clearance rates between the 2 compartments. Additionally, anything that increases systemic clearance or decreases peritoneal cavity clearance will have the positive effect of further augmenting the AUC ratio.

A second factor important in determining the exposure of active drug to the peritoneal cavity compared to the plasma is that of the metabolism of the drug during its passage from the peritoneal cavity to the systemic circulation. Drugs administered directly into the peritoneal cavity can potentially reach the plasma by 1 (or more) of 3 routes. First, the agent may enter the peritoneal lymphatics and reach the venous circulation via the thoracic duct. Second, it may be absorbed directly into capillaries of the parietal peritoneum that drain into the systemic circulation. Finally, the drug may be absorbed into the portal circulation and pass through the liver *before* it reaches the systemic circulation.

Currently available data would strongly suggest that drugs in the molecular weight range of most chemotherapeutic agents will be removed from the peritoneal cavity predominantly by way of the portal circulation.[17,18] Metabolism of an I.P. administered antineoplastic agent into an inactive form during its first pass through the liver will, therefore, have the effect of *reducing* the amount of active drug reaching the plasma and other tissues where it might exert toxic effects. Several lines of experimental evidence support the importance of the portal circulation in clearing I.P. delivered drug from the cavity. Radioactive sodium sulfate placed into the peritoneal cavity of the dog appeared in the portal vein within seconds following instillation, whereas the concentration of the labeled material in the inferior vena cava initially was significantly lower.[17] Also, the radiolabel appeared in the thoracic duct lymph minutes later. In a rat model, similar pharmacokinetics were noted using several drugs including progesterone, caffeine, atropine, glycine, and glucose.[18]

Anatomic considerations also support these experimental observations.[19,20] The structures that make up the greatest part of the surface of the peritoneal cavity—the visceral peritoneum, the omentum, and the mesentary—drain into the portal circulation. The parietal peritoneum, on the other hand, drains directly into the systemic circulation. Also, although there is a network of lymphatics on the undersurface of the diaphrams that communicates directly with the peritoneal cavity by specialized pores,[21] it is known that the flow in these channels is less than that in the portal circulation.[22,23] It is likely that absorption via the lymphatics is significant only for compounds with molecular weights of 1,000 or more.[24]

Investigators at the National Cancer Institute (NCI) attempted to measure directly the absorption of I.P. administered 5-fluorouracil (5-FU).[25] In a group of 4 patients receiving 5-FU I.P., portal vein catheters were placed, and it was calculated that 29–100% of the administered drug was absorbed by the portal circulation.

Similarly, the absorption and distribution of 17 chemotherapeutic agents has been examined in a rat model at the NCI.[26] The percent absorption for 10/17 drugs was 20–37%. L-asparaginase demonstrated the poorest absorption (9%), while hexamethylmelamine exhibited the greatest (92%). Although the clinical relevance is not clear, it should be noted that this study demonstrated a difference in the rate of absorption of I.P. ADR depending on the peritoneal dialysis solution used.

Unfortunately, only limited information is available on the various factors that control absorption of intraperitoneally administered drug into the bloodstream. It is known that initially, the single layer of flattened cells that constitutes the peritoneal membrane proper must be crossed.[27] Following diffusion through a tissue space, the drug must cross the capillary membrane prior to entering the systemic circulation. Torres et al, examining the influence of molecular weight, lipid-water partition coefficient, association constant, and instilled volume of the rate of absorption from the peritoneal cavity in a rat model, made several observations relevant to I.P. chemotherapy.[24] First, is was determined that fluid absorption was most rapid during the first hour following instillation of enough isotonic fluid to fully distend the peritoneal cavity. Second, absorption was demonstrated beyond the first hour, but its rate slowed. With the instillation of small volumes, the percent absorbed during the first hour was greater than with larger volumes, but the absolute volume absorbed was greatest for the largest amount instilled. Third, these investigators demonstrated that the peritoneal cavity was able to buffer 50 ml volumes from pH 3–11, with the solution returning to neutral within 1 hour following instillation. In addition, the ability of the peritoneal cavity to rapidly reconstitute its normal concentration of amino acids within 6 hours of washing of the cavity indicates the rapid transit time for small molecules into the cavity. Finally, it was shown that absorption of water-soluble compounds diminished 5-fold as the molecular weight increased from 18 to 1,000, and the absorption of ionized drugs was found to be slower than the rate of un-ionized agents. The available experimental data would therefore suggest that absorption from the peritoneal cavity occurs principally by passive diffusion, with the major barrier being the presence of a lipid membrane.

The factors important in determining the absorption of toxic waste products and drugs *from* the blood *into* the peritoneal cavity have been studied in much greater detail because of their importance in patients with renal failure who are receiving peritoneal dialysis. For the interested reader, several references pertinent to this issue have been included.[28-32]

The essential initial step in the successful application of I.P. chemotherapy is the delivery of drug to the tumor. Thus, if I.P. chemotherapy is to be effective, then drug-containing fluid *must* be distributed to all involved areas. It has clearly been demonstrated that fluid placed into the peritoneal cavity is not necessarily evenly distributed if only a small volume is instilled.[33-35] Several lines of evidence suggest, however, that if large enough volumes are administered to distend the peritoneal cavity, distribution can be markedly improved. The importance of volume in determining the adequacy of distribution in the peritoneal cavity was initially demonstrated by Rosenshein in an animal model.[36] ^{99}Tc-labeled serum albumin was administered I.P. to monkeys in volumes equivalent to 0.2% (10 ml) or 5% (250 ml) of their body weight. Radioactivity was limited to only a portion of the peritoneal cavity with the small volume, and neither head-up or head-down tilting of the animal nor vigorous massaging of the abdomen improved the fluid distribution. When the larger volume was administered, uniformly good distribution of radioactivity throughout the cavity was observed, and head-down and head-up tilting produced a shift of the distribution.

Most patients who might be considered for I.P. chemotherapy will have had one or more surgical procedures before beginning this treatment approach. Adhesion formation commonly follows such surgery. In addition, certain abdominal tumors (particularly ovarian carcinomas) can elicit an intense fibrous reaction. The formation of fibrous bands in the abdominal cavity can significantly interfere with fluid and drug distribution.

The ability of large treatment volumes to overcome the problem of adhesions interfering with adequate drug distribution has been evaluated by 2 groups of investigators. At the NCI, 10 patients with advanced intra-abdominal malignancies had I.P. Hypaque instilled in large enough volume to distend the peritoneal cavity.[37] In 8 of these patients, distribution was complete and unimpaired when examined by computerized axial tomography (CT). The distribution of ^{99}Tc-sulfur colloid administered I.P. in 2 liters of normal saline to 10 patients with refractory ovarian carcinoma was examined at the University of California, San Diego (UCSD) Cancer Center.[38] In 7 of these patients, the radiolabeled material was found to be distributed in all 4 quadrants when scanned immediately after instillation. We have also noted that even when initial distribution of fluid is not complete, there can be a gradual appearance of contrast material in a larger portion of the peritoneal cavity over a period of several hours. In addition, several individuals scanned following an initial response to the I.P. treatment demonstrated improved fluid distribution, perhaps suggesting that some of the initial poor distribution was due to the presence of tumor rather than adhesions. Thus, available data suggest that during I.P. drug delivery, the distribution of chemotherapeutic agents is adequate in the majority of patients when large treatment volumes are administered. In addition, even in patients with limited distribution, there is often slow exchange of drug into other portions of the peritoneal cavity. One additional important advantage of using large volumes to deliver drugs into the peritoneal cavity would be the ability to avoid the development of extremely high concentration pockets of drug capable of producing serious toxicity.

Although modeling studies may suggest a pharmacokinetic advantage for exposure of the peritoneal cavity to a particular chemotherapeutic agent,[15,16] this does not necessarily mean that tumor present in the cavity will be exposed to the increased drug concentrations. Although the concentration of drug instilled into the peritoneal cavity clearly influences the amount of tumor exposure, a second extremely important factor is the dependence (or lack thereof) of the tumor on free surface diffusion for its nutrients. Thus, free-floating malignant cells or small tumor nodules in the peritoneal cavity are more influenced by the direct instillation of chemotherapeutic agents into the cavity than are large tumor masses.

In addition, tumor exposure is significantly influenced by the ability of the chemotherapeutic agent to penetrate into malignant tissue and cells. Unfortunately, the limited information available would suggest that tissue diffusibility and penetration of chemotherapeutic agents are poor.[39-41] Experimental evaluation of these important issues has been hampered by technical difficulties. The ability to measure ADR-specific intranuclear fluorescence has allowed an evaluation of drug levels in various body tissues of the mouse as well an estimate of tissue penetration of this agent.[42,43] At the NCI, investigators have monitored the penetration of ADR into the murine M5076 tumor model growing intraperitoneally.[44-46] As anticipated, ADR levels were higher in the heart, liver, and kidney following intravenous compared to I.P. therapy, but they were significantly higher in tumor following I.P. drug delivery. Faint ADR-specific fluorescence was seen in a patchy distribution throughout the tumor following I.V. drug administration and bright fluorescence was observed only in the outermost 4–6 cell layers of the tumor with I.P. drug delivery. However, despite what the fluorescence staining might have led one to predict regarding the efficacy of therapy via the 2 treatment routes in this animal model, 70% of mice receiving a single I.P. 10% lethal dose of ADR demonstrated long-term survival (>60 days) when innoculated with 10^6 tumor cells compared to no long-term survivors among mice treated I.V. with a comparable lethal dose of the drug.

It is important to consider factors that can potentially influence tissue or tumor drug penetration. These include plasma and intraperitoneal drug concentrations, intracellular/extracellular drug ratios, surface area available for diffusion, duration of cell surface exposure, diffusion coefficient for the administered drug, rate of cellular uptake, capillary flow, and drug half-life in extracellular fluid and in the tumor cell. Theoretical and experimental models have been developed to predict how these various factors might affect permeability.[27, 47-51] In addition to the issue of direct drug permeability into tumor tissue, the various mechanisms for removal (absorption into capillaries, lymphatics) and inactivation of drug (extracellularly and intracellularly) can significantly influence ultimate clinical activity.

The modeling studies have helped to answer one of the more perplexing questions concerning I.P. chemotherapy. Considering the known susceptibility of the G.I. mucosa to the effects of many chemotherapeutic agents, how is it possible to administer these drugs I.P. without the development of severe G.I. toxicity? As it turns out, while the crypt cells are only about 1 mm from the peritoneal surface, there is a rich capillary network between the mucosa and serosa. This network presumably acts like a sink, drawing off drug diffusing in from the peritoneal cavity and therefore protecting the sensitive mucosal cells. Importantly, it is equally possible that this mechanism of local capillary uptake will also serve to facilitate diffusion of drugs into tumor masses that are relatively less well perfused.

While one might infer from the previous discussion that *large* intra-abdominal tumor masses would be relatively unaffected by I.P. therapy, this may not necessarily be the case. Although it is highly unlikely that free surface diffusion will kill a large fraction of tumor when large masses are present, if drugs are used at near-maximal tolerated doses, then the combination of drug delivery by capillary flow (from absorbed drug) *and* free surface diffusion may still be *more effective* than I.V. treatment alone. It is also possible that repeated courses of therapy may result in sequential layers of tumor being destroyed.

A final important potential advantage of I.P. chemotherapy compared to I.V. chemotherapy with the same agent is the opportunity to use systemically administered neutralizing agents for the I.P. delivered drug. Whether the addition of a neutralizing agent will be advantageous or interfere with the cytotoxic properties of the chemotherapy will depend importantly on the pharmacokinetic and pharmacodynamic characteristics of the antagonist/agonist pair. Ideally, one would wish to work with an antagonist that could be completely excluded from the peritoneal cavity. Unfortunately, once the antagonist is injected I.V. it will begin to diffuse into the peritoneal cavity at a rate determined by local blood flow through the cavity as well as by diffusional characteristics and concentration of the drug.

Therefore, the noncompetitive versus concentration dependence of the agonist/antagonist interactions and the concentration dependence of the antagonism become extremely important. A competitive antagonist, particularly one whose effectiveness is rapidly lost as the concentration of the agonist is increased over a small concentration range, would be the optimal drug to use for this clinical purpose. In theory, such a drug combination would provide protection from toxicity in the systemic circulation (lower agonist concentration) and yet not neutralize the antineoplastic activity in the peritoneal cavity (higher agonist concentration). Conversely, one would *not* wish to select a noncompetitive antagonist that could potentially reverse the cytotoxicity of the agonist irrespective of the latter's higher concentration in the peritoneal cavity. Unfortunately, it is possible that even with the most favorable agonist/

antagonist pairs, sufficient neutralizing agent introduced into the systemic circulation to prevent marrow or other toxicities might compromise both the delivery of active drug to the tumor by capillary flow and by direct penetration of drug instilled into the peritoneal cavity. In addition, any neutralization of the chemotherapeutic agent in the plasma will result in increased dependence on free surface diffusion for the desired cytotoxic effect. The greater the concentration gradient that can be maintained between the peritoneal cavity and the plasma, the less likely that drug neutralization in the plasma or cavity will be a clinical problem.

A second goal in choosing a neutralizing agent would be to select one that acts specifically in the normal tissue exhibiting dose-limiting toxicity and one that does not interfere with the cytotoxic properties of the chemotherapeutic agent. Although it is unlikely that such a specific antagonist will be discovered for any chemotherapeutic agent, even the relative ineffectiveness of a neutralizing agent in interfering with the cytotoxicity in the systemic circulation while providing protection from dose-limiting systemic toxicity might improve the therapeutic index of the I.P. delivered agent.

To date, 2 agonist/antagonist pairs have been clinically evaluated. Both folinic acid[52,53] and sodium thiosulfate,[38,54] neutralizing agents for methotrexate (MTX) and cisplatin (DDP), respectively, appear to be antagonists that fulfill the criteria of steep concentration-dependent antagonism of their respective cytotoxic agents. In addition, sodium thiosulfate appears to act as a relatively specific neutralizing agent, protecting the patient from serious nephrotoxicity while allowing for increased concentrations of active DDP to be delivered both from free surface diffusion and capillary flow. Results of clinical trials employing MTX-folinic acid and DDP-thiosulfate agonist/antagonist pairs will be presented following a discussion of the potential toxicities of I.P. chemotherapy.

Acute and Chronic Toxicities of Intraperitoneal Chemotherapy

The potential toxicities of I.P. chemotherapy can be divided into 2 broad categories: those that would occur with systemic drug administration and those unique to the route of drug delivery. As mentioned in the previous section, these agents enter the systemic compartment and can cause the same side effects as when they are given I.V. For example, when DDP is instilled into the peritoneal cavity, a major toxicity of treatment is the development of significant emesis.[38] Similarly, with 5-FU, mucositis may develop.[55] In addition, it is possible that bone marrow depression may be the dose-limiting toxicity for certain combination regimens.

However, perhaps of more concern is the risk of development of local toxicity due to the route of drug administration. Drugs instilled into the peritoneal cavity can produce a chemical irritation that might be of benefit (if one wishes to produce sclerosis), a hindrance, or a major hazard. Such irritation can lead to pain, fever, adhesion formation, and bowel obstruction. In addition, the symptoms of chemical peritonitis can closely imitate an infectious event, which can make the differential diagnosis of certain clinical situations much more difficult. Adhesion formation can also interfere with the efficacy of therapy by inhibiting adequate drug distribution and can prevent the full use of semipermanent catheters placed to deliver therapy, remove ascites, and monitor peritoneal cavity cytologies. The development of tight, fibrous bands around peritoneal catheters leading to a "one-way valve effect" is a common problem during I.P. chemotherapy and will eventually affect 30–50% of surgically placed semipermanent delivery systems (unpublished data).

We have analyzed our extensive experience with I.P. chemotherapy to assess the seriousness of adhesion formation in the abdominal cavity following I.P. therapy. A group of 115 patients received a total of 435 courses of I.P. treatments on 1 (or 2) of several I.P. chemotherapy programs.[38,56-58] All patients received DDP, while 105 also received cytarabine, 31 ADR, and 19 BLM. The median number of courses/patient was 3 (range 1–18), with a median follow-up of 11 months (range 1–30+ months). The total length of follow-up was 1,103 patient-months. There were 7 episodes of partial small bowel obstruction in this patient population (6%), of which 2 appeared definitely related to extensive adhesion formation (no tumor found at surgery); the other 5 episodes were possibly or probably related to this complication. Although longer follow-up might reveal additional long-term complications of I.P. chemotherapy, all of the episodes of obstruction observed to date have developed within 6 months of completing therapy. To determine whether or not it will be possible to limit the amount of adhesion formation in patients receiving various I.P. chemotherapy regimens through the use of modulating agents that have shown some limited success in preventing postsurgical adhesions will require carefully designed and critically evaluated clinical trials.[59,60] Although we believe that our incidence of clinically relevant chronic complications associated with I.P. chemotherapy is acceptable if such therapy is eventually shown to be more efficacious than systemically administered drugs, it is unknown at present if patients treated via the I.P. route will experience greater difficulty with subsequent abdominal surgery (e.g., second-look laparotomy in ovarian carcinoma).

The potential seriousness of the acute toxicity of I.P. chemotherapy is best exemplified by the limited experience with 2 patients who received vinblastine (VLB) administered I.P. in a small volume during a phase 1 trial.[61] The drug was extremely toxic when delivered by this route, and both patients developed an adynamic ileus within 24 hours of drug instillation. In other situations in which it might be possible to deliver a limited amount of a certain drug via the I.P. route, dose-limiting toxicity could be local pain and chemical irritation rather than the development of systemic side effects. For example, when ADR is administered I.P. either experimentally or therapeutically to patients, dose-limiting toxicity is clearly the production of a chemical peritonitis.[56,62,63]

A second unique acute problem with I.P. chemotherapy is the risk of infectious peritonitis. There is currently greater experience with the management of similar problems in patients receiving peritoneal dialysis for chronic renal insufficiency, and several recent reports on this topic have discussed preventive measures, antibiotic therapy, indications for catheter removal, and the use of prophylactic antibiotics.[64-71] A recent review of our experience with I.P. chemotherapy demonstrates both the similarities and differences between patients receiving this method of treatment for their tumor and patients being treated for kidney failure with peritoneal dialysis.[72]

A total of 32 episodes of infection involving 40 bacterial isolates were observed in a group of 90 patients receiving I.P. chemotherapy as part of our experimental program. Multiple organisms were cultured in 2 episodes of infectious peritonitis in 2 patients treated by the percutaneous placement of a peritoneal dialysis catheter. In neither patient were significant quantities of fluid present when catheter placement was attempted, and it is the author's opinion that this experience demonstrates the extreme importance of establishing safe access to the peritoneal cavity prior to the initiation of treatment. Semipermanent catheters are now surgically placed in all patients receiving I.P. treatment at the UCSD Cancer Center if there are no medical contraindications to surgery. It should also be noted that it is unsafe to deliver a *second* course of I.P. treatment by blind percutaneous catheter placement to patients who initially have ascites and who respond to the first course of therapy with the disappearance of fluid.

In our series, the remaining episodes of peritonitis occurred in patients with semipermanent peritoneal catheters. Two general types of catheters were used: (1) standard peritoneal dialysis catheters (Tenckhoff type) and (2) Tenckhoff-type catheters with a subcutaneous portal delivery system (see figures 1 and 2).[73-76] *Staphlococcus epidermidis* was responsible for 66% of infections not due to bowel perforation, while in 17% of cases *S. aureus* was cultured. This experience is consistent with that reported for patients receiving peritoneal dialysis, where gram positive organisms are usually incriminated as the cause of infection. In addition, the hypothesis that infection develops during manipulation of the catheter is also supported by these clinical data. Although no direct comparison has been made between the 2-catheter delivery system in terms of the incidence of infection, it is our impression that the use of the completely subcutaneous portal system has reduced the incidence of infection. Such a system allows for less catheter manipulation compared to the external Tenckhoff catheter, where the daily instillation of heparin flush has been standard procedure

In our series, 75% of infectious episodes were successfully managed medically without the need for catheter removal. In 25% of episodes, because of persistent positive cultures, fevers, or recurrence of infection, catheter removal was necessary to cure the infection. It would be our recommendation to treat patients with documented I.P. bacterial infections with an I.V. administered antibiotic active against *S. epidermidis* (cephalosporin, vancomycin) for 7 days. If the cultures become negative and the patient remains afebrile, oral antibiotics can be substituted to complete a 14-day course. However, if fever persists, cultures remain positive, or if there is an obvious tunnel infection, catheter removal is required.

Unfortunately, whereas the development of fever, abdominal pain, or an elevated peritoneal cavity white blood cell count in the peritoneal dialysis patient has been demonstrated to be helpful in the differential diagnosis of infection, these findings in patients receiving I.P. chemotherapy may be sec-

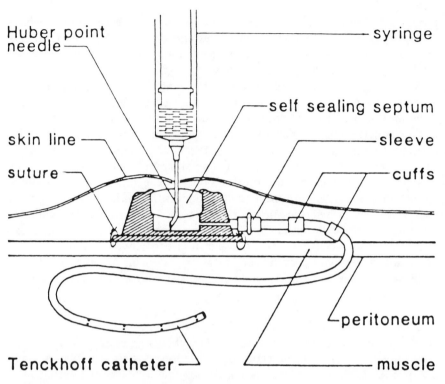

Figure 1.   Diagrammatic representation of subcutaneous portal system.

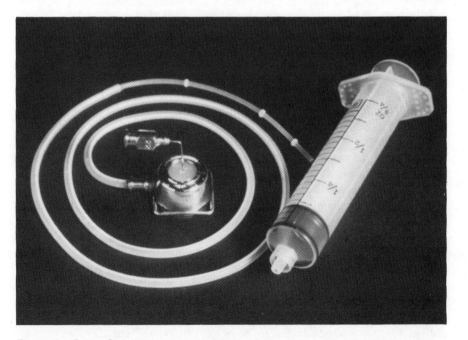

Figure 2.   Port-a-Cath subcutaneous delivery system with inserted Huber needle.

ondary to inflammation only (from drug irritation or lysis of adhesions) and do not necessarily imply the presence of infection. Thus, the documentation of infection with positive cultures becomes extremely important in this clinical setting. In this context it should be noted that in our experience, the initial gram stain on material removed from patients suspected of having bacterial peritonitis has been positive in approximately 40% of situations eventually proven to be infectious in origin. However, in the setting of suspected bacterial peritonitis, it would certainly be appropriate to begin antibiotics pending the results of culture.

Trials of Single-Agent Intraperitoneal Chemotherapy

Methotrexate

Methotrexate (MTX) is an interesting agent to investigate for I.P. chemotherapy, both because it is a cell cycle phase-specific drug whose activity might be significantly enhanced by prolonged exposure to slowly dividing tumor and because the agent has a known safe and effective antagonist. MTX has been evaluated for intracavitary administration at the NCI and the UCSD Cancer Center and has demonstrated a pharmacokinetic advantage when delivered by this route (see table).[52,53,77,78] In a study conducted at the NCI, patients were administered MTX (15–50 μM) via peritoneal dialysis, with the dialysis fluid being changed at 6-hour intervals.[53] Treatment was repeated weekly for 6 weeks. Treatment volume, while initially 2 L, was gradually increased to patient tolerance. Intravenous folinic acid rescue (3.5 mg/kg/hr) was administered as a continuous infusion 40–56 hours after initiation of the MTX instillation. MTX concentrations in the peritoneum were found to be 18–36 times higher than the corresponding values in the plasma. Unfortunately, no definite therapeutic benefit was observed. Toxicity, which was generally mild in this trial, included nausea and vomiting, diarrhea, transient liver function abnormalities, myelosuppression, and chemical and bacterial peritonitis.

The simultaneous intracavitary administration of MTX and I.V. infusion of leucovorin has been evaluated in a trial at the UCSD Cancer Center.[52] MTX was delivered at 30 mg/m^2/day as a constant infusion at 10 mg/hour to patients with ascites or pleural or pericardial effusions. Leucovorin (15 mg/m^2 every 4 hours) was simultaneously administered I.V. in an effort to neutralize the MTX entering the systemic circulation. A single treatment course was delivered to each patient. Treatment duration was successfully escalated from 6 to 120

Chemotherapeutic Agents Investigated for Intraperitoneal Drug Administration for which a Pharmacokinetic Advantage Has Been Demonstrated

Methotrexate	Doxorubicin	Mitomycin-C
5-fluorouracil	Cytarabine	Streptozotocin
Cisplatin	Melphalan	Etoposide

hours. Again, toxicity was mild except for significant thrombocytopenia with infusions lasting longer than 96 hours. In addition, all patients receiving the longest infusions (120 hours) developed laboratory evidence of a chemical serositis. A clinical response observed in all 8 evaluable patients included the disappearance of an effusion in a patient with bronchogenic carcinoma and the complete regression of ascites in a patient with refractory ovarian carcinoma. This latter response lasted 10 months. Of note, thymidylate synthetase activity was found to be inhibited 86% in malignant cells in effusions, whereas bone marrow cells had only a 46% inhibition. In addition, cytokinetic monitoring of marrow demonstrated no abnormalities. Patients receiving I.P., intrapleural, and intrapericardial therapy on this trial experienced a geometric mean steady-state effusion MTX concentration of 24.2 μM, 213 μM, and 434 μM, respectively. This translates into an average cavity-to-plasma ratio of 92, 157, and 470 for the peritoneal, pleural, and pericardial cavities, respectively. Importantly, this study confirmed the possibility of delivering significantly higher levers of MTX to tumors confined to third spaces and also demonstrated the ability to simultaneously administer a neutralizing agent to reduce systemic toxicity.

It should be noted that there is a major difference between the treatment approaches used by NCI and the UCSD investigators. The NCI study demonstrated the safety and pharmacological advantage of administering MTX by the intracavitary route. However, the total duration of exposure had to be limited to 48 hours because of the presence of toxic concentrations of the antineoplastic agent in the plasma. In this study, leucovorin was used in a *rescue* mode to rapidly terminate MTX-induced inhibition of DNA synthesis in the marrow and gut. However, as previously mentioned, MTX is a cell cycle phase-specific agent whose cytotoxicity is a function of both concentration and duration of exposure, and it is unlikely that during a period of 48 hours a larger fraction of cells in a slowly growing tumor will have passed through the sensitive S-phase of the cell cycle. In contrast to this study, in the UCSD trial leucovorin was used in a *neutralizing* mode aimed at extending the total duration of exposure for the body cavity. In this study, the feasibility of maintaining exposure for 5 days with acceptable toxicity was shown, but it remains to be proven that the added cytotoxicity predicted by this approach will make up for the expected antagonism of MTX delivered to the tumor by capillary flow because of the simultaneous I.V. delivery of leucovorin. Finally, as discussed previously, an unknown quantity of intracavitary MTX will also be inactivated by leucovorin entering the body cavity, possibly interfering with the efficacy of therapy.

5-fluorouracil

5-fluorouracil (5-FU) has a long history of I.P. drug delivery for the purpose of preventing the reaccumulation of ascites.[4,79] Studies performed in the 1960s demonstrated a major pharmacological advantage for the I.P. administration of this agent.[80] Pharmacokinetic studies of 5-FU administered I.P. in large volumes have been carried out at the NCI.[25,55,78] A total of 10 patients were treated with 1 of 2 treatment regimens: (1) 8 consecutive instillations of 2 L of drug for

4 hours each (36 hours per course), or (2) once a day instillation of 2 L of fluid for 3–5 days. Treatment was repeated every 2 weeks. 5-FU was administered at concentrations of 5 μM to 8 mM (1.3 to 2,080 mg/^{2} L). Pancytopenia and mucositis were dose-limiting toxicities at 5-FU concentrations of 4.5–5 mM. In addition, bacterial and chemical peritonitis were also observed. Whereas 6 patients demonstrated no response to therapy, 2 (both with ovarian carcinoma) experienced objective evidence of an antineoplastic response, including a surgically defined complete remission (CR) and a partial response (PR) of bulky intra-abdominal disease.

The average 4-hour peritoneal fluid concentration of 5-FU was 298 times the simultaneously measured plasma level. A mean of 82% of the delivered drug was absorbed in 4 hours. The NCI investigators concluded that with I.P. administration of 5-FU, the peritoneal cavity could be exposed to concentrations of this agent 10 times higher (for some finite period of time) than could safely be achieved by the I.V. delivery of the drug.[55]

This same group of investigators have also demonstrated that the total delivery of 5-FU to the liver via the portal circulation during I.P. drug delivery is comparable to that reported following direct intra-arterial (I.A.) administration of this agent.[25] However, it is not possible to draw any conclusions concerning the relative efficacy of this route of drug administration for liver metastasis until a direct comparison with I.A. therapy has been made. This is particularly relevant in view of the fact that it has been shown experimentally that established metastatic liver tumors receive only 5% of their blood supply from the portal circulation, with the remaining 95% coming from the hepatic artery.[81]

An Italian study has confirmed the pharmacokinetic observations made at the NCI.[82] Six patients received a total of 18 courses of I.P. therapy with 5-FU (4–8 mM) in a 2 L treatment volume. Four courses were associated with pain, but narcotic analgesia was not required by any patients. Systemic toxicity was mild. AUC ratios for the peritoneal cavity to plasma ranged from 120 to 1,350. The median absorption of 5-FU from the peritoneal cavity was 83%.

5-FU also has been administered I.P. as a 5-day continuous infusion in a trial at the University of Michigan Medical Center.[83] A total of 20 courses of therapy were delivered to 5 patients. One gram of 5-FU was infused each day at a rate of 42 ml/hour for 5 days. A 2- 3-log difference in steady-state concentrations was observed between the peritoneal cavity and plasma. A single patient who received both an I.P. infusion and bolus of 5-FU demonstrated a doubling of total body clearance with the infusion. This finding would suggest that continuous infusion of 5-FU allows for greater cavity exposure with less systemic toxicity as compared to the bolus technique. Dose-limiting toxicity in this trial was the induction of chemical peritonitis. Systemic toxicity was mild. The single patient with evaluable disease (gastric carcinoma) experienced a PR of metastasis in the liver and conversion of positive peritoneal cytologies to negative.

Finally, a recently completed phase 2 trial of I.P. 5-FU in patients with refractory ovarian carcinoma has demonstrated a response rate of only 7% in a group of heavily pretreated patients.[84]

Doxorubicin

Several groups have examined the I.P. administration of doxorubicin (ADR) both experimentally and clinically.[44–46,62,63,85] There is particular interest in this agent because of its demonstrated activity in ovarian carcinoma, a tumor that remains confined to the peritoneal cavity for most of its natural history.[86] At the Mount Sinai School of Medicine, 2 patients with tumors localized to the abdominal cavity were treated with the I.P. instillation of ADR (20–50 mg in 3 L.).[85] Both patients demonstrated evidence of a clinical response, although they developed complications secondary to the subcutaneous infiltration of the agent.

At the NCI, investigators have treated 10 patients with refractory ovarian carcinoma with 9–54 μM ADR (10–50 in 2 L) delivered via the I.P. route as a single 4-hour dwell every 2 weeks.[63] All patients had failed previous chemotherapy, but had not received I.V. ADR. Two patients experienced significant decreases in ascites, and 3 additional patients demonstrated objective evidence of tumor regression. Unfortunately, as previously mentioned, abdominal pain was the dose-limiting toxicity, occurring along with ascites and adhesion formation at ADR concentrations of greater than 36 μM (40 mg in 2 L). Bone marrow depression was mild at the doses administered.

A significant pharmacokinetic advantage for the peritoneal cavity was shown during this trial. The mean peritoneal cavity level of ADR during the 4-hour dwell was 166 times higher than the corresponding plasma level, with a peak peritoneal concentration to plasma concentration ratio of 474. Finally, it was demonstrated that the peak plasma level following the maximally administered I.P. dose of ADR (54 μM) was only 1/10 that achieved following a 60 mg I.V. dose of the agent. This finding is important in terms of the potential cardiac toxicity of doxorubicin.

Cisplatin

The efficacy and safety of intraperitoneally administered cisplatin (DDP) has been examined by several investigators.[38,87,88] At the UCSD Cancer Center, DDP has been delivered I.P. along with I.V.-administered sodium thiosulfate used as a neutralizing agent for the DDP entering the plasma. Thiosulfate, an agent used clinically for many years for cyanide poisoning, has been shown experimentally to protect against DDP-induced nephrotoxicity and to allow for increased exposure of the peritoneal cavity to active drug with increased efficacy and decreased toxicity.[89,90] Although it was known that there would be loss of activity of the DDP administered directly into the peritoneal cavity from the simultaneous I.V. administration of sodium thiosulfate, this negative factor was predicted to be outweighed by the opportunity to deliver extremely high doses of DDP into the cavity. Doses of DDP up to 270 mg/m^2 could be delivered in a 2 L treatment volume as a 4-hour dwell (with simultaneous I.V. thiosulfate) without evidence of clinical nephrotoxicity in a phase 1 study conducted at the UCSD Cancer Center.[38] Toxicity, except for DDP-induced emesis, was mild during the trial. Importantly, there was no evidence of significant local toxicity due to I.P. DDP administration.

On completion of the 4-dwell, only 7% of the administered DDP could be recovered from the fluid remaining in the peritoneal cavity. The peak peritoneal cavity concentration of free reactive DDP averaged 21-fold higher than peak plasma levels, and the AUC for the peritoneal cavity averaged 12-fold more than the AUC for the plasma. Somewhat surprisingly, despite the presence of thiosulfate, the AUC for the plasma (at a DDP dose of 270 mg/m^2) *increased* 2-fold compared to that reported for native DDP after an I.V. dose of 100 mg/m^2.[91,92] In an effort to explain this unexpected finding, it can be hypothesized that whereas thiosulfate neutralizes DDP, the reaction is slow at the levels of thiosulfate circulating in the plasma but proceeds rapidly in the kidney, where the thiosulfate is concentrated.[93] Regardless of the mechanism of action, thiosulfate, at least clinically, appears to act as a quasi-organ-specific neutralizing agent.

Thirteen patients were evaluable for response to treatment in this phase 1 clinical trial.[38] Of the 7 heavily pretreated patients with ovarian carcinoma entered onto this study, 1 experienced a near CR of extensive nodular disease, which was documented at laparoscopy. A patient with peritoneal mesothelioma demonstrated a significant decrease in ascites and a reduction in the size of an abdominal wall mass. Finally, a patient with a malignant carcinoid tumor had a greater than 50% decrease in ascites and normalization of an elevated 5-hydroxyindoleacetic acid lasting 5 months.

The I.P. administration of DDP (60 mg/m^2) also has been examined in a group of 9 patients with advanced intra-abdominal malignancies and ascites at the Memorial-Sloan Kettering Cancer Center.[87] A systemically delivered neutralizing agent was not employed in this trial. One patient with refractory ovarian carcinoma experienced complete resolution of ascites; a significant pharmacokinetic advantage for the peritoneal cavity also was demonstrated in this trial.

Finally, investigators at the University of California (Los Angeles) Medical Center administered 120–270 mg of DDP to 4 patients with minimal residual ovarian carcinoma following combination I.V. chemotherapy that included DDP.[88] The fluid was left in the peritoneal cavity for 15–20 min. following rapid instillation (10–12 min.) of a 2 L treatment volume and was then removed. Using this technique, 75% of the instilled drug was recoverable, and the peritoneal cavity concentration of DDP was 42–72 times higher than the plasma concentration. Three of the 4 patients responded to this treatment program (1 CR and 2 PR). One patient experienced a significant decrease in creatinine clearance.

At the UCSD Cancer Center, a phase 2 trial of intracavitary DDP has been conducted in malignant mesothelioma, a tumor that remains clinically localized to the peritoneal or pleural cavity for most of its natural history.[58,94] Sixteen previously treated or untreated patients have demonstrated an objective response rate of approximately 50% when treated either intrapleurally or I.P. However, responses generally have been more often observed with tumor confined to the peritoneal cavity. These early results approximate those reported when I.V. ADR, the single most active agent in malignant mesothelioma, is employed.[95] Also, the results in this uncontrolled trial exceed the 10% response rate reported for DDP administered I.V. in this disease.[95]

Cytarabine

Cytarabine (cytosine arabinoside, ara-C) is perhaps the ideal drug to examine for I.P. drug delivery.[15] The agent has an extremely short half-life in the plasma (10–15 min.) because of rapid deamination in the liver, and a significant pharmacokinetic advantage following I.P. drug administration would therefore be predicted.[96,97] Unfortunately, while ara-C is one of the most active agents in acute nonlymphocytic leukemia, it has demonstrated limited activity against solid tumors.[98] It is likely, however, that I.V. administration of ara-C as a bolus or short infusion is not the most rational way to use this cell cycle phase-specific against solid tumors with long doubling times. Although prolonged tumor exposure to ara-C might improve efficacy, such a treatment program would likely result in severe bone marrow toxicity.[99,100]

In order to determine if the theoretical advantage of the I.P. delivery of ara-C could be experimentally confirmed in man, a phase 1 trial of the I.P. administration of this agent was conducted at the UCSD Cancer Center.[101] Three patients were given escalating doses of ara-C during 3 consecutive 5-hour I.P. drug instillations. Peritoneal ara-C levels demonstrated first-order kinetics with half-lives of 70–210 minutes. A 2- 3-log difference between peritoneal cavity and plasma concentrations was demonstrated, and the total peritoneal cavity drug exposure was shown to be 300–1,000 times greater than that of the plasma.

In a phase 2 trial of I.P. ara-C in patients with refractory ovarian carcinoma, 10 patients were treated with 20 consecutive dialysate exchanges (5-hour dwell, 1-hour drainage per exchange) over 5 days with ara-C (30 mg, 60 μM) in each 2 L exchange.[101] In patients not demonstrating evidence of disease progression, treatment was repeated at monthly intervals. WBC nadir counts of $<2,000/mm^3$ developed during only 2 of 25 treatment cycles, whereas thrombocytopenia (platelets $<75,000/mm^3$) occurred following only a single course. A total of 9 episodes of bacterial peritonitis developed in 5 patients participating in this trial. There was no evidence of chemical peritonitis. Objective responses were observed in 2 patients with positive peritoneal cavity cytologies that became negative. Both patients have remained clinically disease-free for $19+$ and $26+$ months.

In view of the major pharmacokinetic advantage demonstrated for the I.P. delivery of ara-C, it is possible that the continuous long-term exposure of tumor in the peritoneal cavity to this agent might be accomplished with minimal systemic drug exposure. As a result of such an approach, it might be possible to continuously expose slowly dividing solid tumor cells to this cell cycle phase-specific agent and allow them to come in contact with the drug when they enter into cycle and are vulnerable to the cytotoxic properties of ara-C. Such a treatment strategy would necessitate the development of a delivery system to administer large treatment volumes (to assure adequate drug distribution), but would also avoid the problem of infection.

Melphalan

Melphalan (MEL), an active agent against ovarian carcinoma, has been investigated by 2 groups for I.P. drug administration.[102,103] Investigators at the Medical College of Wisconsin attempted to increase the activity of this agent by delivering *Acinetobacter* glutaminase-asparaginase (AGA) I.P. shortly before MEL instillation.[102] This trial was based on experimental work demonstrating glutamine to be an active inhibitor of MEL uptake by human ovarian carcinoma cells.[104] A total of 3 patients with ovarian carcinoma were treated with 1–4 courses of MEL plus AGA. In this trial, the dose of MEL ranged from 9 to 40 mg/m^2 in a 2 L treatment volume. The abdomen was drained 24 hours following AGA administration. Plasma MEL was less than 6% of the peritoneal cavity value. Toxicity included nausea and vomiting, fever, abdominal pain, and a single case of ileus. Notably, there was no significant renal or hepatic dysfunction or myelosuppression. One patient experienced disappearance of ascites following 2 courses of therapy.

At the UCSD Cancer Center, 13 patients were administered I.P. MEL in a phase 1 trial.[103] Doses ranged from 30 to 90 mg/m^2 in 2 L of normal saline delivered as a single 4-hour dwell. A major pharmacokinetic advantage for this route of drug delivery was demonstrated. At an I.P. MEL dose of 60 mg/m^2, the mean peritoneal cavity and plasma AUCs were 52.1 and 1.42 µg hr/ml, respectively; the geometric mean ratio of AUCs for the peritoneal cavity to plasma for all courses was 65. Dose-limiting toxicity was myelosuppression, which developed at 70 mg/m^2. Two limited clinical responses were observed.

Mitomycin-C

Two groups have investigated the intraperitoneal delivery of mitomycin-C (MIT).[105,106] In 1 study, 5–30 mg of MIT was administered to 5 patients with advanced intra-abdominal malignancies in a 1.5 L treatment volume, and a 200-fold pharmacokinetic advantage for peritoneal cavity drug exposure was demonstrated.[105] Only at the highest dose level was MIT detected in the plasma. Chemical peritonitis was observed at the 30 mg dose level, but myelosuppression was mild during this trial.

In a second study, MIT was administered I.P. along with floxuridine (FUDR) to 3 patients with colon cancer and to a single patient with gastric cancer.[106] The dose of MIT was 7 mg/m^2 delivered in a 1 L treatment volume, with the drug being left in the peritoneal cavity 24 hours before being drained. The average peritoneal cavity to plasma drug concentration ratio in this study was 71.

Etoposide

Etoposide (VP-16) has undergone limited evaluation for I.P. drug delivery.[107] Investigators administered VP-16 (100 mg/m^2) I.P. along with teniposide (VM-26) to a group of patients with ovarian carcinoma. There was the suggestion of a pharmacokinetic advantage for peritoneal cavity exposure to VP-16 in this trial, with no local toxicity. The question of local toxicity is a particularly relevant issue in terms of the I.P. administration VP-16 because animal data suggest delayed lethal toxicity following its I.P. delivery.[108] The cause of death appeared to be the induction of severe chronic peritonitis.

Streptozotocin

Streptozotocin has been evaluated for I.P. drug administration in a single patient with refractory ovarian carcinoma.[109] While the patient did not demonstrate a clinical response, there was no local or significant systemic toxicity with the dose delivered (1 g, 6 times over a 3-week period), and a major pharmacokinetic advantage for peritoneal cavity exposure to this agent was shown.

Additional Experimental Intraperitoneal Trials

The I.P. administration of chemotherapy in heated dialysis fluid has undergone experimental and preliminary clinical evaluation.[110,111] A patient with pseudomyxoma peritonei was given thio-tepa and MTX I.P. in a hyperthermic perfusion system that heated the peritoneal cavity to 42°C.[111] The treatment program did not appear to result in significant toxicity.

The intraperitoneal use of hypoxic radiosensitizers has been evaluated in a phase 1 trial in an effort to improve the efficacy of abdominal cavity radiotherapy.[112] Six patients with advanced ovarian cancer received misonidazole or demethylmisonidazole in a 2 L treatment volume. Three hours later, any remaining fluid was drained. Concomitant whole abdominal radiation was delivered as part of this treatment program. The concentration of radiosensitizer in the peritoneal fluid was more than 8 times that of the plasma concentration 3 hours after drug administration. The AUC for the peritoneal cavity was 7.6 times greater than the plasma AUC for demethylmisonidazole and 3.2 times greater for misonidazole. Toxicity on this trial included emesis, diarrhea, abdominal pain, and mild paresthesias. The I.P. administration of radiosensitizers has the potential of increasing the efficacy of abdominal radiotherapy while decreasing the systemic toxicity of these neurotoxic agents. In addition, radiosensitizers have also been demonstrated experimentally to be synergistic with several chemotherapeutic agents, including DDP, and it might be interesting to investigate the use of these agents as part of a combination I.P. chemotherapy program.[113]

Combination Intraperitoneal Chemotherapy

Combination I.P. chemotherapy has a sound theoretical basis.[114,115] The I.P. delivery of a combination of drugs potentially allows for the delivery of multiple agents that are active against a particular tumor type and that perhaps will demonstrate nonoverlapping toxicities. As proposed in mathematical model by Goldie and Coldman, the optimal method for reducing the risk of developing tumor resistance (from mutational events) would be the administration of multiple noncross-resistant drug combinations early in the treatment program.[115] These theoretical arguments have been supported in several malignancies in which single-agent therapy has produced lower response rates and shorter survival than combination regimens. A second theoretical advantage for combination chemotherapy is the potential for producing synergy between the administered drugs. If it could be demonstrated that such drug interactions were concentration-dependent, then the I.P. delivery of these agents might be the optimal means for demonstrating clinical synergy because of the significantly higher drug levels that can be achieved and maintained by this treatment technique.

A potentially important experimental observation of drug synergy relevant to I.P. chemotherapy is that demonstrated between DDP and ara-C in the LoVo system.[116-118] In culture with LoVo cells (a human colon carcinoma cell line), DDP alone demonstrates marginal cytotoxicity, while ara-C is totally inactive. However, this drug combination markedly enhances the cell kill produced by DDP in a concentration-dependent manner. At the highest concentration of ara-C tested (4×10^{-2}M), which by itself was nontoxic, the cytotoxicity produced by the 2-drug combination was increased 1,600-fold compared to that produced by DDP alone.[118] It would not be possible to safely achieve in vivo the concentrations tested in vitro with I.V. ara-C. However, the I.P. administration of ara-C will permit these concentrations at least to be approached.

A second interesting drug combination to explore for I.P. therapy is DDP-BLM. In testicular carcinoma, "clinical synergy" has been suggested between these 2 agents because the use of a combination including DDP and BLM has resulted in an extremely high cure rate in advanced disease.[119,120] In addition, both drugs are relatively nonmyelosuppressive, demonstrate non-overlapping toxicities, and can be delivered with more myelosuppresive agents. A theoretically important interaction between DDP and BLM has been shown at the level of DNA-drug binding.[121] Bleomycin has also demonstrated a significant pharmacokinetic advantage for peritoneal cavity exposure when delivered in a 2 L treatment volume (unpublished data), while the systemic absorption of the drug is only 45% of the instilled dose.[122] Finally, the use of BLM in ovarian carcinoma is of particular interest because it has been shown to have definite activity in refractory disease both experimentally and clinically.[123,124]

A third combination containing DDP that has potential utility for I.P. drug delivery includes VP-16. Again, results of experimental and clinical trials suggest possible clinically relevant synergy between these 2 agents.[125-128] In addition, limited clinical experience would suggest that VP-16 can be delivered I.P. with a significant pharmacokinetic advantage for the peritoneal cavity.[107] Clinical trials of DDP and VP-16 administered via the I.P. route will be of major interest.

Clinical Trials of Combination Intraperitoneal Chemotherapy

As previously discussed, investigators at the M. D. Anderson Hospital have reported on a combination I.P. chemotherapy program using MIT and FUDR.[106] Three patients with colon cancer and 1 patient with gastric carcinoma were treated on this trial. MIT (7 mg/m^2) was delivered in a 1 L treatment volume and remained in the abdominal cavity 24 hours. Following drainage, FUDR

(100 mg/m²) was instilled in 1 L and removed 4 hours later. Toxicity of this program included mild peritonitis and limited myelosuppression. A response to treatment was observed in all patients, with decreases in the rate of ascitic fluid accumulation and in CEA levels measured in the peritoneal fluid.

Several combination I.P. chemotherapy regimens have been evaluated at the UCSD Cancer Center. The initial combination program examined the safety and efficacy of DDP, ara-C, and ADR.[56] Because a major focus of our program is on the development of an effective I.P. regimen for ovarian carcinoma, we chose to administer DDP and ADR, 2 drugs demonstrated to possess major activity in this disease.[129-131] In addition, both had been shown to be safe and effective, with a major pharmacokinetic advantage for the abdominal cavity when administered as single agents by the I.P. route.[38,63] Ara-C was selected because of its theorized synergy with DDP and its demonstrated activity in refractory ovarian carcinoma when administered by 5-day dialysis exchange.[101,116-118]

A phase 1 trial of escalating dosages of this treatment combination in patients with refractory ovarian carcinoma or in individuals with other malignancies principally confined to the peritoneal cavity was conducted.[56] The drugs were mixed together in a 2 L treatment volume and infused I.P. with a 4-hour dwell time (see figure 3). Sodium thiosulfate was simultaneously infused, beginning at the time of I.P. drug instillation. It was demonstrated that DDP could be safely escalated from a dose of 100 mg/m² to 200 mg/m² while the concentration of ara-C was increased from 10^{-4}M (50 mg/2 L) to 10^{-3}M (500 mg/2 L). The initial dose of ADR (20 mg/2 L) proved to cause excessive local abdominal discomfort, with 60% of courses being associated with pain lasting longer than 72 hours or requiring narcotic analgesia. The dose of this

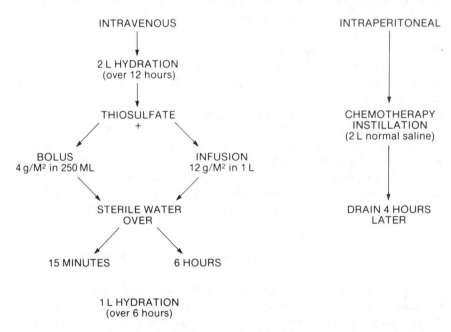

Figure 3.   Treatment plan for patients receiving high-dose intraperitoneal cisplatin with intravenous sodium thiosulfate at the UCSD Cancer Center.

agent was subsequently decreased to 2 mg/2 L, with a marked decrease in the amount of abdominal pain. However, 20% of courses were still associated with significant local discomfort at this lower ADR dose level. Systemic toxicity, with the exception of significant DDP-induced emesis, was not excessive. Eight percent of courses (4/48) administered at 200 mg/m² dose level of DDP were associated with serum creatinine increases to ≥2.0 mg% (normal ≤1.5 mg%). In 37 courses administered at the 100 mg/m² dose level of DDP, there were no creatinine increases to ≥2.0 mg%. In all cases, the serum creatinine returned to baseline within 4 weeks following treatment. Only 4/101 courses were complicated by WBC depressions to <2,000/mm³, with thrombocytopenia (platelet count nadir <75,000/mm³) occurring after only 3 courses. No major neurotoxicity or ototoxicity was observed during this trial.

Eight of 26 evaluable patients demonstrated objective evidence of tumor response, including 7/17 patients with refractory ovarian carcinoma. Several showed significant decreases in ascites lasting 3–7 months. One patient with a vaginal wall mass experienced a PR. Three patients (2 with ovarian carcinoma) had conversions of positive peritoneal cavity cytologies to negative. The responses in these patients lasted 3–6 months following therapy. A single patient with refractory ovarian carcinoma achieved a surgically defined remission lasting 9 months. Finally, a patient with adenocarcinoma of unknown primary site experienced a decrease in ascites, weight gain, and disappearance of signs of partial small bowel obstruction that persisted for 7 months.

In our second I.P. trial, we attempted to reduce local toxicity and take further advantage of the remarkable in vitro synergy demonstrated between DDP and ara-C.[57] ADR was eliminated from the treatment program and the dose of ara-C was significantly escalated. Sixty-two patients (49 with refractory ovarian carcinoma) received a total of 180 courses of DDP administered at 100 mg/m² or 200 mg/m² and ara-C at 4 × 10⁻³M (2000 mg/2 L). In this trial, 4% of courses were associated with a platelet count drop to less than 75,000/mm³, but no patient required platelet transfusions. Following 2 courses, the WBC dropped to <2000/mm³. Four percent of courses were associated with a serum creatinine rise to >1.5 mg%. All patients demonstrating nephrotoxicity had been previously heavily pretreated with DDP. A single patient developed serious nephrotoxicity (serum creatinine 8.0), but dialysis fortunately was not required. There were 3 episodes of bacterial peritonitis, and approximately 20% of courses were associated with fever without evidence of infection. Significant local pain, defined as that lasting longer than 72 hours or requiring narcotic analgesia, occurred in fewer than 10% of courses.

Of the 49 patients with refractory ovarian carcinoma (of whom 47 had previously been treated with DDP), 10 are currently not evaluable for response to therapy. Of the 39 evaluable patients, 14 (36%) demonstrated evidence of a clinical response, including 11/35 patients with bulky intra-abdominal disease and 3/4 patients with minimal or microscopic residual disease. Response in patients with bulky disease included disappearance of ascites, conversion of cytology from positive to negative, and decreases in mass lesions on CT scans. All 3 responses (2 CR, 1 PR) in patients with minimal or microscopic residual disease were defined at laparotomy. Two of 13 patients (15%) with nonovarian malignancies treated on this trial experienced subjective and objective responses that were not surgically defined. The median duration of response on this trial was 5 months (range 2–14+ months).

The current UCSD Cancer Center I.P. trial builds on our experience with the combination of DDP and ara-C and adds BLM to the regimen. The rationale for adding BLM has already been discussed. While this study remains in progress, to date 3/9 evaluable patients have demonstrated an objective response to treatment. Unfortunately, the initial dose of BLM (15 u/m^2) appeared to cause an excessive degree of abdominal pain. With reduction in the dose of this agent to 2 u/m^2, the severity of the local toxicity has decreased. It remains to be determined, however, if the addition of BLM to this treatment program will increase the efficacy of therapy without increasing the incidence of serious chronic complications (secondary to adhesion formation).

Conclusion

In this chapter, the principles, problems, and potential promise of I.P. ("belly bath") chemotherapy have been discussed. As outlined by Myers and Collins, there are several potential applications for I.P. chemotherapy in the treatment of ovarian carcinoma.[132] First, drugs can be administered I.P. in the early stages of this disease as an alternative to radioisotopes or abdominal radiotherapy. Second, the I.P. delivery of chemotherapeutic agents could become part of a frontline approach to the treatment of advanced disease following debulking surgery. Finally, this technique can be applied in patients who have minimal residual or no residual disease (determined at second-look laparotomy) following systemic therapy. For completeness, it should also be mentioned that intrapleural and even intrapericardial administration of chemotherapeutic agents for their cytotoxic properties has been examined, with preliminary results suggesting possible efficacy.[133,134]

However, several important issues remain to be resolved before this treatment approach can become the standard therapy for any tumor type localized to the peritoneal or other body cavities. These include the question of optimal drug combinations and dosages, the adequacy of drug distribution and penetration, and the risks associated with infectious and chemical peritonitis, as well as the appropriate measures to be taken to prevent and treat these potential complications. Finally, carefully designed controlled clinical trials will eventually need to be conducted to define the role of this treatment technique in the therapy of tumors confined to body cavities.

39

INTRAVENTRICULAR CHEMOTHERAPY FOR LEPTOMENINGEAL CARCINOMA

Deborah O. Heros, M.D., and Fred H. Hochberg, M.D.

MENINGEAL CARCINOMATOSIS, OR CARCINOMATOUS meningitis, is the result of diffuse seeding of the subarachnoid space by systemic cancer. The circulation of cerebrospinal fluid (CSF) within the subarachnoid space allows for an excellent application of the concept of regional infusion chemotherapy. An understanding of the clinical presentation, pathophysiology, and historical background of the therapeutic approaches and the associated morbidity of carcinomatous meningitis will help the clinician caring for cancer patients appreciate the necessity of applying innovative techniques in the treatment of this syndrome.

Carcinomatous meningitis may be associated with concomitant intraparenchymal, subdural, or extradural metastasis, or may be the sole site of involvement of the CNS. This disease was once thought to be an uncommon complication of systemic malignancy, but recent reviews suggest an increasing incidence, probably a result of the widespread application of adjuvant chemotherapy (the subarachnoid space acts as a sanctuary site from systemic chemotherapy). In addition, improved methods of detecting malignant cells in the CSF and an increase in clinical awareness of this syndrome may account for some of the apparent increase in incidence. Most patients develop carcinomatous meningitis in the setting of known metastatic cancer. However, 6% of patients may present with the disease without a previously diagnosed underlying malignancy.[4] Several of these patients have no clinical evidence of other organ involvement at the time they present with carcinomatous meningitis. Therefore, the clinician must suspect the diagnosis of the disease when a patient develops the appropriate signs and symptoms, even in the absence of systemic cancer.

Clinical Presentation of Carcinomatous Meningitis

Cancer patients with specific types of systemic cancer may be at particularly high risk for developing carcinomatous meningitis. Five percent of breast cancer patients undergoing therapy have been found to develop the disease. The incidence may be even higher among breast cancer patients receiving adjuvant chemotherapy because the CNS frequently becomes the first site of involvement in these patients.[40,48,49] Development of carcinomatous meningitis in small-cell carcinoma of the lung has been reported in 10% of patients.[3,35] Attempts to prevent CNS relapse by prophylactic craniospinal irradiation did not improve survival, but did decrease the development of metastatic involvement to the CNS.[24] Malignant melanoma, which has a high propensity for metastatic spread to the CNS, results in clinically evident carcinomatous meningitis in 10.6% of patients and may be found postmortem in an additional 41%.[6]

Early reviews demonstrated a male predominance as a result of the previously high incidence of gastric carcinoma. In a more recent review from our institution of 55 patients diagnosed over a 10-year period by CSF cytology or at postmortem examination, breast cancer accounted for greater than 40% of cases, and melanoma and carcinoma of the lung were responsible for the majority of the others. Other less common primary sites causing carcinomatous meningitis include prostate, pancreas, uterus, bladder, ovary, and adrenal glands. In 14.5% of the cases, the primary site was unknown (personal data).

Symptoms and signs of carcinomatous meningitis are the result of involvement at 3 levels of the neuraxis: (1) cortical involvement, resulting in headache, altered level of consciousness, lethargy, and nausea; (2) cranial nerve involvement, most commonly causing diplopia or visual loss and less commonly, facial weakness, facial numbness, deafness, and tongue atrophy;[4,5,25,37,43] and (3) spinal involvement, the most common source of symptoms, accounting for low back pain that frequently radiates into either leg in a radicular pattern, leg weakness, sensory changes, and sphincter dysfunction. Hydrocephalus occurs in 15–25% of patients, and seizures are seen in approximately 15%.[47]

In a patient presenting with neurologic symptoms and signs at various levels of the neuraxis with or without fever, carcinomatous meningitis must be suspected, and the CSF must be studied for malignant cells as well as for evidence of infection.

The diagnosis of carcinomatous meningitis is established by examination of the CSF. Rarely is the CSF normal; however, the literature has stressed the importance of repeated examinations to obtain abnormal cytology. Malignant cells are found in 19–100% of patients.[47] Additional abnormalities may include a lymphocytic pleocytosis, decreased glucose level, elevation of protein, or elevation of pressure. These findings can, of course, also be seen with fungal meningitis; therefore, careful cultures, cryptococcal antigen, and appropriate stains must be done. CSF biochemical markers including carcinoembryonic antigen (CEA), lactic dehydrogenase (LDH) isoenzymes, and beta glucuronidase may indicate early leptomeningeal disease and aid in monitoring the effectiveness of therapy.[38,47] Computerized tomography (CT) may demonstrate parenchymal involvement or communicating hydrocephalus. Administration of contrast frequently demonstrates periventricular or cortical enhancement.[18] Myelography may show thickened spinal roots, nodular deposits near the cauda equina, and irregular filling defects with variable degrees of blocks similar to the findings of arachnoiditis.[26] Studies of CSF flow dynamics by [111]indium-DPTA ventriculography demonstrate abnormalities in 70% of patients with carcinomatous meningitis as a result of tumor or adhesions. These abnormalities include ventricular outflow obstruction and alteration of flow in the spinal canal and over the convexities of the cortex. These findings may provide insight into treatment failure and drug-induced neurotoxicity.[21]

The natural history of carcinomatous meningitis is one of rapid progression to death within weeks or, rarely, months. Untreated, the median life survival is 6 weeks.[27,32,46] The mainstay of therapy has included irradiation of the craniospinal axis and intrathecal chemotherapy. By using these modalities in various combinations, the median survival has been improved to 4–6 months with 10–15% of patients surviving 1 year after diagnosis.[47] Systemic chemotherapy has been ineffective in preventing the development of carcinomatous meningitis or in controlling the disease. Intrathecal chemotherapy is administered by lumbar puncture or through an Ommaya reservoir into the lateral ventricle. Methotrexate (MTX) and, less commonly, cytosine arabinoside (ara-C), thio-tepa, or bleomycin (BLM) have been used in the treatment of carcinomatous meningitis.[9,10,22,50] Administration by lumbar puncture produces variable concentrations of chemotherapy within the subarachnoid space, with epidural and subdural leakage in 10% of patients as shown by radionuclide tracer studies. The preferred method of administration is by an Ommaya reservoir connected to a ventricular catheter. This method produces reliable distribution of the chemotherapy and is better tolerated by the patient.[41] Localized irradiation may be used in combination with chemotherapy for treatment of symptomatic involvement of the spinal cord, spinal roots, cranial nerves, or cerebral cortex.

In spite of intrathecal chemotherapy and craniospinal irradiation, treatment of carcinomatous meningitis remains disappointing, with a median survival of 4–6 months. Some patients die from progression of the systemic cancer despite an apparent response within the CNS. Two factors have been proposed to explain the limitations of present therapy. Abnormalities of CSF flow may result in inadequate distribution of the chemotherapy, allowing for tumor proliferation. In addition, sequestration of chemotherapy, also a result of CSF flow abnormalities, may be related to the development of drug-induced neurotoxicity. The neurotoxicity associated with the treatment of carcinomatous meningitis is usually seen in patients who have received a combination of craniospinal irradiation followed by intrathecal MTX. This results in a leukoencephalopathy that develops acutely or insidiously, manifesting itself clinically as seizures, dementia, and stupor, and that may eventually result in death.[13,21]

The pathologic changes of leukoencephalopathy predominantly involve the white matter, with multifocal necrosis, acute fibrinoid changes in blood vessels, and periventricular calcifications.[1,34,36,42] The mechanism of this encephalopathy remains unknown, but it usually occurs in patients receiving combination therapy. Elevated levels of MTX in the CSF have been correlated with a high risk of developing the syndrome. Total cumulative doses may also be significant in the pathogenesis. Bleyer and his colleagues measured the MTX levels in the CSF after administration of MTX (12–15 mg/m²) in 25 patients receiving therapy for meningeal leukemia. The mean MTX level in 25 patients receiving therapy for meningeal leukemia without evidence of neurotoxicity was 1.7 μM. Five patients with signs of neurotoxicity had CSF concentrations of MTX averaging 13.8 times greater — and the levels were consistently higher — than in patients without symptoms.[12]

'Concentration × Time' Therapy in Carcinomatous Meningitis

The morbidity and mortality associated with current therapy is substantial. Furthermore, the efficacy of this therapy is limited, and the quality of life for a patient with carcinomatous meningitis remains poor. Three goals are to be addressed in considering ways to improve therapy for carcinomatous meningitis: (1) to provide reliable, uniform distribution of the chemotherapy to the entire subarachnoid space within therapeutic levels, with the hope of improving survival; (2) to avoid peak levels of chemotherapy and thus minimize the risk for the development of neurotoxicity; and (3) to provide a convenient form of therapy for improving the quality of life of the cancer patient.

Delivering a low, constant concentration of drug over a prolonged period (C × T) provides such an approach; subtherapeutic trough levels are avoided, thus maximizing the cytotoxic effect of the chemotherapy, and potentially toxic peak drug concentrations are avoided. The total cumulative dose is also reduced by this approach.[2,11] The development of the implantable drug delivery system provides a convenient way to apply this C × T approach to the therapy of carcinomatous meningitis.

An approximation of the C × T schedule was applied to 19 patients with meningeal leukemia in a study by Bleyer et al in which a single injection of MTX (12 mg/m²) was compared to a C × T schedule of 1 mg every 12 hours for 3 days. The mean total cumulative dose necessary to achieve comparable therapeutic levels of the low C × T group was nearly ¹/₃ that of the conventional group. Neurotoxicity occurred in 1 of 8 patients receiving the C × T schedule and in 7/10 patients in the group receiving single intermittent therapy. Clinical responses in the 2 groups were similar in terms of rate of remission, number of relapses, and duration of remission.[11]

Drug Delivery System

The drug delivery system is totally implantable, thus reducing the risk of infection. The system consists of a subcutaneous model 400 Infusaid bellows pump connected to the side arm of an Ommaya reservoir by a small-caliber subcutaneous Silastic catheter. The reservoir is connected to a catheter placed in the right lateral ventricle. The entire system may be implanted in a single procedure under general anesthesia. Alternatively, the procedure may be performed in 2 stages. The first stage consists of placement of the Ommaya reservoir to which a 5 cm piece of Silastic tubing (outside diameter 0.092 in., inside diameter 0.015 in., volume 35 μL per ft.) has been attached to the side arm and plugged with medical Silastic adhesive. This may be performed under local or general anesthesia. The second stage consists of implantation of the pump in a subcutaneous pouch either within the right subclavicular pouch or the abdominal wall inferior to the liver. The Silastic tubing for the outflow system of the pump is then tunneled subcutaneously up to the reservoir, posterior to the ear. The placement of the subcutaneous tubing requires general anesthesia. We choose the subcutaneous infrahepatic location for implantation of the pump in slender, small-statured patients. This is the same location for pumps placed for infusion into the hepatic artery.

Each pump has a capacity of 50 ml, and the flow rate of each pump is calibrated by the manufacturer in vitro at 37°C. Each pump has an individual in vivo flow rate that is calculated each time it is refilled. Flow rates vary minimally as a function of body temperature, altitude, drug viscosity, and pressure fluctuation at the catheter outlet. Flow rates average 3–5 ml per day, requiring a pump refill every 12–14 days.

Drug Administration and Toxicity

Preservative-free MTX is supplied in 20 ml vials. A dose of MTX averaging 20–25 mg/week usually results in CSF levels between 1–20 μM, the accepted therapeutic, tolerable range.[14] Individual patient requirements to obtain CSF levels within this range may be determined by monitoring serial CSF MTX levels. The required dose to achieve levels within this range are quite constant and are independent of individual total body surface area. Serum levels of MTX are undetectable; therefore, the side effects associated with systemic MTX, such as myelosuppression and stomatitis, are not encountered. However, we still prefer to provide systemic rescue by prescribing oral calcium leucovorin 5 mg/day. There is evidence that reduced folate is important for synthesis and metabolism of neurotransmitters. Therefore, although it has not been proven clinically, administration of leucovorin may decrease the risk for the development of neurotoxicity.[1,2,29,41] Thymidine may also offer protection against MTX toxicity.[17] The patient with carcinomatous meningitis often requires concomitant systemic chemotherapy for tumor involvement elsewhere in the body. The absence of systemic toxicity from intrathecal MTX administration allows for the necessary systemic chemotherapy.

The preferred diluent is either lactated Ringer's solution or Elliott's B solution. MTX is chemically stable and compatible at 37°C in this system. We have administered thio-tepa and ara-C through the side port in patients requiring combination chemotherapy for the treatment of carcinomatous meningitis or in patients who have failed MTX therapy. Because these 2 drugs have not been administered by continuous infusion, there are no available data regarding this mode of administration.

The toxicity of continuous intraventricular infusion of MTX may be acute or chronic. Intraventricular infusion may result in headache, vomiting, fever, and meningismus within 24 hours of initiation of MTX infusion. This may be associated with a pleocytosis in the CSF, and it appears to be dose-related. The fever usually resolves within a period of days with continuation of the infusion. Persistent fever should raise concern regarding an underlying infectious process. Occasionally, persistent fever may result from the MTX infusion alone; if this is the case, the fever responds to indomethacin or systemic corticosteroids. Transverse myelitis producing paraplegia has been reported following intrathecal MTX. This reaction is usually attributable to a preservative in the MTX preparation or sustained elevated CSF MTX levels.[10,16] The chronic, progressive leukoencephalopathy that occasionally results in patients receiving intrathecal MTX has been mentioned. Clinically, the syndrome is characterized by dementia, ataxia, spastic quadraparesis, and seizures, progressing to coma and death. The etiology of chronic leukoencephalopathy remains unknown, but, as mentioned earlier, the syndrome appears to be related to radiation therapy and localized elevated levels of MTX in the CNS. The majority of patients received doses of radiation exceeding 2,000 rad.[34] The interaction between the irradiation and MTX remains unclear, and not all patients developing this complication have received radiation. Although unproven clinically, the C × T approach ideally will decrease the risk for development of chronic neurotoxicity.

Clinical Management

The pump is refilled every 12–14 days, depending somewhat upon the individual patient in vivo flow rate. The in vivo flow rate and refill drug concentrations are calculated at the time of each refill. Steady-state lumbar or ventricular CSF levels of MTX are measured periodically during the course of therapy. The pump infusate must be flushed from the reservoir and ventriculostomy catheter to obtain reliable ventricular levels.[28] CSF levels are dependent upon the dose infusion rate and the clearance rate of MTX from the CSF. The clearance rate is proportional to CSF pressure, bulk flow, and state of permeability of the blood/brain barrier. In general, however, the CSF levels have remained rather constant in each patient; therapeutic concentrations are achieved rather consistently with MTX doses of 20–25 mg/week. The previously discussed factors affecting the pump flow rate probably result in only minimal variations in CSF concentrations. The dose may be adjusted at the time of refill based on the sampling of CSF levels of MTX. The aim is to maintain levels of 1–20 μM. Periodic CSF examination, including MTX level, glucose, protein, cytocentrifuge cell count, and cytology, are helpful in assessment of the therapeutic response. When appropriate, biological cell markers may also indicate response or disease progression. Although myelosuppression and peripheral toxicity are not seen with this approach, it is prudent to monitor the peripheral blood count and renal and hepatic chemistry profile periodically. Sequential CT scans with contrast monitor should be done for signs of cortical and periventricular enhancement, hydrocephalus, white matter hypodensity, and other CNS tumor involvement. A radionuclide ^{111}indium cisternogram may be useful in identifying CSF for abnormalities in response failures. Cortical evoked potentials, which reflect function of the white matter, may be used in evaluation of chronic toxicity. Response to treatment is measured in terms of CSF parameters and clinical neurologic examinations; a response is defined as clearing of malignant cells from the CSF, normalization of the glucose, and resolution, improvement, or stabilization in neurologic deficit. Treatment failure may be the result of disease progression or adverse drug reaction. An elevated protein level in the CSF may be the result of drug-induced neurotoxicity and not an indication of disease progression from the meningeal malignancy. Following treatment failure, options include intraventricular ara-C (30 mg/m^2) or thio-tepa (10 mg/m^2) twice weekly through a side port in the Ommaya reservoir or radiation to the craniospinal neural axis or locally for symptomatic therapy. Once the disease is in remission, maintenance or consolidation therapy using intermittent infusion every 4 weeks for a 6-day course or a tapering schedule over 8–12 weeks may be considered. The CSF is then periodically sampled for evidence of recurrence. The optimal schedule for maintenance therapy has not been established. Additional clinical experience will be necessary to determine whether low-dose continuous infusion with a tapering dose or intermittent therapy is more effective.

Clinical Experience

Dakhil et al reported their experience at the University of Michigan using the implanted drug delivery system to infuse intraventricular MTX in 7 patients with various malignancies of the CNS, including 1 patient with meningeal diffuse histiocytic lymphoma, 5 patients with malignant gliomas, and 1 patient with metastatic melanoma to the brain.[16] The patient with meningeal lymphoma, who received an intermittent course of therapy consisting of 6-day courses of continuous infusion every 4 weeks, experienced a complete remission for 10+ months with reversal of neurologic deficit. A retroperitoneal lymph node recurrence was treated with concomitant systemic chemotherapy, demonstrating that the myelosuppressive effect of the C × T therapy is minimal and allows simultaneous use of a systemic myelosuppressive drug. Three of the 5 patients with malignant gliomas had a partial response lasting 2–6 months and then received cranial irradiation, resulting in a total survival of 6–14 months. One patient developed edema acutely following a course of radiotherapy and rapidly deteriorated. The patient received continuous infusion MTX (0.5–10 mg/day) with constant CSF levels in the range of 2–30 μM. Serum MTX levels were undetectable, and systemic toxicity was not seen. Four patients developed fever and meningismus (2 transient and 2 recurrent), but this was resolved with corticosteroids. One patient suffered a transverse myelitis attributed to a preservative in the MTX preparation. White matter hypodensity shown by CT scans developed in 2 patients but was not associated with increased neurologic deficit. The system proved to be a reliable, convenient, and safe means of administering chemotherapy in this group of patients. Pump performance was reliable, and there were no infections or neurologic complications related to the pump system. Intermittent cycles of chemotherapy were administered in 1 patient without blockage of the catheter. The pump, allowed to remain empty, functioned well when later refilled. In all patients who have required temporary discontinuation of chemotherapy, the investigators have elected to keep the pump filled with lactated Ringer's solution to avoid possible catheter blockage.

The authors concluded that the system appears promising for the treatment of meningeal neoplasms; however, the role of chemotherapy delivery into the subarachnoid space for intraparenchymal tumors such as malignant gliomas is unclear. Penetration into brain parenchyma of chemotherapy from the CSF can be achieved with prolonged exposure for 48 to 72 hours, but is approximately 1/10 of the CSF concentration at 1 cm from the surface.[8,9]

The authors of the present review have used this infusion system to treat 4 patients with meningeal malignancies of various origins, including multiple myeloma, esthesioneuroblastoma, and 2 cases of breast cancer. Their histories are presented below to illustrate the complexities of caring for cancer patients suffering from this syndrome.

Case Presentations

Case 1

This 32-year-old female underwent a right radical mastectomy in 1971 for poorly differentiated medullary carcinoma of the breast. A left radical mastectomy was performed in 1981 for malignancy involving the left breast. In 1982, a recurrence in the region of the left surgical scar was found and was treated with radiotherapy. She subsequently developed diffuse metastatic disease to the skeleton and lungs for which she received a course of combination systemic chemotherapy. She then developed headaches in November 1984 and was found to have meningeal carcinomatosis by CSF examination; the CSF glucose was less than 20 mg/dl, the protein 89 mg/dl and several malignant cells were seen on cytologic examination. Her symptoms responded dramatically to twice-weekly intralumbar injections of MTX (15 mg) and corticosteroids. As a result, she underwent placement of an Ommaya reservoir and infusion pump system in January 1985. She received MTX (19–22 mg/week) by continuous infusion, resulting in CSF levels of 4–9 μM. During the course of therapy, she developed persistent fevers for which no infectious etiology could be identified; these were resolved promptly with indomethacin. In April 1984, she developed a progressive right hemiparesis, expressive aphasia, and seizure activity. The CSF showed normalization of glucose without malignant cells. The MTX was discontinued following a diagnosis of MTX neurotoxicity. Two days after the development of headaches, she had an acute episode of elevated intracranial pressure unresponsive to mannitol therapy and expired in April

1985, 6 months following the onset of neurologic symptoms. Postmortem examination showed residual meningeal infiltration of tumor. The deep white matter was abnormal, consistent with MTX leukoencephalopathy.

COMMENT

This patient experienced an excellent initial response to intrathecal MTX therapy. The infusion system provided a reliable, convenient means to administer the chemotherapy, allowing her to remain independent, with biweekly outpatient visits. Her course was complicated by the development of persistent fevers for which no infection could be found. The fever responded promptly to indomethacin. Despite normal evoked potential studies prior to death, postmortem examination demonstrated injury to the deep white matter, consistent with MTX leukoencephalopathy. She had not received prior irradiation to the neuraxis. The fact that residual meningeal tumor and evidence of neurotoxicity were found simultaneously demonstrates the limitations of the available therapy. Intermittent courses of continuous therapy might have decreased the risk for neurotoxicity, but would have been less effective in tumor control.

Case 2

This 47-year-old female underwent a left modified radical mastectomy in 1979 for intraductal carcinoma of the breast. At that time, no nodes were involved. She then suffered a recurrence in 1981 involving the right breast as well as a malignant pleural effusion and metastasis to the lumbar spine. She was treated with a lumpectomy and 2 years of systemic combination chemotherapy that included variable combinations of 5-fluorouracil, cyclophosphamide (CTX), Adriamycin (ADR), and MTX. In September 1983, she developed weakness of the lower extremities. A CSF examination revealed a protein of 260 mg/dl, glucose 36 mg/dl with 32 white blood cells and abnormal cytology. A CT scan demonstrated diffuse cortical enhancement and 2 intraparenchymal metastases. She was treated with 4 courses of intrathecal chemotherapy by way of the lumbar route that included ara-C and MTX. In addition, she received cranial irradiation. Two months later, a CT scan showed progression of the intraparenchymal disease. In addition, her leg weakness progressed. She then developed numbness in the sacral region.

In December 1983, an Ommaya reservoir and drug delivery system were implanted. She received a constant flow of MTX (20 mg/week). She remained neurologically stable, with improvement in the sacral numbness through February 1984. However, she then required systemic chemotherapy, including systemic MTX, CTX, and 5-fluorouracil for systemic dissemination. She expired in February 1984 of pneumonia, 5 months after the onset of neurologic symptoms.

COMMENT

Once again, this patient experienced an initial response to intrathecal MTX. This method of administration allowed for concomitant systemic chemotherapy. The terminal complication from her disease was that of systemic dissemination.

Case 3

This 54-year-old male presented in September 1983 with a right jaw mass, found to be a plasmacytoma on biopsy. Systemic involvement was identified by bone marrow examination. He was treated with a combination of localized irradiation to the jaw and chemotherapy that included melphalan, vincristine, and prednisone. The disease responded with resolution of the Bence Jones protein in his urine.

He then developed low back pain and an episode of speech disturbance associated with confusion in February 1984. A spinal fluid examination disclosed a protein of 925 mg/dl, a glucose of 53 mg/dl, and 566 white blood cells, all of which were plasma cells. He received cranial irradiation and radiation to the lower thoracic spine for multiple lytic lesions. He received intrathecal MTX (10 mg) and thio-tepa (10 mg) by the lumbar route 3 times weekly. His mental status significantly improved. A spinal fluid examination 1 month later was improved, with a protein of 443 mg/dl, glucose 90 mg/dl, and 84 white blood cells, all of which continued to be plasma cells. The chemotherapy was decreased to weekly therapy.

He then noted the acute onset of neck pain and right arm pain with paresthesias suggesting a C6 radiculopathy. A pantopaque myelogram and cervical CT scan suggested spondylosis without evidence of tumor involvement. He initially responded to conservative management, but later required a cervical laminectomy following the development of right arm weakness. The right arm weakness temporarily improved, but he later went on to develop a progressive right hemiparesis.

An Ommaya reservoir was placed with a infusion pump in May 1984 with continuous infusion of MTX (20 mg/week). Levels were maintained in the CSF between 1–10 μM. However, he continued to show neurologic decline, with progressive confusion, quadriparesis, and seizure activity. A spinal fluid examination showed a protein of 994 mg/dl, glucose 58 mg/dl, and 2 plasma cells. Shortly thereafter, he was transferred to a nursing home. He expired following the development of sepsis, 5 months after the development of neurologic symptoms.

COMMENT

This patient's initial response to the meningeal involvement of his multiple myeloma was a result of the combination of intrathecal MTX and thio-tepa. This case illustrates the use of combination chemotherapy for this disorder. Retrospectively, eventual treatment failure may have been the result in part of discontinuing the thio-tepa at the time of the pump system placement. The side port provides a convenient means for administering intermittent injections.

Case 4

This 28-year-old female presented in 1980 with CSF rhinorrhea. A low CSF glucose, elevated protein, and malignant cells were found on examination of the CSF. A dehiscence of the cribiform plate was surgically corrected and an esthesioneuroblastoma was found in the operative material. The postoperative course was complicated by an acute episode of elevated intracranial pressure to 500 mm of water and a generalized seizure. She received a course of craniospinal irradiation of 3,900 rad and an additional 6,600 rad to the nasopharynx. In March 1983, the CSF contained glucose of 57 mg/dl, protein 125 mg/dl, and clusters of malignant cells. A lumbar pantopaque myelogram was normal. The malignant cells disappeared from the CSF following the initiation of twice weekly treatments of intraventricular MTX (15 mg) through an Ommaya reservoir. Chemotherapy was discontinued in July 1983 following the development of nocturnal myoclonus. However, the CSF protein remained elevated and the glucose remained depressed. In February 1984 she developed recurrent headaches, intermittent horizontal diplopia, and partial complex seizures. Malignant cells were once again indentified in the CSF. A subcutaneous continuous infusion drug delivery system was implanted and connected to the Ommaya reservoir on February 16, 1984. She received MTX (20 mg/week) by continuous infusion in lactated Ringer's solution and oral calcium leucovorin 5 mg daily. Lumbar CSF levels of MTX were maintained between 2 and 8 μM. The headaches and diplopia improved.

The flow through the pump was found to be impaired after an attempt to refill the pump produced an inappropriately high residual volume. Testing of the flow through the reservoir, the reservoir pressure, and attempted flushing through the side port suggested that the dysfunction may have been the result of a blockage of the tubing between pump and reservoir. Kinking could not be demonstrated radiographically. However, in view of her deteriorating neurologic course, we did not believe that surgical exploration was indicated to determine the cause of flow impedance. She then received 2 additional courses of MTX and ara-C through the reservoir.

In April 1984, the patient developed progressive paraparesis, urinary retention, and midthoracic back pain, with a sensory level at T8. A metrizamide myelogram and a CT scan did not show abnormalities. Following the development of a progressive encephalopathy characterized by dysarthria, confusion, and seizures, a CT scan showed diffuse low absorption of the white matter with cortical atrophy, and electroencephalography showed diffuse high-amplitude rhythmic delta activity. Chemotherapy was then discontinued on the basis that the encephalopathy may have been the result of the combined therapy, irradiation, and intrathecal MTX. She expired in July 1984, 4 years after diagnosis.

COMMENT

The esthesioneuroblastoma is an uncommon malignancy of the neuroepithelium. Leptomeningeal involvement is uncommon. Experience with chemotherapy in the treatment of this malignant neoplasm is limited. The initial response to intrathecal MTX suggested a promising tumor sensitivity. However, treatment was limited due to the development of neurotoxicity. The radiation of the neuraxis and the high cumulative dose of MTX required in the course of the patient's illness predisposed her to this complication. Dysfunction of the drug delivery system complicated her course of therapy. We were unable to identify the specific cause for this malfunction by noninvasive studies.

Conclusions

The application of C × T therapy by continuous infusion in the treatment of carcinomatous meningitis is in the primary stage. The advantages of this approach include: (1) maintenance of therapeutic levels to prolong cytocidal concentrations of MTX, a cell cycle-specific drug; (2) reduction of neurotoxic peak levels and cumulative amount of drug; and (3) convenience of administration for the patient. Potential uses of this system for neoplastic diseases in the future include prophylactic and symptomatic treatment for acute leukemia; treatment of primary brain tumors in proximity to the leptomeninges, such as medulloblastoma, ependymoma, tumors of the pineal region, and meningeal gliomatosis; and prophylactic treatment of the CNS for solid tumors.

As our understanding of the pharmacokinetics of the chemotherapeutic drugs within the CSF increases, C × T therapy by continuous infusion may be applied using drugs such as ara-C, thio-tepa, and aziridinylbenzoquinone (AZQ).[22,29,50] Insight into the mechanisms of neoplastic cell growth and normal tissue will allow for prevention of neurotoxicity to normal tissue while maximizing the tumoricidal effects. Ara-C is a phase-specific, cycle-dependent chemotherapeutic agent; maximum exposure to tumor cells by C × T therapy would be the most effective method of administration for tumoricidal activity of this drug. Proper sequencing with combination therapy may be advantageous. For example, sequencing a cell cycle-specific drug such as MTX with a noncycle-specific drug such as thio-tepa or AZQ is one possibility. Dosage schedules will undergo modification as our experience with this system grows.

The concept of maintenance or consolidation therapy, in which therapy is continued following an apparent remission, appears to be important in meningeal neoplasms. Tumor cell counts have been estimated to be as high as 10 in the CSF despite negative CSF cytology examinations and normal differential white cell counts. This is supported by the clinical observation that patients with meningeal leukemia treated with maintenance intrathecal MTX following a clinical CSF remission remain without recurrence for a longer period than those patients not receiving maintenance therapy.[44] Consolidation therapy may be administered as continuous low-dose infusion or intermittent courses of therapy for variable periods of time.

As our understanding of the relationship between various non-neoplastic disorders of the CNS and neurochemical mediators increases, this delivery system has obvious additional therapeutic implications. The administration of morphine directly into the CSF has been used to modulate the central pain pathways by stimulating central opiate receptors in patients with intractable pain associated with cancer and various chronic debilitating pain syndromes.[15,31] Intrathecal morphine also has been noted to improve spasticity in patients with a combination of pain and spasticity; thus, it has been applied to the treatment of spasticity in spinal cord injury patients.[19] Preliminary reports of similar implantable drug delivery systems for the treatment of spasticity are promising. This system is useful for patients unable to tolerate oral narcotics or in those who experience excessive side effects from systemically administered narcotics. Newer drugs for the treatment of pain administered intrathecally include the opioid peptides, D-ala d-leu enkephalen (DADL) and beta-endorphin, and the nonopioid drugs clonidine and baclofen.[20] The application of this system in the treatment of various degenerative disorders of the CNS is promising. Decreased cholinergic activity has been documented in patients with Alzheimer's disease by postmortem examination and biopsy of brain tissue. Such tissue has been found to have decreased choline acetyl transferase activity and decreased acetylcholine synthesis as well as loss of cholinergic neurons in the nucleus basalis of Meynert. Attempts to increase the serum levels of acetylcholine precursors have not been effective. Subjective improvement in cognitive function has been reported following the constant intrathecal infusion of bethanechol chloride, a water-soluble muscarinic agent.[23] Intrathecal infusion of thyrotropin-releasing hormone (TRH) appears to improve motor function in some patients with amyotrophic lateral sclerosis, demonstrating the use of neurotransmitter infusion in the treatment of a degenerative disorder.[30]

Long-term intrathecal drug therapy is often necessary in the treatment of various CNS infections. Drugs such as amphotericin-B for fungal meningitis and aminoglycosides for chronic refractory gram-negative meningitis are examples of possible applications of $C \times T$ infusion therapy. Intraventricular lithium by continuous infusion is currently being investigated in animal models to reduce systemic side effects. The results have broad therapeutic implications in various psychiatric and neurologic disorders.[7] The significance of abnormal gamma-aminobutyric acid (GABA) transmission in epilepsy has recently been recognized. Augmentation of GABA activity has been attempted by blocking GABA catabolism. THTP, an antiepileptic agent inhibiting GABA transport of glial cells, may be a candidate for drug infusion in the treatment of epilepsy.[39]

40

INTRAVESICAL CHEMOTHERAPY FOR BLADDER TUMORS

Hugh A. G. Fisher, M.D.

APPROXIMATELY 40,000 NEW CASES of bladder cancer are discovered annually in the United States, with 11,000 bladder cancer-related deaths.[1] Eighty percent of these tumors are superficial at the time of presentation, involving bladder mucosa or submucosa only and thus are potentially curable by transurethral surgical resection.[2] However, following complete excision, 40–80% of patients with superficial papillary carcinoma will develop new growths within 3 years, and up to 30% will progress in grade or stage of disease.[3-5] Prospective longitudinal studies have helped define the natural history of superficial bladder cancer, identifying subgroups within this heterogeneous population who are at higher risk for recurrence and progression. In the past 25 years, the addition of intravesically administered chemotherapeutic or immunotherapeutic agents to transurethral resection has proven effective for both treatment of residual disease in patients undergoing incomplete excision and prophylaxis against new tumor formation in those patients in whom complete resection is possible. This chapter will review the role of intravesical agents in control of this disease.

Characteristics of Superficial Bladder Cancer

Bladder cancer is the sixth most common malignancy, with highest incidence in the sixth decade of life. It is 3–4 times more common in men than women.[1] The transitional cell type accounts for 88% of all urothelial tumors; squamous carcinoma and adenocarcinoma are less common (10% and 2%, respectively), rarely superficial at presentation, and have poorer prognoses.[6] The entire epithelial lining of the urinary tract is at risk for tumor formation of the transitional cell type, including not only the bladder but also the renal collecting systems, ureters, proximal urethra in women, and prostatic urethra in men. Carcinogenesis may involve a multistage process in which exposure to an initiating substance, a known carcinogen whose effects are irreversible, is followed by exposure to a promoting substance that alone is not carcinogenic but acts in synergy to produce frank carcinoma. Several initiating or promoting agents have been identified, including (1) industrial carcinogens, mainly aromatic amines (e.g., betanaphthylamine and para-amino diphenyl in aniline dyes, para-amino phenol in textiles, benzidine in rubber and 3, dichloro-4, 4, diaminodiphenyl methane in plastics;[8] (2) cigarette smoking;[9] (3) phenacetin and other analgesics;[10] and (4) chronic irritation of the bladder by foreign bodies such as an indwelling Foley catheter or infestation with parasites of the *Schistosoma hematobium* species.[11]

Clinical Presentation and Diagnosis

The hallmark of the clinical presentation of bladder cancer is gross, total painless hematuria, i.e., visible discoloration of the urine throughout the urinary stream in the absence of other symptoms. Less commonly, hematuria may occur at initiation or termination of urination or as intermittent spotting, particularly in women in whom vaginal or uterine sources also must be considered. Hematuria may be intermittent, leading to a delay in seeking medical attention, or may be associated with urinary tract infection or calculi, leading to misdiagnosis. Advanced tumors may cause obstructive symptoms, with urinary hesitancy, frequency, and restriction of urinary flow. Obstruction of the ureteral orifices by adjacent or infiltrating tumors may cause upper tract obstruction, with symptoms of flank pain or uremia. Irritative symptoms of frequency, urgency, or suprapubic pain may herald the presence of diffuse carcinoma in situ.[12] Metastatic disease to regional lymph nodes may be associated with lower extremity edema or groin masses. Distant metastatic disease most commonly involves lung, liver, and bone and is associated with anemia, weight loss, and fatigue.[13]

Voided urinalysis, which may detect asymptomatic microscopic hematuria, is a valuable screening test. The persistent presence of even 1–2 red blood cells is significant and demands thorough urologic investigation. When microscopic hematuria is documented or gross hematuria occurs, an I.V. urogram and cystoscopy are performed with retrograde ureteropyelograms, renal ultrasound, computerized tomography (CT) scans and/or renal arteriograms, as indicated, to rule out upper tract lesions arising from the renal parenchyma or collecting systems.

An important adjunctive laboratory test in the evaluation of hematuria of unknown etiology is urinary cytology. Although most bladder tumors are readily visualized by cystoscopic examination, in the case of carcinoma in situ, the bladder mucosa may appear normal or focally or diffusely inflamed.[14] Urine cytology may detect exfoliated malignant cells months or years before the development of visible tumor[14] and is most accurate with high-grade malignancies.[15] Urine cytology is particularly useful and necessary for follow-up of resected transitional cell carcinomas.[15] Persistently positive cytology after tumor resection indicates residual tumor either within the bladder or upper tracts and indicates a much higher risk of subsequent disease. Automated flow cytometry is more sensitive than voided cytology for detection of low-grade lesions and increasingly is being applied in the clinical setting for diagnosis and follow-up of urothelial tumors.[16-18] Refinements in this technology may allow widespread, low-cost screening of high-risk populations.

Staging and Classification

Transurethral resection of visible bladder tumor is used for initial bladder cancer control and for staging purposes. Superficial transitional cell carcinomas are most commonly located on the lateral walls or trigone and are often multiple, with fine vascular stalks and normal surrounding mucosa. Random biopsies are performed adjacent to the tumor base and at distant normal-appearing sites to rule out occult carcinoma or pathologic precursor lesions, e.g., atypia, hyperplasia, or dysplasia, which may predict future tumor occurrences.[19-24] A bimanual examination is performed under anesthesia to detect residual bladder masses or bladder fixation indicating a deeply invasive tumor. Metastatic studies consisting of pelvic CT scan, bone scan, and chest X ray are performed for deeply infiltrating lesions, but are not routinely obtained for superficial disease.

Two staging systems for carcinoma of the bladder currently are in use, the Jewett-Strong-Marshall system, widely used in the United States, and the tumor-node-metastasis (TNM) system of the International Union Against Cancer (see table 1). Superficial bladder carcinoma includes the Jewett-Strong-Marshall stages O, A, and B-1 and the TNM stages TIS, Ta, T1, and T2. The TNM system, which differentiates between flat carcinoma in situ and papillary carcinoma, is the preferred staging system for superficial bladder cancer. Current staging modalities are approximately 80% accurate in differentiating low-

Table 1. Bladder Cancer Staging Systems

Pathologic extent	Jewett-Marshall	UICC* (TNM)
Superficial		
Carcinoma in situ	0	TIS
Papillary tumor confined to mucosa	0	Ta
Submucosal invasion	A	T1
Superficial muscle invasion	B1	T2
Deep		
Deep muscle invasion	B2	T3A
Perivesical fat involved	C	T3B
Invasion of adjacent organs	D	T4
Pelvic lymph nodes	D1	N1-3
Extra pelvic lymph nodes or distant visceral organs	D2	N4-M1

*International Union Against Cancer

stage superficial neoplasms from deeper high-stage lesions, with staging errors highest for deeper penetrating lesions.[25] Inclusion of muscle-invading tumor in the superficial group is controversial because of the higher incidence of recurrence and the difficulty in determining depth of muscle invasion without a full-thickness bladder wall specimen obtained by cystectomy. Conservative treatment of these lesions must be approached with caution, and intravesical chemotherapy has generally not been used for this stage of disease. For purposes of this review, the impact of intravesical agents will be discussed for stages TIS, Ta and T1 only.

Mechanisms of Recurrence

Following complete excision of all visible superficial tumor from the bladder wall, 40–80% of patients will manifest recurrent disease within a 3-year period.[3-5] Common urologic practice calls for repeat cystoscopy every 3 months for the first 2 years, every 6 months in years 2–4, and yearly thereafter. Recurrent tumors may arise from 3 potential sources: (1) *true recurrence*, i.e., incomplete excision of an existing lesion with visible tumor at the site of previous resection; (2) *implantation* of tumor cells from the primary lesion onto inflamed, traumatized, or denuded mucosa with subsequent growth; or (3) a *new occurrence* of tumor arising from the urothelium as part of a generalized carcinogenesis. The incidence of true recurrence remains unquantitiated. The latter 2 hypotheses have support from both laboratory and clinical studies.

McDonald and Thorson[26] transplanted carcinogen-induced bladder cancer to mucosal-lined pouches in dogs. Wallace and Hershfield[27] demonstrated the implantability of sarcoma cells into the bladder when injected through the urethra. Soloway, Wheldon, and associates[28-29] investigated local factors that may enhance tumor cell implantation, including chemical denudation of bladder mucosa by N-methyl-N-nitrosourea and direct trauma to the bladder mucosa with cauterization. Both techniques led to a higher incidence of implantation of viable tumor cells than in normal bladders. Clinical evidence for implantation remains circumstantial, primarily involving analysis of patterns of recurrence following transurethral resection[30-34] or wound recurrence in open procedures.[35] Van der Werf-Messing[36] reported a low incidence of recurrence in solitary bladder tumors treated with transvesical radium needle implantation (12%) as an alternative to transurethral resection, questioning the role of transurethral resection in promoting recurrence through implantation. Conversely, Greene and Yalowitz[37] found no increase in subsequent prostatic urethral recurrence rates in 100 patients undergoing simultaneous transurethral resection of benign prostatic tissue and bladder tumors when compared with 100 patients undergoing bladder tumor resection alone.

Chromosomal studies have provided evidence that successive generations of superficial bladder tumors have similar marker chromosomes, lending support to a monoclonal theory of bladder cancer origin that may recur through implantation of tumor cells shed from a primary lesion.[38,39]

Although tumor implantation may contribute to the high rate of recurrence in superficial bladder cancer, histologic studies support the concept that a new tumor within the bladder is a true occurrence. Since the original observation by Melicow in 1952 of preneoplastic unsuspected urothelial lesions occurring simultaneously with invasive bladder cancer,[40] bladder mapping studies by Cooper et al,[41] Koss et al,[42] Farrow et al,[43] and Soto et al[44] have demonstrated up to an 80% incidence of carcinoma in situ or multifocal carcinoma in bladders removed for invasive disease. Furthermore, abnormal random mucosal biopsies obtained from adjacent or distant areas in the bladder of patients with superficial tumors have correlated with future tumor occurrences,[19-24] and histologic studies of carcinogen-induced changes in animal systems show hyperplasia and dysplasia simultaneously in many separate urothelial areas.[45] Thus, a large body of evidence indicates that urothelial cancers of the transitional cell type represent a field change disease having the potential for multiple areas of involvement over time (polychronotopism). The entire urothelium of the urinary tract is at risk for tumor formation, including the renal collecting systems, ureters, and urethra. These areas must be monitored for concomitant or future occurrences in any patient with superficial bladder cancer.

Risk Factors for Recurrence and Progression of Superficial Bladder Cancer

Superficial bladder cancer stages TIS, Ta, and T1 constitutes a heterogeneous population of tumors with variable capacity to recur and progress to either muscle invasion or metastasis. In order to evaluate the effect of any treatment modality on the recurrence rates and progression rates of this disease, it is paramount to define the natural history and identify risk factors for these events. Through both retrospective and prospective longitudinal studies, a number of factors that affect recurrence and progression have been identified (see table 2).

Retrospective studies have identified the importance of stage, grade, and multiplicity as major determinants of recurrence and progression.[2,3,5,46-48] Solitary papillary noninvasive (stage Ta) grade 1 transitional cell carcinomas, also called papillomas, have the lowest recurrence rates, approximately 30%.[5,48] With multiple tumors at presentation or a history of previous recurrence, the

Table 2. Predictive Factors for Recurrence or Progression of Superficial Bladder Cancer

1. Tumor stage
2. Tumor grade
3. Multiplicity of tumors at presentation
4. Tumor size
5. Status of adjacent epithelium
6. Loss of blood group antigens
7. Presence of marker chromosomes

incidence of subsequent recurrence for noninvasive low-grade tumor rises to 66–94%, but progression to muscle invasion or metastasis is infrequent.[5,46,48] As stage and grade increase, the incidence of recurrence and progression of recurrent tumors increases.[2,3,47,48] Overall survival for patients with superficial tumors is 70–90%,[46-50] with most bladder cancer-related deaths occurring in high-grade tumors.

The National Bladder Cancer Collaborative Group (NBCCG) performed a longitudinal prospective study for patients with stage Ta and T1 tumors at presentation who were treated with transurethral resection alone prior to the first new occurrence of tumor.[3,51] Of 249 patients eligible for recurrence analysis, 175 had tumor confined to the mucosa only, and 74 demonstrated invasion of the lamina propria. Median follow-up was 39 months. For recurrence, stage T1 tumors recurred more frequently (70%) than stage Ta tumors (50%). The interval free of disease was significantly less for patients with grade 3 tumors than for patients with grade 1 or 2 disease. Patients with 4 or more tumors at presentation had significantly higher recurrence rates than patients with 1 tumor at presentation, and patients with tumors 5 cm or more in size had a significantly shorter disease-free interval than patients with tumors less than 5 cm.

The European Organization for Research on Treatment of Cancer (EORTC) analyzed risk factors for recurrence in a group of 308 patients who were treated with transurethral resection alone, intravesical thio-tepa, or teniposide (VM-26).[52] The single most important predictor of recurrence was the number of tumors present at entry into the study. The number of patients with recurrence (percent recurring) increased as the number of tumors present at transurethral resection increased, with the difference among those with 1, 2, and 3 tumors and those with more than 3 being statistically significant. The recurrence rate (the number of recurrences per year) prior to treatment was nearly as important. The recurrence rate for grade 1 tumors was significantly lower than in patients with grades 2 and 3 combined.

Regarding progression to muscle invasion or metastases, in the NBCCG study,[3] by stage alone, of 144 Ta patients 4% progressed, compared to 30% of 63 T1 patients. By grade alone, 2% of grade 1, 11% of grade 2, and 45% of grade 3 tumors had progression. Combining grade and stage, for Ta grade 1, 2% progressed; Ta grade 2, 6%; and Ta grade 3, 25%. For stage T1 grade 2 tumors, 21% of recurrences progressed, compared with 48% of T1 grade 3 tumors. If tumor size was less than 5 cm, 9% progressed, compared with 35% of patients with tumors greater than 5 cm. If a random mucosal biopsy showed moderate to severe dysplasia, 33% of patients progressed, compared with 8% with no abnormalities, hyperplasia, or mild dysplasia. Urine cytology correlated with tumor grade, with a statistically significant difference in progression rates for patients with positive versus negative cytologies.

These studies have helped define groups of patients who are at low, intermediate, or high risk for recurrence and progression of disease. The patient with a solitary stage Ta papillary lesion, grade 1, less than 5 cm in size, with negative cytology and normal random biopsies, is at lowest risk for both recurrence and progression. On the other hand, a patient with multiple stage T1 tumors of higher grade (2–3), with a previous history of recurrence, positive urine cytology, and random biopsy showing moderate dysplasia or carcinoma in situ, has the highest rate of subsequent recurrence and progression to muscle invasion and metastases. These variables should be recorded in any study comparing intravesical agents.

Carcinoma in Situ

Carcinoma in situ is defined as the presence of malignant cells confined to the mucosa.[53] Classically, it appears as a reddened, slightly raised, velvety patch on the bladder wall and may be focal or diffuse.[54] It may exist alone or with previous or synchronous papillary lesions. The natural history of carcinoma in situ is variable and poorly defined, but this lesion is considered a precursor of invasive disease. If existing alone, carcinoma in situ may progress rapidly to invasive disease or remain quiescent for years.[55] Focal carcinoma in situ appears to be less aggressive;[56] however, when associated with papillary carcinoma, progression to invasive disease is more likely to occur in a defined period.[57-59] Althausen et al[59] noted that in patients with normal mucosa adjacent to papillary tumors, only 3/41 (7%) developed invasive carcinoma, but 10/12 (83%) with carcinoma in situ developed muscle invasive disease in 4 years. Carcinoma in situ may also exist at extravesical sites, in distal ureters, or in prostatic ducts, emphasizing the importance of urine cytology and prostate biopsy in the management of patients with this entity. Eradication of diffuse carcinoma in situ by transurethral resection alone is uncommon, and thus these patients should be excluded from prophylactic studies unless urine cytology reverts to negative after resection.

Agents for Intravesical Therapy

Many chemotherapeutic agents have been used for attempted control of recurrent superficial bladder tumors. An ideal agent for intravesical use should have the following characteristics: (1) complete destruction of all tumors, (2) limited number of applications, (3) absence of local side effects, (4) no systemic toxicity, (5) permanent status free of tumor, (6) no local or systemic carcinogenic effects, and (7) low cost. While this ideal agent does not exist, multiple drugs have been tested in the United States and abroad. Bleomycin,[60-62] cyclophosphamide,[63] 5-fluorouracil,[64] and actinomycin-D[64] have been *ineffective* when administered intravesically. Cisplatin has shown limited activity, but anaphylactic reactions have occurred.[65,66] Ethoglucid (Epodyl)[67,68] and VM-26,[52] podophyllum derivatives, have shown activity in European studies, but are not available in the United States. The most active and most commonly used chemotherapeutic agents are thio-tepa, mitomycin-C (MIT), and doxorubicin (ADR). Additionally, immunotherapy with BCG (bacille Calmette-Guerin), although ineffective in other cancer sites, has been singularly effective in superficial bladder cancer. These agents may be used for *ablative treatment* of existing tumors, *long-term prophylaxis* against recurrence after all visible tumor has been eradicated by transurethral resection, or as short-course *adjuvant treatment* after transurethral resection to prevent implantation of tumor cells. Residual disease trials have as their main end point the disappearance of existing tumor, whereas the event of a new tumor occurrence is commonly used for prophylactic or adjuvant studies. The latter type of study may also evaluate the time to tumor recurrence (disease-free interval) and the recurrence rate (e.g., number of tumors per patient month of follow-up) as a measure of treatment efficacy. In early studies, dosage and treatment schedules varied widely, and many studies lacked bona fide control groups or used recurrence rates for patients prior to treatment as controls. Also, urine cytologies and random mucosal biopsies were not routinely done. More recently, randomized prospective studies with appropriate stratification factors comparing intravesical agents with untreated control groups or another intravesical agent have been initiated by large cooperative groups to determine the exact impact of intravesical chemotherapy on recurrence rates, progression rates, and host survival.

Thio-tepa

Thio-tepa, an alkylating agent chemically and pharmacologically related to nitrogen mustard, has a radiomimetic effect, exerting its cytotoxic activity on proliferating cells through the release of ethylenamine radicals.[69] It has been successfully used in body cavities with exposure to normal tissues, with few local adverse effects.[69] It is the most commonly used intravesical agent in the United States.

TREATMENT OF RESIDUAL DISEASE (TABLE 3)

For treatment of existing tumors, early studies showed a 23–41% complete response (CR) rate, 32–85% partial responses (PR), and no response in 15–38%

Table 3. Thio-tepa Treatment of Residual Tumor

Investigator/reference	Dose	No. patients	CR (%)	PR (%)	No response (%)
Jones & Swinney[69] 1961	30 – 90 mg q 2 – 3 days × 4	13	—	11 (85)	2 (15)
Veenema[70] 1962	60 mg weekly × 4 – 8 weeks	10	4 (40)	10 (60)	—
Abassian & Wallace[71] 1966	90 mg every 4 days × 4	13	3 (23)	5 (38)	5 (38)
Veenema[72] 1969	60 mg in 60 ml weekly × 8	46	17 (37)	16 (35)	13 (28)
Edsmyr & Boman[73] 1971	50 mg every other day × 6	29	12 (41)	11 (38)	5 (17)
Pavone & Macaluso[63] 1971	60 mg weekly × 4	25	8 (32)	8 (32)	9 (36)
Koontz[74] 1981	30 – 60 mg weekly × 8	95	45 (47)	—	50 (53)
Heney[142] 1985	30 mg weekly × 8	42	18 (43)	7 (17)	17 (38)

of patients.[69-75] Jones and Swinney[69] used 30–90 mg held for 1–2 hours every 2–3 days for 4 doses, with reduction in size and number of tumors in 11/13 patients (85%). Veenema[70] used weekly doses of 60 mg in 60 ml sterile water for 8 weeks, with either complete disappearance or reduction in size of residual tumors in all 10 patients treated. This same regimen in a larger series (46 patients) produced CR in 17 patients (37%) and PR in 16 (35%).[72] Pavone-Macaluso[63] obtained similar results with this regimen in 25 patients. Abassian and Wallace[71] and Edsmyr[73] noted CR in patients treated with 50 or 90 mg every other day or every 4 days, respectively, but noted fatal toxicity in each series. Low-grade tumors responded best in the above studies.

In a randomized prospective trial, the NBCCG[74] compared 30 mg in 30 ml sterile water with 60 mg in 60 ml sterile water weekly for 8 weeks. Ninety-five patients were treated, 50 with the 30 mg dose and 45 with the 60 mg dose, with CR in 48% and 47%, respectively. Complete responses were more likely with tumors less than 4 cm in diameter. Both low-grade and high-grade tumors responded. Eleven of 20 patients (55%) with carcinoma in situ achieved CR.

TOXICITY

Irritative voiding symptoms, dysuria, and frequency are common, usually subsiding 2–3 days after instillation of the drug.[69-75] The most serious toxic effect with thio-tepa is myelosuppression secondary to absorption of this relatively small molecule (mol wt 189) through the bladder wall. The amount of thio-tepa absorbed varies widely, depending on the extent of tumor involvement. Pavone-Macaluso[76] found that 10.5% of the drug was absorbed from normal bladders, compared to 63% in patients with solid carcinoma and 73% in patients who underwent resection less than 1 week before initiation of thio-tepa. Because of the latter observation, thio-tepa was initially used with caution in the immediate postoperative period, particularly after extensive transurethral resection. Myelosuppression occurs in 2–34% of patients receiving thio-tepa.[69-75,77] Although usually mild (WBC <3,000 but >2,000) and readily reversible by withholding treatment, drug-related deaths have occurred.[71,78] Soloway and Ford,[79] who reviewed their experience and that of others, concluded that the risks of severe acute or chronic myelosuppression appear greater with frequent administration (every 1–2 days) of high doses (60–90 mg). Moderate doses of 30–60 mg 24–48 hours after endoscopic surgery do not appear to expose the patient to high risk. However, WBC and platelet counts should be recorded prior to each instillation and treatment withheld if WBC counts are <3,000 or platelets <100,000.

SHORT-TERM ADJUVANT THERAPY

Instillation of 1–3 doses of thio-tepa in the immediate postoperative period has decreased subsequent recurrence rates without increased toxicity (see table 4). Burnand[80] instilled 90 mg of thio-tepa immediately following resection for 30 minutes and without further therapy noted reduction in the number of patients with recurrence at cystoscopy 3 months later when compared with an untreated control group (58% versus 97%, respectively). Gavrell[81] used 30 mg of thio-tepa in 60 cc sterile water for 30 minutes twice daily for 3 days, with reduction in recurrence rates similar to a second group who received additional thio-tepa weekly for 6 weeks, then monthly. England[82] instilled 30 mg of thio-tepa in 50 cc of saline for 2 hours on postoperative days 1, 3, and 5 in 45 patients, with 70% reduction in the number of new tumors as compared with pretreatment recurrence rates. In these 3 studies, increased myelosuppression was not observed, indicating that thio-tepa can safely be given at these doses and dilutions in the perioperative period. A randomized prospective trial comparing a single instillation of 60 mg within 36 hours of transurethral resection with additional instillations at monthly intervals is currently being performed by the NBCCG.[83] Results are not yet available.

LONG-TERM PROPHYLAXIS

For long-term prophylaxis, thio-tepa has commonly been administered monthly at a dose of 30–60 mg in 30–60 ml of sterile water held for 2 hours (see table 4). Westcott[84] reduced recurrences to 8.3% when compared with a historical control group (75%). Controlled studies, however, have noted a more modest reduction in the number of patients with recurrence and in recurrence rates.[74,80,85,86] The EORTC,[86] in a large randomized controlled study using 30 mg thio-tepa in 30 ml water weekly for 4 weeks, then monthly for 11 months, noted significant reductions in recurrence rates for thio-tepa versus control (8.93 recurrences per 100 patient months of follow-up versus 5.41, respectively). The most important variables for prediction of recurrence were multiple tumors at entry, history of prior recurrence, and tumor size.

The NBCCG compared 30 mg or 60 mg monthly for 2 years in 43 patients compared with 47 untreated controls.[74] Both the control and treatment groups included patients who had responded completely to thio-tepa therapy for residual tumor. With these patients included, 66% of the treatment group were tumor-free at 12 months, compared with 40% of the control group. There was no difference in response between the 30 mg and 60 mg groups. The time to first recurrence was statistically longer in the prophylactic group. Interestingly,

Table 4. Thio-tepa Adjuvant and Prophylaxis: Controlled Studies

Investigator/reference	No. patients	Dose	% Recurring Control	% Recurring Treated
Westcott[84] 1965	12	60 mg in 60 ml weekly × 4, then monthly	75 (historical)	8.3
Pavone & Macaluso[63] 1971	94	60 mg in 60 ml weekly × 4, then monthly	60	23.4
Burnand[80] 1976	51	90 mg for 30 min. × 1 (adjuvant)	97	58
Byar & Blackard[85] 1977	88	60 mg in 60 ml weekly × 4, then monthly	60.4	47.4
Koontz[74] 1981	93	30 – 60 mg monthly × 22	60	34
Schulman (EORTC)[86] 1982	308	30 mg in 30 ml weekly × 4, then monthly × 11	8.93 rec/100 pt. mo. F/U	5.41 rec./100 pt. mo. F/U

patients treated successfully with thio-tepa for ablation of incompletely resected tumor who did not receive additional thio-tepa prophylaxis had fewer long-term recurrences (60% tumor-free at 12 months), implying a prolonged effect of ablative therapy in complete responders. At 48 months follow-up, 52% of the patients treated with 8 weeks of thio-tepa for tumor ablation and additional monthly prophylaxis were tumor-free, compared with 29% of patients who responded to thio-tepa but did not receive additional prophylactic therapy, 23% of patients who received prophylactic therapy only, and 13% of the control patients who never received thio-tepa on any schedule.[87] Progression to muscle invasion, prostatic urethral involvement, or metastases occurred in both treated and untreated groups with equal frequency, in 14/90 patients overall (16%). These events were not detectably inhibited by thio-tepa. Fourteen of 17 deaths (82%) in the prophylaxis group and 5/7 deaths (71%) in the control group were attributed to causes other than bladder cancer. Main toxicity consisted of irritative voiding symptoms, which occurred in 4.3% of the 30 mg group and 39.1% of the 60 mg group. Leukopenia (<3,000/mm) or thrombocytopenia (<100,000 platelets) occurred in 4.3%. Six patients stopped prophylactic therapy because of toxicity. No deaths were attributed to the use of thio-tepa.

In summary, thio-tepa is effective when administered intravesically for both eradication of residual tumors and prophylactic therapy. Thirty mg in 30 ml of sterile water held for 2 hours is as effective as a 60 mg dose, with less toxicity. Patients who respond completely seem to have extended long-term lower recurrence rates, which may be enhanced by additional monthly thio-tepa. The drug is safe for use in the immediate postoperative period for patients with limited resections and with reduced contact time. This agent remains the standard against which other regimens should be compared for efficacy.

Mitomycin-C

Mitomycin-C (MIT) is an antibiotic with antitumor, antibacterial, and antiviral activities. It acts as an alkylating agent, inhibiting DNA synthesis. This large molecule (mol wt 329) is minimally absorbed from the bladder, even in the presence of bladder mucosal injury.[88-90]

TREATMENT OF RESIDUAL TUMOR (TABLE 5)

Early trials for treatment of residual tumor after transurethral resection were conducted in Japan. Mishina[91] treated 50 patients with 20 mg in 20 ml sterile water 3 times weekly for 20 doses. At follow-up cystoscopy, 22/50 (44%) had complete disappearance of tumors and 16 (32%) showed reduction in size or number of tumors. A larger series by Mishina and Watanabe[92] confirmed these CR and PR rates. Harrison et al[93] treated 22 patients with a similar regimen, reporting 17 (77%) CR and 4 (18%) PR. In the United States, Bracken[94] evaluated dose ranges of 20–60 mg administered weekly for 8 weeks, noting a higher overall response rate with doses above 30 mg and CR rates of 33–64%.

Soloway[95] treated 68 patients with 30–40 mg weekly for 8 weeks, with 26 (38%) CR, 26 (38%) PR, and 16 (24%) failures. Criteria for CR included normal cystoscopy, normal bladder biopsy, and negative urine cytology. Partial response was defined as either a greater than 50% reduction in the amount of tumor or complete eradication of visible tumor but with persistent positive cytology. Complete response rates were similar for grade 1 (47%), grade 2 (27%), and grade 3 papillary tumors or carcinoma in situ (43%). Fourteen of 40 (35%) stage O (Ta) patients, 7/16 (43%) stage A (T1) patients, and 5/12 (41%) with carcinoma in situ responded completely. Of 39 patients who had recurrent tumor while under active treatment with thio-tepa, only 20% achieved CR, compared with 62% of patients who had not previously received thio-tepa. Similarly, Issel[96] treated 57 patients who failed thio-tepa treatment, with only 19% CR for patients who never responded to thio-tepa as opposed to 83% CR for patients who responded to prior thio-tepa with subsequent relapse. These data indicate that MIT benefits a relatively small number of patients who have failed thio-tepa by rigid criteria; this is possibly related to common mechanisms of action for these agents.

Soloway[97] reported follow-up recurrence and progression data for 54 patients who responded completely or partially to 8 weekly instillations of MIT. Following a response, these patients were given additional monthly MIT (40 mg) for 1 year. At 28 months mean follow-up, 12/27 (44%) complete responders developed a subsequent tumor, but only 2 (7%) developed muscle

Table 5. Mitomycin-C Treatment for Residual Tumor

Investigator/reference	Dose	No. patients	CR (%)	PR (%)	Overall % resp.
Mishina et al[91] 1975	20 mg/20 ml water 3 × weekly × 20	50	22 (44)	16 (32)	76
Mishina & Watanabe[92] 1979	20 mg/20 ml water 3 × weekly × 20	169	76 (45)	60 (36)	81
Bracken[94] 1980	20 mg/20 ml water	10	4 (40)	2 (20)	60
	25 mg/25 ml water	11	7 (64)	1 (9)	73
	30 mg/30 ml water	6	3 (50)	2 (33)	83
	40 mg/40 ml water	6	2 (33)	3 (50)	83
	60 mg/60 ml water	10	5 (50)	5 (50)	100
Harrison[93] 1983	20 mg/20 ml water 3 × weekly × 20	22	17 (77)	4 (18)	95
Issell[96] 1984	40 mg/40 ml water weekly × 8	57 (thio-tepa failure)	24 (42)	15 (26)	68
Koontz[151] 1984	40 mg/40 ml water weekly × 8	100 (thio-tepa failure)	46 (46)	—	—
Soloway[95] 1984	40 mg/40 ml weekly × 8	62	25 (39)	24 (39)	78
	30 mg/40 ml	6	1 (17)	2 (33)	50
Macfarlane[152] 1985	40 mg/40 ml weekly × 7	25	10 (43)	6 (27)	60
Heney[142] 1985	40 mg/40 ml weekly × 8	46	23 (50)	10 (22)	72

invasion requiring cystectomy. Two complete responders died of transitional cell carcinoma. On the other hand, 21/27 (78%) partial responders developed recurrence, 4 (15%) developed muscle invasive disease, and 8 (30%) required cystectomy. One patient died of transitional cell carcinoma. Thus, both recurrence and progression rates appear to be higher for patients who do not respond completely to induction therapy, but cancer-related deaths remain low.

TOXICITY

The side effects associated with MIT are primarily local, consisting of irritative voiding symptoms, dysuria, frequency, and urgency in up to one-third of cases.[91-98] These symptoms, generally mild, clear within several days. A skin reaction on the hands, genitalia, or both occurs in 4–15% of patients and may represent a contact dermatitis. Occasionally, a generalized rash may occur, possibly due to a generalized allergic phenomenon. Hematologic toxicity, manifested as mild leukopenia, anemia, or thrombocytopenia, occurs in approximately 2%. Bladder contracture, although rare, has been reported.[99] No mutagenesis has been noted clinically.

MITOMYCIN-C PROPHYLAXIS

Following demonstration of response for treatment of residual tumor, many investigators have studied the use of MIT for prophylaxis against new tumor formation[88,100-103] (see table 6). In short-term studies, the dose, dilution, and treatment schedules vary widely, with moderate reduction in recurrences. Fluchter et al[88] used MIT (20 mg in 40 ml saline) daily for 10 days postresection, observing 12% recurrences in 105 patients with average follow-up of 22 months, compared with 26% recurrences in an historical control group treated with transurethral resection alone and followed for an average 36 months.

Table 6. Mitomycin-C for Prophylaxis: Controlled Studies

Investigator/reference	No. patients	Dose	% Recurring Control	% Recurring Treatment	Follow-up
Fluchter et al[88] 1981	105	20 mg/40 ml saline daily × 10 days	26 (historical)	13	22.3 mo. treatment 36 mo. control
Devonec et al[100] 1983	26	40 mg/40 ml water daily × 10	*0.19 rec./pt. mo.	0.11 rec./pt. mo.	28.5 mo.
Niijima et al[101] 1983	139	20 mg/20 ml water twice weekly × 4 weeks	54.4 61.5	38.5 57.6	450 days 540 days
Schutz et al[102] 1984	54	30 mg prior to TUR, 20 mg 8 hours post-op, 20 mg weekly × 12, monthly × 9	*0.076 rec./pt. mo.	0.029 rec./pt. mo.	382 pt. mo.
Huland et al[103] 1984	85	20 mg/20 ml water q. 2 weeks × 1 year q. 4 weeks × 2 years	55.8	11.1	34 mo.

*Clinical course before mitomycin used as control.

Treated patients underwent repeated transurethral resection in the first 10 days, with repeat transurethral resection and a second 10-day course of MIT at 6 weeks. Devonec[100] used 40 mg in 40 ml water for 10 consecutive days starting 48 hours after transurethral resection in 26 evaluable patients, with reduction in recurrences per patient month of follow-up from .19 prior to therapy to 0.11 (median follow-up 28.5 months). Niijima[101] reported a randomized controlled study using 20 mg MIT in 40 cc distilled water twice weekly for 4 weeks. At 450 days, 38.5% of treatment group recurred versus 54.5% of controls. However, at 540 days of follow-up, 57.6% of patients receiving MIT had recurrent disease versus 61.5% of the control group, possibly indicating need for continued long-term prophylaxis.

Schutz,[102] who treated 54 patients with both preoperative and postoperative MIT using 30 mg 2 hours prior to transurethral resection, 20 mg 8 hours postresection and weekly for 12 weeks, then monthly for 9 months, reported a 60% reduction in the recurrence rate from .076 recurrences per month of follow-up to .029 recurrences per month after MIT. Patients were used as their own controls. Huland[103] et al conducted a randomized prospective study comparing no treatment following transurethral resection of stages Ta and T1 to a group receiving MIT. The dose was 20 mg in 20 ml sterile water beginning 4 weeks after transurethral resection and continued every 2 weeks for the first year and every 4 weeks for the second and third year. Patients with positive cytology were omitted from the study and patients with stage T1 lesions underwent repeat cystoscopy and biopsy to assure that no residual tumor was present prior to initiation of therapy. The groups were comparable in stage and grade distribution. With 31 patients in each group and mean follow-up of 30 months (range 12–48 months), recurrence rates were significantly less for the treated group versus controls: 0.37 recurrences per 100 patient months of follow-up versus 3.8 recurrences, respectively. Because of these impressive results, subsequent patients were entered into the treatment arm. Repeat analysis with 54 patients in the treatment arm at 34 months mean follow-up revealed that only 11.1% of treated patients suffered recurrence, compared with 55.8% of the control group. More important, 12 patients in the control group had muscle invasion or metastases, with 6 (19.4%) bladder cancer-related deaths. In contrast, the treated group had 2 patients with muscle invasion and 1 with metastases, with 1 bladder cancer-related death. Progressive disease in these patients occurred in the distal ureter or prostatic ducts, with no progression in noted bladder recurrences. This important study implies that when used as an intensive prophylactic regimen, MIT can modify the rates of progression and possibly improve survival. Side effects of MIT therapy were minimal in this series. No patients suffered myelosuppression. Four patients (7%) had chemical cystitis, with cessation of therapy in 2.

In summary, MIT is effective in eradicating residual tumor in 33–77% of patients at a dose of 40 mg weekly for 8 weeks or 20 mg 3 times per week for 20 doses. It may be marginally more effective than thio-tepa for treatment of residual disease and is effective in carcinoma in situ. Main toxicity has been rash; significant myelosuppression has not been observed. For prophylactic use, long-term, low-dose (20 mg) therapy has produced significant reductions in recurrence rates without cumulative toxicity. The principal drawback to this

drug is its high cost – approximately 6–8 times more than thio-tepa per instillation.

Doxorubicin

Doxorubicin (ADR), an alkylating agent, has been extensively studied in
Europe for both treatment of residual disease and prophylaxis. Absorption of
this large molecule from the bladder at doses of 10–100 mg with contact time
up to 3 hours is minimal.[76,104-107] Concentration of the drug is high in exophytic
papillary tumors, where it exerts its cytotoxic effect through inhibition of
nucleic acid synthesis or interactions at the cell surface membrane.[108]

TREATMENT OF RESIDUAL PAPILLARY TUMORS

In treatment of residual papillary tumors, the dose, dilution, contact time,
and treatment schedules have varied widely (see table 7). Doses range from
10–150 mg, usually at a concentration of 1–2 mg per ml. Concentrations
higher than 2 mg per ml regardless of dose appear to produce more severe local
toxicity. Banks[104] used 50 mg in 150 ml saline held for 1 hour and administered
monthly, with 8 CR in 13 patients (66%) and no toxicity. Fosberg[109] treated 7
T1 tumors with 80 mg in 50 ml saline held for 45 minutes monthly for 3–5
months, with 3 of 7 (42%) CR. Niijima,[110] who administered daily ADR at a

Table 7. Doxorubicin for Treatment of Residual Disease

Investigator/reference	Dose	No. patients	CR (%)	PR (%)	Overall % resp.
Banks et al[104] 1977	50 mg/150 ml saline monthly	13	8 (66)	5 (34)	100
Fosberg[109] 1978	80 mg/50 ml saline × 3–5 months	7	3 (42)	1 (14)	56
Niijima et al[110] 1978	20 mg/30 ml saline	9	—	—	55.6
	50 mg/30 ml saline	25	—	—	72
	60 mg/30 ml saline	46	—	—	73.9
Edsmyr et al[116] 1978	80 mg/100 ml saline monthly × 4 months	6 (CIS)	6 (100)	—	—
		30 (CIS)	20 (67)	—	—
Edsmyr, et al[111] 1980	80 mg/100 ml saline	23	10 (45)	5 (23)	68
Jakse et al[117] 1980	40–50 mg/20–40 ml monthly	15 (CIS)	10 (67)	—	—
Glashan, et al[118] 1981	50 mg/50 ml saline weekly × 6	17 (1° CIS)			88[1]
		38 (2° CIS)			76[2]
Pavone & Macaluso[112] 1982	50–150 mg	98	33 (34)	42 (43)	77
Lamm[113] 1983	Literature summary	521	198 (38)	182 (35)	73

[1]15 patients showed "marked improvement."
[2]29 patients showed "marked improvement."

dose of 20, 50, or 60 mg in 30 ml saline daily for 3 days with repeat treatment in 2–3 weeks, noted a 56%, 72%, and 74% overall response rate (PR + CR), respectively. Twenty-four of 80 (30%) patients experienced dysuria or urgency. Edsymr[111] treated 23 patients with stage T1 disease with monthly doses of 80 mg in 100 ml saline, held for 1 hour, noting 10/23 (45%) CR and minimal local toxicity. In a summary of several studies, Pavone-Macaluso,[112] at dose ranges of 50–150 mg during varying treatment schedules in 98 patients, noted a 34% CR rate and a 43% PR rate. Lamm[113] summarized 12 therapeutic studies with 521 patients, with an overall CR rate of 38% and PR rate of 35%.

PROPHYLACTIC TREATMENT

For prophylaxis, 50 mg in 50 ml of water or saline has been the most commonly used dose. In an efficacy versus toxicity study, a multicenter, uncontrolled European trial studied recurrence rates in 110 patients treated with both early and continued ADR following complete resection of all visible tumor.[114] The dose was 50 mg in 50 ml of saline given within 24 hours after transurethral resection, again on days 3 and 7, then weekly × 4 and monthly for 1 year. The 1-year recurrence rate was 39% (32/82 evaluable patients). At 2 to 3 years, 51% recurred. This regimen produced a 21.8% incidence of severe local side effects. Pavone-Macaluso[112] reported on 289 patients treated with 50 mg in 50 ml water or saline for 1 hour weekly for 4 weeks, then monthly for 1 year, with a 35% recurrence rate at 1 year, a cystitis rate of 16.6%, and 5% of patients stopping treatment because of toxicity. Abrams et al[115] reported lowered recurrence rates at 6-month follow-up cystoscopy with a single dose of 50 mg held for 30 minutes within 24 hours or resection; there were 8.3 tumors/patient prior to treatment versus 5.2 after ADR.

A randomized, controlled prospective study was performed by the EORTC and reported by Kurth et al.[68] Patients were treated with 50 mg ADR in 50 ml saline for 1 hour weekly for 1 month and then monthly thereafter for 1 year. There were 86 patients in the treated group and 69 patients in the control group treated with transurethral resection only. Mean follow-up was 11–12 months in both groups. Recurrence rate in terms of number of recurrences per 100 patient months of follow-up were 4.11 for the ADR group and 7.58 for the control group. The mean interval between recurrences (disease-free interval) was 24.3 months for the treatment group versus 13.2 months for the control group. These results show significant prolongation of the disease-free interval, reduction in the number of patients recurring, and the recurrence rate for ADR versus transurethral resection alone. Irritative symptoms were noted in 4% of patients. Systemic toxicity, such as allergic reaction, mild nausea, diarrhea, and vomiting, was noted in 5%. Neither leukopenia nor thrombocytopenia was seen in this study.

TREATMENT OF CARCINOMA IN SITU

Doxorubicin has been effective in the treatment of carcinoma in situ at doses of 40–80 mg administered weekly or monthly for up to 11 months. Edsmyr,[116] using 80 mg in 100 cc monthly for 4 months, noted 6 CR in 6 patients, with no side effects. A similar regimen in 30 patients with persistently positive cytologies produced 20 cytology remissions (67%) requiring 4 treatments for previously untreated carcinoma in situ and up to 11 monthly treatments for recurrent carcinoma in situ.[111] Jakse and Hofstadter[117] used 40–80 mg at a concentration of 2 mg per ml every 2–4 weeks, with 67% CR in 15 patients. Chemocystitis and hematuria were noted with this concentration. Glashan[118] used a dose of 50 mg in 50 ml saline held for 2 hours weekly for 6 weeks, noting 15 cytologic regressions in 17 patients with primary carcinoma in situ, "marked improvement" in bladder appearance in 20/22 patients with secondary carcinoma in situ with prior history of superficial tumors, and "marked improvement" in 9/16 patients with secondary carcinoma in situ associated with simultaneous superficial lesions.

BCG Immunotherapy

Nonspecific immune stimulation using BCG, although unsuccessful in other human tumor systems, has definite activity in superficial bladder cancer. Effectiveness of the vaccine depends on several factors, including ability of the host to react to mycobacteria antigens, small tumor load, and adequate numbers of living bacilli in close contact with tumor cells. Superficial bladder cancer fulfills these criteria. The mechanism of action remains unknown. BCG may exert its effect through a local inflammatory reaction that denudes mucosa, or responses may be secondary to the development of a systemic immune response to BCG antigens.[120-122] Shapiro[123] initially showed increases in circulating interferon after BCG instillation into animal bladders, but elevated levels in patients receiving intravesical BCG were not noted. Lamm[124] and Catalona[125] have correlated the conversion of cutaneous P.P.D. from negative to positive with bladder responses, although Herr[126] noted good responses in patients with persistently negative skin tests as well. The finding of noncaseating granulomas within bladder biopsy specimens following treatment correlates well with response.[124,125]

TREATMENT OF RESIDUAL DISEASE (TABLE 8)

Morales[127] reported the first clinical use of BCG in bladder cancer in 1976, treating 5 patients for prevention of recurrence and 4 for residual tumor. BCG was administered both intravesically (120 mg [Pasteur strain] in 50 ml saline for 2 hours) and intradermally (5 mg with a Heaf gun) weekly for 6 weeks. All patients responded, and subsequent follow-up revealed only 1 tumor recurrence in 41 patient months of follow-up, compared with 22 recurrences in 77 patient months prior to treatment. Five additional patients with metastatic disease had no response to treatment. Morales et al[128] treated 17 additional patients with residual tumor with the same regimen, with CR in 59%. Schellhammer[129] noted 71% CR in 24 patients without addition of intradermal BCG. DeKernion[130] treated 22 patients with Tice strain weekly for 8 weeks followed by monthly maintenance for 12 months, with 8 (36%) CR. Intradermal BCG was not used.

The most dramatic results have been obtained in carcinoma in situ, with or without associated papillary lesions. Morales[131] noted responses in 10/17 patients (60%) treated with 6 weekly intravesical doses of BCG with simultaneous intradermal injection. Herr and associates[132] compared transurethral resection alone with transurethral resection + BCG in 41 patients with carcinoma in situ associated with papillary superficial tumors. BCG-treated patients were given 6 weekly bladder instillations (120 mg Pasteur strain) with intradermal injection simultaneously. Complete response was defined by negative biopsy of any residual suspicious lesions, negative urine cytology, and distinct improvement in the severity of voiding complaints by 3–6 months after treatment. Cystoscopy was repeated every 3 months. With mean follow-up of 18 months, 11/17 (65%) patients in the transurethral resection + BCG group had no clinical or pathological evidence of carcinoma in situ, compared with only 2/24 (8%) patients in the transurethral resection alone group. Three of the BCG-treated patients (17%) required cystectomy 12–18 months after BCG, compared with 12/24 (50%) control patients.

Herr[133] reported additional experience with BCG in carcinoma in situ associated with papillary tumors in 47 patients. One-half of the group received intravesical BCG (120 mg Pasteur strain in 50 ml saline) weekly for 6 weeks, while the other half received both intradermal injections and bladder instillations. Thirty-four patients (72%) were free of disease after 2+ years (median 36 months, range 24–60 months), 15 of 23 (65%) after intravesical and

Table 8. BCG for Treatment of Residual Disease

Investigator/reference	Strain	Dose	No. patients	CR (%)	PR (%)	Follow-up
Morales et al[127] 1976	Pasteur	120 mg/50 ml saline + 5 mg I.D. weekly × 6	4	4 (100)		One rec. in 47 mo.
Morales et al[128]	Pasteur	120 mg/50 ml saline + 5 mg I.D. weekly × 6	17	10 (59)		Mean F/U 19 mo.
Herr[132] 1983	Pasteur	120 mg/50 ml saline weekly × 6	17 (CIS) 24 (control)	11 (65) 2 (8)		
Schellhammer[129] 1984	Pasteur	120 mg/50 ml saline weekly × 6	24	17 (75)		
Herr[133] 1984	Pasteur	120 mg + 5 mg I.D. weekly × 6	23 (CIS)	15 (65)		Median 45 mo.
		120 mg weekly × 6 (no intradermal)	24 (CIS)	19 (79)		Median 30 mo.
Morales et al[153] 1984	Pasteur	120 mg/50 ml saline + 5 mg I.D. weekly × 6	23	14 (60)		Mean F/U 51 mo.
DeKernion et al[130] 1985	Tice	2–8 × 10^8 organisms/ 60 ml saline weekly × 8, then monthly × 12	22 19 (CIS)	8 (36) 13 (68)	5 (23) 3 (16)	
Brosman[131] 1985	Tice	2–8 × 10^8/60 ml saline weekly × 12, q. 2 weeks × 6, monthly × 3, q. 3 mo. × 5	33 (CIS)	31 (94)		

intradermal BCG, and 19/24 (79%) with intravesical BCG alone. This study provides evidence that both long-term remission of carcinoma in situ and delay in progression may be possible with intravesical BCG alone. Brosman[134] treated 33 patients with biopsy-proven carcinoma in situ with an intensive regimen using Tice strain BCG ($2-8 \times 10^8$ colony-forming units in 60 ml saline) intravesically weekly for 12 consecutive weeks. If response was complete, maintenance therapy was begun with biweekly BCG for 6 doses, then monthly for 18 months. If follow-up cystoscopy or urine cytology was not negative, weekly treatments continued for an additional 6–12 weeks until biopsies were negative. Eighteen of 27 evaluable patients became tumor-free after 12 weeks of therapy. An additional 6 patients were free of tumor after 18 weeks of therapy, and 3 patients became tumor-free after 24 weeks of therapy. Overall, 31/33 patients (94%) were rendered tumor-free. No patient received intradermal BCG. Average followup was 4.16 years. Recurrences were seen in four of 31 patients (13%). One patient died of bladder cancer.

BCG FOR PROPHYLAXIS

Randomized prospective trials of BCG for prophylaxis of new tumor formation when compared with transurethral resection alone have been reported. Camacho and associates[135] compared recurrence rates in 51 patients randomized to transurethral resection alone or transurethral resection + BCG (Pasteur strain, 120 mg in 50 ml saline) weekly for 6 weeks, held for 2 hours, with simultaneous intradermal administration. All gross tumor was removed from the bladder prior to treatment. The groups were comparable for grade and stage. Prior to therapy, the rates of tumor formation (tumors per patient month of follow-up) in the BCG and control groups were 3.6 and 2.97, respectively. Following therapy, the BCG group had a recurrence rate of 0.75 tumors per patient month compared with 2.37 for the control group, a statistically significant difference. Lamm and associates,[136] using a similar schedule, treated 57 patients with either transurethral resection plus BCG or transurethral resection alone. Of 54 evaluable patients, 13/26 (50%) control patients and 6/28 (21%) treated patients experienced recurrence in 3–30 months. At 30 months median follow-up (range 3–60 months), the mean interval to recurrence was 24 months in the control group and 48 months in the BCG group.

Brosman[137] used the Tice strain of BCG (6×10^8 organisms in 60 ml saline) prophylactically weekly for 6 weeks, every 2 weeks for 6 treatments, then monthly for 21 months without intradermal injection. Twenty-five patients who completed this rigorous BCG schedule had no evidence of recurrence with a minimum follow-up of 24 months. Eleven patients (28%) suffered significant toxicity. One refused therapy after 6 weekly instillations because of severe bladder irritability. Six patients had prolonged episodes of fever, chills, anorexia, malaise, and bladder irritability, but improved on treatment with isoniazid. Four patients required hospitalization and triple-drug antituberculin therapy. These patients had abnormal liver function studies and evidence of pulmonary infection. Thirteen of 16 patients converted P.P.D. skin test to positive after intravesical BCG alone. This series was recently expanded and updated, with 53 patients in the prophylactic group followed from 6–15 months (mean 21 months).[138] Four of 53 patients (8%) have shown recurrent tumors. Although these excellent results indicate a cumulative therapeutic effect with an intense regimen, the toxicity has been high.

The role of maintenance therapy with BCG following complete remission of residual tumor or for prophylaxis remains unclear. Huffman and associates[139] noted no advantage to maintenance BCG therapy in a controlled study. On the other hand, Lamm has demonstrated increased protection by repeated administration of BCG in an animal model.[140] Further clinical trials with and without maintenance therapy are necessary.

TOXICITY

Irritative symptoms are the most commonly encountered toxicity.[141] The most common are dysuria (91%), frequency (90%), hematuria (46%), transient fever (24%), malaise (18%), nausea (8%), and chills (8%). These are generally mild, self-limiting, and well tolerated.

Comparative Studies

Few prospective randomized studies with appropriate stratification factors and long-term follow-up comparing these agents have been reported. Such studies are necessary to determine the most effective agent for intravesical use.

The NBCCG studied 2 groups to compare the efficacy of thio-tepa versus MIT for treatment of residual disease.[142] Patients were stratified by grade and stage. A total of 156 patients were accessioned, including 34 with papilloma, 56 with carcinoma in situ only, and 10 with carcinoma in situ and papillary tumors. These patients were equally distributed in both groups. Complete response criteria included negative cystoscopy, negative cytology, and negative biopsy. Analysis of 88 patients who received 8 weekly instillations of thio-tepa (60 mg in 60 ml water) or MIT (40 mg in 40 ml water) showed a CR rate of 43% in patients treated with thio-tepa and 50% patients given MIT. Mild leukopenia occurred in 14% of the thio-tepa patients and anemia in 9%. Fifteen percent of the MIT patients had rash, 4% anemia, and 2% mile leukopenia.

Randomized studies comparing thio-tepa with MIT for prophylaxis have shown no significant differences in recurrence rates. Zincke and colleagues[143] treated 63 patients with disease confined to the mucosa (stage Ta or CIS) with either 60 mg thio-tepa in 60 ml water or with MIT (40 mg in 40 ml water), beginning shortly after transurethral resection, then every 2 weeks for 3 months, and monthly for an additional 6 months. Seven of 31 (22%) patients given thio-tepa developed a subsequent tumor, compared with 9/32 (28%) treated with MIT (mean follow-up 14 months). No differences in actuarial progression rates at 3 months and 12 months were noted. Flanigan et al[144] treated 40 patients prophylactically with either thio-tepa (60 mg in 60 ml) or MIT (40 mg in 40 ml) weekly for 8 weeks, then monthly for 22 cycles. There was 1 recurrence in 220 patient months of follow-up in 15 thio-tepa patients and 4 recurrences in 337 patient months of follow-up in 25 MIT-treated patients. No significant difference between the 2 groups was seen. Seven patients could not tolerate MIT, primarily because of cutaneous reaction, and were changed to thio-tepa.

Zincke et al[145] compared thio-tepa (60 mg) with ADR (50 mg in 60 ml water) for prophylaxis following transurethral resection of all obvious tumor, with instillation immediately after transurethral resection and held 25–30 minutes. A control group received sterile water only. Approximately half of the patients in each of the treatment arm received subsequent thio-tepa every 10–14 days. All treatment groups, whether immediate treatment only or immediate treatment plus delayed treatment, showed significant reductions in rates of new occurrence of bladder tumor compared with placebo, but showed no differences when compared with one another. This implies that a single dose of ADR or thio-tepa in the immediate postoperative period may be as effective as a more intensive regimen, a finding reported by others as well.[80,115]

The EORTC[146] compared thio-tepa (50 mg) with ADR (50 mg) in a prophylactic study for stage TIS, Ta, and T1 tumors. Treatment commenced within 14 days of tumor ablation, with 4 weekly instillations followed by 11 monthly instillations. With 328 patients entered, there were no significant differences in disease-free interval or recurrence rate between thio-tepa and ADR.

Two studies have shown BCG to be superior to thio-tepa when used for prophylaxis. Brosman[137] randomized 49 patients to receive thio-tepa (60 mg in 60 ml water) or Tice strain BCG 6×10^8 organisms given in an intensive regimen of weekly instillations for 6 weeks, every 2 weeks for 6 treatments, then monthly for 21 months. Intradermal BCG was not used. At 21 months mean follow-up, no patients had recurrence in the BCG-treated group, while 9/19 thio-tepa patients (40%) developed recurrent tumors. Netto and Lemos[147] treated 26 patients with either thio-tepa (60 mg in 60 ml saline) or oral BCG, beginning 2 days after tumor resection, then daily for 7 days, monthly for 3 months, every third month for 1 year, twice yearly for 2 years, and yearly for 2 years. At 30–39 months median follow-up, the statistical recurrence rate was significantly lower for BCG compared with either controls or thio-tepa. Thio-tepa was slightly more effective than no treatment. This interesting study is the only reported use of oral BCG for prophylaxis.

Lamm and associates[148] reported preliminary results of a Southwest Oncology Group study comparing BCG with ADR for prophylaxis. BCG (120 mg Connaught) was given intravesically and percutaneously weekly for 6 weeks, at 3 months, at 6 months and every 6 months thereafter. The ADR dose was 50 mg intravesically weekly for 4 weeks and then monthly for 1 year. Twelve of 52 patients (23%) receiving BCG developed tumor recurrence, compared with 34/52 patients (65%) receiving ADR (median follow-up 6 months).

The above studies indicate that for treatment of residual disease, MIT is not more effective than thio-tepa. Thio-tepa, MIT, and ADR have equal efficacy in comparative prophylaxis trials, whereas BCG appears to be clearly superior to thio-tepa or ADR. BCG is the most effective agent for treatment of carcinoma in situ. All 4 agents are superior to transurethral resection alone.

Future Considerations

Randomized prospective studies comparing these commonly used agents with one another in varying dose schedules with and without maintenance therapy in order to determine optimal dose and timing are now under way. The simultaneous or sequential administration of multiple intravesical agents, similar to combination chemotherapy for I.V. use, needs to be explored.[149] New agents, such as interferon, have produced regressions in carcinoma in situ and must be tested in comparative trials.[150] In vivo or in vitro techniques of tissue culturing may help to determine the best drugs for an individual patient, correlating with clinical response. Improved biochemical parameters to predict invasion and metastases in superficial bladder cancer may allow the identification of high-risk groups who should not undergo intensive intravesical therapy but rather have immediate bladder removal.

The impact on short-term control of superficial disease by intravesical chemotherapy has been well documented. The long-term effect of these treatments on progression rates to muscle invasion or metastases and, ultimately, survival from this disease remains less clear.

41

COMBINATION CHEMOTHERAPY AND
INFUSIONAL SCHEDULES

Jacob J. Lokich, M.D.

APPLYING THE PRINCIPLES FOR combining multiple drugs in cancer chemo-therapy is unique in infusional delivery systems. The rationale for the use of multiple drugs has been based upon effecting multiple metabolic processes within the tumor cell to increase the likelihood of lethal damage and to prevent the early emergence of resistant cell lines. The principles involve using noncross-resistant agents and agents that do not overlap in terms of host toxicities. The use of multiple agents has had a substantial impact on response rates, particularly in the treatment of acute leukemia, Hodgkin's disease and non-Hodgkin's lymphoma, and testicular cancer.

The standard form of chemotherapy today is the use of multiple agents simultaneously on a bolus schedule. Many of the standard combination chemotherapy regimens (see table 1) have not necessarily been studied in the context of prospective comparative trials with single-agent therapy. In fact, the combined simultaneous use of multiple agents as opposed to sequential application of the individual agents may not be advantageous in terms of survival, although response rates are substantially higher when multiple agents are delivered simultaneously.

Considering the number of chemotherapeutic agents for cancer, the potential number of combinations of drugs that could be administered is enormous. Most of the standard regimens involve 2 or 3 agents, and as the number of potentially active drugs is expanded, as is the case for very few tumors, the combined application of 6 or even 8 drugs may be evoked. Two special types of combination chemotherapy are biochemical modulation and the use of alternating noncross-resistant drugs based on the Goldie Coldman hypothesis (see table 2). The Goldie Coldman hypothesis suggests that the delivery of alternating noncross-resistant regimens containing multiple drugs will minimize the likelihood of development of tumor cell resistance or isolation of the resistant clone.[1] Tumor cell resistance remains a substantial problem in the use of chemotherapy for cancer in that even in patients who achieve a complete clinical response, the likelihood of recurrence and unlikelihood of cure are high.

Biochemical modulation refers to the interaction of 2 chemotherapeutic substances not necessarily in the context in which each agent induces lethal cell damage, but rather that one agent facilitates or enhances the effectiveness of the other agent. In this setting, the use of a relatively ineffective agent in terms of single-agent activity may have a meaningful impact on the tumor when employed with a second agent. This concept is substantially different from the usual approach to combination chemotherapy, in which each of the component drugs in a combination should demonstrate some intrinsic single-agent activity.

Table 1. Standard Combination Chemotherapy Bolus Regimens for Solid Tumors

Tumor	Regimen
Breast	CMF, CAF
Lung	
Small-cell	ACE
Nonsmall-cell	CAP
Gastric	FAMi
Pancreas	S MiF
Testicular	VPB
Ovarian	CHAP, CAP

C = cyclophosphamide; M = methotrexate; F = 5-fluorouracil; A = Adriamycin;
E = etoposide; P = cisplatin; Mi = mitomycin-C; V = vinblastine; B = bleomycin;
H = hexamethylmelamine; S = streptozotocin

Table 2. Combination Chemotherapy and Alternating Noncross-Resistant (Goldie-Coldman) Agents or Biochemical Modulation

	Drug regimen
Goldie Coldman principle	
Small-cell lung cancer	CAV alternating MEP
Ovarian	CAP alternating TM
Biochemical modulation	
Breast cancer	5-FU and MTX
Colon cancer	5-FU and PALA
	5-FU and LCV
	5-FU and thymidine
Leukemia	Ara-C and hydroxyurea

Tactics of Combination Chemotherapy

The pragmatic issues of employing multiple agents simultaneously in bolus schedules have been developed over the past 2 decades. Individually active agents are delivered on a bolus schedule intermittently on a day 1 and 14 or a day 1 and 8 schedule, with cycles repeated at 28-day intervals. For component agents that have overlapping toxicities, such as dose-limiting marrow suppression, the optimal single-agent dose is proportionately reduced in keeping with the number of drugs that share that toxicity.

In developing combination chemotherapy in which an infusion schedule to deliver the drug for 24 hours or more is planned, there are distinctive practical issues, depending on the type of tactic employed. Three tactical approaches to the infusion schedule for combination chemotherapy may be considered:

1. An infusion schedule may be employed for only one of the component agents, and the other agents may be administered on the standard bolus regimen. Because the infusion schedule may be associated with an altered toxicity, the interdigitation of the component drugs may behave differently, permitting dose adjustments.

2. The component agents may be all infused simultaneously through use of multiple access sites and multiple infusion devices. This method is clearly unwieldly and not suitable for outpatient delivery of chemotherapy. For the most part, the constraints are related to technology, but the recent development of double-lumen venous access ports, implanted devices, miniaturized portable pumps, and multiple chambers could permit this method to be used in the future.

3. Drug admixtures may be infused simultaneously through a single site. The compatibility of a number of 2-drug combinations has been demonstrated, and preliminary clinical trials have been carried out for combinations that involve doxorubicin (ADR)–based admixtures and a 5-flourouracil (5-FU)-based admixture.

The following review of the first and third methods of delivering continuous infusion chemotherapy is based on ongoing clinical trials.

Combination Chemotherapy with Single-Agent Infusions

The infusion schedule delivery in combination chemotherapy has been employed only rarely or not at all in the more responsive solid tumors and hematologic malignancies, but it is becoming an increasingly common application against generally poorly responsive tumors or relatively uncommon tumors.

A selected summary of trials in which one or more of the agents of a combination is delivered on a continuous infusion schedule is presented in table 3. Most experience has been with 5-FU 2-drug combinations and with durations of infusion of 5 days or less. The combination of 5-FU and cisplatin (DDP) has been particularly effective in head and neck cancer and esophageal cancer. One study by Kish et al was a prospective randomized trial of 5-FU delivered as a bolus or as an infusion with DDP as a bolus.[2] Statistically, response rates in head and neck cancer were significantly higher in the group receiving the infusion schedule for 5-FU. In esophageal cancer, a study reported by Cary et al yielded a $> 50\%$ response rate, with approximately 40% of patients achieving a complete response.[3]

The same combination of 5-FU and DDP has been administered to patients with nonsmall-cell lung cancer, with the DDP delivered on a continuous infusion schedule for 24 hours only in conjunction with a 5-day continuous infusion of 5-FU. A response rate of 40% was achieved in a preliminary report by Hein et al.[4]

Five-day infusion of 5-FU in conjunction with bolus mitomycin-C (MIT) has similarly been applied in esophageal cancer, anal cancer, and colon cancer.[5,6,7] The addition of MIT to 5-FU infusions in esophageal and anal cancer may not be essential in that one study of infusional 5-FU with bolus MIT in the anus indicated that MIT did not contribute to the effectiveness of the combination.[8] In colon cancer, there has been no reported advantages of infusional 5-FU and MIT by bolus (or methyl CCNU replacing MIT) over standard bolus 5-FU in prospective trials when survival was the primary determinant of effectiveness. Response rates are somewhat higher with the combination, however.

Vinblastine (VLB) as a single-agent infusion for 5 days has demonstrated activity in advanced breast cancer as second- and third-line therapy. This has prompted the evaluation of the infusion schedule in combination with bolus DDP in nonsmall-cell lung cancer. A series of 6 studies of the VLB-DDP combination have been reported and summarized by Huberman et al.[9] A response rate of 35% was achieved for the infusion schedule, but compared to other phase 2 trials in which VLB is delivered as a bolus, no advantage was clearly discernible for the infusion schedule. Because of the heterogeneity of the study populations, however, it would be necessary to evaluate infusional versus bolus VLB in a comparative trial prospectively.

Bleomycin (BLM) may be administered either as a bolus or an infusion as part of the standard VPB program for testicular cancer. With some evidence of

Table 3. Combinations for which 1 Agent Is Generally Infused for 24 Hours or More

Combination	Infusion drug/dose rate	Tumor
5-fluorouracil + cisplatin	5-FU 1,000 mg/M²/d × 5	Head and neck, esophagus
5-fluorouracil + cisplatin	5-FU 900 mg/M²/d × 5 d CDDP 120 mg/M² over 24 h	Nonsmall-cell lung
5-fluorouracil + mitomycin C	Same	Esophagus, anus, colon
5-fluorouracil + methotrexate	5-FU 62.5 mg/M²/h × 24 h MTX 15 mg/M²/h × 36 h	Phase 1
Vinblastine + cisplatin	VLB 1.5 mg/M²/d × 5 d	Nonsmall-cell lung
Bleomycin + VLB + CDDP	BLM 10 – 15 U/M²/d × 5 – 7 d	Testicular
Cisplatin + cyclophosphamide	Cisplatin 20 mg/M²/d × 5 d	Ovarian
Adriamycin + 5-FU + CTX	ADR 15 mg/M²/d × 4 d	Breast

a decrease in pulmonary toxicity at the clinical level, and with improved tumor cell kill in experimental systems, the infusional delivery of BLM seems justified. However, logistical and cost considerations may dictate the use of bolus delivery. No prospective comparative trials have been performed to clarify any potential advantage for infusion delivery of this agent.

DDP has been delivered on an infusion schedule for 5 days or longer in many phase 1 and phase 2 studies. The combination of DDP and cyclophosphamide (CTX) in ovarian cancer yields response rates of >60% employing the bolus schedule.[10,11] In a trial by Lokich et al, DDP delivered as an infusion for 5 days in conjunction with oral daily CTX had a response rate of 62%. This is comparable to the response rate reported in the bolus delivery trials.[12] Although the response rates are comparable and adverse gastrointestinal effects are ameliorated by the infusion of DDP, peripheral neuropathy and DDP-related anemia appeared to be accentuated on the infusion schedule.

A common first-line regimen for treating advanced breast cancer involves a 3-drug regimen of 5-FU, ADR, and CTX (FAC). In studies reported by Benjamin et al, this 3-drug combination delivered on a bolus schedule achieves responses of 65–75%.[13] Subsequent reports of the same regimen with ADR administered as a 96-hour infusion yielded comparable response rates.[14] Although these consecutive studies do not represent prospective randomized comparisons of the infusion and bolus schedule, they were nonetheless performed at a single institution. The infusion schedule for ADR resulted in less G.I. toxicity and chronic cardiac toxicity; in addition, response and duration of response rates were comparable, with more than 100 patients on the study.

A number of "standard" combination chemotherapy regimens have not incorporated an infusion schedule for any of the component drugs. These standard regimens include CTX, methotrexate (MTX) and 5-FU (CMF) for breast cancer; 5-FU, ADR, and MIT (FAM) for gastric carcinoma; and ADR, CTX, and etoposide (VP-16) (ACE) for nonsmall-cell lung cancer. For the hematologic malignancies, standard combinations include MOPP (nitrogen mustard, oncovin, procarbazine, and prednisone); ABVD (ADR, BLM, VLB, and DTIC); and CHOP (CTX, ADR, oncovin, and prednisone). MOPP would not lend itself to an infusional system of delivery because of the instability of nitrogen mustard following reconstitution. In addition, the procarbazine and prednisone are administered orally, but if these 2 agents are administered on a divided daily dose over 14 days, a continuous exposure comparable to that of continuous infusion is achieved.

Table 4 summarizes these 5 combination regimens involving 3 or more drugs and the usual standard bolus dose schedule. A possible infusion dose schedule for each of the component drugs is indicated as well, although with one exception, no pilot studies have been reported to date in which the infusion schedule for any component drug has been employed. ACE (ADR, CTX, and VP-16) has become one of the standard first-line regimens for small-cell lung cancer. ADR could be administered as a 5-day infusion, as also could CTX. The advantage of the infusion schedule for VP-16 has not been demonstrated, although in a single prospective comparative trial of the infusion versus the bolus schedule in advanced breast cancer, activity was demonstrated for this agent on an infusion schedule.[15] In one trial of ACE in SCCL, VP-16 was administered as a 5-day infusion without improving the effectiveness of the regimen compared to other reports of bolus delivery.[16]

5-FU, ADR, and MIT (FAM) has become a standard regimen in gastric cancer, although prospective comparative trials have failed to demonstrate a superiority for this 3-drug bolus regimen over 5-FU alone.[17] Each of the component agents can be delivered as an infusion, although MIT is somewhat less stable in solution over time than the other 2 components.

CTX, MTX, and 5-FU (CMF) is the standard treatment not only for advanced breast cancer but also for adjuvant treatment of primary breast cancer. Bolus schedules for each of the component drugs are variable, however, in some instances involving weekly induction periods of 4–6 weeks; at the other end of the spectrum, all 3 drugs are administered at 21–day intervals. The most common regimen is a day 1 and 8 schedule with CTX administered orally for 14 days. The possibility of an infusion delivery system for MTX and 5-FU is particularly intriguing. Experimental studies have demonstrated that MTX may facilitate incorporation of 5-FU, resulting in greater tumor cell kill. A phase 1 study of MTX administered as a 36-hour infusion, overlapping with 5-FU administered as a 24-hour infusion at hour 12, indicated that the regimen was feasible and was associated with clinical tumor responses.[18] The potential for interdigitating the infusions of the 2 antimetabolites in a rational sequence in conjunction with CTX has some appeal, but no clinical trials of this regimen have been initiated.

Both ABVD and CHOP are standard regimens employed in the treatment of Hodgkin's disease and non-Hodgkin's lymphoma, respectively. Both regimens are associated with a substantial response rate and potential cure rate in these

Table 4. Standard Combinations that Potentially Could Be Delivered with an Infusion for One or More Components

Combination	Bolus dose schedule		Infusion dose schedule*
ACE	A	50 mg/M^2/dl	15 mg/M^2/d $\times$ 5
	C	500 – 750 mg/M^2/dl	150 mg/M^2/d $\times$ 5
	E	100 – 150 mg/M^2/d $\times$ 3	60 mg/M^2/d $\times$ 5
FAM	5-FU	500 mg/M^2/dl,8,28,35	1,000 mg/M^2/d $\times$ 5
	A	30 mg/M^2/dl,8,28,35	15 mg/M^2/d $\times$ 5
	Mi	10 mg/M^2/dl,42	3 mg/M^2/d $\times$ 5
CMF	C	400 – 600 mg/M^2/dl,8	150 mg/M^2/d $\times$ 5
	M	40 – 60 mg/M^2/dl,8	1.0 mg/M^2/d $\times$ 5
	F	400 – 600 mg/M^2/dl,8	1,000 mg/M^2/d $\times$ 5
ABVD	A	30 mg/M^2/dl,14	15 mg/M^2/d $\times$ 5
	B	10 mg/M^2/dl,14	15 mg/M^2/d $\times$ 5
	V	5 mg/M^2/dl,14	1.5 mg/M^2/d $\times$ 5
	DTIC	250 mg/M^2/dl,14	—
CHOP	C	1,000 mg/M^2/dl	150 mg/M^2/d $\times$ 5
	A	50 mg/M^2/dl	15 mg/M^2/d $\times$ 5
	O	1.4 mg/M^2/dl	1.0 mg/M^2/d $\times$ 5

*No established pilot studies reported; potential programs in which one or more of component agents could be administered as continuous infusion

diseases. Possibly for these reasons, there has been reluctance to investigate an infusion schedule for the component drugs. Nonetheless, as indicated in table 4, a number of the component drugs lend themselves to an infusion schedule, and the possibilities and potential usefulness of the infusion schedule in these regimens remain an open question.

Combination Chemotherapy Using Drug Admixtures

Drug-drug interactions both in vitro and in vivo are common phenomena. In vitro mixing of 2 agents may result in alterations of the individual drugs or creation of a new chemical moiety. Cancer chemotherapeutic agents are generally reconstituted with inert diluents and administered as a bolus or an infusion with a flush of the I.V. catheter between drug administrations. The well-known incompatibility of ADR with heparin, which results in drug precipitation, has reinforced concerns regarding drug admixtures. This is particularly true with cancer chemotherapeutic agents, which are often classified as highly reactive, unstable compounds prone to interact with additive agents. The scarcity of studies of drug compatibility for cancer chemotherapeutic agents is related to the fact that chemotherapy is traditionally delivered on a bolus schedule. However, isolated reports of clinical trials employing cancer chemotherapeutic drugs delivered on an infusion schedule in multidrug admixture solutions have appeared.

ADR has been the agent most commonly employed (see table 5). This agent is stable in solution for up to 14 days, with a less than 10% degradation of the parent compound over that time.[19] Four clinical trials in which ADR was admixed with vincristine (VCR),[20] CTX,[21] VLB,[21] or DTIC[22] have been reported. The compatibility and stability data for admixtures of ADR-VCR or ADR-DTIC have not been reported in detail. For the other ADR-containing admixtures, several studies have established that ADR is stable and compatible in solution for a minimum of 14 days with CTX and VLB. The additive agents are stable in solution for 6 and 7 days, respectively.[21,23] The compatibility of ADR with DDP

Table 5. Reported Infusional Admixture Studies

Combination	Dose rate	Tumor category
Adriamycin + vincristine	$10-15$ mg/M^2/d $\times$ 4 d 1.0 mg/M^2/d $\times$ 4 d	Multiple myeloma
Adriamycin + cyclophosphamide	3 mg/M^2/d $\times$ 14 d 50 mg/M^2/d $\times$ 14 d	Mixed phase I
Adriamycin + vinblastine	3 mg/M^2/d $\times$ 14 d 0.5 mg/M^2/d $\times$ 14 d	Mixed phase I
Adriamycin + DTIC	15 mg/M^2/d $\times$ 4 d 250 mg/M^2/d $\times$ 4 d	Sarcoma
5-fluorouracil + methotrexate	300 mg/M^2/d $\times$ 28 d 0.75 mg/M^2/d $\times$ 14 d	Gastrointestinal

has been studied, and ADR is stable in the admixture.[24] DDP was not evaluated, however.

In a study of 52 patients treated with either ADR-CTX or ADR-VLB delivered as a continuous infusion for protracted intervals, dose-limiting toxicity was leukopenia.[21] Tumor responses were observed in 6/13 breast cancer patients; 2/2 hepatoma; and 2/4 soft tissue sarcoma. The contribution of the agent added to ADR is unclear in that responses were observed exclusively in tumors known to be responsive to ADR.

The admixture of 5-FU and MTX is particularly stable, with neither drug degrading over a period of 28 days.[25] This combination of agents is of special interest because of the emerging concept of biochemical modulation, in which MTX represents the modulating agent increasing the incorporation of 5-FU into DNA and RNA. In a phase 1 study of protracted infusion 5-FU admixed with MTX, dose-limiting toxicity for the infusion was related to the MTX component,[26] manifested as thrombocytopenia and stomatitis as well as chemical hepatitis. The optimal dose and schedule for a protracted infusion was 5-FU (300 mg/m^2/day) administered for 28 days combined with MTX (0.75 mg/m^2/day) for the first 14 days. The staggered schedule for the MTX was based upon the development of dose-limiting toxicity that was unaffected by the continuation of 5-FU while interrupting the MTX infusion. Tumor responses were observed in this phase 1 study in both esophageal and colon cancer.

The use of admixtures to develop multiple-agent infusions has a potentially important role in cancer chemotherapy. There are a number of other admixtures for which compatibility studies are pending and which may represent important areas of exploration (see table 6). DDP-based combinations are of particular appeal in that this agent has particular pharmacologic and toxologic rationale for administration by the infusion schedule. DDP combined with ADR would bring together 2 agents with a broad spectrum of activity. 5-FU and DDP is a combination being applied in the treatment of lung cancer, head and neck cancer, esophageal cancer, and other tumors, and extensive experience in short-term infusion of each agent individually has accumulated. CTX-DDP is a combination particularly applied in the treatment of ovarian cancer and could be explored in lung cancer as well as in lymphomas.

Three-drug admixtures would appear to be feasible, inasmuch as 2-drug admixtures have had a remarkable track record for compatibility. The 3-drug

Table 6. Potential Chemotherapy Admixtures for which Stability and Compatibility Studies Are Pending

2-drug admixtures	
Adriamycin + cisplatin	
5-fluorouracil + cisplatin	
Cyclophosphamide + cisplatin	
3-drug admixtures	
CMF	Cyclophosphamide, methotrexate, 5-fluorouracil
CAP	Cyclophosphamide, Adriamycin, cisplatin
CAV	Cyclophosphamide, Adriamycin, vinblastine
FAM	Fluorouracil, Adriamycin, mitomycin-C.

admixtures generally are based on the addition of an alkylating agent. This agent may be administered as an I.V. infusing agent or, alternatively, one may emulate an infusion by oral administration. Other alkylating agents such as thio-tepa may also come to be more useful on an infusion schedule.

Summary

In addition to increasing the response rates to cancer chemotherapy, combination chemotherapy may prevent the development of tumor cell resistance. Infusional chemotherapy, particularly for protracted periods with single agents, theoretically may cultivate the development of tumor cell resistance similar to bacteria resistance to antibiotics. Therefore, the development of strategies to employ multiple agents on an infusion schedule may be important.

Dose-limiting toxicity for the infusion schedule of single agents is distinctive from bolus delivery, and the absence of overlapping toxicity may accentuate and augment the capability of combining agents. Specifically, the lack of dose-limiting marrow suppression for most drugs delivered as an infusion may permit the use of a maximal dose. This possibility, is not uniform, however, as evidenced by the combination of MTX and 5-FU, in which the thrombocytopenia induced by MTX limits employing an optimal dose in combination with 5-FU.

42

CONTINUOUS INFUSION ANTIBIOTIC THERAPY FOR NEUTROPENIC PATIENTS

Gerald P. Bodey, M.D.

THE SCHEDULE OF ANTIBIOTIC administration has not been considered to be an important consideration in the therapy of most infections. Usually, antibiotic schedules have been selected rather arbitrarily and often as a matter of convenience. The serum half-life and serum concentrations have had some impact on the selection of conventional dosage schedules, but few clinical studies have addressed the issue of the optimum dosage schedule. Attention has been focused on dosage schedule primarily for those infections in which perfusion of antibiotic to the site of infection is a concern, as in meningitis and large abscesses. Whether continuous or intermittent therapy is superior was a subject of controversy in the management of meningitis for many years. Because most antibiotics do not freely permeate the blood/brain barrier, at issue was the question of how to maximize the concentration of antibiotic in the CSF. The current consensus is that intermittent injections provide adequate CSF concentrations, and it is unlikely that clinical studies will be designed to further evaluate this question.

High antibiotic concentrations are difficult to achieve in large abscesses for several reasons. Blood supply to the area may be compromised, substances within the abscess may inactivate some antibiotics, and diffusion may be inadequate throughout the area of infection. A wide variety of experimental animal models have been developed to determine the optimal antibiotic schedule for these infections. Most studies have indicated that higher antibiotic concentrations can be achieved at the site of infection when antibiotics are administered on an intermittent rather than continuous schedule. The high peak concentrations achieved in the serum ensure better perfusion into the abscess.[1] Continuous infusion therapy fails to provide peaks and thus may represent suboptimal therapy.

569

Infection in Neutropenic Patients

Although many studies of antibiotic therapy have been conducted in neutropenic patients, few have been designed to address the question of what is the optimal schedule. There are several reasons to believe that the schedule of antibiotic administration could be important in these patients (see table 1). The neutrophil is the primary defense mechanism to localize infection. The importance of this function of the neutrophil is illustrated in a study of children with cancer who contracted pneumonia documented at autopsy examination.[2] None of the 18 children with adequate neutrophil counts ($>1,000$ mm^3) developed bacteremia whereas 8/10 children with severe neutropenia (< 100/mm^3 developed bacteremia in association with their pneumonia. Hence, the absence of neutrophils permits the dissemination of localized infection. Presumably, bloodstream invasion and dissemination is less likely to occur in the presence of adequate combinations in neutropenic patients.

The neutropenic patient is unable to mount an adequate inflammatory response at the site of primary infection and usually does not form abscesses despite extensive infection.[3] Consequently, antibiotic perfusion is a lesser consideration in these patients, the possible exception being those infections causing substantial tissue necrosis. Because the inflammatory response is insufficient, adequate antibiotic concentrations at the site of the infection are more critical in these patients than in normal hosts. Intermittent schedules of antibiotic administration may result in intervals between doses when the serum concentration is too low to inhibit the growth of the infecting organism. Some in vitro studies indicate that gram-negative bacilli quickly recover the ability to proliferate once an antibiotic is no longer present. Animal studies have emphasized the importance of antibiotic schedule in eradicating experimental infections.

In Vitro Studies

The conventional method for measuring the effects of an antibiotic on a bacterial organism is to determine the minimum inhibitory concentration

Table 1. Reasons that Schedule of Antibiotic Administration May Be Important in Neutropenic Patients

1. Lack of inflammatory response in neutropenic patients.

2. Intermittent schedules of antibiotic administration result in intervals when serum concentrations are suboptimal.

3. In vitro studies indicate rapid recovery of gram-negative bacilli after exposure to some antibiotics.

4. Animal infections treated with intermittent schedules that provide inadequate serum concentrations are not cured.

5. Clinical studies in neutropenic patients suggest that continuous infusion therapy is superior.

(MIC), i.e., the lowest concentration that prevents the growth of the organism in vitro. The methodology of these studies requires that the bacteria be exposed to a constant concentration of antibiotic for 18–24 hours. The conditions of these laboratory studies do not mimic the clinical situation, in which the intermittent injection of the antibiotic results in changing serum concentrations rather than a steady concentration.

Several investigators have attempted to develop laboratory models that would reproduce the clinical situation of fluctuating antibiotic concentrations. Unfortunately, no model can accurately duplicate the dynamics of antibiotic administration and elimination that occur in the human. However, it is possible to determine how quickly bacteria can recover from the effects of temporary exposure to an antibiotic. The usual methodology is to incubate rapidly proliferating organisms in the presence of the MIC of the antibiotic (or multiples thereof) for several hours, after which the antibiotic is destroyed. The concentration of organisms present at different times is determined by subculturing aliquots on antibiotic-free agar plates and counting the number of colonies growing after 18 hours. The β-lactam antibiotics have been studied most extensively because they are easily destroyed by the addition of β-lactamases, which do not affect the bacterial organisms. Other methods are to dilute the antibiotic by the addition of more culture media or to centrifuge the organisms and resuspend them in antibiotic-free medium. These latter methods are less satisfactory because the methods themselves may adversely affect the growth of the organisms.

After the introduction of penicillin, many investigators conducted studies of its effect on gram-positive cocci. The most extensive studies were conducted by Eagle et al.[4,5] They exposed strains of *Streptococcus pyogenes* and *Streptococcus pneumoniae* to inhibitory concentrations of penicillin for $1\frac{1}{2}$ hours and then destroyed the antibiotic with penicillinase. They found that the surviving bacteria did not begin to multiply for 2–3 hours thereafter. They believed that this postantibiotic effect was due to antibiotic-induced cell damage that had to be repaired before the bacteria could proliferate again. Parker and Luse reported similar observations with strains of *Staphylococcus aureus*.[6]

Gram-negative bacilli are able to recover more rapidly from the inhibitory effects of antibiotics than gram-positive cocci. Rolinson compared the effects of carbenicillin on *S. aureus* and *Pseudomonas aeruginosa*.[7] The strain of *P. aeruginosa* began to proliferate within $\frac{1}{2}$ hour after the carbenicillin was destroyed by penicillinase, whereas *S. aureus* required $2\frac{1}{2}$ hours to recover. In a second study, Wilson and Rolinson exposed a strain of *Escherichia coli* to 100 times the MIC of ampicillin for $1\frac{1}{2}$ hours.[8] The organism was able to proliferate again approximately $\frac{1}{2}$ hour after the ampicillin was destroyed. Bodey et al evaluated the effects of cephalothin on strains of *E. coli, Proteus mirabilis, Klebsiella pneumoniae*, and *S. aureus*.[9] Approximately $\frac{1}{2}$ hour after the cephalothin was destroyed by β-lactamase, the gram-negative bacilli began to proliferate at the same rate as control organisms that were not exposed to the antibiotic (see figure 1). However, *S. aureus* did not begin to proliferate for more than 4 hours after the cephalothin was destroyed.

Bundtzen et al evaluated a variety of antibiotics for their postantibiotic effects on gram-positive cocci and gram-negative bacilli.[10] In most of their experiments, antibiotic removal was accomplished by dilution with fresh media. The duration of postantibiotic effect and the drug concentrations (multiples of the MIC) required to produce this effect varied with the organism and the antibiotic. They also noted that gram-negative bacilli recovered more quickly after exposure to β-lactam antibiotics than gram-positive cocci. Furthermore, much higher antibiotic concentrations were required to achieve a postantibiotic effect against gram-negative bacilli. They found that the aminoglycoside gentamicin had a brief postantibiotic effect against strains of

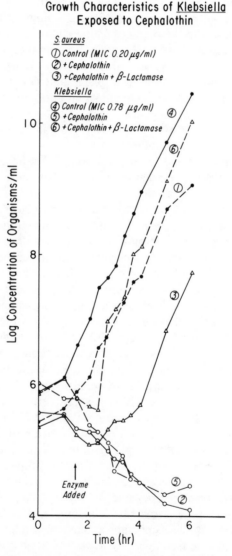

Figure 1.   Growth characteristics of an isolate of *Staphylococcus aureus* and of *Klebsiella pneumoniae* exposed to cephalothin. (Reprinted with permission from *Journal of Antibiotics* [ref. 9])

S. aureus and *E. coli*, whereas the postantibiotic effect against strains of *P. aeruginosa* lasted 1.6–2.6 hours. Interestingly, gentamicin had a longer postantibiotic effect against strains of *P. aeruginosa* than ticarcillin, cefoperazone, or moxalactam.

Experimental Animal Studies

Most of the animal studies that evaluated the impact of the schedule of antibiotic administration on response to therapy used penicillin G against gram-positive cocci. Unfortunately, these studies are not very relevant to the treatment of infections in neutropenic patients. In vitro studies have shown that gram-positive cocci recover slowly from the effects of antibiotics; therefore, longer intervals between doses would be of less consequence than with gram-negative bacilli, which recover more rapidly. Furthermore, normal host defense mechanisms can be mobilized to destroy residual organisms during the interval between doses of antibiotics. Despite these differences, several studies have suggested that an antibiotic schedule does have an impact on therapeutic efficacy.

Jawetz studied the effect of penicillin against *S. pyogenes* in infections in mice.[11] Serum concentrations of penicillin diminished very rapidly after penicillin administration in these animals. A single dose of 500,000 u/kg cured 95% of animals, whereas 3 doses of 5,000 u/kg given at 4-hour intervals cured 85% of animals. He concluded that ". . .the success of parenteral penicillin therapy for mice depends on both the quantity of penicillin administered and the interval between injections." The need for frequent dosing could be obviated by administering higher doses. Gibson was unable to demonstrate any difference in efficacy between an every 8 hours schedule and an every 3 hours schedule of penicillin for the treatment of pneumococcal infection in mice.[12]

Eagle et al conducted numerous studies of the effect of dose, interval, and duration of penicillin therapy on recovery from streptococcal and pneumococcal infections in mice.[4,5,13–15] Only a few of these studies will be described. A *S. pyogenes* infection induced in the muscles of mice was treated with doses of 0.2 to 50 mg/kg penicillin. The rate of bactericidal activity was independent of the dose of penicillin administered as long as the serum concentration (SC) was adequate. Organisms continued to die as long as the SC was maintained above 0.02–0.05 μg/ml. Once the SC fell below 0.02 μg/ml, the bactericidal effect ceased. The important difference between varying doses of penicillin was not the rate of the bactericidal action, but rather the duration of time that an effective serum concentration was maintained.

Table 2 summarizes a study of the effect of total dose and interval between doses on duration of time required to cure *S. pyogenes* infection in mice.[16] At any interval, the time required to cure the infection was inversely related to the total dose of penicillin administered. However, the longer the interval between doses of penicillin, the longer the time required to cure the infection. Hence, smaller doses of penicillin administered at more frequent intervals were more effective than larger doses administered at less frequent intervals. These authors concluded that ". . .penicillin is most rapidly effective if the concentration at the focus of infection remains continuously in excess of that necessary to kill the particular organism at the maximum rate."

In a related study, these authors demonstrated that the greater the number of doses of penicillin, the lower the cumulative dose required to cure the infection (see table 3). Furthermore, there was an optimal interval between doses (3 hours); shortening or lengthening this interval increased the dose of drug necessary to cure the infection. For example, the curative dose was higher when 8 doses were given at intervals of 12 hours than when 3 doses were given at intervals of 3 hours. They further concluded from their series of experiments that ". . .the factor that primarily determines its [penicillin] therapeutic efficacy is the total time for which the drug remains at effective levels at the focus of infection. The number of streptococci or pneumococci surviving . . . was found to decrease rapidly only as long as the penicillin remained at effective levels. Extremely large doses . . . were initially no more rapidly bactericidal than much lower dosages; the difference lay merely in the time for which that bactericidal effect continued. However, the aggregate 'penicillin time' required to cure a given infection . . . was largely independent of the method of administration, provided the penicillin-free interval between injections had not been so prolonged so as to permit the interim remultiplication of the surviving bacteria."[15]

Penicillin is less effective against pneumococcal pneumonia in rats given cobra venom factor because it suppresses phagocytosis as a result of complement depletion.[16] Normal animals were cured by doses of 2 mg/kg every

Table 2. Effect of Interval between Penicillin Doses and Time to Cure of Streptococcal Infection in Mice

Dose	Time (hrs) to cure at treatment interval of				
(mg/kg)*	0.75 hr	1.5 hr	3 hr	6 hr	12 hr
50	1.5 – 2.25	3 – 4.5	3 – 6	6 – 12	12 – 24
12.5	3 – 4.5	6	6 – 9	6 – 12	24 – 72
3.2	4.5 – 6.0	6 – 9	6 – 9	12 – 18	36 – 48
0.8	6 – 9	9 – 12	9 – 12	24 – 36	> 144

*Cumulative dose
Source: Eagle et al, New Engl J Med 1953; 248: 481

Table 3. Effect of Interval between Penicillin Doses on the Curative Dose for Streptococcal Infection in Mice

	Total curative dose (mg/kg) when given at intervals of				
No. doses	0.75 hr	1.5 hr	3 hr	6 hr	12 hr
3	133	62	6.3	9.6	9.9
4	68	31	3.0	6.0	7.6
6	49	4.8	4.3	< 4.8	5.4
8	5.5	0.5	1.9	4.1	8.0

Source: Eagle et al, New Engl J Med 1953; 248: 481

12 hours for 4 days, whereas it required 50 mg/kg doses to sterilize the lungs of all animals treated with cobra venom factor. However, a dose of 34 mg/kg was sufficient if the interval between doses was reduced from 12 to 8 hours.[17] This difference in the dosage requirements could be related to the duration of time when the plasma concentration exceeded the estimated minimal effective plasma concentration of penicillin.

Rolinson induced a *P. aeruginosa* infection in the thigh muscle of mice.[7] With this animal model, it was possible to quantitate the number of organisms at the site of infection (see figure 2). An intermittent schedule of carbenicillin was used to treat this infection. When the SC of carbenicillin was high, the number of organisms at the site of infection decreased, but when the SC decreased substantially, the number of organisms at the site of infection increased and the infection was never eradicated. A more frequent schedule, which maintained adequate SC for a longer period, successfully eradicated the infection. This animal model extended the in vitro observation that surviving gram-negative bacilli recover quickly from the effects of β-lactam antibiotics.

Gerber et al evaluated the effect of dosing intervals of gentamicin and ticarcillin against an experimental *P. aeruginosa* infection in the thigh muscle

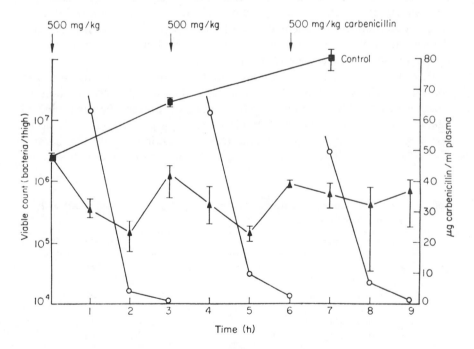

Figure 2.   Effects of repeated subcutaneous injections of carbenicillin on
            Pseudomonas aeruginosa infection in the thigh of muscle of mice. Viable
            organisms at side of infection:
            ■ = Control animals
            ▲ = Carbenicillin treated animals
            o = Plasma concentration of carbenicillin (μg/ml)
(Reprinted with permission from MacMillan Co. [ref. 7])

of neutropenic mice.[18] Animals were treated at 1-hour or 3-hour intervals for at least 12 hours and then sacrificed, and the concentration of organisms was determined at the site of infection. With ticarcillin, they found that 1-hour injection schedules were 7–10 times more effective than 3-hour injection schedules, providing the same total doses were given. Gentamicin was less effective than ticarcillin, but the opposite effect was observed. Gentamicin was more effective when given by an every 3 hours schedule than by an every 1 hour schedule. When the 2 antibiotics were used in combination, the most effective regimen was ticarcillin every 1 hour and gentamicin every 3 hours.

The effect of schedule of administration of ticarcillin and amikacin was evaluated against an experimental model of *P. aeruginosa* peritonitis in neutropenic rats.[19] The MIC of amikacin was 40 μg/ml, and the MIC of ticarcillin was 160 μg/ml against the strain of *P. aeruginosa* used for these experiments; the combination interacted synergistically. Both drugs were administered I.M.; the intermittent schedule for amikacin was every 3 hours and for ticarcillin, every 2 hours. The continuous schedule was every $^1/_2$ hour for both drugs. Survival rates for rats treated with amikacin alone by either schedule were no different than for untreated controls (see table 4). Survival rates for rats treated with ticarcillin alone were superior to untreated controls; the difference was statistically significant only for those rats receiving the continuous schedule. The most effective regimen was the continuous schedule of both drugs. It should be emphasized that neither schedule of amikacin ever produced SC that exceeded the MIC, and only the intermittent schedule of ticarcillin produced SC (only at the peak) that exceeded the MIC of the organism.

Powell et al compared once daily administration of aminoglycosides to continuous infusions in several experimental Pseudomonas infections, none of which used neutropenic animals.[20] The efficacy of tobramycin was evaluated against acute Pseudomonas pneumonia in guinea pigs. Survival at 72 hours was 25% for controls, 25% for animals receiving continuous infusion therapy, and 42% for animals receiving single dose therapy, a difference that was not

Table 4. Effect of Schedule of Antibiotics on Survival of Neutropenic Rats with Pseudomonas Peritonitis

Dose and schedule	Mortality rate (%)
Controls	68
Amikacin—Continuous (C)	67
Amikacin—Intermittent (I)	63
Ticarcillin—Continuous (C)	37
Ticarcillin—Intermittent (I)	47
Amikacin—I Ticarcillin—I	30
Amikacin—C Ticarcillin—I	23
Amikacin—I Ticarcillin—C	17
Amikacin—C Ticarcillin—C	0

30 animals treated in each group with 60 controls
Continuous; q 0.5 hr
Intermittent; q 2 hr for ticarcillin, q 3 hr for amikacin

Source: Mordenti J, Thesis, Ph.D., U of Conn, 1983.

statistically significant. However, the concentration of viable organisms in the lung at the end of therapy was significantly higher in the group of animals treated with continuous infusion to bramycin than in the animals treated with the single-dose regimen. The 2 methods of administration of tobramycin were equally efficacious in treating chronic Pseudomonas pneumonia in rats. They also studied Pseudomonas endocarditis in rabbits, finding similar survival rates with the single-dose and continuous infusion regimens. However, after 7 days of therapy, blood cultures remained positive in 32% of animals receiving the single-dose schedule, compared to 10% of animals receiving the continuous infusion schedule (p = 0.18).

The relevance of in vitro and in vivo models to the clinical situation is uncertain. Most in vitro studies are in agreement that the postantibiotic effect in gram-negative bacilli is short-lived. The pharmacokinetics of antibiotics are distinctly different in different animal species; therefore, it is inappropriate to rely excessively on animal models as a guide to therapy in humans. Furthermore, some of the above-mentioned studies were conducted in animals with normal host defenses, and these models are certainly not relevant to neutropenic patients.

The effect of schedule of aminoglycosides on their toxicity has also been evaluated in animals. Dogs were given 10 days of gentamicin, tobramycin, or netilmicin by single dose, every 4 hours, or continuous infusion schedules.[20] The continuous infusion regimens were associated with greater decrements in glomerular filtration rate than the every 4 hours schedules (p = 0.01) or the single-dose schedules (p = 0.003). Aminoglycoside concentrations in the kidney cortex were not significantly influenced by drug or schedule.

Rats were given gentamicin for 10 days by a once, twice, or 3 times daily schedule.[21] At 2 days, the single-dose schedule produced the highest SC during the first hour after administration, whereas the 3 times daily schedule produced the lowest SC. At 10 days, the twice daily schedule produced the lowest SC. The greatest increase in serum creatinine concentrations after 10 days was observed with the 3 times daily schedule (p = <0.001). Rabbits were given gentamicin for 4 weeks by a once or 3 times daily schedule.[22] After 4 weeks, the serum creatinine increased significantly with the 3 times daily schedule but not with the once daily schedule. Also, the serum half-life of gentamicin increased with the 3 times daily schedules.

The relevance of these observations to humans is questionable. All animal species are not equally susceptible to the nephrotoxicity of aminoglycosides. Dosages and serum concentrations in these studies far exceed those in humans. Also, the pharmacokinetics of aminoglycosides vary in different species.

Human Pharmacology Studies

Several factors would be expected to influence the importance of the schedule of administration of antibiotics in humans.[23] The toxicity of the antibiotic and its relation to serum concentration could limit the amount of drug that could safely be administered. The serum half-life is an important consideration. If the half-life is long, then it is easier to maintain adequate SC with infrequent dosing. If the half-life is short, repeated doses at short intervals would likely be advantageous. The MIC of the infecting organism could affect the dosing schedule. If it is high, it might only be possible to achieve an adequate SC by intermittent dosing. The peak SC could exceed the MIC, but for much of the interval between doses, the SC would be inadequate. Under these circumstances, it would not be possible to achieve an adequate SC by the continuous infusion schedule if the antibiotic had any substantial toxicity that was dose-related.

A major advantage of the β-lactam antibiotics is their minimal toxicity. This permits the administration of doses of these drugs that provide high SC with little risk of serious side effects. When carbenicillin first became available, the dosage schedule of 5 g administered over a 2-hour period every 4 hours was arbitrarily selected for neutropenic patients.[24] This dosage schedule produced an average peak SC of more than 200 μg/ml and maintained a mean SC of 145 μg/ml. When administered in this fashion, carbenicillin cured 75% of 59 Pseudomonas infections, including 38 episodes of bacteremia.[25] There was no correlation between the response rate and the initial neutrophil count, nor with changes in the neutrophil count during therapy.

Because ticarcillin was about twice as active as carbenicillin in vitro, a dose of 5 g over 2 hours every 6 hours was selected initially. Of the 5 patients with Pseudomonas infections who were treated with this regimen, only 2 were cured of their infection (an additional patient's infection responded but relapsed when the drug was discontinued). With this schedule of administration, the average SC at the end of 6 hours was only 19 μg/ml.[26] Thereafter, the dose was changed to 3.5 g over 2 hours every 4 hours. This dosage schedule was selected so that the total daily dose was not changed substantially. Using this schedule, the average peak SC was 210 μg/ml, and the SC was maintained at approximately 50 μg/ml. Among 42 patients with Pseudomonas infections who were treated with this schedule, 74% were cured.[27] As with carbenicillin, response was independent of the patient's neutrophil counts.

Table 5 lists the dosage schedules for neutropenic patients in pharmacokinetic studies of various β-lactam antibiotics.[25,27,28-34] Two schedules have

Table 5. Schedules of β-Lactam Antibiotics

Antibiotic	Dosage schedule	Infusion period	Mean maintained concent. (μg/ml)	Reference
Carbenicillin	5 g q4h	2 hr	145	24
Ticarcillin	3.5 g q4h	2 hr	50	26
Mezlocillin	3 g q4h	2 hr	>50	28
Cefamandole	2 g q6h	cont.inf.	>20	29
Moxalactam	2 g q6h	cont.inf.	33 – 42	30
Cefoperazone	2 g q6h	cont.inf.	77 – 100	31
Ceftriaxone	2 g q8h	cont.inf.	117 – 151	32
Ceftazidime	1 g q4h	2 hr	30	33
Aztreonam	1.5 g q4h	2 hr	26 – 31	34

Continuous infusions preceded by loading dose of 1 – 2 g over 30 min.

been used arbitrarily. Either the antibiotic was administered over a 2-hour period at 4-hour intervals or by continuous infusion, preceded by a loading dose given over 30 min. Both methods maintain high SC. The 2-hour schedule is more practical and also provides a peak SC that may be advantageous. Generally, there are only minimal variations in corresponding SC on consecutive days of therapy. For example, figure 3 shows the daily fluctuations when moxalactam was administered by a continuous infusion of 2 g every 6 hours. Mean 10 a.m. SC varied between 33.8 and 42.1 μg/ml, whereas mean 4 p.m. SC varied between 33.2 and 41.5 μg/ml during days 2 through 9 of the study.[30] In another study, aztreonam was administered at a dose of 1.5 g over 2 hours every 4 hours. The mean daily peak SC varied from 75.0 to 85.3 μg/ml, and then the mean daily trough SC varied from 25.6 to 31.2 μg/ml during the 7 days of the study.[34]

A recent study has suggested that a more rapid infusion may be more desirable than a 2-hour infusion as long as the interval between doses is 4 hours. Ticarcillin 4 g (in combination with clavulanic acid) was administered over $^1/_2$ hour or over 2 hours and SC were measured.[35] The mean peak SC were 341 and 210 μg/ml, respectively, and the mean trough SC before the next dose

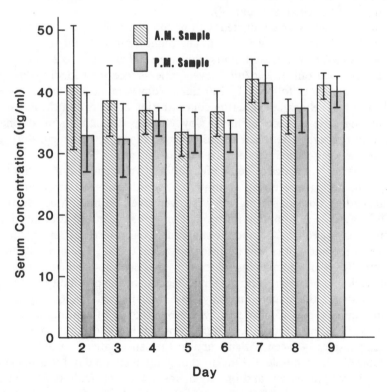

Figure 3.   Mean morning and afternoon serum concentrations of moxalactam obtained with continuous I.V. infusion of 2 g over 6 hr every 6 hr after a 1 g loading dose in 11 patients. Bars indicate standard errors of the means.

were 37 and 42 μg/ml, respectively. Thus, the more rapid administration resulted in higher peak SC but did not compromise the trough SC.

Aminoglycosides are usually administered at 6-, 8-, or 12-hour intervals. When gentamicin was administered at a dose of 30 mg/m^2 (0.75 mg/kg) over a 2-hour period every 6 hours, the average SC at the end of the infusion was 4.2 μg/ml.[36] Immediately before the initiation of the next infusion, the average SC was 1.1 μg/ml.[37] The corresponding average SC after the administration of tobramycin at a dose of 50 mg/m^2 (1.25 mg/kg) by the same schedule were 3.6 μg/ml and 1.1 μg/ml.[37] This type of schedule results in intervals between doses when the SC decreases below the MIC for some infecting organisms. The longer the interval between doses, the longer the period of inadequate SC.

The pharmacokinetics of amikacin have been studied in patients receiving intermittent and continuous I.V. schedules for therapy of infections.[38] Five patients received a dose of 150 mg/m^2 (3.75 mg/kg) administered over ^{1}/$_2$ hour every 6 hours and serum concentrations were determined on day 3 and 7 of therapy (see figure 4). On day 7, the initial mean SC was 4.1 μg/ml. The highest mean SC (at the end of the infusion) was 20.6 μg/ml and decreased to 3.9 μg/ml immediately before the next infusion. Five patients received a loading dose of 150 mg/m^2 over 30 min. followed by 800 mg/m^2/day administered as a continuous infusion. The mean serum concentrations were maintained above 8 μg/ml with this schedule (figure 4).

Similar studies were conducted with netilmicin.[39] Nine patients received 60 mg/m^2 over 30 min. every 6 hours. The highest mean SC (at the end of the infusion) was 7.8 μg/ml. At 4 hours, the mean SC had fallen to 2.0 μg/ml, and by 6 hours it was only 0.9 μg/ml. Eleven patients received a loading dose of 60 mg/m^2 over ^{1}/$_2$ hour followed by 240 mg/m^2/day administered as a continuous I.V. infusion. The mean peak serum concentration at the end of the infusion of the loading dose was 6.6 μg/ml; it slowly declined to 2.9 μg/ml during the following 6 hours. The mean serum concentrations of netilmicin during the subsequent week varied between 2.1 and 3.1 μg/ml.

The pharmacokinetics of gentamicin, tobramycin, and sisomicin have been studied in patients receiving continuous I.V. infusions.[40] For sisomicin, an initial loading dose of 40 mg/m^2 was given over ^{1}/$_2$ hour followed by 240 mg/m^2 day as a continuous infusion. For gentamicin and tobramycin, the loading dose was 60 mg/m^2 and the subsequent daily dose was 300 mg/m^2. The dosage of the antibiotics was adjusted based on the SC. The objective was to maintain the SC of gentamicin and tobramycin between 4 and 6 μg/ml and the SC of sisomicin between 3 and 4 μg/ml. Because of the possibility of excessive nephrotoxicity, the maximum daily dose was limited to 360 mg/m^2, 360 mg/m^2, and 200 mg/m^2, respectively. Despite the use of continuous infusions and dosage adjustments, there were considerable variations in the SC of aminoglycosides between patients and in the same patient on different days (see table 6). For example, the mean SC of gentamicin on day 1 was 4.4 μg/ml, on day 3 was 5.6 μg/ml, and on day 5 was 4.4 μg/ml. On day 3, the SC for different patients varied from 3.3 to 11.0 μg/ml. The widest variation in the same patient on different days was 1.6–8.2 μg/ml, even though the dosage was adjusted to try to maintain a constant SC and an infusion pump was used to maintain a constant infusion.

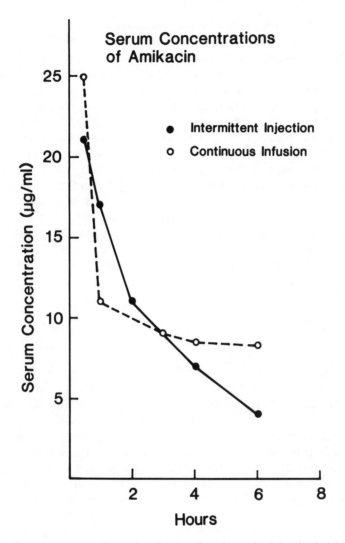

Figure 4.   Serum concentrations of amikacin related to schedule of administration.

Table 6. Observed Serum Concentrations (μg/ml) During Continuous Infusions of Aminoglycoside Antibiotics

	Gentamicin	Tobramycin	Sisomicin	Netilmicin
Range, day 1	2.6 – 6.2	1.0 – 3.7	1.3 – 3.6	0.8 – 4.1
Range, day 7	1.6 – 5.6	2.6 – 4.5	1.1 – 3.5	1.6 – 6.2
Widest range in same patient	1.6 – 8.2	1.7 – 5.4	1.7 – 7.2	1.9 – 4.8

Table 7 lists the recommended loading doses and initial schedule for continuous infusion therapy with the various aminoglycosides. Serum concentrations should be measured on day 2 and at least every 2 days thereafter. Drug dosage should be adjusted to try to maintain the SC in the optimum therapeutic range rather than relying upon a fixed dosage schedule.

Because it is inconvenient to administer drugs by continuous I.V. infusion, an attempt was made to develop a more optimal intermittent schedule that would maintain adequate SC. Ten patients were given a loading dose of tobramycin of 60 mg/m^2 over 30 min. followed immediately by 60 mg/m^2 over 2 hours every 4 hours.[41] The highest mean SC (at the end of the loading dose) was 6.0 μg/ml and the mean SC 2 hours after the end of the initial 2-hour infusion was 3.0 μg/ml. This schedule of tobramycin was used to treat 117 patients with presumed or proven infection. On day 3 of therapy, only 48% of patients had an adequate trough SC ($>$ 3.0 μg/ml), and 22% had an excessive peak SC ($>$10.0 μg/ml). Although only 3 patients developed nephrotoxicity, it was concluded that this was an unsatisfactory alternative to the continuous infusion schedule.

Clinical Therapeutic Studies

The broad-spectrum activity of the aminoglycosides made them appealing antibiotics for the treatment of infections in neutropenic patients. Early studies of gentamicin used a total daily dose of 3 mg/kg. Bodey et al were the first to evaluate I.V. gentamicin, using a dosage schedule of 30 mg/m^2 over 2 hours every 6 hours.[42] The overall cure rate in 63 infections caused by single gram-negative bacilli was 52%. Among patients with adequate neutrophil counts, the cure rate was 79%, whereas among patients with severe neutropenia, the cure rate was only 23% (see table 8). The response rate was also related to whether the patients' neutrophil counts increased or decreased during their infection. It was possible to culture the infecting organism from the blood of some neutropenic patients for several days during therapy, even though the organism was sensitive to gentamicin in vitro and the serum concentration 1 hour after infusion was higher than the MIC.

Subsequently, almost identical results were obtained in a study of tobramycin.[43] The same schedule was used, but the dose was increased to 50 mg/m^2.

Table 7. Recommended Schedules for Continuous Infusions of Aminoglycoside Antibiotics

Antibiotic	Loading dose (mg/m²)	Daily dose (mg/m²)	Maximum dose given (mg/m²)	Estimated optimum serum concent. (μg/ml)
Gentamicin	60	300	360	4 – 6
Tobramycin	60	360	400	4 – 6
Sisomicin	40	160	200	3 – 4
Amikacin	150	800	1,000	12 – 16
Netilmicin	60	240	240	4 – 5

The cure rate for the 59 infections caused by a single gram-negative bacillus was 58% (table 8). Response was related to initial neutrophil count and to changes in neutrophil count during therapy. The suboptimal results in neutropenic patients were not due to the emergence of resistant bacteria nor to inadequate serum concentrations.

Jackson and Riff determined the effects of dose and SC on response of Pseudomonas bacteremia to gentamicin.[44] None of 7 patients with rapidly fatal underlying diseases responded to gentamicin, whereas 6/14 patients without rapidly fatal underlying diseases responded. Five of the former 7 patients had persistent bacteremia regardless of peak SC varying from <1 μg/ml to >4 μg/ml gentamicin. Among the remaining patients, bacteremia persisted in 4/5 patients whose peak SC was <2 μg/ml, but in none of 6 patients whose peak SC was at least 4 μg/ml. Of these 14 patients without rapidly fatal underlying diseases, none of 3 whose SC of gentamicin was <1 μg/ml survived, 2/6 whose SC was 1-2 μg/ml survived, and 4/5 patients whose SC exceeded 4 μg/ml survived. The majority of patients with rapidly fatal underlying diseases had acute leukemia and most likely were neutropenic. Hence, the peak SC was only an important determinant in patients who were not neutropenic; the intermittent schedule was ineffective in neutropenic patients regardless of the peak SC.

The poor results with aminoglycosides in neutropenic patients led to an assessment of potential responsible factors. It was postulated that intermittent schedules resulted in intervals between doses when the SC was inadequate. There are no data defining the adequate SC required to achieve maximum efficacy with an antibiotic in neutropenic patients. Because these patients lack normal host defense mechanisms, it is reasonable to assume that the SC should always exceed the MIC of the infecting organism. Because those gram-negative bacilli that survive after being exposed to antibiotic recover their ability to proliferate shortly after the antibiotic is destroyed in vitro, it seems likely that similar events can occur in neutropenic patients if the interval between doses of antibiotics permits the SC to fall below the MIC for the infecting organism. Based upon this rationale, studies of continuous infusion therapy with aminoglycosides were initiated.

The first study was conducted with amikacin.[45] Patients with adequate neutrophil counts were treated with 150 mg/m² amikacin administered I.V. over

Table 8. Response of Gram-Negative Bacillary Infections to Aminoglycoside Antibiotics

Initial neutrophils/mm³	Neutrophil trend	Gentamicin		Tobramycin		Amikacin		Netilmicin	
		Episodes	% cure	Episodes	% cure	Episodes	% cure	Episodes	% cure
<100	Total	22	23	21	24	13	69	11	73
101–1,000	Total	17	53	10	70	14	79	8	50
>1,000	Total	24	79	28	79	43	74	34	59
<100	Increased	6	33	14	29	7	100	6	83
<100	Unchanged	16	19	7	14	6	33	5	60
Total	Decreased	32	31	23	39	—	—	15	47
Total	Increased	31	74	36	69	—	—	38	66
Total	Total	63	52	59	58	70	74	53	62

$^1/_2$ hour every 6 hours. Neutropenic patients received a loading dose of 150 mg/m^2 over $^1/_2$ hour followed immediately by 800 mg/m^2/day given as a continuous infusion. Serum concentrations were determined daily in these latter patients, and the dose of amikacin was adjusted to try to maintain a SC of 15 µg/ml. The overall response rate for infections caused by a single gram-negative bacillus was 74% (table 8). Unlike the experience with intermittent gentamicin and tobramycin therapy, the results with amikacin in neutropenic patients were as good as those observed in patients with adequate neutrophil counts. Daily SC were determined in 45 patients with identified infections. The response rate was 63% for those 16 infections in which the patients' SC of amikacin was maintained at < 10 µg/ml. The response rate was 83% for those 29 infections in which the patient's SC was maintained at > 10 µg/ml. However, toxicity was unacceptably high when the SC was maintained above 15 µg/ml.

A total of 173 patients treated for presumed or proven infection had normal renal function at the onset of therapy. Nephrotoxicity occurred during therapy in 6% of the 86 patients who received continuous infusion therapy and in 21% of the 87 patients who received intermittent therapy (p = 0.008). This difference occurred despite the fact that the total daily dose was substantially higher with the continuous infusion schedule.

Among those patients who received the continuous infusion schedule, the frequency of nephrotoxicity was related to the maximum SC. Azotemia occurred in none of the patients whose SC was maintained below 10 µg/ml, in 14% at 10–20 µg/ml, and in 56% above 20 µg/ml.[46]

Subsequently, further studies were conducted with netilmicin using the same therapeutic design.[47] Patients who had adequate neutrophil counts received 60 mg/m^2 over $^1/_2$ hour every 6 hours. Neutropenic patients received a loading dose of 60 mg/m^2 over $^1/_2$ hour followed immediately thereafter by 240 mg/m^2/day as a continuous infusion. The response rate for the 53 infections caused by a single gram-negative bacillus was 62% (table 8). Netilmicin proved to be as effective in neutropenic patients when given by continuous infusion as it was in patients with adequate neutrophils when given by intermittent injection. Ratios of mean SC/MIC were calculated for patients who received continuous infusion therapy. The response rate was substantially higher in patients whose ratio was greater than 3 when compared to patients whose ratio was less than 3 (80% versus 20%). In this study, transient azotemia occurred more frequently with the continuous infusion schedule (12% versus 2%).

The first prospective randomized study of the impact of schedule on the efficacy of antibiotic therapy in neutropenic patients used sisomicin to compare intermittent I.V. injection with continuous infusion therapy.[48] All patients entered on this study had failed to respond to carbenicillin plus a cephalosporin. Patients received either 30 mg/m^2 sisomicin over $^1/_2$ hour every 6 hours or a loading dose of 30 mg/m^2 over $^1/_2$ hour followed by 120 mg/m^2/day as a continuous infusion. Apart from the loading dose, both groups received the same total daily dose of sisomicin. The results of this study are summarized in table 9. Although the results favored the continuous infusion schedule, there were no statistically significant differences. However, in this study, the dose of sisomicin was not adjusted to maintain a fixed SC, which might have adversely affected the results. Among those patients with normal renal function prior to the onset of therapy, the frequency of azotemia was less when the drug was administered by continuous infusion, but the difference was not statistically significant.

Subsequently, sisomicin was combined with carbenicillin as initial therapy for presumed or proven infection in neutropenic patients.[49] Patients were randomized to receive either intermittent or continuous infusion schedules of sisomicin. Inasmuch as no differences could be detected, the randomization was changed to fixed-dose continuous infusion versus adjusted-dose continuous infusion. In the latter group of patients, the dose of sisomicin was modified to maintain the serum concentration at 3–4 μg/ml. There was no advantage observed with the adjusted dose schedule in this study.

Feld et al compared intermittent injection to continuous infusion tobramycin in combination with cefamandole as initial therapy for presumed or proven infection in neutropenic patients.[50] The dose of tobramycin was either 75 mg/m² over 30 min. every 6 hours or a loading dose of 60 mg/m² over 30 min. followed by 300 mg/m²/day as a continuous infusion. Dosage adjustments were made with the continuous infusion schedule to maintain the SC at 4–5 μg/ml. There were no differences in the response rates for the 2 regimens among patients with fever of unknown origin (67% for both regimens) or among patients with documented infection (83% for continuous infusion, 77% for intermittent injection). However, because only 9 infections were caused by gram-negative bacilli in this study, it would have been difficult to detect any differences in tobramycin efficacy. It is of some interest that 6/6 patients with severe neutropenia responded to continuous infusion tobramycin, whereas only 6/11 responded to intermittent tobramycin. Continuous infusion therapy was not more toxic than conventional therapy. These authors concluded that "although there is a suggestion that aminoglycosides given by continuous infusion, at least in patients with neutropenia, may be superior to intermittent administration when given alone, the results of our study would suggest that this benefit is probably lost when the aminoglycosides are used in combination." This conclusion may be correct, but it has not been adequately demonstrated in any clinical study.

Table 10 summarizes the results of several large studies of antibiotic therapy of infections in neutropenic patients in which aminoglycosides were

Table 9. Prospective Randomized Study of Intravenous Sisomicin for Therapy of Infections in Neutropenic Patients

	Intermittent		Continuous	
	Episodes	% cure	Episodes	% cure
Total episodes	61	47,	60	65
Fever of unknown origin	26	50	22	73
Documented infection	35	46	38	61
Gram-negative bacilli	18	44	21	62
<100 neutrophils/mm³	15	40	20	50
Nephrotoxicity	57	21	61	13

administered by continuous infusion. One of these studies was a randomized comparative trial of gentamicin, amikacin, and sisomicin in combination with carbenicillin.[53] Response rates for documented infections varied from 67% to 84%. Even in patients with severe neutropenia, more than 60% of infections responded to these regimens. In the comparative trial, the efficacy of the aminoglycosides was evaluated against infections caused by gram-negative bacilli that were resistant to carbenicillin. Because there were no significant differences between the aminoglycosides, the results could be combined. Considering only these infections, the overall response rate in patients with severe neutropenia was 58%. Even in patients whose neutrophil count remained < 100 per mm^3 throughout their infection, the response rate was 53%. This response rate compared favorably with the 67% response rate among similar patients who were infected by gram-negative bacilli sensitive to both antibiotics. In this study, it was demonstrated that the response rate correlated with the ratio between the serum concentration of the aminoglycoside and the MIC.

Only a few studies have examined the effect of schedule on response to β-lactam antibiotics in neutropenic patients. Cephalothin and cefazolin proved to be suboptimal when administered by intermittent schedule in combination with carbenicillin for the therapy of infections caused by carbenicillin-resistant gram-negative bacilli in neutropenic patients.[54,55] The cephalosporins were administered over 1/2 hour at 6-hour intervals. The cure rates for these infections among patients with severe neutropenia were only 15% and 30%. In one of these studies, only 12% of 26 Klebsiella infections were cured.[55] Since the serum half-lives of cephalothin and cefazolin are less than 1 hour, this dosage schedule results in intervals between doses when the serum concentrations are suboptimal.

Only 1 prospective randomized trial has evaluated the role of schedule on response rates with cephalosporins.[56] In this study, patients were randomly assigned to receive carbenicillin plus intermittent cefamandole (3 g over 30 min. every 6 hours) or continuous infusion cefamandole (3 g loading dose over 30 min. followed by 12 g over 24 hours). A third group of patients included in this study who received carbenicillin plus tobramcyin will not be

Table 10. Antibiotic Regimens Using Continuous Infusion Aminoglycosides

Regimen	Documented infections		GNB infections		Septicemia		Neutrophils (<100/mm³)		Reference
	Episodes	% cure	Episodes	% cure	Episodes	% cure	Episodes	% cure	
Carb + tobra	125	70	62	69	26	76	439	62	51
Ceph + amik*	38	84	9	78	8	100	13	92	52
Carb + gent	115	67	55	67	27	44	56	63	53
Carb + amik	102	68	44	64	29	72	47	62	53
Carb + siso	93	67	43	74	24	75	55	64	53

*Carbenicillin substituted for cephalothin in Pseudomonas infections

Carb = carbenicillin; Ceph = cephalothin; Gent = gentamicin; Tobra = tobramycin; Amik = amikacin; Siso = sisomicin discussed here. The results of this study consistently favored the group of patients who received cefamandole by the continuous infusion schedule, although most of the differences were not statistically significant (see table 11). However, among the patients with the poorest prognosis, i.e., patients whose initial neutrophil count of < 100 mm^3 did not increase during their infection, the continuous infusion schedule of cefamandole was significantly more effective than the intermittent schedule (65% versus 21%, p = 0.03). Although the numbers are small, a substantial difference in the response rate was also observed among patients with severe neutropenia who were infected by carbenicillin-resistant gram-negative bacilli (71% versus 0%, p = 0.06). Thus, the continuous infusion schedule of cefamandole proved to be more effective in those situations where it was anticipated to be advantageous.

The complexities of infection in the neutropenic patient make it difficult to design studies that will conclusively demonstrate whether or not the schedule of antibiotic administration is an important consideration. Even prospective randomized comparative studies are unsatisfactory because of the large number of patient entries required and the lack of comparability of groups. Most of the available data suggest that the schedule of antibiotic administration is important in neutropenic patients. It is hoped that future studies will be designed to further explore this potentially important aspect of antibiotic therapy.

Table 11. Prospective Randomized Trial of Carbenicillin Plus Intermittent Cefamandole Versus Continuous Infusion Cefamandole

	Intermittent cefamandole		Continuous cefamandole	
	Episodes	% Resp.	Episodes	% Resp.
Total febrile episodes	170	60	160	69
Fever of unknown origin	78	64	86	73
Documented infections	92	57	74	65
Total septicemia	23	65	27	78
GNB infections	29	59	31	74
Carbenicillin-resistant	7	43	8	88
Neutrophils < 100/mm^3	36	56	35	74
No increase	14	21	20	65
Carbenicillin-resistant GNB	5	0	7	71

43

DEGRADABLE STARCH MICROSPHERES INFUSION: BASIC CONSIDERATIONS FOR TREATMENT OF HEPATIC NEOPLASIA

Leif Håkansson, M.D., Ph.D., Hans Starkhammar, M.D., Stefan Ekberg, M.Sc., Olallo Morales, M.D., Rune Sjödahl, M.D., Ph.D., and John Svedberg, Ph.D.

THE RATIONALE FOR GIVING cytostatic drugs by the intra-arterial (I.A.) route is to achieve a regionally high concentration of drug while limiting systemic toxicity. This method can be employed for the majority of clinically detectable liver tumors, since they mainly depend on arterial blood supply, whereas small metastases are mainly supplied by the portal blood flow.[1-4] The effect of I.A. administered chemotherapeutic agents has generally not been as good as expected,[5-8] to some extent because of rapid washing out by the arterial flow. With the aim of reinforcing the advantages of this route of administration, manipulation of the arterial blood flow has been tried in several ways. Permanent ligation of the hepatic artery alone or combined with infusion of a cytostatic drug into an arterial catheter generally results in short-lasting tumor regression owing to the rapid development of collateral arteries to the liver.[9,10]

Degradable starch microspheres (DSM) can be used to induce temporary vascular occlusion. Currently available microspheres have a mean diameter of 45 μM, providing vascular occlusion at the arteriolar level.[11] They are degraded by serum alpha-amylase, and have a half-life in human serum of about 20 min. at 37°C in vitro. During degradation by the normal alpha-amylase activity of human serum, the microspheres maintain their size and shape until they finally collapse. They are then forced into thinner capillary vessels, and the blood flow recommences. It has been shown that this mode of degradation is due to the higher density at the periphery of the spheres. However, if degradation takes place at a higher alpha-amylase concentration, the size of the micro-spheres gradually decreases.[12]

Different types of DSM have been used in experimental studies. Efficient vascular occlusion was achieved in organs such as intestine,[13,14] liver,[15] and kidney.[16] Several studies have shown that this type of transient ischemia is fully reversible[13-15,17,18] even after repeated administration of the microspheres.[15]

Drugs injected with DSM should become lodged in the arterial microcircula-tion while occlusion lasts. Increased uptake in the tissue of the target organ has been demonstrated for various substances, such as inulin[19] and 5-fluorouracil[19,20] in the liver, actinomycin-D in the kidney,[16] and ^{99m}Tc-DTPA in tumors transplanted to the rabbit hind leg.[21] Parallel to increased retention of the drug in the target organ, the systemic concentration and/or systemic side effects were reduced. Reduction of the systemic concentration of carmustine (BCNU),[22] doxorubicin (ADR),[23] and mitomycin-C (MIT)[24] was achieved when these drugs were injected into the hepatic artery with DSM. In a study by Gyves et al,[24] the reduction in systemic MIT concentration was roughly the same irrespective of the dose of DSM (900 mg or 360 mg). At first glance, this seems surprising, but within a certain range of DSM concentration, the same fraction of co-administered drug should be retained in the blood vessel compartment occluded by the microspheres. Obviously, this type of determination gives no information about the degree of vascular occlusion in the target organ.

To achieve optimal effect on the tumor, the blood flow in the entire liver tumor should be temporarily blocked by DSM. Because the flows through the normal liver tissue and the liver tumor cannot be interrupted separately, DSM must be given until the circulation through the whole organ has stopped. However, if more than this optimum amount of DSM is given, there will be an overflow of microspheres and cytostatic drug to other organs such as the stomach and duodenum. This may result in acute pain and mucosal lesions. Thus, it is critical that the degree of vascular occlusion be determined continu-ously throughout each treatment session. The arterial blood flow cannot be measured directly because treatment is given via a surgically inserted indwell-ing catheter or a catheter introduced via the femoral or brachial artery. Alter-natively, the passage of the cytostatic drug or radio-labeled low-molecular-weight substance can be traced through the liver to the systemic circulation.

Choice of Tracer for Continuous Monitoring of DSM Treatment

If it is desired to study the effect of DSM on the systemic concentration of a co-injected cytostatic drug, then this drug must be measured, because its metabolism and uptake by the liver cells are of great importance. Schematic curves based on the finding of several groups[22-24] concerning the systemic concentration of cytostatic drugs (such as BCNU, MIT, and ADR) given alone or mixed with DSM are shown in figure 1-A. DSM obviously reduces the systemic concentration. However, from these results it cannot be decided to what extent the effect is due to vascular occlusion alone, to metabolism, or to uptake of the drug by the liver cells. But because no late increase (corresponding to release of the drug when the microspheres are degraded) is seen, the 2 last-named mechanisms are probably of importance for the reduced systemic concentration. This view is further supported by the less pronounced effect of DSM on the systemic concentration of co-injected ^{99m}Tc-DTPA, a substance with a slower metabolism that is not specifically taken up by the liver cells (figure 1-B). These results (in figure 1-A and 1-B) were obtained by analyzing blood samples for drug concentration. However, the systemic concentration of technetium-labeled substances can be continuously measured by a detector placed over suitably large vessels.[25] Under such circumstances, the curves are smoothed, permitting measurements soon after the injection (figure 1-C). As will be discussed below, this form of registration can be used to monitor continuously the effect of DSM on the passage of low-molecular-weight substances through the liver during each treatment session. Also, the kinetics of the passage of this type of tracer through the liver can yield valuable information about the development of arteriovenous (AV) shunting and the degree of vascular occlusion obtained by the DSM injections.

Monitor for Continuous Registration of the Effect of DSM on the Passage of Low-Molecular-Weight Substances

In these studies, the passage of ^{99m}Tc-MDP through the liver into the systemic circulation was continuously registered by a Naj-detector placed over the left

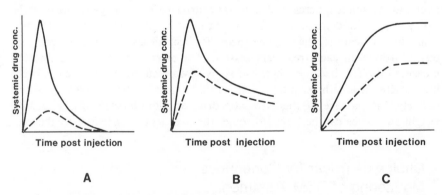

A   **B**   **C**

Figure 1.   Effect of DSM on the systemic concentration of intra-arterially co-injected drugs. A—Cytostatic agents such as BCNU, mitomycin C, or Adriamycin, determined in blood samples collected during the first 30 minutes post injection. B—^{99m}Tc-DTPA determined in blood samples collected during the first 30 minutes post injection. C—^{99m}Tc-MDP continuously determined for 5 minutes post injection by a detector placed over the infraclavicular area.
— — — — — with DSM
_____ without DSM

Source: Svedberg et al (ref. 25)

subclavian area.[25] The pulse rate (counts per seconds) was recorded in a multis-cale mode by a multichannel analyzer (Nuclear Data, ND 66), allowing instant graphical and numerical monitoring. The data were later transferred to a computer (see figure 2).

The passage of each dose of ^{99m}Tc-MDP through the liver into the systemic circulation was compared with that of an initially given reference dose of ^{99m}Tc-MDP. A typical recording of a treatment session is shown in figure 3. A reference dose of ^{99m}Tc-MDP is given at the arrows shown in the figure. The passage through the liver to the systemic circulation is very rapid, and the systemic concentration reaches a plateau in 60–90 seconds. The cytostatic drug mixed with DSM and the labeled tracer is then given in repeated injections. The plateau reached after each injection is calculated as a percent of the plateau of the reference dose. The rapidity of the passage of the tracer is calculated as increased systemic concentration per 10 seconds. This increase is expressed in percent of the initially registered reference plateau.

The existence or development of AV shunting before or during DSM treat-ment was measured by recording the passage of I.A. injected, ^{99m}Tc-labeled macroaggregated albumin (^{99m}Tc-MAA) through the liver to the lung capillaries. This passage was calculated in the following way: Because some of the technetium dose not become bound to the macroaggregates during the labeling pro-cedure, a certain amount will pass to the systemic circulation as free technetium. In order not to overestimate the AV shunting, a limit for the passage of free technetium was set at 20%. The amount of technetium passing through the liver is thus compared with the initially given reference dose. If more than 20% passes through, this should be due to the passage of labeled macroaggregates that have become lodged in the lung capillaries (AV shunting). There is obviously no reason to compare technetium trapped in the lungs with the reference dose, but for the sake of simplicity, the calculated percent values are used as arbitrary units for the passage of ^{99m}Tc-labeled macroaggregates to the lung capillaries.

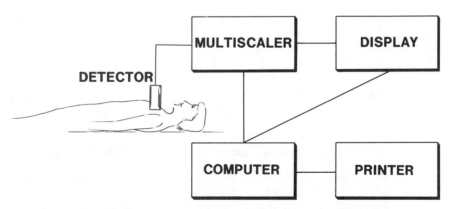

Figure 2.   Monitor used to register continuously the effect of DSM on the passage of a co-injected labeled tracer, ^{99m}Tc-MDP, through the liver into the systemic circulation.

Effect of DSM on the Passage of Low-Molecular-Weight Substances in the Treatment of Liver Tumors

In a pilot study of 18 patients,[26,27] the intention was to give 900 mg of DSM mixed with MIT (15 mg/m^2) at each treatment session. In the first 4 sessions, 2 patients were given 900 mg over a period of 2–4 min. Because of the risk of back flow into the gastroduodenal area, the dose was subsequently fractionated and was, as a rule, mainly given according to 1 of 2 dose schedules: (1) an initial injection of 360 mg followed by repeated 180 mg doses (schedule 1); (2) repeated doses of 150–180 mg given from the start (schedule 2). In 3 patients, the dose had to be reduced (150–540 mg) owing to abdominal pain and nausea and vomiting, whereas in 3 others it was further increased (1,080–1,350 mg) because no unpleasant side effects appeared.

The effect of DSM on the passage of ^{99m}Tc-MDP through the liver when given after or mixed with DSM and MIT was studied in 7 schedule 1 sessions. DSM (360 mg) mixed with MIT was injected into the hepatic artery. Immediately thereafter, ^{99m}Tc-MDP in a small volume (1 ml) was administered through the catheter, and the fraction passing the liver was compared with the initial reference dose. In 5/7 patients, less than 75% of the marker passed into the systemic circulation, indicating a flow reduction induced by DSM. Sixty seconds

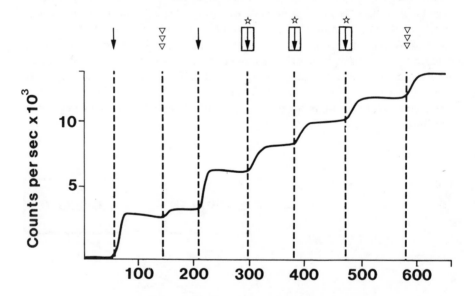

Time after start of measurement (sec)

Figure 3. Cumulative systemic concentration after intra-arterial injection of
^{99m}Tc-MDP given alone (↓) or with DSM and cytostatic drug (⬇).
↯ indicates administration of ^{99m}Tc-MAA. The time of each injection is
shown by a broken vertical line.

Source: Svedberg et al (ref. 25)

later, the passage of a second, identical ^{99m}Tc-MDP injection was close to 100% of the reference dose in all patients. Two to 4 minutes later, a mixture of 180 mg DSM, MIT, and the labeled tracer was injected. In 2 patients who had shown a high passage of the tracer immediately after injection of 360 mg of DSM, the passage was still very high when the tracer was given mixed with the microspheres; in the others, the passage was reduced to about 60% or less.

The variation in the passage of the labeled tracer when given with DSM was further studied in 6 patients who had their first treatment according to schedule 2. The passage of the marker varied greatly among different patients, both in the first and in later injections. In 2 of these patients, repeated injections of ^{99m}Tc-MDP mixed with DSM resulted in a gradual reduction of the fraction of the marker passing to the systemic circulation. In these 2, only about 40% of the marker passed after the final injection, whereas in the other 4 patients, 64–87% passed. In the patients in whom reduction of blood flow was demonstrated by angiography, the passage of ^{99m}Tc-MDP was also reduced. However, even if vascular occlusion was almost total on angiography, the passage of ^{99m}Tc-MDP given mixed with DSM was still about 40%.

From this pilot study,[27] it was concluded that (1) the effect of DSM on the passage to the systemic concentration of low-molecular-weight substances injected into the hepatic artery showed great individual variations; (2) new vascular passages were opened after initial occlusion during the first injection; and (3) even if total vascular occlusion was achieved, when mixed with DSM some of the tracer passed into the systemic circulation.

Effect of Portal Blood Flow on the Passage of ^{99m}Tc-MDP Injected Intra-Arterially with DSM

To further analyze this complex situation, an experimental model using the liver of the pig was developed. The model was characterized by determining the dose of DSM needed to cause maximum vascular occlusion. A catheter was inserted into the gastroduodenal artery, the hepatic artery was ligated, and the liver was perfused with buffered Ringer's solution. The perfusion pressure was measured during injection of DSM. The pressure in the hepatic artery increased with increasing doses of DSM up to 240 mg, after which a plateau was reached.[28]

The effects of arterial perfusion and portal blood flow were studied separately by shutting off one or the other or both of these flows. The portal flow turned out to be of great importance for the passage of low-molecular-weight substances injected into the hepatic artery.[28] In one series of experiments using this model, a reference dose was given as described above. The portal vein was then clamped and a second reference dose was given. As shown in figure 4, the passage into the systemic circulation was considerably reduced as long as the portal vein was clamped; when the vessel was reopened, however, the remaining amount of the tracer entered the systemic circulation. The passage of ^{99m}Tc-MDP through the liver was only moderately affected when the substance was injected together with DSM while the arterial perfusion and portal flow were in progress (not shown in the figure). However, if the portal vein was clamped and ^{99m}Tc-MDP was injected with DSM, a very marked dose-dependent reduction of the tracer was recorded. Here again, much of the injected tracer became lodged in a vessel compartment that was drained by the portal vein, as demonstrated by the increase in systemic concentration of the tracer when the portal vein was reopened.[29,30]

Because the portal flow is of importance for drainage of normal liver vessels, it can be anticipated that most of the drug that becomes lodged distal to the microspheres will rapidly pass into the systemic circulation via the portal pathway. This could explain why, in most of the treatment sessions in the pilot series described previously, the passage of ^{99m}Tc-MDP could not be reduced below 40% even when the arterial flow was almost completely occluded. In contrast, however, in liver tumors with no portal circulation, injected drugs will most likely be retained also in the capillary vessels.

Several explanations can be put forward for the great individual variations in the effect of DSM on the passage of the labeled tracer through the liver of patients in the pilot series. These include differences in the blood flow in the hepatic artery, resulting in differences in the dilution of injected DSM, tracer, and drugs; the existence of or opening of AV shunts; the use of a too-small dose of DSM with respect of the size of the vascular bed in the liver and the tumor; or the use of a too-high dose, resulting in overflow of DSM and labeled tracer to the vessels of the gastroduodenal area.

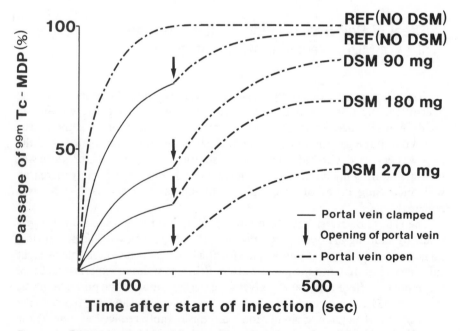

Figure 4. Effect of portal blood flow on the passage of ^{99m}Tc-MDP injected with DSM into the hepatic artery in a pig liver model.

Source: Starkhammar et al (ref. 29)

Importance of AV Shunting to the Effect of DSM

To investigate further these possibilities, a new series of treatments[29] was set up according to the following protocol: The blood flow through the liver was checked by angiography immediately before and after each treatment session. The injections were started with a reference dose of only ^{99m}Tc-MDP (10 ml given over 20 seconds). Arteriovenous shunting was determined by injecting technetium-labeled macroaggregated albumin (^{99m}Tc-MAA), and the amount passing the liver and lodging in the lung capillaries was measured by placing the detector over the subclavian vessel and the apex of the lung. Next, a new reference dose was given, followed by 3 doses, each consisting of 300 mg of DSM mixed with MIT and ^{99m}Tc-MDP. A new injection of ^{99m}Tc-MAA was now given. If less than 20% passed to the lungs, the shunting was considered to be of no clinical importance. In this situation, and provided the patient had experienced no epigastric pain, nausea, or vomiting, and if more than 50% of ^{99m}Tc-MDP injected with the third DSM injection passed the liver, further mixed injections were given until only 40% of the ^{99m}Tc-MDP passed to the systemic circulation.

An example of a treatment session according to the above schedule is illustrated in figure 5. Shunting was not registered, neither initially nor after administration of 900 mg of DSM (mixed with MIT). The passage of the co-administered ^{99m}Tc-MDP was about 50% in the first injections. It then increased to about 70%, after which it gradually fell to about 35%. In the light of present knowledge, this treatment session ought to have ended here, but unfortunately, a further 150 mg of DSM mixed with [99m]TcMDP was injected. The passage of the labeled tracer in this injection was about 60%, probably indicating overflow to the gastroduodenal vascular bed. This interpretation is consistent with the appearance of epigastric pain, nausea and vomiting, and also with symptoms of gastritis during the following 2–3 weeks.

In patients showing an initially large passage of ^{99m}Tc-MAA or with increased ^{99m}Tc-MAA passage after the injection of DSM, ^{99m}Tc-MDP generally passed into the systemic circulation to the same extent with all injections given during the same treatment session.

As pointed out above, overestimation of AV shunting was avoided by setting a 20% limit for passage of unbound technetium in the preparation of labeled macroaggretates. Defined in this way, 4/19 patients showed measurable AV shunting before treatment. After administration of DSM, significant passage of ^{99m}Tc-MAA to the lungs was demonstrated in 12/17 patients.[29,31] In other words, passage through AV shunts increased in about half of the patients during the treatment session. This increase in AV shunting took place to the same extent irrespective of the degree of passage of ^{99m}Tc-MAA through the liver before DSM administration (see figure 6).

Kinetics of the Passage of ^{99m}Tc-MDP Injected With DSM

The rate of passage of the tracer (flow rate) through the liver to the systemic circulation was calculated as the maximum passage during 10 seconds corrected for the plateau value of each injection. This flow rate showed a considerable individual variation. A correlation emerged between the angiographically shown flow reduction and the difference in flow rate between the reference and the first or second DSM injection. The treatment sessions were grouped arbitrarily. When the flow rate difference was less than 10, over 80% of the co-injected tracer in the first injection as a rule passed to the systemic circulation (figure 7-A). The passage of the tracer was roughly the same in the subsequent injections. When the flow rate difference exceeded 10, the passage of the labeled tracer was much more variable. The posttreatment angiography generally showed considerable back flow of the contrast medium. The patients in this group either had a remarkable increase in AV shunting during the treatment sessions (passage of MAA after treatment was more than 20 arbitrary units; figure 7-B) or had no AV shunting at all (figure 7-C). In the latter group, a gradual decrease in the passage of the tracer was generally observed when the DSM injections were repeated. During some sessions, the passage was greater with the second injection than with the first. In 2 of the sessions, this could have been due to overflow to the gastroduodenal area, because the patient

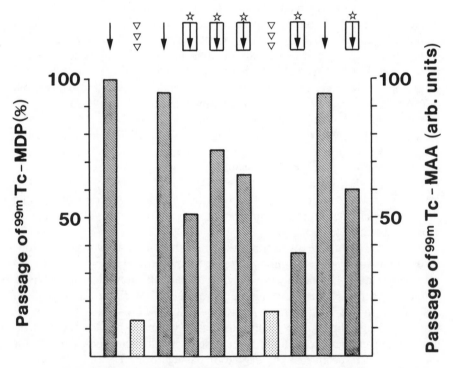

Figure 5. The effect of DSM on the passage of intra-arterially co-injected 99mTc-MDP through the liver into the systemic circulation. The passage of 99mTc-MAA before and after administration of 900 mg DSM is also shown. The results of the injections are shown in the order they were given, from left to right. Symbols as in figure 3.

Source: Starkhammar et al (ref. 29)

experienced intense pain and nausea and vomiting; as noted above, a total vascular occlusion is achieved in some patients with a normal-sized liver after only 450 mg of DSM. However, in patients who experience no unpleasant side effects, the greater passage with the second than with the first injection of DSM might be the result of the opening of new vascular areas (see pilot study above). A gradual decrease in passage of the tracer, which occurred in several treatment sessions, indicates increasing vascular occlusion, as confirmed by angiography. In some situations, there was an increase in the passage of the labeled tracer between the penultimate and final injections. In these sessions, the patient always experienced intense epigastric pain and nausea and vomiting. We therefore interpret this increased passage with the final injection as indicating an overflow of injected DSM tracer and cytostatic drug to a new vascular area where the blood flow was previously unaffected.

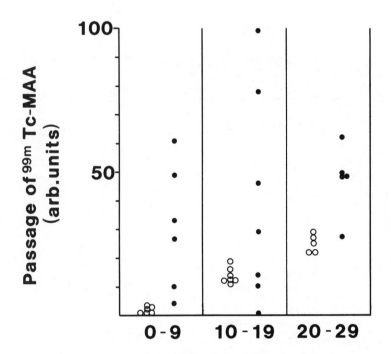

Passage of ^{99m}Tc-MAA before DSM treatment (arb.units)

Figure 6. Passage of ^{99m}Tc-MAA before (o) and after (•) DSM treatment. The patients are divided into 3 groups according to the passage of ^{99m}Tc-MAA before DSM treatment. Increased passage after the session was found in all groups.

Source: Starkhammar et al (ref. 29)

Conclusion

The model described for continuous monitoring of DSM treatment can be used to identify patients showing different effects of DSM on the passage of low-molecular-weight substances through the target organ. In one group of patients, mainly those with AV shunts, almost no retention of co-injected drugs was achieved. In another group, about 30% retention was obtained despite the presence of AV shunting. In a third group, in which most patients had no AV shunts in the tumor, a gradual decrease in the passage of the tracer could generally be used as an indicator of the degree of vascular occlusion, and an overflow of DSM and co-injected drugs to the gastroduodenal area could therefore be avoided.

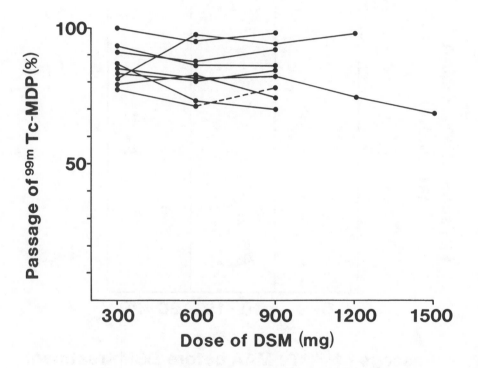

Figure 7A. Relationship between reduction of flow rate of ^{99m}Tc-MDP and the passage of this labeled marker given together with DSM in repeated doses. Each line represents 1 treatment session, involving several repeated injections. The cumulative dose of DSM at each treatment session is shown. The figure above shows flow rate reduction < 10.

Source: Starkhammar et al (ref. 29)

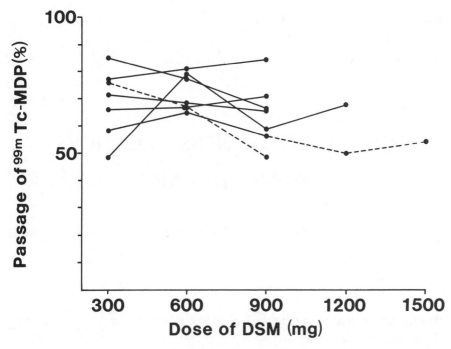

Figure 7B.   Flow rate reduction ≥ 10 and AV shunting.

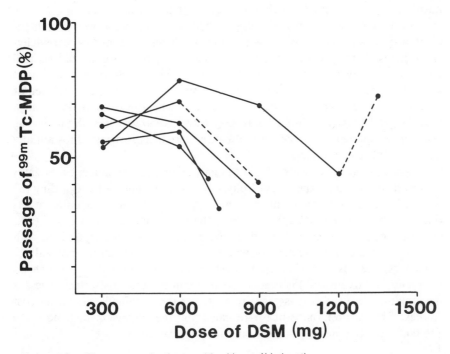

Figure 7C.   Flow rate reduction ≥ 10 without AV shunting.

44

COST-EFFECTIVENESS IN CANCER CHEMOTHERAPY

Jacob J. Lokich, M.D.

THE COST OF HEALTH care in the United States is an enormous political and social issue. The health care industry, second only to the military in annual budget needs, is being subjected to extraordinary regulation in an attempt to restrain growth and limit costs. In 1980, the overall medical costs for patients with cancer was $10.8 billion. At the established rate of rise of 20% per year, that cost by 1985 had doubled. The major portion (two-thirds) is spent for hospital care and approximately one-fourth for physicians' fees.

Cost-effectiveness is stressed today in medical education as well as in high-technology business operations. It is pervasive throughout medical care delivery systems, from private practice to health maintenance organizations and from community hospitals to tertiary care centers. Cost-effectiveness as it applies to the treatment of cancer is particularly complex for a number of reasons. First, cancer is an area of medicine in which research at the clinical level in particular is essential because effective treatment is so limited. The research component in the delivery of cancer care increases costs substantially and is not always definable.

A second issue making it difficult to analyze the costs of cancer care relates to the attitudes and perspectives of physicians and patients alike regarding the disease itself. Cancer treatment, particularly when given in a noncurative setting, may be considered inappropriate in the sense that an optimal goal (i.e., cure) cannot be achieved with existing modalities of treatment. In patients with advanced disease in particular, for whom palliative goals are the only realistic objectives, the absence of symptoms represents a circumstance in which no intervention ("treatment") is best. In such circumstances, cost-effectiveness is maximized, since the cost is zero. In fact, for the terminally ill, actual cost studies of the last 6 months of life revealed that the average medical cost was $16,000, with the major portion going for hospital costs.

It is clear that the disease itself will substantially influence the cost issue. Many clinical aspects of the disease have an impact on cost-effectiveness considerations, including the stage of disease, the effectiveness of the treatment or the likelihood of the response, the patient's age, the effect of the disease complications on life expectancy, and the effect of treatment complications on life-style.

The cost of cancer care is much more easily defined than cost-effectiveness. In the cancer circumstance, "effectiveness" is burdened by definitional problems with regard to effective treatment end points and by philosophical perspectives on the disease. The focus of the present chapter, therefore, will be on defining the costs for chemotherapy in terms of actual costs, and it will be left to readers to apply the formulation that is most appropriate for their own perspective in determining cost-effectiveness. The costs cited throughout the chapter are actual for the year 1985 and were confirmed by the manufacturer or distributor or by the department of pharmacy at a university teaching hospital.

Defining the Cost Basis

Following is a listing of the individual issues to be addressed in quantifying the cost of chemotherapy treatment. This list of cost categories for chemotherapy is by no means comprehensive, but it does represent the spectrum of quantifiable costs as well as "nondollar costs":

- Chemotherapeutic agents costs
- Administration cost (clinic fee)
- Physician's fee
- Treatment complications costs
- Nonmedical costs
- Nondollar costs

Chemotherapeutic Agents

There is a substantial range of costs for the individual cancer chemotherapeutic agents, with 5-fluorouracil (5-FU) priced at less than one cent per mg and cisplatin (DDP) at \$3.64/mg. When described in such a fashion, however, the therapeutic dose must be factored in. Furthermore, most standard chemotherapy involves delivery of multiple agents in combination chemotherapy regimens in which the component drug doses are adjusted for the combination.

Table 1 details the drug costs alone to the patient (or the third-party carrier) for delivery of a number of common cancer chemotherapeutic regimens. The costs are based upon the optimal dose rate of delivery for each of the component agents in a 1.7 m^2 individual and include a standard pharmacy markup of 300%. The latter is representative of the markup in a teaching institution; the increment may be modified for the administration of such drugs in a physician's office or other setting.

Some of the drug costs should be put in perspective. High-dose cytosine arabinoside (ara-C) is an experimental program with no established role — but an interesting potential — in the treatment of malignancy. For 12 doses of high-dose ara-C, a drug cost of approximately $6,000 is reached. Although for some programs, 4 or even 2 doses have been administered, and repeated cycling of therapy is necessary; therefore, $6,000 probably represents a minimum cost.

CMF and AV represent standard regimens for the treatment of breast cancer, both in an adjuvant setting and for metastatic disease. The cost of adjuvant CMF delivered for a minimum of 7 courses is more than $1,200. Again, this represents drug cost only; therefore, it represents only a portion of the cost for adjuvant therapy, excluding laboratory tests and the other components listed at the beginning of this section. It is clear that the definition of the necessity for adjuvant therapy and its impact on disease-free interval or — more important — survival, must be established if the dollar costs are to be justified.

A standard regimen for small-cell carcinoma of the lung is a combination of cyclophosphamide, Adriamycin, and VP-16. The impact of this drug combination on response is unquestionable, but the curability of this tumor with this combination is essentially nil. FAM, at a cost of $900/cycle, may be compared to 5-FU at a cost of $30/cycle. The comparison is particularly poignant in that FAM has become standard therapy for advanced gastric cancer in spite of the lack of superiority of this regimen in prospective randomized controlled studies against 5-FU, at least as measured by survival.[1]

VBP represents a chemotherapeutic regimen that is curative in patients with even advanced testicular cancer; it involves a patient population that is youthful and therefore has a productive period of life possible with effective treatment. Generally, 4 courses of VBP are administered, at a cost of approximately

Table 1. Standard Cancer Chemotherapeutic Regimens and Drug Costs for Each Cycle of Bolus Therapy

Regimen		Drug schedule	Total drug cost cycle ($)
FAM	5-FU	300 mg/M^2 days 1, 8, 28, 35	899
	Adriamycin	30 mg/M^2 days 1, 8, 28, 35	
	Mitomycin-C	10 mg/M^2 day 1	
CMF	Cyclophosphamide	100 mg/M^2 daily 10 days oral	201
	Methotrexate	60 mg/M^2 day 1, 8 I.V.	
	5-FU	600 mg/M^2 day 1, 8 I.V.	
CAV	Cytoxan	600 mg/M^2	633
	Adriamycin	60 mg/M^2	
	VP-16	150 mg/M^2	
AV	Adriamycin	50 mg/M^2 I.V.	454
	Vincristine	2 mg/M^2 I.V.	
High-dose ara-C	Ara-C	3 g/M^2 × 12 doses continuous infusion	6,029

$2,400 per course. The adjuvant application of VBP should be placed in perspective in this setting, in which salvage therapy is successful and the costs of adjuvant treatment enormous. For VBP, the drug costs represent a relatively small portion of the overall costs for delivery because almost all patients treated with this regimen will develop treatment-related complications requiring hospitalization.

Administration Costs

These costs depend to some extent on the treatment to be administered. Generally, the total cost is a combination of the cost of syringes, I.V. solutions, and catheter materials and the cost of the time spent in administration by the nurse or physician. Thus, agents that require hydration prior to administration, e.g., DDP, or agents that require infusion over 30 minutes to 2 hours will be associated with higher costs. In comparison, 5-FU delivered as a bolus injection has a minimal cost.

Physician's Fee

Reimbursement for the professional component in the delivery of chemotherapy is variable. In 1985, a minimum fee of $50 per administration was relatively standard; it included an assessment of the appropriateness of the chemotherapy program and a brief physical examination.

Treatment Complications

The area of treatment complications represents a major and important part of a determination of cost-effectiveness. The development of complications is related to host factors that may reflect the sensitivity of normal tissues to the drugs. For standard bolus chemotherapy the dose is the most important determinant of treatment complications. Chemotherapeutic dose is generally maximized to induce a toxic effect, manifested by leukopenia or thrombocytopenia in the majority of patients, in order to validate the fact that cytocidal levels of the drug are achieved.

The potential complications of chemotherapeutic treatment are indicated in table 2, along with the general approach to management. These complications are the acute toxicities related to the administration of most, but not all, chemotherapeutic agents; excluded are chronic toxicities, such as renal failure, cardiac toxicity, infertility, and even second neoplasms due to chemotherapy exposure, that may result from chemotherapy.

Nausea and vomiting are the most common complications one deals with in bolus-oriented chemotherapy. For DDP, the use of high-dose Decadron at a dose of 20 mg pretreatment and every 6 hours for 24 hours after treatment incurs a substantial cost, as does the use of newer antiemetics. Hospitalization, with its attendant services needed to provide supervision during the period of acute toxicity, increases the cost of this complication substantially.

The major costs of treatment of complications are linked with those patients in whom severe or life-threatening leukopenia or thrombocytopenia can occur, with risk of actual development of infection or hemorrhage. Hospitalization as a consequence of these 2 complications is generally for at least 7 days, perhaps for an average of 10–14 days. A major cost of the hospitalization is related particularly to the use of antibiotics, especially combinations of antibiotics (see table 3). Broad-spectrum antibiotic coverage is often provided for in the neutropenic patient by using a combination of ticarcillin and tobramycin; in a standard 14-day course, the cost for antibiotics alone is $2,400 or more. Moxalactum alone for a 14-day course may cost $2,400.

Nonmedical Costs

The definition of nonmedical costs has been infrequently addressed in the literature. Hodgson describes the economic costs of cancer in a chapter of a book on cancer epidemiology published in 1975.[2] Houts et al discussed a method for data collection on medical expenses for cancer patients in a conference on cancer control in 1982,[3] specifically addressing the issue of nonmedical costs.[4] In the latter study, outpatients receiving cancer chemotherapy were studied in an attempt to estimate costs to patients receiving chemotherapy,

Table 2. Treatment Complications Related to Chemotherapy and Management Costs

Complication	Management cost options
Nausea/vomiting	Hospitalization Decadron Antiemetics
Stomatitis	Viscous Xylocaine Mycostatin
Hair loss	Wig
Leukopenia	Hospitalization Antibiotics
Thrombocytopenia	Platelet transfusion

Table 3. Antibiotic Therapy: Cost to Patient for 14-Day Course

Drug	Average dose	No. doses/day	Daily cost ($)	Total cost/ 14 days ($)
Kefzol	500 mg – 1 g	3	19 – 33	277 – 476
Ticarcillin	3 g	6	117	1646
Piperacillin	3 g – 4 g	4	119 – 148	1666 – 2075
Moxalactam	2 g	2 – 3	116 – 174	1627 – 2441
Amikacin	500 mg (7.5 mg/kg)	2	84	1181
Gentamicin	80 mg	3	13	181
Tobramycin	80 mg	3	51	718
Amphotericin	(Max. 1.5 mg/kg)	1	74	1044

separating the components into treatment weeks and nontreatment weeks and defining the out-of-pocket versus other costs.

The major categories of nonmedical costs were transportation, food, family care, and lost wages. Transportation, which represents the largest out-of-pocket cost after lost wages, is clearly related to the distance from a treatment center. Transportation cost also included the cost of trips to pharmacies or for follow-up blood counts. In the study by Houts et al, transportation also included the cost of trips to visit individuals or places that would not have been taken if the patient had not had cancer. Transportation costs were about $16 in a treatment week, compared to about $2.60 in a nontreatment week.

Food costs, which represent the second highest cost for both treatment or nontreatment weeks, included the use of vitamin supplements, special foods and protein supplements necessitated by the patient's condition, and meals necessarily bought away from home. Food costs during a treatment week were approximately 2½ times those during a nontreatment week, coming to about half of the transportation costs.

Family care is a potential cost that would vary with family circumstances but could involve the cost of baby-sitters to care for children or companions to care for the elderly in the absence of the patient during outpatient treatment time or hospitalization.

Lost wages represent a substantial portion of nonmedical costs; in fact, in the study by Houts et al, this cost was 49% of the total nonmedical cost during a treatment week. Income loss is an overlooked issue for patients and their families. Disability insurance may or may not be a part of the patient's portfolio, and supplemental income from employers or from social agencies is often delayed or involves frustrating paperwork. Lost wages must also include those lost by individuals who provide transportation to the hospital or clinic.

An application of the methodology employed by Houts et al is included in their paper in a discussion of the nonmedical costs for the adjuvant treatment of breast cancer. By extrapolating the data from their study and applying a formula for calculating cost on treatment weeks and nontreatment weeks, they were able to identify a savings of $1,427 in nonmedical costs per patient if adjuvant therapy was reduced from 12 months to 6 months.

Nondollar Costs

Describing the costs of therapeutic modality in terms of dollars alone is inadequate. To these quantifiable costs must be added the intangible costs related to life-style modifications, altered interpersonal and family relationships, and lowered self-image and self-esteem. These nondollar costs of having cancer represent the biased perspective of the author and certainly are not intended to be all-encompassing.

Major life-style alterations are experienced by most, if not all, cancer patients. The treatment as well as the disease requires availability to a treatment center and thereby restricts the mobility of patients. Individuals prone to travel need, therefore, to restrict that activity, sometimes with a substantial effect on their work pattern. Treatment complications may substantially affect physical appearance, thus restricting work activities for individuals who interface with the public as a major part of their life-style.

The commonly observed impact of cancer and its treatment on interpersonal and family relationships is sometimes subtle. An anecdote will serve to suggest the range of effects that chemotherapy can have on such relationships. A young married male with acute leukemia was placed on chemotherapeutic program and promptly entered complete remission. He subsequently was treated as an outpatient and tolerated therapy quite well except for intermittent thrombocytopenia. On one visit to the outpatient department, the patient was extraordinarily agitated and fearful. In an interview, the patient expressed his fear that he was soon going to die. On further questioning, it was learned that the patient had avoided sexual relationships with his recent bride for the previous 3 months, but the night before had renewed them with vigor. He also said that he had been admonished by his physician to be careful in contact sports while on chemotherapy because of the possibility of hemorrhage. The warning was interpreted by the patient as including sexual activity, and as a consequence of this misperception he had become celibate and had, in his view, risked the possibility of death the night before.

The myths and misunderstandings regarding chemotherapy may contribute to the impact in terms of cost on interpersonal relationships; therefore, clear communication between physician and family as well as physician and patient is essential.

There are potentially positive benefits from the delivery of chemotherapy in these settings as well. The tragedy of cancer often brings families together in a united way to share feelings openly, something that can be cathartic and emotionally satisfying. Many anecdotal experiences of patients receiving infusional chemotherapy have suggested that the necessary involvement of family members and close friends has permitted an expanded relationship with patients.

Self-image and self-esteem are two often-ignored but costly secondary effects of cancer chemotherapy. Not infrequently, the development of cancer is regarded by the patient as a punishment for some obscure deed of the past. The disease may be perceived as something foul or dirty for which the patient feels guilty, making him unwilling to share his life with others. The consequent impact on self-esteem can be substantial to the point of inducing withdrawal from activities and regression and depression. The self-image impact of chemotherapy is clear, with its induction of hair loss and cutaneous changes as well as nutritional effects, all of which work together to alter one's appearance.

These nondollar costs may in fact be more costly than the treatment itself, or at least more costly than the drugs that are used. It is most important that care givers in particular be aware of and sensitive to these issues in dealing with the patient receiving chemotherapy.

Comparative Costs of Infusion Chemotherapy

As with bolus chemotherapy, the dollar cost of infusion schedules is complex and obscured by confounding factors. In comparing infusion chemotherapy to bolus chemotherapy, one should restrict such a comparison to infusion chemotherapy delivered on an outpatient basis and compare it to outpatient bolus chemotherapy. Any comparison between outpatient and inpatient chemotherapy is clearly weighted by hospitalization costs; therefore, the focus of this section will be on infusion chemotherapy administered on an outpatient basis.

Another confounding variable is the type of infusion administered—either short-term or protracted infusion. These 2 categories are also associated with different possibilities in terms of treatment complications as well; therefore, costs incurred for the whole treatment cycle will be necessarily different. Furthermore, regional infusion, a third category of infusion chemotherapy, is associated with costs related to the operative procedure, and the extraordinary cost of the implanted pump system clearly adds substantially to total cost. For this reason, the type of infusion employed should be considered in an analysis of cost whenever possible.

The cost categories presented above, which are similar for bolus or infusion chemotherapy, include drug costs, treatment complications, and nonmedical and nondollar costs. Extra costs for infusion chemotherapy involve the technology applications and hardware employed in delivery. This section will address the cost categories for infusion chemotherapy as well as the cost of the extraordinary aspects of infusion delivery.

Chemotherapeutic Agents

Tables 4 and 5 list the drug cost for delivery of single agents on an infusion schedule administered on a short-term infusion for 4–5 days or for 30 days. Short-term infusion 5-FU is comparable on a bolus or infusion schedule at $38 and $30, respectively, for a standard course. Adriamycin is substantially less in drug costs when administered by short-term infusion with a similar or slightly higher cumulative dose. For protracted duration infusion of 30 days, the costs are substantially higher than when the same agents are delivered on a 4- or 5-day schedule (table 5).

Treatment Complications

The cost of treatment complications is substantially altered with infusion chemotherapy. Specific drug-related complications are eliminated or modified, but complications related to the catheter system and the pump system

Table 4. Drug Cost For 5-Day Course of Continuous Infusion Chemotherapy

Drug	Schedule*	Drug cost to patient ($)
5-FU	1 mg/M^2/d × 5 d	38
Vinblastine	1.5 mg/M^2/d × 5 d	88
Adriamycin	10–15 mg/M^2/d × 4 d	214–320
Cisplatin	20 mg/M^2/d × 5 d	567

*Assume M^2 = 1.7

may contribute to treatment costs. The most frequent complications of infusion chemotherapy to be dealt with are catheter occlusion and subclavian vein thrombosis. In the former complication, the use of urokinase or streptokinase to clear the catheter may be necessary. With subclavian vein thrombosis, hospitalization and consequent heparinization and oral anticoagulation may be in order. This complication occurs in 15% of patients with venous access of chronic nature. Other potential treatment-related complications include infection developing as a consequence of placement of a chronic access catheter; this complication is infrequent, however, occurring in fewer than 3% of the largest reported series.

Hardware and Management Costs

The costs that are unique to infusion chemotherapy are related to venous access and the portable infusion pumps.

VENOUS ACCESS

Chronic venous access is best obtained by the placement of a permanent or semipermanent access through the subclavian vein. The use of the Broviac or Hickman catheter has recently been complemented by the development of implanted access devices. The costs of the established access devices are listed in Table 6. The costs given are for 1985 and may vary according to the region of the United States or from country to country. Added to this cost is the surgical fee, which is also variable but is generally between $200–$500. The vascular access devices may be inserted in an outpatient setting, but require a

Table 5. Drug Cost to Patient for 30-Day Course of Continuous Infusion Chemotherapy

Drug	Daily dose	Total drug cost to patient ($)
5-FU	300 mg/M^2	209
FUDR	0.125–0.15 mg/kg	262
Vinblastine	0.5 mg/M^2	327
Adriamycin	3 mg/M^2	892
Mitomycin-C	0.5 mg/M^2	695
Cisplatin	5 mg/M^2	1,921
Cytoxan	50 mg/M^2	374

Table 6. Costs of Vascular Access Devices

Device	Cost ($)
Infusaport	250
Mediport	295
Port-a-Cath	330

surgery center facility or operating room and recovery room time as an added hospital cost.

Additional costs for the use of vascular access for the implanted devices are specifically the Huber point needles. These specially designed needles, which promote the longevity of the access device, cost $2.50 each. The cost for needles may be quite variable, depending upon the institution's policy on the frequency of needle exchange.

AMBULATORY INFUSION PUMPS

Technical issues relating to the various infusion devices are reviewed in a previous chapter. The costs of such infusion pumps, competitive with syringe pumps, range from $1,200–$1,300; rotary drum pumps cost from $1,300–$2,100 (table 7). Newer pump designs incorporating unique mechanisms of delivery and microchip components may substantially raise the costs of such devices. The pumps are paid for by the individual patient or third-party payer or, alternatively, patients may rent pumps for the duration of the infusion. The daily rental rate generally is $10–$12 per day. For a protracted infusion, the cost of the pump alone would be approximately $360 per month. For a 5-day infusion, the pump rental fee would approximate $60. Because the ambulatory infusion pumps can be used by multiple patients in sequence (in contrast to the implanted devices and implanted pump systems), the pump cost may be spread among patients to reduce costs over time.

Additional costs for infusion chemotherapy involve the necessity for dressing changes, the use of heparin to maintain the catheter, and the cost of the drug reservoir. For protracted infusion, a weekly dressing change is employed with the use of the implanted access devices. For other types of access, biweekly changes of dressing are generally the policy. Heparin flush may be necessary at 4- to 6-week intervals for the implanted vascular access device, with heparinization of the external devices, including the Hickman catheter, as often as once a day. Finally, the contribution of the drug reservoirs to cost may be related to the type of pump used, the duration of the infusion, and the stability of the drug to be used. The 50 cc reservoir employed with the rotary drum pump may result in a cost to the patient of $20–$30 each.

Table 7. Costs of Portable Infusion Pump*

Type of pump	Cost ($)
Syringe pump	
Autosyringe (AS2F)	1,345
Graseby	1,150
Rotary drum pump	
Cormed I	1,325
Cormed II	1,595
Deltec CADD I	2,195
Pancreatic IV 2000	1,850
Parker	2,000

*Quoted for 1985; may vary according to manufacturer's policies

Cost Comparisons: Bolus Versus Infusion Chemotherapy

With the exception of a brief report by Stagg et al describing the relative costs of hepatic arterial infusion and systemic venous infusion,[5] there is virtually no literature on the total cost of infusion chemotherapy. Furthermore, it is clear from the previous discussions that the costs of infusion chemotherapy vary considerably according to such factors as geographical location and prevailing economic determinants. Table 8 attempts to describe the comparative costs of infusion and bolus chemotherapy. There are inherent fixed costs for the hardware involved with infusion chemotherapy that are not applicable to bolus delivery. Drug costs are clearly at least comparable between the 2 methods. Venous access is not included here as a difference because bolus chemotherapy not infrequently requires some type of venous access as well. However, the clinic time spent in setting up a patient on an infusion translates to a $100 fee per session. Pump costs, which may be minimized by distributing the cost among patients, vary with the duration of infusion. Similarly, drug reservoir costs in infusion chemotherapy vary according to whether syringes or polyvinyl collapsible pouches are used.

Administration costs are comparable for both bolus and infusion delivery, but the use of infusion chemotherapy may permit the therapy to be initiated by family members at home, thereby diminishing the costs. Venous access maintenance costs depend upon the type of venous access employed and may be applicable to bolus chemotherapy as well. Nonmedical costs have not been addressed in any studies of infusion chemotherapy reported to date. For bolus chemotherapy, however, in the singular study by Houts et al the costs were approximately $72/week during treatment weeks.

Other costs include the nondollar costs and the costs of complications. The positive reinforcement provided by the absence of toxicity and the involvement of patient and family and friends in the infusion system suggests a shift in the balance favoring infusion chemotherapy in this column. Similarly, the absence

Table 8. Relative Costs of Bolus Versus Infusion Chemotherapy

Cost item	Bolus		Infusion
Drug	—	comparable	—
Pump	N/A*		$1,200 – $1,800
Reservoir	N/A		$3 – $30
Venous access	—	comparable	—
Administration	Variable		Variable
Maintenance of venous access	N/A		$50/mo.
Nonmedical costs	$72/wk		N/A
Nondollar costs	—	comparable	—
Complication costs	Major		Minimal

*N/A = Not applicable

of drug-related complications with infusion chemotherapy suggests that infusion delivery may be superior to bolus in this category as well.

Quantitative comparisons are difficult. However, even a single drug-related episode of leukopenia or thrombocytopenia calling for a protracted hospitalization will add substantial cost to the chemotherapy experience; the absence of such complications with infusion chemotherapy eliminates that cost. In addition, the fact that no work time is lost because of toxicity among patients receiving infusion therapy permits one in a qualitative sense to infer that infusion chemotherapy has an economic advantage for the patient as well as for industry.

Comparison of External and Implanted Pump Infusion Programs

The only study reported relating to this question is by Stagg et al.[5] The study represented a retrospective analysis of 32 patients, half of whom were treated with an external pump administering the drug either I.V. or I.A. The cost of I.V. therapy was comparable for both the external and the implanted pumps, totaling approximately $5,800 for 6 months of outpatient care. Intra-arterial chemotherapy costs were substantially higher—approximately $15,000 for the same period—but again were comparable for both the external and implanted pump devices. The authors conclude that there are specific roles for either the external or the implanted pump, depending upon the drug to be infused and the patient prognosis. The issue of comparative costs for implanted and external infusion devices will certainly be addressed more comprehensively over time as technology advances.

Summary

Cost-effective chemotherapy depends in part on the efficacy of the delivery system, but in the context of cancer care, cost-effectiveness may be a complex formulation involving the therapeutic index as well as issues relative to lifestyle. In fact, the traditional concept of the therapeutic index may be modified in the context of cost-effectiveness concerns.

One suggestion for a new design of the traditional formula for therapeutic index (TI) is as follows:

$$\text{Therapeutic Index} = \frac{\text{Antitumor Effect} \times \text{Survival}}{\text{Toxicity} + \text{Cost}}$$

The TI balances the therapeutic effect or antitumor effect observed in the numerator against a denominator represented by the toxicity or adverse effects incurred as a consequence of the treatment. One may consider introducing survival into the formulation; this component would reasonably be a multiplying factor in the numerator, especially if survival is translated into cure. To the denominator one may reasonably add the fiscal costs of treatment delivery. Adding dollar cost rather than multiplying it seems reasonable in that costs in dollars at least philosophically should be counted for less than the extension of life.

It is clear that infusion delivery of chemotherapy substantially reduces toxicity and possibly costs, thus influencing the TI of the old design as well as the proposed new design. The specific quantitative impact of infusion chemotherapy on the TI awaits future prospective studies.

45

ADJUVANT APPLICATIONS OF
INFUSIONAL CHEMOTHERAPY

Jacob J. Lokich, M.D., and Paul H. Sugarbaker, M.D.

ADJUVANT APPLICATIONS OF CHEMOTHERAPY represent one of the more important developments of cancer treatment in the decade of the 1970s. The concepts of multidisciplinary treatment in primary cancer management have been expanded to employ chemotherapy as the initial modality, followed in sequence by definitive local treatment to permit less radical approaches and to provide for expeditious treatment of occult metastases systemically. In fact, multimodality or multidisciplinary approaches to primary cancer may be the more appropriate terminology in the cancer lexicon. "Adjuvant" implies a modality of secondary importance, and it is most likely the optimal interdigitation of each modality that results in the most effective treatment and the best chance for cure.

One might reasonably separate categories of "adjuvant" chemotherapy as outlined in table 1. In category 1, involving postoperative delivery of chemo-

Table 1. Categories of 'Adjuvant' Chemotherapy or Chemoradiotherapy

Category/reference	Regimen
1. Postoperative therapy	
Breast cancer[1]	CMF, LPAM + FU
Gastric cancer[2]	5-FU + MeCCNU
Pancreas cancer[3]	5-FU + radiation
Rectal cancer[4]	5-FU + MeCCNU + radiation
2. Protochemotherapy	
Esophagus, Anus	5-FU + MIT + radiation
Head & Neck[7]	5-FU + DDP
Lung[8]	CAP
Ovary	CAP

therapy, prospective randomized trials in breast cancer, gastric cancer, and pancreas cancer in which untreated control groups were employed have all demonstrated a survival advantage for various subsets for a treatment regimen.[1-3] An advantage has also been demonstrated for postoperative administration of chemotherapy (in conjunction with radiation) in rectal cancer[4] but not in colon cancer.[5]

In category 2, defined as "protochemotherapy," chemotherapy or chemotherapy combined with radiation has been employed as the initial treatment, followed by surgery. Two tumors are now routinely approached in this fashion. In esophageal and anal cancer, the delivery of chemotherapy in combination with radiation as the initial modality has resulted in a substantial change in the management of the primary tumor.

For example, for anal cancer, an abdominoperineal resection with colostomy construction is no longer routinely employed.[6] For head and neck cancer involving T3 and T4 tumors and N1 nodes, 3-year survival is uncommon; however, up to 30% of patients may now achieve that goal with primary chemotherapy followed by regional radiation.[7] For each of these tumor categories, the "adjuvant" chemotherapy is most often delivered on an infusion schedule. Other tumors in which primary chemotherapy is employed include Stage 3 Mo nonsmall-cell lung cancer,[8] ovarian cancer, and testicular cancer. In the latter 2 tumors, secondary debulking is applied either before or after chemotherapy for advanced disease. Preoperative application of chemotherapy for primary breast cancer is also being investigated.[9]

The present discussion will review the ongoing adjuvant trials employing infusion chemotherapy. Trials in colon cancer in particular will be reviewed in depth, including regional and systemic infusional chemotherapy as well as intraperitoneal chemotherapy. Adjuvant applications of infusional chemotherapy in the treatment of other G.I. tumors, breast cancer, and lung cancer will be conceptually explored in an attempt to identify future applications of infusional chemotherapy.

Colon and Rectal Cancer

The adjuvant chemotherapy approaches to colorectal cancer over the past 15 years may be described as having demonstrated no impact on this tumor. The trials have involved bolus chemotherapy using antipyrimidines in a variety of schedules and drug combinations. Nonetheless, important information has been derived from these studies, including the fact that the experimental design and staging is critical. For example, patients with B2 colon cancer have an excellent prognosis with surgery alone and are not, as a rule, candidates for additional therapy. Furthermore, separation of patients into subgroups according to the number of positive nodes allows for an important substaging for stratification of treatment groups. Finally, the inclusion of control groups (surgical treatment only) within the experimental design continues to be absolutely essential. In at least one controlled study, a disadvantage for a treatment secondary to the induction of leukemia as a consequence of one of the component agents in a combination chemotherapy regimen was uncovered.[10]

Clinical trials of adjuvant treatment of colon cancer employing an infusion schedule have focused particularly on regional delivery. Administration techniques have included:

- Intraluminal chemotherapy
- Portal vein infusion
- Hepatic arterial infusion
- Intraperitoneal infusion
- Systemic (venous) infusion

Intraluminal "infusion" is included because it represents the early conceptual orientation leading to several other local/regional chemotherapy strategies. Four of the 5 infusion trials are directed at regional disease.

Intraluminal 5-FU Administration

The local/regional concept of 5-fluorouracil (5-FU) drug administration was initiated by 2 groups. Grossi et al[11] and Lawrence et al[12] pursued intraluminal 5-FU chemotherapy instillations at the time of surgery as an adjuvant treatment. Both groups used untreated control groups by which to measure the effects of the intraluminal 5-FU. One study used I.V. 5-FU to supplement the intraluminal drug, and the other used immediate postoperative I.V. 5-FU and then oral 5-FU as part of the intensive adjuvant chemotherapy course.

The technique of intraluminal chemotherapy involved isolating with surgical tapes the segment of bowel that contained the malignancy. 5-FU at a dose of 30 mg/kg was placed in 50 cc of saline and injected into the bowel; at least 30 minutes was allowed to pass prior to resection of the bowel segment. Neither study showed an advantage in survival for the intraluminally treated patient groups. Although these studies were not successful in their attempt to improve survival, they served as a model for subsequent attempts to test local/regional 5-FU administration as an adjuvant to surgery.

Portal Vein Infusion

A number of controlled clinical trials of portal vein infusion with 5-FU have been reported or are ongoing (see table 2). The rationale for portal vein drug delivery is based upon the fact that in "early stage" cancer with microscopic disbursement of tumor, the blood supply to that tumor in the liver is provided by the portal system. Second, there is a substantial frequency of liver metastases from colorectal cancer, and the liver is often the limiting organ in terms of life-style and longevity. The initial study by Taylor et al reported in 1977 on 50 consecutive patients.[13] Twenty-four of the 50 patients received 5-FU (1 g/day) as a continuous infusion for 7 days through the portal venous system. An interesting observation at a mean follow-up time of 15.5 months was that no patient in the infusion group developed clinical evidence of hepatic metastases. This provocative report fostered subsequent trials by Taylor and by others. The follow-up study by Taylor, reported in 1984, included a much larger patient entry, with a total of 257 patients at a median follow-up of 48 months.[14] In this study, there appeared to be an advantage in terms of the reduction of liver metastases in patients with Duke's B colorectal cancer and an improvement in survival as well. There was, however, no survival benefit in patients with Duke's C colon cancer or with rectal cancer.

In an initial report by Metzger et al on a study of 170 patients, a 50% reduction in overall metastases resulted for a treated group, with only 6 patients developing liver metastases. In an updated report on 390 patients, only 14% of patients have relapsed compared to 27% in the control group, with a median follow-up of 22 months.[15] This is the only study in which mitomycin-C (MIT) is added to the 5-FU regimens.

Conflicting data have been reported from the group at St. Mary's and in Rotterdam. These studies are 3-arm protocols in which an anticoagulant infusion serves as an additional control. The St. Mary's study suggests that the frequency of liver metastases is reduced by more than 50%; a group receiving heparin without 5-FU infusion also had a reduced frequency of metastases. In contrast, the Rotterdam group could demonstrate no difference in the frequency of metastases for the treated versus the control group at a median follow-up of 18 months.

Three ongoing studies are employing similar regimens in terms of dose and duration of infusion for 5-FU, and in one, a heparin infusion control arm is included. It is anticipated that these trials will definitely answer the question of the role of portal vein infusion in the adjuvant therapy of colon and rectal cancers.

Table 2. Prospective Randomized Trials with Adjuvant Portal Infusion

Institution	No. patients	Entry	Primaries	Treatment (vs. control)	Results
Liverpool	257	1976–80	C + R*	1 g 5-FU + heparin/d × 7	4-year survival 70% vs. 92%
St. Mary's	317	1978–83	C + R	1 g 5-FU + heparin/d × 7 or 10,000 u heparin/d × 7	Frequenty liver mets: 6.5% vs. 8% vs. 15.3%
Rotterdam	303	1981–84	C + R	1 g 5-FU + heparin/d × 7 or 240,000 u urokinase/24 hr	Frequenty liver mets: 4.9% vs. 7% vs. 4.9%
Mayo/NCCTG	?	1980–	C	1 g 5-FU + heparin/d × 7	No data
NSABP	250	1984–	C	600 mg/M² 5-FU + heparin/d × 7	No data
EORTC	150	1983–	C	500 mg/M² 5-FU + heparin/d × 7 or 5,000 u heparin/d × 7 alone	No data
SAKK	390	1981–	C + R	500 mg/M² 5-FU + heparin/d × 7 + 10 mg/M² mitomycin C d 1	Relapses 14% vs. 27%

Source: Metzger U. Adjuvant treatments for primary colorectal cancer. Eur J Surg Oncol (in press)
*C = colon; R = rectum

Intra-Arterial Infusion

The regional delivery of arterial chemotherapy to the liver has been extensively employed for the management of hepatic metastases from colorectal cancer in particular. In patients with Duke's C carcinoma, however, adjuvant applications have not been previously explored, with the exception of the ongoing clinical trials developed at the M. D. Anderson Hospital. The rationale for such a trial is similar to that for portal vein infusion in that the liver represents a dominant site of metastases. Two pilot studies were carried out at the M. D. Anderson Hospital and within the Southwest Oncology Group (see table 3). The first study by Patt et al administered floxuridine (FUDR) and MIT in short-term infusions over multiple courses in 40 patients.[16] In the pilot study, 14 patients with Duke's C carcinoma relapsed, and 4 relapses were in the liver (10%). The results are in contrast to the usual 30% incidence of liver-only metastases, but the number of patients accrued was small. The study by McCracken et al[17] employed 5-FU plus MIT and added hepatic radiation to the program. In a pilot study involving 19 patients, 2/13 evaluable patients developed hepatic recurrence but, most important, the treatment regimen was associated with a substantial toxicity. Eleven patients developed radiation hepatitis and 1 of the 19 patients died of liver failure. The severity of the hepatic toxicity is surprising considering the fact that these patients presumably did not have a poor performance status (they had no evidence of metastases). Other clinical trials employing combined arterial infusion plus radiation for patients with sometimes extensive liver metastases have failed to identify serious adverse effects.

In 1985, Patt et al inaugurated a prospective comparative trial in patients with Duke's C carcinoma only in which patients would receive intermittent course FUDR and MIT administered via a percutaneously placed catheter for a total of 3 courses. An untreated control group in this second generation study should establish the role of hepatic arterial infusion as an adjuvant approach to colorectal cancer.

Hepatic Resection and Adjuvant Chemotherapy

The use of chemotherapy in an attempt to prevent recurrence following resection of hepatic metastases from colorectal cancer has been referred to as "semi"- or "pseudoadjuvant" therapy.

O'Connell et al[18] reported on the use of systemic 5-FU following hepatic resection of colorectal metastases in 26 patients. Nineteen of the 26 patients

Table 3. Clinical Trials of Adjuvant Hepatic Arterial Infusion

Trial/reference	Chemotherapy	No. patients	Relapsed/liver
Patt et al[16]	FUDR + MIT	40	14 / 4
McCracken et al[17]	5-FU + MIT + radiation	19	ND* / 2
Patt et al	Controlled trial	ND	ND

*ND = No data

had progressed; the median survival was 34 months, with a projected 5-year survival of 15%. A watched but not randomized control group had a similar 5-year survival.

In uncontrolled studies, several investigators have added intra-arterial (I.A.) or intraportal fluorinated pyrimidines to the surgical treatment of hepatic metastases. Fortner et al reported on their experience with I.A. and intraportal 5-FU,[19] and Kemeny et al instituted a study comparing I.A. chemotherapy with the implanted pump and no added therapy in patients with resected hepatic metastases.[20] This latter trial has not accrued enough patients to permit a definitive statement concerning efficacy. Patt et al have treated a pilot group of 28 patients with I.A. FUDR before and after hepatic resection.[21] As expected, complications with surgery following I.A. FUDR were high, but treatment was suggestively successful in that few intrahepatic sites of treatment failure developed, and patients with positive margins seemed to do as well as patients with clear resections.

Intraperitoneal Chemotherapy

Intraperitoneal (I.P.) administration of chemotherapy for patients with colorectal cancer became an attractive route of drug administration as the natural history of treatment failures following surgical resection became clear. Treatment failures occur at the resection site, but the second and third most frequent areas for treatment failure are the peritoneal surfaces and, finally, the liver. Intraperitoneal administration of 5-FU was found to yield high levels of drug both on peritoneal surfaces and within the liver.[22] Figure 1 shows the intraportal levels of 5-FU after 1 g of the drug is placed in the abdominal cavity in 2 L of dialysis fluid. Levels of 5-FU within the peritoneum are about 2,000 times greater than in the circulation, and drug levels in the portal vein are 10–40 times greater than with systemic infusion of 5-FU.

Sugarbaker et al reported the results of a randomized controlled trial of I.V. versus I.P. 5-FU in patients with advanced primary colon or rectal cancer.[23] When 5-FU was delivered by the I.P. route, the tolerable dose of drug was markedly increased without an increase in adverse side effects (see figure 2).

The toxic side effects of I.P. or I.V. 5-FU administration were seen in the same proportion of patients. Toxicity was experienced in virtually all patients on this study because the dose of drug was escalated in all patients until toxicity was observed. However, the toxic manifestations of the drug were markedly different when the 2 routes of 5-FU administration were compared. Toxicities with I.V. 5-FU were primarily hematologic. Patients also reported diarrhea and more mucositis than those receiving drug I.P. The limiting factor for I.P. 5-FU administration was abdominal pain.

Perhaps the most interesting results of this trial revolve around an analysis of treatment failures following I.P. or I.V. drug administration. The natural history of surgically treated disease was changed by reducing the incidence of peritoneal carcinomatosis (see table 4). Unfortunately, the survival and time to relapse in these 2 patient groups did not differ significantly.

The precise role for I.P. 5-FU in patients with large-bowel malignancy has not been defined. These are patients who are at extremely high risk for recurrent disease on peritoneal surfaces. There are patients with perforated colon cancer, and there are those with adjacent organ involvement in whom lysis of adhesions between a tumor mass and a vital structure is required for removal of the primary tumor. It has been shown that viable tumor cells are nearly always present within tumor adhesions. Intraperitoneal 5-FU could be used to prevent peritoneal implants in these patients.

Another adjuvant application of I.P. chemotherapy is in patients undergoing hepatic resection. A randomized controlled study comparing I.P. 5-FU to no further treatment has been instituted at the National Institutes of Health in patients undergoing successful resections of hepatic metastases from colorectal cancer. It is yet too early to assess the results of this protocol.

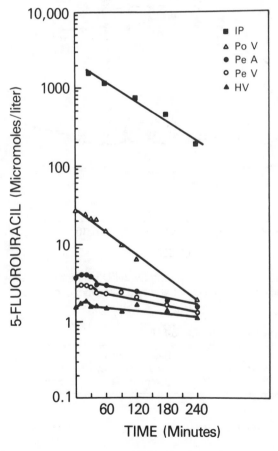

INTRAPERITONEAL 5-FU CHEMOTHERAPY
(1040 mg/2L)

Figure 1.   5-FU blood levels after 1 g of 5-FU in 2 L of dialysis fluid are placed in the abdominal cavity. (From ref. 22.)

Systemic Adjuvant Infusion Trials

Systemic approaches to adjuvant chemotherapy of colon cancer have been based on delivery of bolus 5-FU. Systemic infusional fluoropyrimidines have not been reported in the adjuvant setting. However, if the enthusiasm for and track record of infusional 5-FU and FUDR are maintained as a consequence of ongoing prospective clinical trials in advanced disease, an adjuvant application may be feasible and realized in the near future.

Lokich et al did initiate a prospective randomized controlled trial in Duke's C carcinoma of the colon in 1980, but an insufficient number of patients have accrued for a meaningful analysis. This study employed the prerandomization concept to enter patients, and only those patients who had positive lymph nodes (Duke's C lesion) were eligible. The rationale for the study was based upon pharmacologic issues related to 5-FU and on tumor cytokinetic consider-

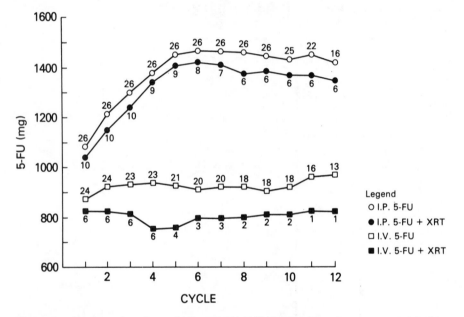

Figure 2.   Comparative dose of I.P. and I.V. 5-FU when drug dose was escalated to toxicity. (From Gianola et al, Am J Clin Oncol, in press.)

Table 4. Sites of Treatment Failure for I.V. and I.P. 5-FU

	No. patients	No. (%) of recurrence	Peritoneal surface	Liver	Retroperitoneal and/or pelvic lymph nodes	Abdominal incision	Lung	Bone marrow
I.P. 5-FU	36	13 (36)	2/10	3/11	7/11	2/11	2/11	3/13
I.V. 5-FU	30	11 (37)	10/11	4/11	3/10	1/11	4/11	0/11
Statistical analysis p =		NS	.003	1.0	.27	1.0	.64	.57

ations suggesting that the tumor doubling time in early stage colon cancer may be about 30 days. The design of the program was such that patients would be assigned to either the control group (surgical therapy only) or receive a 30-day continuous infusion of 5-FU at a dose of 300 mg/m^2/day administered via the subclavian vein. On completion of therapy, no additional treatment was introduced, and patients were followed at 3- 4-month intervals thereafter.

Table 5 summarizes the data in this trial, which accrued a total of 22 patients over the 2½-year period June 1980 through February 1982. The imbalance in numbers of patients entered and treated in the control group relates to 2 patients who were randomized to receive a 30-day infusion but refused. They have been included in the control group. The site of the primary tumor was relatively balanced across the groups, although the treated group had a higher frequency of transverse colon lesions and the untreated group had a larger proportion with sigmoid lesions. Two patients in each group had 4 or more positive nodes. Three relapses have occurred in the treated group (33%), 2 of which were in the liver alone. In the untreated group, 9 patients have relapsed (70%), 5 in the liver and 1 in the lung. With a median follow-up of 33 months, the median survival of the treated group is 39+ months, and for the untreated control group, 36+ months.

Rectal Cancer

Cancers of the rectum are defined as lesions occurring below the peritoneal refection. The biologic history of these tumors is distinctive from that of colon cancer in that they have a greater tendency to recur locally, depending upon the initial stage. Multiple studies have indicated that augmented local treatment using radiation has an advantage, at least in terms of local control.

When added to radiation in the treatment of virtually all G.I. tumors, including esophageal cancer, gastric cancer, and pancreatic cancer, chemotherapy consistently demonstrates an additive and possibly a synergistic effect. Improvement in survival was demonstrated in a report by the Gastrointestinal

Table 5. Summary of Data from Randomized Trial of Adjuvant 30-Day 5-FU Infusion

	Treated group	Untreated group
Number of patients	9	13*
Relapsed	3 (33%)	9 (70%)
Metastatic sites:		
Liver	2	4
Peritoneum	0	1
Lung	0	2
Unknown	1	4
Survival:		
Number alive	6	7
NED	6	3
Median	39 mo.	36 mo.

*Includes 2 patients randomized to treatment but refused

Tumor Study Group indicating that 5-FU and methyl CCNU delivered as a bolus with radiation was superior as compared to a control group treated by surgery alone.[4] The advantage was achieved in both local control and disease-free interval. A second-generation study is comparing radiation combined with bolus 5-FU to radiation combined with bolus 5-FU plus methyl CCNU. If, in fact, the bolus 5-FU added to the radiation continues to be the important component in the combined modality approach to rectal cancer, a potential future program could be as outlined in figure 3. Such a study has been proposed by Mayer.[24] In it, patients would receive either bolus 5-FU in conjunction with radiation or continuous infusion 5-FU in conjunction with radiation, employing the same dose of radiation but a different delivery schedule (and a different dose of 5-FU). A pilot study of continuous infusion 5-FU in conjunction with radiation has already demonstrated the feasibility of the combination.[25] Clearly, the continuous infusion of 5-FU, which may function as a radiation sensitizer, is the much more rational interdigitation of the 2 modalities, since the constant availability of 5-FU must be important to radiation sensitization.

Applications of Adjuvant Infusional Chemotherapy to Other Tumors

Adjuvant chemotherapy has an established role for such tumors as breast cancer and osteogenic sarcoma. Isolated clinical trials, however, have suggested that adjuvant chemotherapy may also play a role in gastric cancer, pancreatic cancer, and ovarian cancer. Although no clinical trials of infusional chemotherapy in an adjuvant setting have been reported for these tumors, it is reasonable to consider infusional delivery schedules for chemotherapeutic agents that have been established in adjuvant applications for a specific tumor. This section will address the role of infusional adjuvants according to tumor categories in which a potential or real adjuvant role for chemotherapy has been established.

Breast Cancer

The adjuvant application of the 3-drug regimen cyclophosphamide (CTX), methotrexate (MTX), and 5-FU (CMF) has become standard for patients with pathologic stage 2 breast cancer. In addition, doxorubicin (ADR)-containing multidrug regimens such as CTX plus ADR (CA) or CTX, ADR, and 5-FU (CAF) have been employed.

Each of the component drugs of either the CMF or the CA regimen can be administered as an infusion and could therefore be delivered as an adjuvant infusion. In addition, admixtures of MTX and 5-FU,[26] as well as CTX and ADR,[27] are possible, and would permit the infusion of all or most of the component drugs in a combination.

Osteogenic and Soft Tissue Sarcoma

It has been suggested only recently that adjuvant therapy could have an effect on these rare tumors. The chemotherapy employed generally has been an ADR-based program. As indicated in other chapters, ADR can be administered by a continuous infusion and has been employed in an infusional setting in these tumors, showing a response rate comparable to bolus delivery. Thus, the use of ADR infusions in an adjuvant setting is possible.

Gastric Cancer

Although a host of adjuvant trials in gastric cancer have employed 5-FU-based regimens, only a single clinical trial (by the Gastrointestinal Tumor Study Group) has indicated that the adjuvant application of 5-FU delivered as a bolus combined with methyl CCNU may increase the cure rate for surgically resected cancer of the stomach by as much as 20%.[2] In addition, a number of Japanese trials using MIT as an intraperitoneal bath have indicated a possible benefit in survival.[28] Adjuvant chemotherapy in gastric cancer therefore has a modest clinical experience with survival benefit, and systemic infusion of these agents (5-FU, MIT) can be explored.

ADJUVANT RECTAL CANCER PROTOCOL

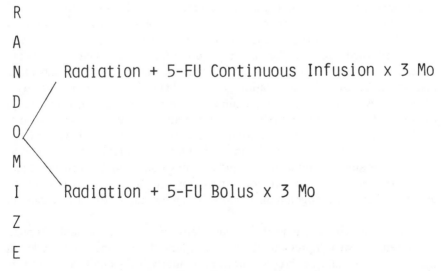

Figure 3.   Proposed trial of adjuvant fluoropyrimidine administered as a bolus or infusion in conjunction with "adjuvant radiation."

Pancreas Cancer

A single trial of adjuvant chemotherapy consisting of 5-FU combined with radiation therapy has demonstrated an advantage for this therapy over a control group.[3] In addition, a study comparing chemotherapy to no therapy in a prospective randomized study from Great Britain has also demonstrated an advantage for the chemotherapy group in terms of survival.[29] Infusional delivery of 5-FU in conjunction with radiation, as well as infusion of components of the complex multidrug regimen employed without radiation, could be studied in prospective trials on this tumor.

Ovarian Cancer

In contrast to the tumors cited previously, ovarian tumors are exquisitely responsive to chemotherapy. For advanced disease, combination chemotherapy involving an alkylating agent (generally CTX) and cisplatin (DDP) achieves responses in up to 70% of patients. Cisplatin on a continuous infusion schedule for 5 days in conjunction with CTX has demonstrated substantial activity in advanced disease and could reasonably be applied to an adjuvant setting.[30] Infusional I.P. DDP has been effective in advanced ovarian cancer, and the use of I.P. DDP following induction chemotherapy to the point of complete pathologic response is being evaluated in clinical trials.

Protochemotherapy

The concept of applying chemotherapy as the initial treatment for some cancers was named "neoadjuvant chemotherapy" by Frei, and as the concept has become more intriguing and applied more broadly, the term "protochemotherapy" has been promulgated. With this concept, chemotherapy is moved from a palliative mode for patients with terminal disease to a primary modality for treating local and regional tumor as well as distant micrometastatic disease. The basic ingredients for applying a program of protochemotherapy are predicated on the identification of effective chemotherapy in the advanced disease setting and the application of such chemotherapy to patients with earlier stages of disease. Candidate tumors for protochemotherapy include (1) tumors with poor prognosis related to intermediate or advanced stage of disease, (2) tumors with poor prognosis related to biological behavior of the tumor, and (3) tumors with major morbidity for regional treatment related to surgical therapy (see table 6). Excluded from consideration for protochemotherapy would be those tumors with poor prognoses but no established effective therapy; malignant melanoma is representative of such a case in point.

The tumors for which protochemotherapy might be reasonably applied have been reviewed in previous chapters, but other tumors may be included in the future. For example, breast cancer, particularly if regionally advanced, is increasingly being treated with primary chemotherapy followed by either surgery or radiation or a combination of both. The delivery of chemotherapy on an infusion schedule has not been explored in this patient population, but for this stage of disease, primary infusional chemotherapy and subsequent surgery may be advantageous.

For lung cancer, effective treatment for advanced disease has been an elusive goal. Nonetheless, combination chemotherapy employing CTX and ADR in conjunction with DDP or other agents in patients with stage 3 nonsmall-cell lung carcinoma as initial treatment prior to surgery or radiation has demonstrated an improved 2- and 3-year survival compared to nonrandomized controls.[8] Infusional trials using DDP and 5-FU have achieved similar response rates[31] and may be applied in a neoadjuvant setting in the future.

Table 6. Candidate Tumors for Protochemotherapy

Tumors	Infusional trials/reference
Tumors with poor prognosis related to stage	
Breast cancer — Stage 3	None
Lung cancer — Stage 3	None
Ovarian cancer — Stage 3 and 4	None
Tumors with poor prognosis related to biologic behavior	
Esophageal cancer	5-FU + DDP[32]
Tumors with major morbidity related to surgical therapy	
Anal cancer	5-FU + MIT[33]
Extremity sarcoma	Adriamycin[34,35]
Head and neck	Cisplatin
	Bleomycin[7,36]
	5-FU
Tumors with poor prognosis but no effective chemotherapy	
Malignant melanoma	None

Summary

Infusional chemotherapy, if it becomes established as superior to standard bolus chemotherapy, will enter the arena of adjuvant applications. The most readily apparent application has been in the multimodality approach, with radiation for esophageal and anal cancer as well as head and neck cancer. However, the spectrum of tumors for which adjuvant therapy has become or is becoming standard practice is expanding. The variety of infusional delivery systems being employed in ongoing prospective trials, including regional intra-arterial, I.P., and systemic delivery, will, along with the experimental designs incorporated into the trials, have the potential to answer the question of the specific role for infusion chemotherapy in the adjuvant setting.

REFERENCES

References—Chapter 1

1. Frei E III, Canellos GP. Dose: a critical factor in cancer chemotherapy. Am J Med 1980; 69:585–94.

2. Brindley CO et al. Further comparative trial of thio-phos-phoro-amide and mechlorethamine in patients with melanoma and Hodgkin's disease. J Chronic Dis 1964; 17:19.

3. Frei E III, Spurr CL, Brindley CO, et al. Clinical studies of dichloromethotrexate (NSC 29630). Clin Pharmacol Ther 1965; 6:160–171.

4. O'Bryan RM, Baker LH, Gottleib JE, et al. Dose response evaluation of Adriamycin in human neoplasia. Cancer 1977; 39:1940–48.

5. McVie JG, Dalesio O, Smith IE, eds. Autologous bone marrow transplantation and solid tumors. 14, Raven Press, 1984.

6. Richards MA, Barnett MJ, Waxman JH, et al. The use of high dose cytosine arabinoside for non-Hodgkins lymphoma. Seminars in Onc. 1985; 12(2) Supplement 3:223–26.

7. Ozols RF, Ostchega Y, Myers CE, Young RC. High dose cisplatin in hypertonic saline in refractory ovarian cancer. J Clin Oncol 1985; 3(9):1246–50.

8. Scheving LE, Burns ER, Pauly JE, Halberg F. Circadian bioperiodic response of mice bearing advanced L1210 leukemia to combination therapy with Adriamycin and cyclophosphamide. Cancer Res 1980; 40:1511–15.

9. Focan C. Sequential chemotherapy and circadian rhythm in human solid tumors. A Randomized Trial. Cancer Chemother Pharmacol 1979; 3:197–202.

10. Ludwig R, Alberts DS, Miller TP, Salmon SE. Evaluation of anticancer drug schedule dependency using an in vitro human tumor clonogenic assay. Cancer Chemother Pharmacol 1984; 12:135–41.

11. Lokich JJ, Zipoli T, Moore C, Sonneborn H, Paul S, Greene R. Doxorubicin/vinblastine and doxorubicin/cyclophosphamide combination chemotherapy by continuous infusion. J Clin Oncol (in press).

12. Lokich JJ, Phillips D, Greene R, et al. 5-fluorouracil and methotrexate administered simultaneously as a continuous infusion: a phase I study. Cancer 1985; 56:2395–98.

References—Chapter 2

1. Bruce WR, Meeker BE, Valeriote FA. Comparison of the sensitivity of normal hematopoietic and transplanted lymphoma colony-forming cells to chemotherapeutic agents administered in vivo. J Natl Cancer Inst 1966; 37:233–45.

2. Shimoyama M. Cytocidal action of anticancer agents: evaluation of the sensitivity of cultured animal and human cancer cells. Bibl Haemat 1975; 40:711–22.

3. Drewinko B., Roper PR, Barlogie B. Patterns of cell survival following treatment with anticancer agents in vitro. Eur J Cancer 1979; 15:93–99.

4. Powis G. Anticancer drug pharmacodynamics. Cancer Chemother Pharmacol 1985; 14:177–83.

5. Eichholtz H, Trott KR. Effect of methotrexate concentration and exposure time on mammalian cell survival in vitro. Br J Cancer 1985; 41:277–84.

6. Rupniak HT, Whelan RDH, Hill BT. Concentration and time-dependent inter-relationships for antitumour drug cytotoxicities against tumour cells in vitro. Int J Cancer 1983; 32:7–12.

7. Johnson RK, Garibjanian BT, Houchens DP, et al. Comparison of 5-fluorouracil and ftorafur. I. Quantitative and qualitative differences in toxicity to mice. Cancer Treat Rep 1976; 60:1335–45.

8. Himmelstein KJ, Bischoff KB. Mathematical representations of cancer chemotherapy effects. J Pharmacokin Biopharm 1973; 1:51–69.

9. Shackney SE. A computer model for tumor growth and chemotherapy, and its application to L1210 leukemia treated with cytosine arabinoside (NSC-63878). Cancer Chemother Rep 1970; 54:399–429.

10. Jusko WJ. A pharmacodynamic model for cell cycle-specific chemotherapeutic agents. J Pharmacokin Biopharm 1973; 1:175–200.

11. Simpson-Herren L, Lloyd HH. Kinetic parameters and growth curves for experimental tumor systems. Cancer Chemother Rep 1970; 54:143–174.

12. Lira AK. The dynamics of tumour growth. Br J Cancer 1966; 28:490–502.

13. Goldin A, Venditti JM, Humphreys SR, Mantel N. Modification of treatment schedules in the management of advanced mouse leukemia with amethopterin. J Natl Cancer Inst 1956; 17:203–12.

14. Chabner BA, Young RC. Threshold methotrexate concentration for in vivo inhibition of DNA synthesis in normal and tumorous target tissues. J Clin Invest 1973; 52:1804–11.

15. Dahl WN, Oftebro R, Pettersen EO, Brustad T. Inhibitory and cytotoxic effects of Oncovin (vincristine sulfate) on cells of human line NHIK 3025. Cancer Res 1976; 36:3101–05.

16. Ludwig R, Alberts DS. Chemical and biological stability of anticancer drugs used in a human tumor clonogenic assay. Cancer Chemother Pharmacol 1984; 12:142–45.

17. Drewinko B, Novak JK, Barranco SC. The response of human lymphoma cells in vitro to bleomycin and 1,3-Bis (2-chloroethyl)-1-nitrosourea. Cancer Res 1972; 32:1206–08.

18. Alberts DS, Chen H-SG. Tabular summary of pharmacokinetic parameters relevant to in vitro drug assay. In: Salmon SE, ed. Cloning of human tumor stem cells. New York: Alan R. Liss, 1980; 351–359.

19. Vogelzang NJ. Continuous infusion chemotherapy: a critical review. J Clin Oncol 1984; 2:1289–1304.

20. Lister TA, Rohatiner AZS. The treatment of acute myelogenous leukemia in adults. Semin Hematol 1983; 19:172–92.

21. Wisch JS, Griffin JD, Kufe DW. Response of preleukemic syndromes to continuous infusion low-dose cytarabine. N Engl J Med 1983; 309:1599–1602.

22. Ho DHW, Frei E. Clinical pharmacology of 1-β-D-arabinofuranosylcytosine. Clin Pharmacol Ther 1971; 12:944–54.

23. Wu P-C, Ozols RF, Hatanaka M, Boone OW. Anticancer drugs: effect on the cloning of Raji lymphoma cells. J Natl Cancer Inst 1982; 68:115–21.

24. Greenberg PL, Van Kersen I, Moshy S. Cytotoxic effects of 1-β-D-arabinofuranosylcytosine and 6-thioguanine in vitro on granulocytic progenitor cells. Cancer Res 1976; 36:4412–17.

25. Kline I, Venditti JM, Tyrer DD, Goldin A. Chemotherapy of leukemia L1210 in mice with 1-β-D-arabinofuranosylcytosine hydrochloride. I. Influence of treatment schedules. Cancer Res 1966; 26:853–59.

26. Skipper HE, Schabel FM, Mellett LB, et al. Implications of biochemical, cytokinetic, pharmacologic, and toxicologic relationships in the design of optimal therapeutic schedules. Cancer Chemother Rep 1970; 54:431–50.

27. Venditti JM. Treatment schedule dependency of experimentally active antileukemic (L1210) drugs. Cancer Chemother Rep 1971; 2:35–59.

28. Skipper HE, Schabel FM, Wilcox WS. Experimental evaluation of potential anticancer agents. XXI. Scheduling of arabinosylcytosine to take advantage of its S-phase specificity against leukemia cells. Cancer Chemother Rep 1967; 51:125–65.

29. Volger WR, Miller DS, Keller JW. 5-azacytidine (NSC 102816): a new drug for the treatment of myeloblastic leukemia. Blood 1976; 48:331–37.

30. Covey JM, Zaharko DS. Effects of dose and duration of exposure on 5-aza-2'-deoxycytidine cytotoxicity for L1210 leukemia in vitro. Cancer Treat Rep 1984; 68:1475–81.

31. Momparier RL, Gonzales FA. Effect of intravenous infusion of 5-aza-2'-deoxycytidine on survival time of mice with L1210 leukemia. Cancer Res 1978; 38:2673–78.

32. Zimm S, Collins JM, Riccardi R, et al. Variable bioavailability of oral mercaptopurine: is maintenance chemotherapy in acute lymphoblastic leukemia being optimally achieved? N Engl J Med 1983; 308:1005–09.

33. Venditti JM, Sheldon DR, Goldin A. Evaluation of antileukemic agents employing advanced leukemia L1210 in mice. VII. Cancer Res 1964; 24:145–96.

34. Venditti JM, Kline I, Goldin A. Evaluation of antileukemic agents employing advanced leukemia L1210 in mice. VIII. Cancer Res 1964; 24:827–79.

35. El Sayed YM, Sadee W. In: Ames MM, Powis G, Kovach JS, eds. Pharmacokinetics of anticancer agents in humans. New York: Elsevier, 1983; 209–227.

36. Kufe DW, Majors PP. 5-fluorouracil incorporation into human breast carcinoma RNA correlates with cytotoxicity. J Biol Chem 1981; 256:9802–05.

37. Calabro-Jones PM, Byfield JE, Ward JF, Sharp TR. Time-dose relationships for 5-fluorouracil cytotoxicity against human epithelial cancer cells in vitro. Cancer Res 1982; 42:4413–20.

38. Drewinko B, Yang LY, Ho DHW, Benvenuto J, Loo TL, Freireich EJ. Treatment of cultured human colon carcinoma cells with fluorinated pyrimidines. Cancer 1980; 45:1144–58.

39. Matsushima Y, Kanzawa F, Hoshi A, et al. Time-schedule dependency of the inhibiting activity of various anticancer drugs in the clonogenic assay. Cancer Chemother Pharmacol 1985; 14:104–07.

40. Ferguson T. Prevention and delay of spontaneous mammary and pituitary tumors by long- and short-term ingestion of 5-fluorouracil in Wistar-Furth rats. Oncology 1980; 37:353–356.

41. Lin H. Schedule-dependent effect of phase-specific cytotoxic agents on production of hemolytic plaque-forming cells. J Natl Cancer Inst 1976; 56:95–99.

42. Henry MC, Blair WH, Sheffner AM, Schein P. Beagle dog as predictor of schedule-dependent toxicity of 5-fluoro-2-deoxyuridine. Toxicol Appl Pharmacol 1972; 23:532–34.

43. Collins JM. Pharmacokinetics of 5-fluorouracil infusions in the rat: comparison with man and other species. Cancer Chemother Pharmacol 1985; 14:108–11.

44. Schilsky RL. Clinical pharmacology of methotrexate. In: Ames MM, Powis G, Kovach JS, eds. Pharmacokinetics of anticancer agents in humans. New York: Elsevier, 1983; 187–208.

45. Keefe DA, Capizzi RL, Rudnick SA. Methotrexate cytotoxicity for L5178Y/Asn⁻ lymphoblasts: relationship of dose and duration of exposure to tumor cell viability. Cancer Res 1982; 42:1614–45.

46. Johnson LF, Fuhrman CL, Abelson HT. Resistance of resting 3T6 mouse fibroblasts to methotrexate cytotoxicity. Cancer Res 1978; 38:2408–12.

47. Pinedo HM, Chabner BA. Role of drug concentration, duration of exposure, and endogenous metabolites in determining methotrexate cytotoxicity. Cancer Treat Rep 1977; 61:709–19.

48. Zaharko DS, Dedrick RL, Peale AL, Drake JC, Lutz RJ. Relative toxicity of methotrexate in several tissues of mice bearing Lewis lung carcinoma. J Pharmacol Exp Ther 1974; 189:585–92.

49. Pinedo HM, Zaharko DS, Bull J, Chabner BA. The relative contribution of drug concentration and duration of exposure to mouse bone marrow toxicity during continuous methotrexate infusion. Cancer Res 1977; 37:445–50.

50. Krakoff IH, Brown NC, Reichard P. Inhibition of ribonucleoside diphosphate reductase by hydroxyurea. Cancer Res 1968; 28:1559–65.

51. Fishbein WN. Excretion and hematologic effects of single intravenous hydroxyurea infusions in patients with chronic myeloid leukemia. Johns Hopkins Med J 1967; 121:1–8.

52. Sinclair WK. Hydroxyurea: differential lethal effects on cultured mammalian cells during the cell cycle. Science 1965; 150:1729–31.

53. Plager J. The induction of transient increases in mitotic rate in murine tissues following prolonged intravenous infusions of hydroxyurea. Cell Tissue Kinet 1975; 8:517–28.

54. Ross W, Rowe T, Glisson B, Yalowich J, Liu L. Role of topoisomerase II in mediating epipodophyllotoxin-induced DNA cleavage. Cancer Res 1984; 44:5857−60.

55. Minocha A, Long BH. Inhibition of the DNA catenation activity of type II topoisomerase by VP-16-213 and VM-26. Biochem Biophys Res Commun 1984; 122:165-70.

56. Creasey WA. The vinca alkaloids and similar compounds. In: Crooke ST, Prestayko AW, eds. Cancer and chemotherapy (Vol. III, Antineoplastic agents). New York: Academic Press, 1981; 79-96.

57. Nelson RL. The comparative clinical pharmacology and pharmacokinetics of vindesine, vincristine, and vinblastine in human patients with cancer. Med Pediatr Oncol 1982; 10:115-27.

58. Lau ME, Hansen HH, Niessen NI, Pedersen H. Phase 1 trial of a new form of an oral administration of VP-16-213. Cancer Treat Rep 1979; 63:485-87.

59. Gout PW, Noble RL, Bruchorsky N, Beer CT. Vinblastine and vincristine-growth-inhibitory effects correlate with their retention by cultured No2 node lymphoma cells. Int J Cancer 1984; 34:245-48.

60. Jackson DV, Bender RA. Cytotoxic thresholds of vincristine in a murine and a human leukemia cell line in vitro. Cancer Res 1979; 39:4346-49.

61. Ludwig R, Alberts DS, Miller TP, Salmon SE. Evaluation of anticancer drug schedule dependency using an in vitro human tumor clonogenic assay. Cancer Chemother Pharmacol 1984; 12:135-41.

62. Wells J, Berry RJ, Laing AH. Reproductive survival in vitro of recently explanted human tumour cells following exposure to vinblastine. A suggestion for improved clinical dose schedules. Europ J Cancer 1976; 12:793-96.

63. Mujagic H, Chen S-S, Geist R, et al. Effects of vincristine on cell survival, cell cycle progression, and mitotic accumulation in asynchronously growing sarcoma 180 cells. Cancer Res 1983; 43:3591-97.

64. Bruce WR, Meeker BE, Powers WE, Valeriote FA. Comparison of the dose- and time-survival curves for normal hematopoietic and lymphoma colony-forming cells exposed to vinblastine, vincristine, arabinosylcytosine, and amethopterin. J Natl Cancer Inst 1969; 42:1015-23.

65. Feaux de Lacroix W, Klein M. Comparative investigations on the effect of the phase-specific drug vincristine (VCR) on the proliferation kinetics of a solid experimental tumor. J Cancer Res Clin Oncol 1983; 106:187-91.

66. Feaux de Lacroix W, Mallmann H. Comparative investigations on the effect of different dose schedules of the phase-specific drug vincristine (VCR) on the proliferation kinetics of a solid experimental tumour. Cell Tissue Kinet 1984; 17:583-91.

67. Jackson DV, Bender RA. The clinical pharmacology of the vinca alkaloids, epipodophyllotoxins, and maytansine. In: Pinedo HM, ed. Clinical pharmacology of anti-neoplastic drugs. Amsterdam: Elsevier, 1978; 277-93.

68. Drewinko B, Barlogie B. Survival and cycle-progression delay of human lymphoma cells in vitro exposed to VP-16-213. Cancer Treat Rep 1976; 60:1295-1306.

69. Vietti TJ, Valeriote FA, Kalish R, Coulter D. Kinetics of cytotoxicity of VM-26 and VP-16-213 on L1210 leukemia and hematopoietic stem cells. Cancer Treat Rep 1978; 62:1313-20.

70. Broggini M, Colombo T, D'Incali M. Activity and pharmacokinetics of teniposide in Lewis lung carcinoma-bearing mice. Cancer Treat Rep 1983; 67:555-59.

71. Dombernowsky P, Nissen NI. Schedule dependency of the antileukemic activity of the podophyllotoxin-derivative VP-16-213 (NSC-141540) in L1210 leukemia. Acta Pathol Microbiol Scand 1973; 81:715-24.

72. Traganos F, Staiano-Loico L, Dorzynkiewicz Z, Melamed MR. Effects of ellipticine on cell survival and cell cycle progression in cultured mammalian cells. Cancer Res 1980; 40:2390-99.

73. Takemura Y, Ohnuma T, Chou T-C, Okano T, Holland JF. Biologic and pharmacologic effects of harringtonine on human leukemia-lymphoma cells. Cancer Chemother Pharmacol 1985; 14:206-10.

74. Colvin M. Molecular pharmacology of alkylating agents. In: Crooke ST, Prestayko AW, eds. Cancer and chemotherapy (Vol. III, Antineoplatic agents). New York: Academic Press, 1981; 287-302.

75. Grochow LB, Colvin M. Clinical pharmacokinetics of cyclophosphamide. In: Ames MM, Powis G, and Kovach JS, eds. Pharmacokinetics of anticancer agents in humans. New York: Elsevier, 1983; 135-54.

76. Williamson CE, Kirby JG, Miller JI, et al. Enzyme-alterable alkylating agents. IX. The enzymatic

transformation of some nitrogen mustards in the presence of carbon dioxide: Implications in respiration. Cancer Res 1966; 26:323–30.

77. Bruce WR, Meeker BE, Valeriote FA. Comparison of the sensitivity of normal hematopoietic and transplanted lymphoma colony-forming cells to chemotherapeutic agents administered in vivo. J Natl Cancer Inst 1966; 37:233–45.

78. Drewinko B, Novak JK, Barranco SC. The response of human lymphoma cells in vitro to bleomycin and 1,3-bis(2-chloroethyl)-1-nitrosourea. Cancer Res 1972; 32:1206–08.

79. Wheeler KT, Tel N, Williams ME, Sheppard S, Levin VA, Kabra PM. Factors influencing the survival of rat brain tumor cells after in vitro treatment with 1,3-bis(2-chloroethyl)-1-nitrosourea. Cancer Res 1975; 35:1464–69.

80. Schmidt V, Zapol W, Prenoky W, Wonders T, Wodinsky I, Kitz R. Continuous cancer chemotherapy: nitrosourea diffusion through implanted silicone rubber capsules. Trans Amer Soc Artif Int Organs 1972; 18:45–52.

81. Crooke ST. Mitomycin C – an overview. In: Crooke ST, Prestayko AW, eds. Cancer and chemotherapy (Vol. III, Antineoplastic agents). New York: Academic Press, 1981; 49–60.

82. Choi KE, Sinkule JA, Crom W, Thompson E, Evans W. HPLC assay of mitomycin C in biological fluids. J Chromatogr (in press).

83. Barlogie B, Drewinko B. Lethal and cytokinetic effects of mitomycin-C on cultured human colon cancer cells. Cancer Res 1980; 40:1973–80.

84. Bergerat J-P, Barlogie B, Golde W, Johnston DA, Drewinko B. In vitro cytokinetic response of human colon cancer cells to cis-dichlorodiammineplatinum(II). Cancer Res 1979; 39:4356–63.

85. Patton TF, Repta AJ, Sternson LA. Clinical pharmacology of cisplatin. In: Ames MM, Powis G, Korach JS, eds. Pharmacokinetics of anticancer agents in humans. New York: Elsevier, 1983; 155–186.

86. Drewinko B, Brown BW, Gottlieb JA. The effect of cis-diamminedichloroplatinum (II) on cultured human lymphoma cells and its therapeutic implications. Cancer Res 1973; 33:3091–95.

87. Bergerat J-P, Barlogie B, Drewinko B. Effects of cis-dichlorodiammineplatinum (II) on human colon carcinoma cells in vitro. Cancer Res 1979 39:1334–38.

88. Niell HB, Wood CA, Mickey DD, Soloway MS. Time- and concentration-dependent inhibition of the clonogenic growth of N-[4-(5-nitro-2-furyl)-2-thiazoly] formamide-induced murine bladder tumor cell lines by cis-diamminedichloroplatinum (II). Cancer Res 1982; 42:807–11.

89. Moran RE, Straus MJ. Effects of pulse and continuous intravenous infusion of cis-diamminedichloroplatinum on L1210 leukemia in vivo. Cancer Res 1981; 41:4993–96.

90. Drewinko B, Yang L-Y, Barlogie B, Trujillo JM. Comparative cytotoxicity of bisantrene, mitoxantrone, ametantrone, dihydroxyanthracenedione, dihydroxyanthracenedione diacetate, and doxorubicin on human cells in vitro. Cancer Res 1983; 43:2648–53.

91. Nguyen-Ngoc T, Vrignaud P, Robert J. Cellular pharmacokinetics of doxorubicin in cultured mouse sarcoma cells originating from autochthonous tumors. Oncology 1984; 41:55–60.

92. Krishan A, Frei E. Effect of adriamycin on the cell cycle traverse and kinetics of cultured human lymphoblasts. Cancer Res 1976; 36:143–50.

93. Barlogie B, Drewinko B, Johnston DA, Freireich EJ. The effect of adriamycin on the cell cycle traverse of a human lymphoid cell line. Cancer Res 1976; 36:1975–79.

94. Eichholtz-Wirth H. Dependence of the cytostatic effect of adriamycin on drug concentration and exposure time in vitro. Br J Cancer 1980; 41:886–91.

95. Zirvi KA, Masui H, Giuliani FC, Kaplan NO. Correlation of drug sensitivity on human colon adenocarcinoma cells grown in soft agar and in athymic mice. Int J Cancer 1983; 32:45–51.

96. Bailey-Wood R, Dallimore CM, Whittaker JA. Effect of adriamycin on CFU_{GM} at plasma concentrations found following therapeutic infusions. Br J Cancer 1984; 50:351–55.

97. Ensminger WD, Greenberger JS, Egan EM, Muse MB, Moloney WC. Technique for preclinical evaluation of continuous infusion chemotherapy with the use of WF rat acute myelogenous leukemia. J Natl Cancer Inst 1979; 62:1265–68.

98. Goldin A, Johnson RK. Experimental tumor activity of adriamycin (NSC-123127). Cancer Chemother Rep 1975; 6:137–45.

99. Sandberg JS, Howsden FL, DiMarco A, Goldin A. Comparison of the antileukemic effect in mice of adriamycin (NSC-123127) with daunomycin (NSC-82151). Cancer Chemother Rep 1970; 54:1-7.

100. Pacciarini MA, Barbieri B, Colombo T, Broggini M, Garattini S, Donelli MG. Distribution and antitumor activity of adriamycin given in a high-dose and a repeated low-dose schedule to mice. Cancer Treat Rep 1978; 62:791-800.

101. Jensen RA, Acton EM, Peters JH. Doxorubicin cardiotoxicity in the rat: comparison of electrocardiogram, transmembrane potential, and structural effects. J Cardiovasc Pharmacol 1984; 6:186-200.

102. Solcia E, Ballerini L, Bellini O, et al. Cardiomyopathy of doxorubicin in experimental animals. Factors affecting the severity, distribution and evolution of myocardial lesions. Tumori 1981; 67:461-72.

103. Young RC, Ozols RF, Myers CE. The anthracycline antineoplastic drugs. N Engl J Med 305:139-153.

104. Hill BT, Dennis LY, Li X-T, Whelan RDH. Identification of anthracycline analogues with enhanced cytotoxicity and lack of cross-resistance to adriamycin using a series of mammalian cell lines in vitro. Cancer Chemother Pharmacol 1985; 14:194-201.

105. Andersson B, Beran M, Peterson C, Tribukait B. Significance of cellular pharmacokinetics for the cytotoxic effects of daunorubicin. Cancer Res 1982; 42:178-83.

106. Tanabe M, Miyamoto T, Nakajima Y, Terasima T. Lethal effect of aclacinomycin A on cultured mouse L cells. Gann 1980; 71:699-703.

107. Bhuyan BK, Blowers CL, Crampton SL, Shugars KD. Cell kill kinetics of several nogalamycin analogs and adriamycin for chinese hamster ovary, L1210 leukemia, and B16 melanoma cells in culture. Cancer Res 1981; 41:18-24.

108. Hellmann K, Carter SK, eds. Cancer treatment reviews—mitoxantrone (novantrone). New York: Academic Press, Vol. 10 (Suppl B), Dec. 1983.

109. Fountzilas G. Gratzner H, Lim LO, Yunis AA. Sensitivity of cultured human pancreatic carcinoma cells to dihydroxyanthracenedione. Int J Cancer 1984; 33:347-53.

110. Vosika G, Cooper MR, Vogelzang N, et al. Severe toxicity and death associated with zinostatin administration. Cancer Treat Rep 1982; 66:410-411.

111. Citarella RV, Wallace RE, Murdock KC, Angier RB, Durr FE, Forbes M. Activity of a novel anthracenyl bishydrazone, 9,10-anthracenedicarboxaldehyde Bis [4,5-dihydro-1H-imidazol-2-yl) hydrazone] dihydrochloride, against experimental tumors in mice. Cancer Res 1982; 42:440-44.

112. Von Hoff DD, Myers JW, Kuhn J, et al. Phase 1 clinical investigation of 9,10-anthracenedicarboxaldehyde Bis [4,5-dihydro-1H-imidazol-2-yl) hydrazone] dihydrochloride (CL216,942). Cancer Res 1981; 41:3118-21.

113. Peng Y-M, Alberts DS, Davis TP. In vivo and in vitro metabolism of the new anticancer drug bisantrene. Cancer Chemother Pharmacol 1985; 14:15-20.

114. Powis G, Kovach JS. Disposition of bisantrene in humans and rabbits: Evidence for intravascular deposition of drug as a cause of phlebitis. Cancer Res 1983; 43:925-29.

115. Umezawa H, Meada K, Takeuchi T, Toshioka O. New antibiotics: bleomycin A and B. J Antibiot[A] (Tokyo) 1966; 19:200-06.

116. Yagoda A, Mukherji B, Young C, et al. Bleomycin, an antitumor antibiotic: Clinical experience in 274 patients. Ann Intern Med 1972; 77:861-70.

117. Bennett JM, Reich SD. Diagnosis and treatment: Drugs five years later. Ann Intern Med 1979; 90:945-48.

118. Sausville EA, Stein RW, Peisach J, Horwitz SB. Properties and products of the degradation of DNA by bleomycin and iron. Biochemistry 1978; 17:2746-54.

119. Pratt WB, Ruddon RW. The anticancer drugs. Oxford: Oxford University Press, 1979.

120. Krakoff IH, Cvitkovic E, Currie V, Yeh S, LaMonte C. Clinical pharmacologic and therapeutic studies of bleomycin given by continuous infusion. Cancer 1977; 40:2027-37.

121. Broughton A, Strong JE, Holoye PY, Bedrossian WM. Clinical pharmacology of bleomycin following intravenous infusion as determined by radioimmunoassay. Cancer 1977; 40:2772-78.

122. Yee GC, Crom WR, Lee FH, Smyth RD, Evans WE. Bleomycin disposition in children with cancer. Clin Pharmacol Ther 1983; 33:668-73.

123. Haas CD, Coltman CA, Gottlieb JA, et al. Phase 2 evaluation of bleomycin. Cancer 1976; 38:8–12.

124. Cooper KR, Hong WK. Prospective study of the pulmonary toxicity of continuously infused bleomycin. Cancer Treat Rep 1981; 65:419–25.

125. Drewinko B, Novak JN, Barranco SC. The response of human lymphoma cells in vitro to bleomycin and 1,3-Bis(2-chloroethyl)-1-nitrosourea. Cancer Res 1972; 32:1206–08.

126. Terasima T, Takabe Y, Katsumata T, Watanabe M, Umezawa H. Effect of bleomycin on mammalian cell survival. J Natl Cancer Inst 1972; 49:1093–1100.

127. Takabe Y, Miyamoto T, Watanabe M, Terasima T. Bleomycin: Mammalian cell lethality and cellular basis of optimal schedule. J Natl Cancer Inst 1977; 59:1251–55.

128. Sikic BI, Collins JM, Mimnaugh EG, Gram TE. Improved therapeutic index of bleomycin when administered by continuous infusion in mice. Cancer Treat Rep 1978; 62:2011–17.

129. Peng YM, Alberts DS, Chen H-SG, Mason N, Moon TE. Antitumour activity and plasma kinetics of bleomycin by continuous and intermittent administration. Br J Cancer 1980; 41:644–47.

130. Waksman SA, Woodruff HB. Bacteriostatic and bactericidal substances produced by a soil actinomyces. Proc Soc Exp Biol Med 1940; 45:609.

131. Glaubiger D, Ramu A. Anti-tumor antibiotics. In: Chabner B, ed. Pharmacologic principles of cancer treatment. Philadelphia: WB Saunders, 1982; 402–15.

132. Bhuyan BK, Fraser TJ, Day KJ. Cell proliferation kinetics and drug sensitivity of exponential and stationary populations of cultured L1210 cells. Cancer Res 1977; 37:1057–62.

133. Valeriote F, Vietti T, Tolen S. Kinetics of the lethal effect of actinomycin D on normal and leukemic cells. Cancer Res 1973; 33:2658–61.

134. Galbraith WM, Mellett LB. Disposition of [^{3}H]actinomycin D in tumor-bearing mice. Cancer Res 1976; 36:1242–45.

135. Capizzi RL, Bertino JR, Steel RT et al. L-asparaginase: clinical, biochemical, pharmacological and immunological studies. Ann Intern Med 1971; 24:893–901.

136. Sutow WW, George S, Lowman JT, et al. Evaluation of dose and schedule of L-asparaginase in multidrug therapy of childhood leukemia. Med Pediatr Oncol 1976; 2:387–95.

137. Russell D. The roles of the polyamines, putrescine, spermidine and spermine in normal and malignant tissues. Life Sci 1973; 13:1635–47.

138. Warrell RP Jr, Burchenal JH. Methylglyoxal-bis(guanylhydrazone) (methyl-GAG): current status and future prospects. J Clin Oncol 1983; 1:52–65.

139. Scher HI, Yagoda A, Ahmed T, Watson RC. Methylglyoxal-Bis(guanylhydrazone) in hormone-resistant adenocarcinoma of the prostate. J Clin Oncol 1985; 33:224–28.

140. Ethridge B, Von Hoff D. Activity of one-hour and continuous exposure of acivicin in a human tumor cloning system. Proc Am Soc Clin Oncol 1985; 4:30.

141. O'Dwyer PJ, Alonso MT, Leylane-Jones B. Acivicin: a new glutamine antagonist in clinical trials. J Clin Oncol 1984; 2:1064–71.

References—Chapter 3

1. Legha SS, Benjamin RS, MacKay B, et al. Reduction of doxorubicin cardiotoxicity by prolonged continuous intravenous infusion. Ann Intern Med 1982; 133–139.

2. Weiss AJ, Manthal RW. Experience with the use of adriamycin in combination with other anticancer agents using a weekly schedule, with a particular reference to lack of cardiac toxicity. Cancer 1977; 46:2046–52.

3. Chlebowski RT, Paroly WS, Pugh RP, et al. Adriamycin given as a weekly schedule without a loading dose: clinically effective with reduced incidence of cardiac toxicity. Cancer Treat Rep 1980; 64:47–51.

4. Garnick MB, Weiss GR, Steele GD, et al. Clinical evaluation of long-term, continuous-infusion doxorubicin. Cancer Treat Rep 1983; 67:133–42.

5. Sikic BI, Collins JM, Mimnaugh EG, Gram TE. Improved therapeutic index of bleomycin when administered by continuous infusion in mice. Cancer Treat Rep 1978; 62:2011–17.

6. Krakoff IH, Cuitkovic E, Currie V, Yeh S, LaMonte C. Clinical pharmacologic and therapeutic studies of bleomycin given by continuous infusion. Cancer 1977; 40:2027–37.

7. Cooper KR, Hong WK. Prospective study of the pulmonary toxicity of continuously infused bleomycin. Cancer Treat Rep 1981; 65:419–25.

8. Salem P, Khalyl M, Jabboury K, Hashimi L. *Cis*-diamminedichloroplatinum (II) by five-day continuous infusion. A new dose schedule with minimal toxicity. Cancer 1984; 53:837–40.

9. Lokich JJ. Phase 1 study of *cis*-diamminedichloroplatinum(II) administered as a constant five-day infusion. Cancer Treat Rep 1980; 64:905–08.

10. Seibert K, Golub G, Smiledge P, Nystram JN. Continuous streptozotocin infusion: a phase 1 study. Cancer Treat Rep 1979; 63:2035–37.

11. Warvell RP, Coonley CJ, Straus DJ, Young CW. Treatment of patients with advanced malignant lymphoma using gallium nitrate administered as a seven-day continuous infusion. Cancer 1983; 51:1982–87.

12. Seifert P, Baker LH, Reed M, Vaitkevicius VK. Comparison of continuously infused 5-fluorouracil with bolus injection in treatment of patients with colorectal adenocarcinoma. Cancer 1975; 36:123–28.

13. Hum CJ, Bateman JR. Five-day I.V. infusion with 5-fluorouracil for gastroenteric carcinoma after failure on weekly 5-FU therapy. Cancer Chemother Rep 1975; 59:1177–79.

14. Lokich J, Bothe A Jr, Fine N, Perri J. Phase 1 study of protracted venous infusion of 5-fluorouracil. Cancer 1981; 48:2565–68.

15. Lokich J, Fine N, Perri J, Bothe A Jr. Protracted ambulatory venous infusion of 5-fluorouracil. Am J Clin Oncol 1983; 6:103–08.

16. Yap HY, Blumenschein GR, Keating MJ, et al. Vinblastine given as a continuous five-day infusion in the treatment of refractory advanced breast cancer. Cancer Treat Rep 1980; 64:279–83.

17. Shackney SE, Ritch PS. Cell kinetics. In: Chabner BA, ed. Pharmacologic principles of cancer treatment. Philadelphia: WB Saunders, 1982; 45–76.

18. Wan SH, Huffman DH, Azarnoff DL, et al. Effect of route of administration and effusion on methotrexate pharmacokinetics. Cancer Res 1974; 34:3487–91.

19. Bleyer WA. The clinical pharmacology of methotrexate. Cancer 1978; 41:36–51.

20. Isacoff WH, Morrison PF, Aroesty J, et al. Pharmacokinetics of high-dose methotrexate with citrovorum factor rescue. Cancer Treat Rep 1977; 61:1665–74.

21. Jolivet J, Cowan KH, Curt GA, et al. The pharmacology and clinical use of methotrexate. N Engl J Med 1983; 309:1094–1104.

22. Chan KK, Cohen JF, Gross JF, et al. Prediction of adriamycin disposition in cancer patients using a physiologic pharmacokinetic model. Cancer Treat Rep 1978; 62:1161–66.

23. Reich SD. Clinical correlations of adriamycin pharmacology. Pharmacol Ther 1978; 2:239–45.

24. Bagley CM, Batich FW, DeVita VT. Clinical pharmacology of cyclophosphamide. Cancer Res 1973; 33:226–31.

25. Juma FD, Rodgers HJ, Trounce JR. The pharmacokinetics of cyclophosphamide, phosphoramide mustard, and nor-nitrogen mustard studied by gas chromatography in patients receiving cyclophosphamide therapy. Br J Clin Pharmacol 1980; 10:327.

26. Nelson RL, Dyke RW, Root MA. Comparative pharmacokinetics of vindesine and vinblastine in patients with cancer. Cancer Treat Rev 1980; 7:17–24.

27. Litterst CL, LeRoy AF, Guarino AM. The disposition and distribution of platinum following parenteral administration to animals of *cis*-dichlorodiammineplatinum (II). Cancer Treat Rep 1979; 63:1485–92.

28. Patton TF, Himmelstein KJ, Belt R, et al. Plasma levels and urinary excretion of filterable

platinum species following bolus injection and I.V. infusion of *cis*-dichlorodiammineplatinum-II in man. Cancer Treat Rep 1979; 63:1359–63.

29. Ho DH, Frei E. Clinical pharmacology of arabinofuranosylcytosine. Clin Pharmacol Therap 1971; 12:944–47.

30. Harris C. Pharmacokinetics of cytosine arabinoside in patients with acute myeloid leukemia. Br J Clin Pharmacol 1979; 81:219–22.

31. Kirkwood JM, Ensminger W, Rosowsky A. Comparison of the pharmacokinetics of 5-fluorouracil and 5-fluorouracil with concurrent thymidine infusions in a phase 1 clinical trial. Cancer Res 1980; 40:107–13.

32. Curt GA, Clendeninn NJ, Chabner BA. Drug resistance in cancer. Cancer Treat Rep 1984; 68:87–99.

33. Collins JM. Pharmacologic rationale for regional drug delivery. J Clin Oncol 1984; 2:498–504.

34. Vogelzang NJ. Continuous infusion chemotherapy: a critical review. J Clin Oncol 1984; 2:1289–1304.

References—Chapter 4

1. Goldman P. Rationale for continuous infusion drug therapy. 13th annual cancer course—infusional cancer chemotherapy. Harvard Medical School, Boston, Mar. 1–3, Part 1.

2. Blackshear PJ. Implantable drug-delivery systems. Scientific American 1979 Dec. 241:6; 66–73.

3. Albisser AM, Leibel BS, et al. Clinical control of diabetes by the artificial pancreas. Diabetes 1974 May 23:5; 397–404.

4. Soeldner S. Treatment of diabetes mellitus by devices. Am J Med 1981; 70:183–94.

5. Bothe A Jr, Piccione W, et al. Implantable central venous access system. Am J Surg 1984; 147:565–69.

6. Lokich JJ, Bothe A, Yanes L, Moore C. Continuous infusion chemotherapy with an ambulatory pump. 13th Int Cong of Chemother, Vienna 1983.

7. Watkins E Jr. Chronometric infusor—an apparatus for protracted ambulatory infusion therapy. N Engl J Med 1963; 269:850–51.

8. Watkins E Jr, Khazei AM. Arterial infusion chemotherapy of liver cancer. Bull Societe Internationale De Chirurgie, No. 3, 1966.

9. Watkins E Jr, Khazei AM. Surgical basis for arterial infusion chemotherapy of disseminated carcinoma of the liver. Surg Gynecol Obstet 1970; 130:580–605.

10. Oberfield RA. Current status of regional arterial infusion chemotherapy. Med Clin of N Am 1974; 59:2.

11. Lokich JJ. Portable external and implanted pump infusion devices. 13th Ann Cancer Course—infusional cancer chemother. Harvard Medical School, Boston, March 1–3, 1984, Part 1.

12. Drug infusion system uses inflatable rubber reservoirs. C&EN 1977; July 11:30.

13. Dorr RT, Trinca C, et al. Limitations of a portable infusion pump in ambulatory patients receiving continuous infusions of anticancer drugs. Cancer Treat Rep 1979; 63:2.

14. Ansman RK, Caballero GA, et al. Long-term ambulatory continuous intravenous infusion of 5-fluorouracil for the treatment of metastatic adenocarcinoma in the liver. Wis Med J 1982; 81:25–28.

15. Carlson RW, Branimer IS. Continuous infusion or bolus injection in cancer chemotherapy. Ann Intern Med 1983; 99:823–33.

16. Blackshear PJ, Dorman F, et al. The design and initial testing of an implantable infusion pump. Surg Gynecol Obstet 1972; 134:51–56.

17. Rohde T, Blackshear PJ, et al. One year of heparin anticoagulation. Minn Med 1977; 60:719–22.

18. Ensminger W, Niederhuber J, et al. Totally implanted drug delivery system for hepatic arterial chemotherapy. Cancer Treat Rep 1981; 65:393.

19. Buchwald H, Rohde T. Implantable infusion pumps, Adv Surg 1984; 18:177–221.

20. Prestele K, Funke H, et al. Development of remotely controlled implantable devices for programmed insulin infusion. 1983 Eur Soc Artif Organs, Life Support Syst 1983; 23–38.

21. Mirouse J, Selam J, et al. Clinical experience in human diabetics with portable and implantable insulin mini pumps. Eur Soc Artif Organs, Life Support Syst 1983; 39–50.

22. Comben R, Bartelt K, et al. Experimental and clinical studies using Medtronic's programmable implantable drug administration device. Artif Organs 1983; 7A:107.

23. Kowaluk E, Roberts M, Polack A. Interactions between drugs and intravenous delivery systems. Am J Hosp Pharm 1982; 39:460–67.

24. Benvenuto J, Anderson R, et al. Stability and compatibility of antitumor agents in glass and plastic containers. Am J. Hosp Pharm 1981; 38:1914–18.

25. Tangen O. Stability of drugs in plastic drug delivery systems. Pharmacia Nu Tech, Inc. 1984 (internal design notes).

26. Robinson L. Volume accuracy versus rate precision. Infusion Tech and Ther, Tech Assess Rep No. 5-83, AAIM, 1983.

27. Carlson R, Branimir I. Continuous infusion or bolus injection in cancer chemotherapy. Ann Intern Med 1983; 99:823–33.

References—Chapter 5

1. Daly JM, Lawson M, Speir A, et al. Angioaccess in cancer patients. Curr Probl Cancer 1981; 5:9, 1–37.

2. Lokich JJ, Bothe Jr A, Fine N, et al. The delivery of cancer chemotherapy by constant venous infusion. Cancer 1982; 50:2731–35.

3. Vogelzang NJ. Continuous infusion chemotherapy. J Clin Oncol 1984; 2:1289–1304.

4. Scribner BH, Cole JJ, Christopher TG. Long-term total parenteral nutrition. JAMA 1970; 212:457–63.

5. Hickman RO, Buckner CD, Clift RA, et al. A modified right atrial catheter for access to the venous system in marrow transplant recipients. Surg Gynec Obstet 1979; 148:871.

6. Bothe Jr A, Blackburn GL. Septic thrombophlebitis and venous catheter-related infections. In: Current therapy in internal medicine. B.C. Decker/Mosby, 1984; 218–20.

7. Raaf JH. Results from use of 826 vascular access devices in cancer patients. Cancer 1985; 55:1312–21.

8. Newsome HH, Armstrong CW, Mayhall GC, et al. Mechanical complications from insertion of subclavian venous feeding catheters. Comparison of de novo percutaneous venipuncture to change of catheter over guidewire. JPEN 1984; 8:560–62.

9. Benotti PN, Bothe Jr A, Miller JB, et al. Safe cannulation of the internal jugular vein for long-term hyperalimentation. Surg Gynec Obst 1977; 144:574–76.

10. Bland KI, Woodcock T. Totally implantable venous access system for cyclic administration of cytoxic chemotherapy. Am J Surg 1984; 147:815–16.

11. Bothe Jr A et al. Implantable central venous access system. Am J Surg 1984; 147:565–69.

12. Khoury MD, Lloyd LR, Burrows J, et al. Totally implanted venous access system for the delivery of chemotherapy. Cancer 1985; 56:1231–34.

13. Soo KC, Davidson TI, Selby P, et al. Long-term venous access using a subcutaneous implantable drug delivery system. Ann R Coll Surg Eng 1985; 67:263–65.

14. Davis SJ, Thompson JS, Edney JA. Insertion of Hickman catheters. Comparison of cutdown and percutaneous techniques. Am Surg 1984; 50:673–76.

15. Bern MM, Bothe Jr A, Bistrian BR, et al. Prophylaxis against thrombosis with low-dose warfarin. Surgery Feb. 1986.

16. Lokich JJ, Bothe Jr A, Benotti P, et al. Complications and management of implanted venous access catheters. J Clin Oncol 1985; 3:710–17.

17. Harley DP, White RA, Nelson RJ. Pulmonary embolism secondary to venous thrombosis of the arm. Am J Surg 1984; 147:221–24.

18. Fabri PJ, Mirtallo JM, Ebbert ML, et al. Clinical effect of nonthrombotic total parenteral nutrition catheters. JPEN 1984; 8:705–07.

19. Glynn MFX, Langer B, Jeejeebhoy KN. Therapy for thrombotic occlusion of long-term intravenous alimentation catheters. JPEN 1984; 8:705–07.

20. Hurtubise MR, Bottini JC, Lawson M, et al. Restoring patency of occluded central venous catheters. Arch Surg 1980; 115:212–13.

21. Begala JE et al. Risk of infection associated with the use of Broviac and Hickman catheters. Am J Infect Control 1982; 10:17–23.

22. Bozzetti F. Central venous catheter sepsis. Surg Gynec Obstet 1985; 161:293–301.

23. Press OW, Ramsey PG, Larson EB, et al. Hickman catheter infections in patients with malignancies. Medicine 1984; 63:189–200.

24. Reed WP, Newman KA, Applefield MM, et al. Drug extravasation as a complication of venous access ports. Ann Intern Med 1985; 102:788–90.

25. Conces Jr DJ, Holden RW. Aberrant locations and complications in initial placement of subclavian vein catheters. Arch Surg 1984; 119:293–95.

26. Rubenstein RB, Altery RE, Michals LG, et al. Hickman catheter separation. JPEN 1985; 9:754–57.

27. Fisher WB. Complication of Hickman catheter. Cutaneous erosion of the Dacron cuff. JAMA 1985; 254:2934.

28. Neiderhuber J, Enzminger WD. Surgical considerations in the management of hepatic neoplasia. Sem Oncol 1983; 10:135–47.

29. Cohen AM, Kaufman SD, Wood WC, et al. Regional hepatic chemotherapy using an implantable drug infusion pump. Am J Surg 1983; 145:529–33.

30. Kemeny M, Goldberg D, Beatly JD, et al. Results of a prospective randomized trial of continuous regional chemotherapy and hepatic resection as treatment of hepatic metastases from colorectal primaries. Cancer 1986; 57:492–98.

31. Hohn DC, Rayner AA, Economou JS, et al. Toxicities and complications of implanted pump hepatic arterial and intravenous floxuridine infusion. Cancer 1986; 57:465–70.

32. Hohn D, Melnick J, Stogg R, et al. Biliary sclerosis in patients receiving hepatic arterial infusions of floxuridine. J Clin Oncol 1985; 3:98–102.

33. Neiderhuber J, Enzminger WD, Gyves J, et al. Regional hepatic chemotherapy for colorectal cancer metastatic to the liver. Cancer 1984; 53:1336–43.

34. Balch CM, Urist MM, Soong SJ, et al. A prospective phase 2 trial of continuous FUDR regional chemotherapy for colorectal metastases to the liver using a totally implantable infusion pump. Am J Surg 1983; 198:567–73.

35. Kemeny N, Daly J, Oderman P, et al. Hepatic artery pump infusion: toxicity and results in patients with metastatic colorectal carcinoma. J Clin Oncol 1984; 2d:595–600.

References—Chapter 6

1. Goodman MS, Wickman R. Venous access devices: an overview. Oncology Forum 1984; 11:5,16–23.

2. Lokich JJ, Becker B. Subclavian vein thrombosis in patients treated with infusion chemotherapy for advanced malignancy. Cancer 1983; 52 (9):1586–89.

3. Lokich JJ, Bothe A, Benotti P, Moore C. Complications and management of implanted venous access catheters. J Clin Oncol 1985; 3:5.

4. Goldman ML, Bilboa MK, Rosch J, Dotter CT. Complications of indwelling chemotherapy catheters. Cancer 1975; 36:1983–90.

5. Perri J, Erikson KA. Nursing issues for hepatic arterial infusion therapy. Seminars in Oncol 1983; 10:2, 191–98.

6. Clouse ME, Ahmed R, Ryan RB, Oberfield RA, McAffrey JA. Complications of long-term transbrachial hepatic arterial infusion chemotherapy. Am J Roentgenol 1977; 129:799–803.

7. Cohen AM, Wood AC, Greenfield, et al. Transbrachial hepatic arterial chemotherapy using an implantable infusion pump. Dis Colon Rectum 1980; 23:223–27.

8. Lee RGL, Hill TC, Lokich JJ, et al. Use of Technetium-^{99M} macroaggregated albumin to evaluate the position and condition of totally implanted venous and arterial access devices. Radiol 1984; 150(2):593–94.

References—Chapter 7

1. Benvenuto JA, Anderson RW, Kerkhof K, Smith RG, Loo TL. Stability and compatibility of antitumor agents in glass and plastic containers. Am J Hosp Pharm 1981; 39:1914–18.

2. Tunbridge LJ, Lloyd TV, Penhall RK, Wise AL, Maloney T. Stability of diluted heparin sodium stored in plastic syringes. Am J Hosp Pharm 1981; 38:1001–04.

3. Chen ML, Chiou WL. Adsorption of methotrexate onto glassware and syringes. J Pharm Sci 1982; 71:129–31.

4. Tomlinson H, Malspeis L. Concomitant adsorption and stability of some anthracycline antibiotics. J Pharm Sci 1982; 71:1121–25.

5. Quebbeman EJ, Hamid AAR, Hoffman NE, Ausman RK. Stability of fluorouracil in plastic containers used for continuous infusion at home. Am J Hosp Pharm 1984; 41:1153–56.

6. Gannon PM, Sesin GP. Stability of cytarabine following repackaging in plastic syringes and glass containers. Am J I.V. Ther Clin Nutr 1983 (June); 11–16.

7. Bosanquet AC. Stability of solutions of antineoplastic agents during preparation and storage for in vitro assays: general considerations, the nitosoureas and alkylating agents. Cancer Chemother Pharmacol 1985; 14:83–95.

8. Hirsch JI, Wood JH, Thomas RB. Insulin adsorption to polyolefin infusion bottles and polyvinyl chloride administration sets. Am J Hosp Pharm 1981; 38:995–97.

9. Kowaluk EA, Roberts MS, Polack AE. Interactions between drugs and intravenous delivery systems. Am J Hosp Pharm 1982; 39:460–67.

10. Trissel LA. Avoiding common flaws in stability and compatibility studies of injectable drugs. Am J Hosp Pharm 1983; 40:1159–60.

11. Nedich RL. Selection of containers and closure systems for injectable products. Am J Hosp Pharm 1983; 40:1924–27.

12. Newton DW. Physiochemical determinants of incompatibility and instability of drugs for injection and infusion of drugs for injection. In: Trissel LA. Handbook on injectable drugs, 3rd ed. Bethesda: American Society of Hospital Pharmacists, 1983.

13. Moorhatch P, Chiou WL. Interactions between drugs and plastic intravenous fluid bags. Am J Hosp Pharm 1974; 31:72–78.

14. Trissel LA. Handbook on injectable drugs, 3rd ed. Bethesda: American Society of Hospital Pharmacists, 1983.

15. Pavlik EJ, Van Nagell JR, Hanson MB, Donaldson ES, Powell DE, Denady DE. Sensitivity of anticancer agents in vitro: standardizing the cytotoxic response and characterizing the sensitivities of a reference cell line. Gyn Oncol 1982; 14:243–61.

16. Pavlik EJ, Kenady DE, Van Nagell JR, et al. Properties of anticancer agents relevant to in vitro determinations of human cancer cell sensitivity. Cancer Chemother Pharmacol 1983; 11:8–15.

17. Bjannister SJ, Sternson LA, Repta AJ. Urine analysis of platinum species derived from cis-dichlorodiommine platinum (II) by high performance liquid chromatography following derivation with sodium diethyl-dithiocorbamate. J Chromatogr 1979; 173:333–42.

18. Turco SJ. The stability of frozen antibiotics (injectable medication). Am J I.V. Ther Clin Nutr 1982 (Sep) 9–10.

References—Chapter 8

1. Duschinsky R, Pleven E, Heidelberger C. The synthesis of 5-fluoropyrimidines. J Amer Chem Soc 1957; 79:4559–60.

2. Heidelberger C. Pyrimidine and Pyrimidine Nucleoside Antimetabolites. In: Holland JF, Frei E III, eds. Cancer medicine. Philadelphia: Lea & Febinger, 1973; 768–91.

3. Chabner BA, Myers CE. Clinical Pharmacology of Cancer Chemotherapy. In: DeVita VT Jr, Hellman S, Rosenberg SA, eds. Principles and practice of oncology, 2nd ed. Philadelphia: Lippincott, 1985; 287–328.

4. Clarkson B, O'Connor A, Winston L, et al. The physiologic disposition of 5-fluorouracil and 5-fluoro-2'-deoxyuridine in man. Clin Pharmacol Ther 1964; 5:581–610.

5. Myers CE, Diasio R, Eliot HM, et al. Pharmacokinetics of the fluoropyrimidines: implications for their clinical use. Cancer Treat Rev 1976; 3:175–83.

6. Keller JH, Ensminger WD. Stability of cancer chemotherapeutic agents in a totally implanted drug delivery system. Am J Hosp Pharm 1982; 39:1321–23.

7. Fraile RJ, Baker LH, Buroker TR, et al. Pharmacokinetics of 5-fluorouracil administered orally, by rapid intravenous, and by slow infusion. Cancer Res 1980; 40:2223–28.

8. Moertel CG, Schutt AJ, Reitemeier RJ, et al. A comparison of 5-fouorouracil administered by slow infusion and rapid injection. Cancer Res 1972; 32:2717–19.

9. Moertel CG, Reitemeier RJ, Hahn RG. Slow versus rapid administration of the fluorinated pyrimidines. In: Advanced gastrointestinal cancer clinical management and chemotherapy. New York: Harper, 1969; 108–18.

10. Moertel CG, Reitemeier RJ, Hahn RG. A controlled comparison of 5-fluoro-2'-deoxyuridine therapy administered by rapid intravenous injection and by continuous intravenous infusion. Cancer Res 1967; 27:549–52.

11. Sullivan RG, Miller E, Chryssochos T, et al. The clinical effects of the continuous intravenous and intra-arterial infusion of cancer chemotherapeutic compounds. Cancer Chemother Rep 1962; 16:499–510.

12. Seifert P, Baker LH, Reed ML, et al. Comparison of continuously infused 5-fluorouracil with bolus injection in treatment of patients with colorectal adenocarcinoma. Cancer 1975; 36:123–28.

13. Curreri AR, Ansfield FJ. Comparison of 5-fluorouracil and 5-fluoro-2'-deoxyuridine in the treatment of far-advanced breast and colon lesions. Cancer Chemother Rep 1962; 16:387–88.

14. Young CW, Ellison RR, Sullivan RD, et al. The clinical evaluation of 5-fluorouracil and 5'-fluoro-2'-deoxyuridine in solid tumors in adults. Cancer Chemother Rep 1960; 6:17–20.

15. Reitemeier RJ, Moertel CG, Hahn RG. Comparison of 5-fluorouracil (NSC-19893) and 2'-deoxy-5-fluorouridine (NSC-27640) in treatment of patients with advanced adenocarcinoma of the colon or rectum. Cancer Chemother Rep 1965; 44:39–43.

16. Buroker T, Kim PN, Groppe C, et al. 5FU infusion with mitomycin-C versus 5FU infusion with methyl-CCNU in the treatment of advanced colon cancer. Cancer 1978; 42:1228–33.

17. DeConti RC, Kaplan SR, Papac RJ, et al. Continuous intravenous infusion of 5-fluoro-2'-deoxyuridine in the treatment of solid tumors. Cancer 1973; 31:894–98.

18. Spiers ASD, Kasimis BS, Janis MG. High-dose intravenous infusions of 5-fluorouracil for refractory solid tumors—the HI-FU regimen. Clin Oncol 1980; 6:63–69.

19. Lokich JJ, Sonneborn H, Paul S, et al. Phase 1 study of continuous venous infusion of floxuridine (5-FUDR) chemotherapy. Cancer Treat Rep 1983; 67:791–93.

20. Lokich JJ, Bothe A, Fine N, et al. Phase 1 study of protracted venous infusion of 5-fluorouracil. Cancer 1981; 48:2565–68.

21. Spicer D, Ardalan B, Silberman H, et al. Phase 1 trial of prolonged continuous intravenous infusion of 5-fluorouracil (5-FU) with pharmacokinetics. Proc Am Soc Clin Oncol 1984; 41.

22. Lokich JJ, Fine N, Perri J, et al. Protracted ambulatory venous infusion of 5-fluorouracil. Am J Clin Oncol (CCT) 1983; 6:103-07.

23. Faintuch J, Shepard KV, O'Laughlin K, et al. Toxicity of continuous infusion 5-FU. Proc ASCO 1985; 4:92.

24. Leichman L, Leichman CG, Kinzie J, et al. Long-term low-dose 5-fluorouracil (5-FU) in advanced measurable colon cancer: no correlation between toxicity and efficacy. Proc ASCO 1985; 4:86.

25. Ausman R, Caballero G, Quebbeman E, et al. Response of metastatic colorectal adenocarcinomas to long-term continuous ambulatory intravenous infusion of 5-fluorouracil. Proc ASCO 1985; 4:86.

26. Belt RJ, Davidner ML, Myron MC, et al. Continuous low-dose 5-fluorouracil for adenocarcinoma: confirmation of activity. Proc ASCO 1985; 4:90.

References—Chapter 9

1. Farber S, Diamond CK, Mercer RD, Sylvester RF, Wolff VA. Temporary remissions in acute leukemia in children produced by folic acid antagonist 4-amethopteroylglutamic acid (aminopterin). N Engl J Med 1948; 238:787-93.

2. Hertz R, Ross GT, Lipsett MB. Primary chemotherapy of nonmetastatic trophoblastic disease in women. Am J Obstet Gyn 1963; 86:808-14.

3. Selawry OS. New treatment schedule with improved survival in childhood leukemia. Intermittent parenteral versus daily oral administration of methotrexate for maintenance of induced remission. JAMA 1965; 194:75-81.

4. Selawry O, James D. Therapeutic index of methotrexate as related to dose schedule and route of administration in children with acute lymphocytic leukemia. Proc Am Assoc Cancer Res 1965; 6:56.

5. Djerassi I. Continuous infusions of methotrexate in children with acute leukemia. Cancer 1967; 20:233-42.

6. DeVita VT, Hellman S, Rosenberg SA, eds. Cancer: principles and practice of oncology. Philadelphia: JB Lippincott, 1985.

7. Penta JS. Overview of protocols on clinical studies of high-dose methotrexate (NSC-740) with citrovorum factor. Cancer Chemother Rep 1975; 6:7-12.

8. Pinedo HM, Chabner BA. The role of drug concentration, duration of exposure, and endogenous metabolites in determining methotrexate cytotoxicity. Cancer Treat Rep 1977; 61:709-14.

9. Eichholtz H, Trott KR. Effect of methotrexate concentration and exposure time on mammalian cell survival in vitro. Br J Cancer 1980; 41:277-84.

10. Chabner BA. Methotrexate. In: Chabner BA, ed. Pharmacologic principles of cancer treatment. Philadelphia: WB Saunders, 1982; 229-55.

11. McGuire JT, Bertino JR. Enzymatic synthesis and function of folylpolyglutamates. Mol Cell Biochem 1981; 38:19-48.

12. Allegra CJ, Drake JC, Jolivet J, Chabner BA. Inhibition of AICAR transformylase by methotrexate and dihydrofolic acid polyglutamates. Proc Natl Acad Sci USA 1985; 82:4881.

13. Allegra CJ, Chabner BA, Drake JC, Lutz R, Rodbard DA, Jolivet J. Enhanced inhibition of thymidylate synthase by methotrexate polyglutamates. J Biol Chem 1985; 260:9720-26.

14. Matthews RG, Baugh CM. Interactions of pig liver methylene tetrahydrofolate reductase with methylene tetrahydro pteroyl polyglutamate substrates and with dihydropteroyl polyglutamate inhibitors. Biochemistry 1980; 19:1036-41.

15. Rosenblatt DS, Whitehead VM, Vera N, Pottier A, Dupont M, Vuchich MJ. Prolonged inhibition of DNA synthesis associated with the accumulation of methotrexate polyglutamates by cultured human cells. Mol Pharmacol 1978; 14:1143-47.

16. Posner RG, Sirotnak FM, Chello PL. Differential synthesis of methotrexate polyglutamates in normal proliferative and neoplastic mouse tissues in vivo. Cancer Res 1981; 41:4441–46.

17. Schilsky RL, Bailey BD, Chabner BA. Methotrexate polyglutamate synthesis by cultured human breast cancer cells. Proc Natl Acad Sci USA 1980; 77:2919–22.

18. Jolivet J, Schilsky RL, Bailey BD, Drake JC, Chabner BA. Synthesis, retention and biological activity of methotrexate polyglutamates in cultured human breast cancer cells. J Clin Invest 1982; 70:351–69.

19. Cowan KH, Jolivet J. A novel mechanism of resistance to methotrexate in human breast cancer cells: lack of methotrexate polyglutamate formation. J Biol Chem 1984; 259:10793–10800.

20. Curt GA, Jolivet J, Carney DN, et al. Determinants of the sensitivity of human small-cell lung cancer cell lines to methotrexate. J Clin Invest (in press).

21. Jolivet J, Chabner BA. Intracellular pharmacokinetics of methotrexate polyglutamates in human breast cancer cells: selective retention and less dissociable binding of 4-NH$_2$-10-CH$_3$-PteGlu$_4$ and $_5$ to dihydrofolate reductase. J Clin Invest 1983; 72:773–78.

22. Goldman ID, Lichtenstein NS, Oliverio VT. Carrier-mediated transport of the folic acid analogue methotrexate in the L1210 leukemia cell. J Biol Chem 1968; 243:5007–17.

23. Sirotnak FM, Donsbach RL. Further evidence for a basis of selective activity and relative responsiveness during antifolate therapy of murine tumors. Cancer Res 1975; 35:1737–44.

24. Warren RD, Nichols AP, Bender RA. Membrane transport of methotrexate in human lymphoblastoid cells. Cancer Res 1978; 38:668–71.

25. Curt GA, Carney DN, Cowan KH, et al. Unstable methotrexate resistance in human small-cell carcinoma associated with double-minute chromosomes. N Engl J Med 1982; 308:199–202.

26. Horns RC, Dower WJ, Schimke RT. Gene amplification in a leukemic patient treated with methotrexate. J Clin Oncol 1984; 2:2–7.

27. Carman MD, Schornagel JH, Rivest RS, et al. Resistance to methotrexate due to gene amplification in a patient with acute leukemia. J Clin Oncol 1984; 2:16–20.

28. Trent JM, Buick RN, Olson S, Horns RC, Schimke RT. Cytologic evidence for gene amplification in methotrexate-resistant cells obtained from a patient with ovarian adenocarcinoma. J Clin Oncol 1984; 2:8–15.

29. Chabner BA, Young RC. Threshold methotrexate concentration for in vivo inhibition of DNA synthesis in normal and tumorous target tissues. J Clin Invest 1973; 52:1804–11.

30. Ettinger LJ, Chervinsky DS, Freeman AI, Creaven PJ. Pharmacokinetics of methotrexate following intravenous and intraventricular administration in acute lymphocytic leukemia and non-Hodgkin's lymphoma. Cancer 1982; 50:1676–82.

31. Shapiro WR, Young DF, Mehta BM. Methotrexate: distribution in cerebrospinal fluid after intravenous, ventricular and lumbar injections. N Engl J Med 1975; 293:161–66.

32. Janka GE, Mack R, Helmig M, Haas RJ, Bidlingmaier F. Prolonged methotrexate infusions in children with acute leukemia in relapse and in remission and with medulloblastoma. Oncology 1984; 41:225–32.

33. Bleyer WA, Poplack DG. Clinical studies on the central nervous system pharmacology of methotrexate. In: Pinedo HM, ed. Clinical pharmacology of antineoplastic drugs. Amsterdam: Elsevier/North Holland, 1978; 115–131.

34. Liguori VR, Giglio JJ, Miller E, Sullivan RD. Effects of different dose schedules of amethopterin on serum and tissue concentrations and urinary excretion patterns. Clin Pharmacol Therap 1961; 3:34–40.

35. Cohen HJ, Jaffe N. Pharmacokinetic and clinical studies of 24-hour infusions of high-dose methotrexate. Cancer Chemother Pharmacol 1978; 1:61–64.

36. Rosen G, Nirenberg A. Chemotherapy for osteogenic sarcoma: an investigative method, not a recipe. Cancer Treat Rep 1982; 66:1687–97.

37. Jaffe N, Paed D. Recent advances in the chemotherapy of metastatic osteogenic sarcoma. Cancer 1972; 30:1627–31.

38. Mitchell MS, Wawro NW, DeConti RC, Kaplan SR, Papac R, Bertino JR. Effectiveness of

high-dose infusion of methotrexate followed by leucovorin in carcinomas of the head and neck. Cancer Res 1968; 28:1088–95.

39. Levitt M, Mucher M, DeConti RC, et al. Improved therapeutic index of methotrexate with "leucovorin rescue." Cancer Res 1973; 33:1729–34.

40. Taylor SG, McGuire WP, Hauck WW, Showel JL, Lad TE. A randomized comparison of high-dose infusion methotrexate versus standard-dose weekly therapy in head and neck squamous cancer. J Clin Oncol 1984; 2:1006–11.

41. Woods RL, Fox RM, Tattersall MHN. Methotrexate treatment of advanced head and neck cancers: a dose response evaluation. Cancer Treat Rep 1981; 65:155–59.

42. DeConti RC, Schoenfield D. A randomized prospective comparison of intermittent methotrexate, methotrexate with leucovorin and a methotrexate combination in head and neck cancer. Cancer 1981; 48:1061–72.

43. Vogler W, Jacobs J, Moffitt S, et al. Methotrexate therapy with or without citrovorum factor in carcinoma of the head and neck, breast and colon. Cancer Clin Trials 1979; 2:227–36.

44. Sullivan RD, Miller E, Zurek WZ, Oberfield RA, Ojima Y. Re-evaluation of methotrexate as an anticancer drug. Surg Gynecol Obstet 1967; 121:819–24.

45. Pratt CB, Roberts D, Shanks E, Warmath EL. Response, toxicity, and pharmacokinetics of high dose methotrexate (NSC-740) with citrovorum factor rescue for children with osteosarcoma and other malignant tumors. Cancer Chemother Rep 1975; 6:13–18.

46. Lokich JJ, Curt G. Phase 1 and pharmacology study of continuous infusion low-dose methotrexate. Cancer 1985; 56:2391–94.

References—Chapter 10

1. Von Hoff DD, Layard MW, Basa P, et al. Risk factors for doxorubicin-induced congestive heart failure. Ann Intern Med 1979; 91:710–17.

2. Haq MM, Legha SS, Choksi J, et al. Doxorubicin-induced congestive heart failure in adults. Cancer 1985; 56:1361–65.

3. Unverferth DV, Jagadeesh JM, Unverferth BJ, Magorien RD, Leier CV, Balcerzak SP. Attempt to prevent doxorubicin-induced acute human myocardial morphologic damage with acetylcysteine. J NCI 1983; 71:917–20.

4. Legha SS, Wang Y-M, Mackay B, et al. Clinical and pharmacologic investigation of the effects of α-tocopherol on adriamycin cardiotoxicity. Ann N Y Acad Sci 1982; 393:411–18.

5. Weiss AJ, Manthel RW. Experience with the use of adriamycin in combination with other anticancer agents using a weekly schedule with particular reference to lack of cardiac toxicity. Cancer 1977; 40:2046–52.

6. Chlebowski RT, Paroly WS, Pugh RP, et al. Adriamycin given as a weekly schedule without a loading course: clinically effective with reduced incidence of cardiotoxicity. Cancer Treat Rep 1980; 64:47–51.

7. Valdivieso M, Burgess MA, Ewer MS, et al. Increased therapeutic index of weekly doxorubicin in the therapy of non-small cell lung cancer: a prospective, randomized study. J Clin Oncol 1984; 2:207–14.

8. Torti FM, Bristow MR, Howes AE, et al. Reduced cardiotoxicity of doxorubicin delivered on a weekly schedule. Ann Intern Med 1983; 99:745–49.

9. Legha SS, Benjamin RS, Mackay B, et al. Adriamycin therapy by continuous intravenous infusion in patients with metastatic breast cancer. Cancer 1982; 49:1762–66.

10. Legha SS, Benjamin RS, Mackay B, et al. Reduction of doxorubicin cardiotoxicity by prolonged continuous intravenous infusion. Ann Intern Med 1982; 96:133–39.

11. Garnick MB, Weiss, GR, Steele Jr GD, et al. Clinical evaluation of long-term, continuous-infusion doxorubicin. Cancer Treat Rep 1983; 67:133–42.

12. Hoffman DM, Grossano DD, Damin LA, Woodcock TM. Stability of refrigerated and frozen solutions of doxorubicin hydrochloride. Am J Hosp Pharm 1979; 36:1536–38.

13. Hickman RO, Buckner CD, Clift RA, et al. A modified right atrial catheter for access to the venous system in marrow transplant recipients. Surg Gynecol Obstet 1979; 148:871–75.

14. Gyves JW, Ensminger WD, Niederhuber JE, et al. A totally implanted injection port system for blood sampling and chemotherapy administration. JAMA 1984; 251:2538–41.

15. Gyves J, Ensminger W, Niederhuber J, et al. Totally implanted system for intravenous chemotherapy in patients with cancer. Am J Med 1982; 73:841–45.

16. Yap BS, Baker LH, Sinkovics JG, et al. Cyclophosphamide, vincristine, adriamycin and DTIC (CYVADIC) combination chemotherapy for the treatment of advanced sarcomas. Cancer Treat Rep 1980; 64:93–98.

17. Hortobagyi G, Frye D, Blumenschein G, et al. FAC with adriamycin by continuous infusion for treatment of advanced breast cancer. Proc Am Soc Clin Oncol 1983; 2:105.

18. Legha SS, Blumenschein GR. Systemic therapy of metastatic breast cancer: a review of the current trends. Oncology 1982; 39:140–45.

19. Lokich JJ, Becker B. Subclavian vein thrombosis in patients treated with infusion chemotherapy for advanced malignancy. Cancer 1983; 52:1586–89.

20. Legha SS, Haq M, Rabinowits M, Lawson M, McCredie K. Evaluation of silicone elastomer catheters for long-term intravenous chemotherapy. Arch Intern Med 1985 (in press).

21. Bristow MR, Mason JW, Billingham ME, Daniels JR. Doxorubicin cardiomyopathy: evaluation by phonocardiography, endomyocardial biopsy, and cardiac catheterization. Ann Intern Med 1978; 88:168–75.

22. Legha S, Benjamin R, Ewer M, et al. Reduction of adriamycin cardiotoxicity by continuous I.V. infusion: the effect of duration of infusion on cardiotoxicity. Proc Am Soc Clin Oncol 1982; 23:127(499).

23. Legha SS, Benjamin RS, Ewer M, Mackay B, et al. Continuous intravenous infusion of adriamycin: evaluation of its efficacy and toxicity. In: Adriamycin. Its expanding role in cancer treatment. M. Ogawa, FM Muggia and M Rozencweig, eds. Amsterdam: Excerpta Medica, 1984; 378–86.

24. Benjamin RS, Chawla SP, Ewer MS, et al. Cardiac toxicity of high-cumulative-dose adriamycin by rapid or 24- 96-hour continuous infusion. Proc Am Soc Clin Oncol 1983; 2:40(C-159).

25. Green MD, Speyer JS, Blum R, Wernz J, Muggia FM. The effect of 6-hour infusions of adriamycin on anthracycline cardiotoxicity. Proc Am Soc Clin Oncol 1983; 2:26 (C-100).

26. Bowen J, Rosenthal CJ, Gardner B. Phase 1 study of adriamycin by 5-day continuous intravenous infusion. Proc Am Assoc Cancer Res 1981; 22:354 (C-84).

27. Lokich JJ, Bothe A, Zipoli T, et al. Constant infusion schedule for adriamycin: a phase 1–2 clinical trial of a 30-day schedule by ambulatory pump delivery system. J Clin Oncol 1983; 1:24–28.

28. Vogelzang NJ, Ruane M, O'Drobiniak J, DeMeester T. Continuous doxorubicin infusion using an implanted lithium battery-powered drug administration device system (DADS, Medtronic, Inc.). Proc Am Soc Clin Oncol 1984; 3:263 (C-1030).

29. Legha S, Benjamin R, Mackay B, et al. Reutilization of adriamycin in previously treated patients. Proc Am Assoc Cancer Res 1981; 22:534 (C-791).

30. Benjamin RS, Keating MJ, Swenerton KD, Legha S, McCredie KB. Clinical studies with rubidazone: Cancer Treat Rep 1979; 63:925–29.

31. Benjamin RS, Keating MJ, McCredie KB, Bodey GP, and Freireich EJ. A phase 1 and 2 trial of rubidazone in patients with acute leukemia. Cancer Res 1977; 37:4623–28.

32. Aboud A, Yap HY, Esparza L, et al. Carminomycin: a new anthracycline analog in the treatment of advanced breast cancer. Cancer 1984; 53:9–12.

33. Ogawa M, Inagaki J, Horikoshi N, et al. Clinical study of aclacinomycin A. Cancer Treat Rep 1979; 63:931–34.

34. Oka S, Mathe G, Mitrou PS. Aclacinomycin A. Cancer Treat Rev 1984; 11:299–302.

35. Garnick MB, Griffin JD, Sack MJ, Blum RH, Israel M, Frei II E. Phase 2 evaluation of N-trifluoroacetyladriamycin-14-valerate (AD32). In: Anthracycline antibiotics in cancer therapy. FM Muggia, CW Young, SK Carter, eds. Boston: Martinus Nijhoff, 1982; 541–48.

36. Ganzina F. 4'-epi-doxorubicin, a new analogue of doxorubicin: a preliminary overview of preclinical and clinical data. Cancer Treat Rev 1983; 10:1–22.

37. Jain KK, Casper ES, Geller NL, et al. A prospective randomized comparison of epirubicin and doxorubicin in patients with advanced breast cancer. J Clin Oncol 1985; 3:818–26.

38. Kaplan S, Martini A, Varini M, Togni P, Cavalli F. Phase 1 trial of 4-demethoxydaunorubicin with single I.V. doses. Eur J Cancer Clin Oncol 1982; 18:1303–06.

39. Berman E, Wittes RE, Leyland-Jones B, et al. Phase 1 and clinical pharmacology studies of intravenous and oral administration of 4-demethoxydaunorubicin in patients with advanced cancer. Cancer Res 1983; 43:6096–6101.

40. Daghestani AN, Zalmen AA, Leyland-Jones B, et al. Phase 1 and 2 clinical pharmacological study of 4-demethoxydaunorubicin (idarubicin) in adult patients with acute leukemia. Cancer Res 1985; 45:1408–12.

41. Stanton GF, Raymond V, Wittes RE, et al. Phase 1 and clinical pharmacological evaluation of 4'-deoxydoxorubicin in patients with advanced cancer. Cancer Res 1985; 45:1862–68.

42. Rozencweig M, Nicaise C, Dodion P, et al. Preliminary experience with marcellomycin: preclinical and clinical aspects. In: Anthracycline antibiotics in cancer therapy. FM Muggia, CW Young, SK Carter, eds. Boston: Martinus Nijhoff, 1982; 549–67.

43. Jacquillat C, Auclerc MF, Weil M, et al. Clinical activity of detorubicin: a new anthracycline derivative. Cancer Treat Rep 1979; 63:889–93.

44. Chawla SP, Legha SS, Benjamin RS. Detorubicin — an active anthracycline in untreated metastatic melanoma. J Clin Oncol (in press).

45. Ogawa M, Miyamoto H, Inigaki J, et al. Phase 1 clinical trial of a new anthracycline: 4'-o-tetrahydropyranyl adriamycin. Invest New Drugs 1983; 1:169–72.

46. Ogawa M. New anthracyclines in Japan. In: Adriamycin: its expanding role in cancer treatment. M Ogama, FM Muggia, M Rozencweig, eds. Princeton: Excerpta Medica, 1983; 491–505.

47. Dodion P, Sessa C, Gerard B, et al. Phase 1 trial of menogaril. Proc Am Soc Clin Oncol 1985; 4:26(C-95).

48. Dorr A, Von Hoff D, Kuhn J, Kisner D. Phase 1 clinical trial of menogaril. Proc Am Soc Clin Oncol 1985; 4:39(C-148).

49. Long HJ, Powis G, Schutt AJ, Moertel CG, Kovach JS. Menogaril by 72-hour continuous intravenous infusion: a phase 1 study with pharmacokinetics. Proc Am Soc Clin Oncol 1985; 4:28(C-102).

References—Chapter 11

1. Rosenberg B, Van Camp L, Krigas T. Inhibition of cell division in E. coli by electrolysis products from a platinum electrode. Nature 1965; 205:698.

2. Rosenberg B, Van Camp L, Trosko JE, et al. Platinum compounds: a new class of potent antitumor agents. Nature 1969; 222:385.

3. Higby DJ, Wallace HJ, Holland JF. Cis-diammine dichloro-platinum (NSC-119875): a phase 1 study. Cancer Chemother Rep 1973; 57:459.

4. Higby DJ, Wallace HJ, Albert DJ, et al. Diammine dichloroplatinum: a phase 1 study showing responses in testicular and other tumors. Cancer 1974; 33:1219.

5. Rossof AH, Slayton RE, Perlia CP. Preliminary clinical experience with cis-diamminedichloroplatinum (II)(NSC-119875, CACP) Cancer 1972; 30:1451.

6. Talley RW, O'Bryan RM, Gutterman JU, et al. Clinical evaluation of toxic effects of cis-diamminedichloroplatinum (NSC-119875) — a phase 1 clinical study. Cancer Chemother Rep 1973; 57:465.

7. Einhorn LH, Donohue J: Cis-diamminedichloroplatinum, vinblastine and bleomycin combination chemotherapy in disseminated testicular cancer. Ann Intern Med 1977; 87:293.

8. Sampson MK, Rivkin SE, Jones SE, et al. Dose-response and dose-survival advantage for high versus low-dose cisplatin combined with vinblastine and bleomycin in disseminated testicular cancer: a Southwest Oncology Group study. Cancer 1984; 53:1029.

9. Peckman MJ, Barrett A, Liew KW, et al. The treatment of metastatic germ-cell testicular tumors with bleomycin, etoposide and cisplatin (BEP). Br J Cancer 1983; 47:613.

10. Katz ME, Schwartz PE, Kapp DS, et al. Epithelial carcinoma of the ovary; current strategies. Ann Intern Med 1981; 95:98.

11. Ozols RF, Young RC: Chemotherapy of ovarian cancer. Semin Oncol 1984; 11:251.

12. Kish J, Drelichman A, Jacobs J, et al. Clinical trial of cisplatin and 5-FU infusion as initial treatment for advanced squamous cell carcinoma of the head and neck. Cancer Treat Rep 1982; 66:471.

13. Hong WK, Schaefer S, Issel B, et al. A prospective randomized trial of methotrexate versus cisplatin in the treatment of recurrent squamous cell carcinoma of the head and neck. Cancer 1983; 52:206.

14. Klastersky J, Nicaise C, Longeval E, et al. Cisplatin, adriamycin and etoposide (CAV) for remission induction of small cell bronchogenic carcinoma. Cancer 1982; 50:652.

15. Klastersky J, Sculier JP, Nicaise C, et al: Combination chemotherapy with cisplatin, etoposide and vindesine in non-small cell lung carcinoma: a clinical trial of the EORTC lung cancer working party. Cancer Treat Rep 1983; 67:727.

16. Hoffman PC, Bitran JD, Golomb HM. Chemotherapy of metastatic non-small cell bronchogenic carcinoma. Semin Oncol 1984; 10:111.

17. Soloway MS, Einstein A, Corder MP, et al. A comparison of cisplatin and the combination of cisplatin and cyclophosphamide in advanced urothelial cancer. Cancer 1983; 52:767.

18. Hogan WN, Young RC. Gynecologic malignancies. In: Pinedo HM, ed. Cancer chemotherapy. Amsterdam: Excerpta Medica, 1982; 309–38.

19. Kelsen D. Chemotherapy of esophageal cancer. Semin Oncol 1984; 11:159.

20. Creagan ET, O'Fallon JR, Woods JE. Cis-diamminedichloroplatinum (II) administered by 24-hour infusion in the treatment of patients with advanced aerodigestive cancer. Cancer 1983; 51:2020.

21. Vogl SE, Comacho FJ, Engstrom PF, et al. Phase 2 trial of cisplatin in advanced gastric cancer. Cancer Treat Rep 1984; 68:1497.

22. Beer M, Cocconi G, Ceci G, et al. A phase 2 study of cisplatin in advanced gastric cancer. Eur J Cancer Clin Oncol 1983; 19:717.

23. Zwelling LA, Kohn KW. Mechanism of action of cis-dichlorodiammine platinum (II). Cancer Treat Rep 1979; 63:1439.

24. Rosenberg B. Anticancer activity of cis-dichlorodiammine-platinum (II) and some relevant chemistry. Cancer Treat Rep 1979; 63:1433.

25. Drobnick J, Horacek P. Specific biological activity of platinum complexes. Contribution to the theory of molecular mechanism. Chem Biol Interact 1973; 7:223.

26. Zwelling LA, Anderson T, Kohn KW. DNA-protein and DNA interstrand cross-linking by cis and trans-platinum (II) diamminedichloride in L1210 mouse leukemia cells and relation to cytotoxicity. Cancer Res 1979; 39:365.

27. Fraval HNA, Roberts JJ. Excision repair of cis-diamminedichloroplatinum (II)-induced damage to DNA of chinese hamster cells. Cancer Res 1979; 39:1793.

28. Fraval HNA, Roberts JJ. G1 phase chinese hamster V79-379A cells are inherently more sensitive to platinum bound to their DNA than mid S-phase or asynchronously treated cells. Biochem Pharmacol 1979; 28:1575.

29. Bergerat JB, Barlogie B, Gohde W, et al. In vitro cytokinetic response of human colon cancer cells to cis-dichlorodiammine platinum (II). Cancer Res 1979; 39:4356.

30. Moran RE, Straus MJ. Effects of pulse and continuous intravenous infusion of cis-diamminedichloroplatinum on L1210 leukemia in vivo. Cancer Res 1981; 41:4993.

31. Bergerat JP, Barlogie B, Drewinko B. Effects of cis-dichlorodiammineplatinum (II) on human colon carcinoma cells in vitro. Cancer Res 1979; 39:1334.

32. DeConti RC, Toftness BR, Lange RC, et al. Clinical pharmacological studies with cis-diamminedichloroplatinum (II). Cancer Res. 1973; 33:1310.

33. LeRoy AF, Wehling ML, Sponseller HL, et al. Analysis of platinum in biological materials by flameless atomic absorption spectrophotometry. Biochem Med 1977; 18:184.

34. Daley-Yates PT, McBrien DCH. Cisplatin metabolites in plasma, a study of their pharmacokinetics and importance in the nephrotoxic and antitumor activity of cisplatin. Biochem Pharmacol 1984; 33:3063.

35. Bannister SJ, Sternson LA, Repta AJ. Measurement of free-circulating cis-dichlorodiammineplatinum (II) in plasma. Clin Chem 1977; 23:2258.

36. Bannister SJ. Chang Y, Sternson LA, et al. Atomic absorption spectrophotometry of free circulating platinum species in plasma derived from cis-dichlorodiommine platinum (II). Clin Chem 1978; 24:877.

37. Daley-Yates PT, McBrien DCH. Cisplatin metabolites: a method for their separation and for measurement of their renal clearance in vivo. Biochem Pharmacol 1983; 32:181.

38. Andrews PA, Wung WE, Howell SB. An HPLC analysis of active cisplatin in plasma ultrafiltrate. Proc Am Assoc Cancer Res 1984; 25:647.

39. Litterst CL, Gram TE, Dedrick RL, et al. Distribution and disposition of platinum following intravenous administration of cis-diamminedichloroplatinum II (NSC-119875) to dogs. Cancer Res 1976; 36:2340.

40. Himmelstein KJ, Patton TF, Belt RJ, et al. Clinical kinetics of intact cisplatin and some related species. Clin Pharmacol Ther 1981; 29:658.

41. Gullo JJ, Litterst CL, Maguire PJ, et al. Pharmacokinetics and protein binding of cis-dichlorodiammine platinum (II) administered as a one-hour or as a twenty-hour infusion. Cancer Chemother Pharmacol 1980; 5:21.

42. LeRoy AF. Some quantitative data on cis-dichlorodiammineplatinum (II) species in solution. Cancer Treat Rep 1979; 63:231.

43. Gormley PE, Bull JM, LeRoy AF, et al. Kinetics of cis-dichlorodiammine-platinum. Clin Pharmacol Ther 1979; 25:351.

44. Vermorken JB, Vander Vijgh WJF, Klein I, et al. Pharmacokinetics of free and total platinum species after short-term infusion of cisplatin. Cancer Treat Rep 1984; 68:505.

45. Patton TF, Himmelstein KJ, Belt R, et al. Plasma levels and urinary excretion of filterable platinum species following bolus injection and IV infusion of cis-dichlorodiammineplatinum (II) in man. Cancer Treat Rep 1978; 62:1359.

46. Belt RJ, Himmelstein KJ, Patton TF, et al. Pharmacokinetics of nonprotein-bound platinum species following administration of cis-dichlorodiammineplatinum (II). Cancer Treat Rep 1979; 63:1515.

47. Williams CJ, Stevenson KE, Buchanan RB, et al. Advanced ovarian carcinoma: a pilot study of cis-dichlorodiammineplatinum (II) in combination with adriamycin and cyclophosphamide in previously treated patients. Cancer Treat Rep 1979; 63:1745.

48. Vermorken JB, Vander Vijgh WJF, Klein I, et al. Pharmacokinetics of free platinum species following rapid, 3-hr, and 24-hr infusions of cis-diamminedichloroplatinum (II) and its therapeutic implications. Eur J Cancer Clin Oncol 1982; 18:1069.

49. Sasaki K, Murakami T, Fujimoto T. Clinical pharmacokinetics of cis-platinum in children. Proc Am Assoc Cancer Res 1985; 26:641.

50. Bajorin D, Bosl GJ, Alcock N, et al. Pharmacokinetics of free platinum and total platinum after administration of cisplatin in hypertonic saline. Proc Am Assoc Cancer Res 1985; 26:620.

51. Litterst CL, LeRoy AF, Guarino AM. The disposition and distribution of platinum following parenteral administration to animals of cis-dichlorodiammine platinum (II). Cancer Treat Rep 1979; 63:1485.

52. Nelson JA, Santos G, Herbert BH. Mechanisms for the renal excretion of cisplatin. Cancer Treat Rep 1984; 68:849.

53. Daley-Yates PT, McBrien DCH. The mechanism of renal clearance of cis-platin (cis-dichlorodiammineplatinum (II)) and its modification by furosemide and probenecid. Biochem Pharmacol 1982; 31:2243.

54. LeRoy AF, Lutz RJ, Dedrick RL, et al. Pharmacokinetic study of cis-dichlorodiammineplatinum (II) (DDP) in the beagle dog: thermodynamic and kinetic behavior of DDP in a biologic milieu. Cancer Treat Rep 1979; 63:59.

55. Casper ES, Kelson DP, Alcock NW, et al. Platinum concentrations in bile and plasma following rapid and six-hour infusion of cis-dichlorodiammenplatinum (II). Cancer Treat Rep 1979; 63:2023.

56. DiSimone PA, Yancey RS, Coupal JJ, et al. Effect of a forced diuresis on distribution and excretion (via urine and bile) of [195m] platinum when given as [195m] platinum cis-dichlorodiammine platinum. Cancer Treat Rep 1979; 63:951.

57. Stewart DJ, Mikhael N, Nanji S, et al. Human tissue cisplatin pharmacology: clinical implications. Proc Am Assoc Cancer Res 1985; 26:608.

58. Posner MR, Belliveau JF, Ferrari L, et al. Clinical and pharmacokinetic study of 5-day continuous infusion cis-platinum. Proc Am Soc Clin Oncol 1985; 4:C145.

59. Leonard BJ, Eccleston E. Jones et al. Antileukemic and nephrotoxic properties of platinum compounds. Nature 1971; 234:43.

60. Ward JM, Fauvie KA. The nephrotoxic effects of cis-dichloroplatinum (II) (NSC-119875) in male F344 rats. Toxicol Appl Pharmacol 1976; 38:535.

61. Kociba RJ, Sleight SD. Acute toxicologic and pathologic effects of cis-diamminedichloroplatinum (NSC-119875) in the male rat. Cancer Chemother Rep 1971; 55:1.

62. Dentino M, Luft FL, Yum MN, et al. Long-term effect of cis-diamminedichloro platinum (CDDP) on renal function and structure in man. Cancer 1978; 41:2174.

63. Gonzalez-Vitale JC, Hayes DM, Cvitkovic E, et al. The renal pathology in clinical trials of cis-platinum (II) diamminedichloride. Cancer 1977; 39:1362.

64. Schilsky RL, Anderson T. Hypomagnesemia and renal magnesium wasting in patients receiving cisplatin. Ann Intern Med 1979; 90:929.

65. Vogelzang NJ, Torkelson JL, Kennedy BJ. Hypomagnesemia renal dysfunction and Raynaud's phenomenon in patients treated with cisplatin, vinblastine and bleomycin. Cancer 1985; 56:2765.

66. Cvitkovic E, Spaulding J, Bethune V, et al. Improvement of cis-dichlorodiammineplatinum (NSC-119875) therapeutic index in an animal mode. Cancer 1977; 39:1357.

67. Chary KK, Higby DJ, Henderson ES, et al. Phase 1 study of high dose cis-dichlorodiammineplatinum (II) with forced diuresis. Cancer Treat Rep 1977; 61:367.

68. Hayes DM, Cvitkovic E, Golbey RB, et al. High dose cisplatinum diamminedichloride: amelioration of renal toxicity by mannitol diuresis. Cancer 1977; 39:1372.

69. Merrin C. A new method to prevent toxicity with high doses of cis-diammine platinum (therapeutic efficacy in previously treated widespread and recurrent testicular tumors). Proc Am Soc Clin Oncol 1976; 17:243.

70. Pera MF, Harder MC. Effects of mannitol and furosemide diuresis on cis-dichlorodiammine platinum (II) antitumor activity and toxicity to host renewing cell populations in rats. Cancer Res 1979; 39:1279.

71. Holdener EE, Park CH, Belt RJ, et al. Effect of mannitol and human plasma on cytotoxicity of cis-dichlorodiammineplatinum. Clin Res 1978; 26:4364.

72. Poore GA, Todd GC, Grindey GB. Effect of sodium thiosulfate (S_2O_3) on intravenous cisplatin (DDP) toxicity and antitumor activity. Proc Am Assoc Cancer Res 1984; 25:1466.

73. Iwatmoto Y, Kawano T, Uozumi J. 'Two-route chemotherapy' using high-dose ip cisplatin and IV sodium thiosulfate, its antidote, for peritoneally disseminated cancer in mice. Cancer Treat Rep 1984; 68:1367.

74. Dedon PC, Borch RF. Diethyldithiocarbamate (DDTC) reversal of cisplatin (DDP) nephrotoxicity. Proc Am Assoc Cancer Res 1984; 25:1470.

75. Pfeifle CE, Howell SB, Felthouse RD, et al. High-dose cisplatin with sodium thiosulfate protection. J Clin Oncol 1985; 3:237.

76. Juckett DA, Parham DM, Schonbaum GR, et al. A new treatment for prevention of cisplatin nephrotoxicity: adjunct therapy using polar dithiocarbamates. Proc Am Assoc Cancer Res 1984; 25:1274.

77. Glover D, Glick JH, Weiler C, et al. Phase 1 trials of WR-2721 and cis-platinum. Proc Am Assoc Cancer Res 1984; 25:720.

78. Roemeling R, Wick M, Berestka J, et al. Disulfiram and cisplatin chronotherapy allows safe and effective megadose therapy. Proc Am Assoc Cancer Res 1985; 26:1038.

79. Levi F, Hrushesky WJM, Borch RF, et al. Cisplatin urinary pharmacokinetics and nephrotoxicity: a common circadian mechanism. Cancer Treat Rep 1982; 66:1933.

80. Hruskesky WJM: Circadian chronopharmacokinetics and chronotoxicology of doxorubicin and cisplatin in human beings with cancer. In: Reinberg A, Smolensky M. Labreque G, eds. Annual review of chronopharmacology. Elmsford, NY: Pergamon Press 1984.

81. VonHoff DD, Schilsky R, Reichert CM, et al. Toxic effects of cis-dichlordiammineplatinum (II) in man. Cancer Treat Rep 1979; 63:1527.

82. Gagen M, Gochnour D, Young D, et al. A randomized trial of metoclopramide and a combination of dexamethasome and lorazepam for prevention of chemotherapy-induced vomiting. J Clin Oncol 1984; 2:696.

83. Reddel RR, Kefford RF, Grant JM, et al. Ototoxicity in patients receiving cisplatin: importance of dose and method of drug administration. Cancer Treat Rep 1982; 66:19.

84. Thompson SW, Davis LE, Kornfeld M, et al. Cisplatin neuropathy: clinical, electrophysiologic, morphologic and toxicologic studies. Cancer 1984; 54:1269.

85. Mollman JE, Glover DJ, Hogan WM, et al. Cis-platin neuropathy: a possible protective agent. Proc Am Assoc Clin Oncol 1985; 4:C127.

86. Hadley D, Herr HW. Peripheral neuropathy associated with cis-dichlorodiammineplatinum (II) treatment. Cancer 1979; 44:2026.

87. Drewinko B, Brown BW, Gottlieb JA. The effect of cis-diamminedichloroplatinum (II) on cultured human lymphona cells and its therapeutic implications. Cancer Res 1973; 33:3091.

88. Sigdestad CP, Grdina DJ, Peters LF, et al. Cell cycle phase preferential killing of fibrosarcoma tumor cells by cis-DDP or Adriamycin. Proc Am Assoc Cancer Res 1979; 20:1278.

89. Repta AJ, Long DF, Hincal AA. Cis-dichlorodiammineplatinum (II) stability in aqueous vehicles. Cancer Treat Rep 1979; 63:229.

90. Mariani EP, Southard BJ, Woolever JT, et al. Physical compatibility and chemical stability of cisplatin in various diluents and in large-volume parenteral solutions. In: Prestayko AW, Crooke ST, Carter SK, eds. Cisplatin: current status and new developments. New York: Academic Press, 1980.

91. Lokich JJ. Phase 1 study of cis-diamminededichloroplatinum (II) administered as a constant 5-day infusion. Cancer Treat Rep 1980; 64:905.

92. Jacobs C, Bertino JR, Goffinet DR. 24-hour infusion of cisplatinum in head and neck cancers. Cancer 1978; 42:2135.

93. Amrein P, Weitzman S. 24-hour infusion cisplatin and 5-day infusion 5-fluorouracil in squamous cell carcinoma of the head and neck. Proc Am Soc Clin Oncol 1985; 4:C519.

94. Bozzino JM, Prasad V, Koriech OM. Avoidance of renal toxicity by 24-hour infusion of cisplatin. Cancer Treat Rep 1981; 65:351.

95. Richardson RL, Hahn RG, Kvols LK, et al. Bleomycin, etoposide and continuous-infusion cisplatin in metastatic testicular cancer. Proc Am Assoc Cancer Res 1985; 4:C410.

96. Salem P, Hall SW, Benjamin RS, et al. Clinical phase 1-2 study of cis-dichlorodiammine platinum II given by continuous IV infusion. Cancer Treat Rep 1978; 62:1553.

97. Salem P, Khalyl M, Jabboury K, et al. Cis-diamminedichloroplatinum (II) by 5-day continuous infusion: a new dose schedule with minimal toxicity. Cancer 1984; 53:837.

98. Tisman G, Flener V, Hsu MYK, et al. Outpatient high-dose cis-platinum continuous infusion chemotherapy Proc Am Soc Clin Oncol 1984; 3:C104.

99. Sand J, Rosenthal CJ, Rotman M, et al. Lack of toxicity of cisplatin administered as a radiosensitizer by long-term continuous infusion. Proc Am Assoc Clin Oncol 1984; 3:C172.

100. Loh SH, Choi K, Aziz H, et al. Cis-platinum by continuous infusion with concomitant radiation effective in the therapy of primary advanced squamous cell carcinoma of the lung. Proc Am Soc Clin Oncol 1985; 4:C741.

101. Lokich JJ, Zipoli TE. Phase 1 study of protracted infusion of cisplatin. Cancer Drug Deliv 1984; 1:247.

102. Lokich JJ, Becker B. Subclavian vein thrombosis in patients treated with infusion chemotherapy for advanced malignancy. Cancer 1983; 52:1586.

103. Chen HSG, Gross JF. Intra-arterial infusion of anticancer drugs: theoretic aspects of drug delivery and review of responses. Cancer Treat Rep 1980; 64:31.

104. Campbell TN, Howell SB, Pfeifle CE, et al. Clinical pharmacokinetics of intra-arterial cisplatin in humans. J Clin Oncol 1983; 1:755.

105. Stewart DJ, Benjamin RS, Zimmerman S, et al. Clinical pharmacology of intra-arterial dis-diammedichloroplatinum (II). Cancer Res 1983; 43:917.

106. Lehane DE, Bryan RN, Horowitz B, et al. Intra-arterial cis-platinum chemotherapy for patients with primary and metastatic brain tumors. Cancer Drug Deliv 1983; 1:69.

107. Feun LG, Wallace S, Stewart DJ, et al. Intracarotid infusion of cis-diamminedichloroplatinum in the treatment of recurrent malignant brain tumors. Cancer 1984; 54:794.

108. Khan AB, D'Souza BJ, Wharam MD, et al. Cisplatin therapy in recurrent childhood brain tumors. Cancer Treat Rep 1982; 66:2013.

109. Walker RW, Allen JC. Treatment of recurrent primary intracranial childhood tumors with cis-diamminedichloroplatinum. Ann Neurol 1983; 14:371.

110. Kapp JP, Vance RB. Supraophthalmic arterial infusion of cisplatinum and BCNU for recurrent malignant glioma. Proc Am Soc Clin Oncol 1984; 3:C710.

111. Stewart DJ, Grahovic Z, Maroun J, et al. Intra-arterial chemotherapy for brain tumors, Proc Am Soc Clin Oncol 1985; 4:C513.

112. Vance RB, Kapp JP. Supraophthalmic arterial infusion of low-dose cisplatin and BCNU for malignant glioma. Proc Am Soc Clin Oncol 1985; 4:C525.

113. Purvis J, Bay J. Intracarotid chemotherapy with BCNU and cisplatin for recurrent glioma. Proc Am Soc Clin Oncol 1985; 4:C546.

114. Feun LG, Lee YY, Yung WKA, et al. Phase 2 trial of intracarotid BCNU and cisplatin in malignant brain tumors. Proc Am Soc Clin Oncol 1985; 4:C585.

115. Frustaci S, Tumolo S. Veronesi A, et al. Intra-arterial cisplatin (IA-CDDP) in head and neck cancer. Proc Am Soc Clin Oncol 1984; 3:C697.

116. Mortimer J, Cummings C, Laramore G, et al. Selective intra-arterial (IA) cisplatin for localized (Stage 3 and 4) unresectable head and neck cancer. Proc Am Soc Clin Oncol 1985; 4:C577.

117. Calvo DB, Patt YZ, Wallace S, et al. Phase 1–2 trial of percutaneous intra-arterial cis-diammine-dichloroplatinum (II) for regionally confined malignancy. Cancer 1980; 45:1278.

118. Jaffe N, Bowman R, Wang Y, et al. Chemotherapy for primary osteosarcoma by intra-arterial infusion. Cancer Bull 1984; 36:37.

119. Benjamin RS, Murray JA, Wallace S. Intra-arterial preoperative chemotherapy for osteosarcarma—a judicious approach to limb salvage. Cancer Bull 1984; 36:32.

120. Stewart DJ, Leavens M, Maor M, et al. Human central nervous system distribution of cis-diamminedichloroplatinum and use as a radiosensitizer in malignant brain tumors. Cancer Res 1982; 42:2474.

121. Lee FH, Canetta R, Issell BF, et al. New platinum complexes in clinical trials. Cancer Treat Rev 1983; 10:39.

122. Wolpert-DeFillipes MK. Antitumor activity of cisplatin analogues. In: Prestayko AW, Crooke ST, Carter SK, eds. Cisplatin: current status and new developments. New York: Academic Press, 1980; 183.

123. Lilieveld P, Van der Vijgh WJF, Veldhuizen RW, et al. Principal studies on toxicity, antitumor activity and pharmacokinetics of cisplatin and three recently developed derivatives. Eur J Cancer Clin Oncol 1984; 20:1087.

124. Cleare MJ, Hydes PC, Hepburn DR, et al. Antitumor platinum complexes: structure activity relationships. In: Prestayko AW, Crooke ST, Carter SK, eds. Cisplatin: current status and new developments. New York: Academic Press, 1980; 149.

125. Harrap KR, Jones M, Wilkinson CR et al. Antitumor toxic and biochemical properties of cisplatin and eight other platinum complexes. In: Prestayko AW, Crooke ST, Carter SK, eds. Cisplatin: current status and new developments. New York: Academic Press, 1980; 163.

126. Wilkinson R, Cox PF, Jones M, et al. Selection of potential second generation platinum compounds. Biochimie 1978; 60:851.

127. Calvert AH, Harland SJ, Newell DR, et al. Early clinical studies with cis-diammine -1,1-cyclobutane dicarboxylate platinum (II). Cancer Chemother Pharmacol 1982; 9:140.

128. Curt GA, Grygiel JJ, Corden BJ, et al. A phase 1 and pharmacokinetic study of diamminecyclo-butane dicarboxylato platinum (NSC 241 240). Cancer Res 1983; 43:4470.

129. Egorin MJ, Van Echo DA, Whitacre MY, et al. Phase 1 study and clinical pharmacokinetics of carboplatin (CBDCA) (NSC 241 240). Proc Am Soc Clin Oncol 1983; 2:C109.

130. Lassus M, Ohnuma T, Leyvraz S, et al. A phase 1 study of CBDCA (carbo platin). Proc Am Soc Clin Oncol 1983; 2:C-144.

131. Koeller JM, Earhart RH, Davis TE, et al. Phase 1 trial of carboplatin (NSC 241 240) by bolus intravenous injection. Proc Am Assoc Cancer Res 1983; 24:643.

132. Evans BD, Raju KS, Calvert AH, et al. Phase 2 study of JM-8, a new platinum analog, in advanced carcinoma. Cancer Treat Rep 1983; 67:997.

133. Kaplan S, Joss R, Sessa C, et al. Phase 1 trials of cis-diammine -1,1-cyclobutane dicarboxylate platinum (II) (CBDCA) in solid tumors. Proc Am Assoc Cancer Res 1983; 24:520.

134. Kelsen D, Sternberg C, Einzig A, et al. Phase 2 study of carboplatin (CBDCA) in advanced upper gastrointestinal tract (UGIT) malignancy. Proc Am Soc Clin Oncol 1984; 3:C-552.

135. Ten Bokkel Huinink WW, van der Burg MEL, Vermorken JB, et al. Carboplatin in combination chemotherapy for ovarian cancer, a feasibility study. Proc Am Soc Clin Oncol 1984; 3:C-690.

136. Rozencweig M, Nicaise C, Beer M, et al. Phase 1 study of carboplatin given on a five-day intravenous schedule. J Clin Oncol 1983; 1:621.

137. Ohnuma T, Leyvraz S, Coffey V, et al. Carboplatin: activity in patients with head and neck (H&N), renal cell (RC) and ovarian carcinomas. Proc Am Assoc Cancer Res 1984; 25:710.

138. Creekmore SP, Micetich KC, Vogelzang N. Low toxicity and significant tumor responses in phase 2 trials of carboplatin (CBDCA) in head and neck, nonsmall F-cell lung, urothelial and ovarian cancers. Proc Am Soc Clin Oncol 1985; 4:C562.

139. Siddik ZH, Newell DR, Jones M, et al. Pharmacokinetics of cis-diammine -1,1-cylobutanedicarboxylato platinum (II) (CBDCA, JM 8) in mice and rats. Proc Am Assoc Cancer Res 1982; 23:659.

140. Priego V, Luc V, Bonnem E, et al. A phase 1 study and pharmacology of diammine (1,1) cyclobutane dicarboxylato (2-1-0-) platinum (CBDCA) administered on a weekly schedule. Proc Am Soc Clin Oncol 1983; 2:C-117.

141. Tauer K, Bosl GJ, Golbey RB, et al. A phase 2 trial of cis-diammine -1,1-cyclobutane dicarboxy-late platinum II in patients with cisplatin-resistant germ cell tumors. Proc Am Soc Clin Oncol 1985; 4:C406.

142. Ozols RF, Ostchega Y, Curt G, et al. High-dose cisplatin and high-dose carboplatinum in refractory ovarian cancer: salvage drugs with different toxicities. Proc Am Soc Clin Oncol 1985; 4:C462.

143. Wiltshaw E, Evans B, Harland S. Phase 3 randomized trial cisplatin versus JM8 (carboplatin) in 112 ovarian cancer patients, stages 2 & 4. Proc Am Soc Clin Oncol 1985; 4:C471.

144. Evans BD, Weston C, Smith IE. Carboplatin (JM8) and VP-16 combination chemotherapy for untreated small lung cell carcinoma. Proc Am Soc Clin Oncol 1985; 4:C734.

145. Egorin MJ, Van Echo DA, Tipping SJ, et al. Pharmacokinetics and dosage reduction of cis-diammine-1,1-cyclobutane-dicarboxylatoplatinum in patients with impaired renal function. Cancer Res 1984; 44:5432.

146. Harland SJ, Newell DR, Siddik ZH, et al. Pharmacokinetics of cis-diammine-1,1-cyclobutane dicarboxylate platinum (II) in patients with normal and impaired renal function. Cancer Res 1984; 44:1693.

147. Bitran JD. Personal communication.

148. Mihich E, Bullard G, Pavelic Z, et al. Preclinical studies of dihydroxy-cis-dichloro-bis-isopropylamine platinum (IV) (CHIP). Proc Am Soc Clin Oncol 1983; 2:C559.

149. Yap BS, Tenney DM, Yap HY, et al. Phase 1 clinical evaluation of cis-dichloro-trans-dihydroxy-bis-isopropylamine platinum IV (CHIP, JM9) Proc Am Assoc Cancer Res 1983; 24:658.

150. Ginsberg SJ, Lee F, Issell B, et al. A phase 1 study of cis-dichloro-trans-dihydroxy-bis (isopropylamine) -platinum IV (CHIP) administered by intravenous bolus daily for 5 days. Proc Am Clin Oncol 1983; 2:C139.

151. Creaven PJ, Madajewicz S, Pendyala L, et al. Phase 1 clinical trial of cis-dichloro-trans-dihydroxy-bis-isopropylamine platinum IV (CHIP). Cancer Treat Rep 1983; 67:795.

152. Sessa C, Cavalli F, Kaye S, et al. Phase 2 study of cis-dichloro-trans-dihydroxy-bis-isopropylamine platinum IV (CHIP) in advanced ovarian carcinoma. Proc Am Soc Clin Oncol 1985; 4:C452.

153. Pendyala L, Cowens JW, Creaven PJ, et al. Studies on the pharmacokinetics and metabolism of cis-dichloro-trans-dihydroxy-bis-isopropylamine platinum IV in the dog. Cancer Treat Rep 1982; 66:509.

154. Pfister M, Pavelic Z, Bullard GA, et al. Dichloro-dihydroxy-bis-isopropylamine platinum IV, a new antitumor platinum complex. Pharmacokinetics in the rat; relation to renal toxicity. Biochimie 1978; 60:1057.

155. Pendyala L, Cowens JW, Mittelman A, et al. Clinical pharmacokinetics of cis-dichloro-trans-dihydroxy-bis-isopropylamine platinum IV (CHIP). A new platinum drug in phase 1 trial. Proc Am Assoc Cancer Res 1982; 23:497.

156. Kriesman H, Ginsberg S, Feldstein M, et al. Iproplatin (CHIP) or carboplatin (CBDCA) in extensive nonsmall-cell lung cancer. Proc Am Soc Clin Oncol 1985; 4:C725.

157. Edwards CL, Hayes RL. Tumor scanning with ^{67}Ga-citrate. J Nucl Med 1969; 10:103.

158. Bekerman C, Hoffer PB, Bitran JB. The role of gallium -67 in the clinical evaluation of cancer. Semin Nucl Med 1984; 14:296.

159. Hart M, Adamson R. Antitumor activity and toxicity of salts of inorganic group III A metals: aluminum, gallium, indium and thallium. Proc Natl Acad Sci (USA) 1971; 68:1623.

160. Adamson RH, Canellos GP, Seiber SM, et al. Studies on the antitumor activity of gallium nitrate (NSC-15200) and other group III A metal salts. Cancer Treat Rep 1975; 59:599.

161. Rubin H, Koide T. Mutual potentiation by magnesium and calcium of growth in animal cells. Proc Natl Acad Sci (USA) 1976; 73:168.

162. Vallabhajosula SR, Harwig JF, Siemsen JK, et al. Radiogallium localization in tumors: blood binding and transport and the role of transferrin. J Nucl Med 1980; 21:650.

163. Larson SM, Rasey JS, Allen DR, et al. Common pathway for tumor cell uptake of gallium-67 and iron-59 via a transferrin receptor. J Nat Cancer Inst 1980; 64:41.

164. Hall SW, Yeung K, Benjamin RS, et al. Kinetics of gallium nitrate, a new anticancer agent. Clin Pharmacol Ther 1979; 25:82.

165. Krakoff IH, Newman RA, Goldberg RS. Clinical toxicologic and pharmacologic studies of gallium nitrate. Cancer 1979; 44:1722.

166. Kelsen DP, Alcock N, Yeh S, et al. Pharmacokinetics of gallium nitrate in man. Cancer 1980; 46:2009.

167. Bedikian AY, Valdivieso M, Bodey GP. Phase 1 clinical studies with gallium nitrate. Cancer Treat Rep 1978; 62:1449.

168. Warrell RP, Coonley CJ, Straus DJ, et al. Treatment of patients with advanced malignant lymphoma using gallium nitrate administered as a seven-day continuous infusion. Cancer 1983; 51:1982.

169. Danieu L, Atkins C, Sykes M, et al. Gallium nitrate, methyl-GAG (MGBG), and etoposide: an effective investigational combination for relapsed lymphoma. Proc Am Soc Clin Oncol 1985; 4:C815.

170. Leyland-Jones B, Bhalla RB, Farag F, et al. Administration of gallium nitrate by continuous infusion: lack of chronic nephrotoxicity confirmed by studies of enzymuria and β-microglobulinuria. Cancer Treat Rep 1983; 67:941.

171. Casper ES, Stanton GF, Sordillo PP. Phase 2 study of gallium nitrate infusion in patients with advanced malignant melanoma. Proc Am Soc Clin Oncol 1985; 4:C567.

172. Weick JK, Stephens RL, Baker LH, et al. Gallium nitrate in malignant lymphoma: a Southwest Oncology Group study. Cancer Treat Rep 1983; 67:823.

173. Keller JW, Johnson L, Raney M, et al. Phase 2 study of gallium nitrate (GaNO₃)(NSC- 15200) in refractory lymphoproliferative diseases. A Southeastern Cancer Study Group (SCSG) study. Proc Am Soc Clin Oncol 1984; 3:C967.

174. Samson MK, Fraile RJ, Baker LH, et al. Phase 1-2 clinical trial of gallium nitrate (NSC-15200). Cancer Clin Trials 1980; 3:131.

175. Saiki JH, Baker LH, Stephens RL, et al. Gallium nitrate in advanced soft tissue and bone sarcomas: a Southwest Oncology Group study. Cancer Treat Rep 1982; 66:1673.

176. Scher H, Tauer K, Alcock N, et al. Preliminary evaluation of gallium nitrate on bone turnover and antitumor activity in patients with hormone resistant prostatic cancer metastatic to bone. Proc Am Soc Clin Oncol 1985; 4:C407.

177. National Cancer Institute. CTEP, Annual report to the FDA: gallium nitrate NSC 15200. March 1981.

178. Decker DA, Costanzi JJ, McCracken JD, et al. Evaluation of gallium nitrate in metastatic or locally recurrent squamous cell carcinoma of the head and neck: a Southwest Oncology Group study. Cancer Treat Rep 1984; 68:1047.

179. Warrell RP, Bockman RS, Coonley CJ, et al. Gallium nitrate inhibits calcium resorption from bone and is effective treatment for cancer related hypercalcemia. J Clin Invest 1984; 73:1487.

180. Rice LM, Slavik M, Schein P. Clinical brochure. Spriogermanium (NSC-192965) Bethesda: National Cancer Institute, 1977.

181. Hill BT, Whatley SA, Bellamy AS, et al. Cytotoxic effects and biological activity of 2-aza-8-germanspiro (4,5)-decane-2-propanamine-8,8-diethyl-N,N-dimethyl dichloride (NSC-19265, spirogermanium) in vitro. Cancer Res. 1982; 42:2852.

182. Larsson H, Trope C, Mattsson W, et al. Clinical pharmacokinetics of intravenously administered spirogermanium. Proc Am Soc Clin Oncol 1980; 21:C62.

183. Schein PS, Slavik M, Smythe T, et al. Phase 1 clinical trial of spirogermanium. Cancer Treat Rep 1980; 64:1051.

184. Legha SS, Ajani JA, Bodey GP. Phase 1 study of spirogermanium given daily. J Clin Oncol 1983; 1:331.

185. Mattson W. A phase 1 study of spirogermanium. Proc Am Assoc Cancer Res 1980; 21:778.

186. Budman DR, Schulman P, Vinciguerra V, et al. Phase 1 trial of spirogermanium given by infusion in a multiple dose schedule. Cancer Treat Rep 1982; 66:173.

187. Budman DR, Ginsberg S, Perry M, et al. Phase 2 study of spirogermanium in breast adenocarcinoma: a cancer and leukemia group B study. Cancer Treat Rep 1982; 66:1667.

188. Pinnamaneni K, Yap HY, Legha SS, et al. Phase 1 study of spirogermanium in the treatment of metastatic breast cancer. Cancer Treat Rep 1984; 68:1197.

189. Falkson G, Falkson HC. Phase 1 trial of spirogermanium for treatment of advanced breast cancer. Cancer Treat Rep 1983; 67:189.

190. Kuebler JP, Tormey DC, Harper GR, et al. Phase 2 study of spirogermanium in advanced breast cancer. Cancer Treat Rep 1984; 68:1515.

191. Trope C, Mattsson W, Gynning I, et al. Phase 2 study of spirogermanium in advanced ovarian malignancy. Cancer Treat Rep 1981; 65:119.

192. Weiselberg L, Budman DR, Schulman P, et al. Phase 2 trial of spirogermanium in advanced epithelial carcinoma of the ovary. Cancer Treat Rep 1982; 66:1675.

193. Schulman P, Davis RB, Rafla S, et al. Phase 2 trial of spirogermanium in advanced renal cell carcinoma: a Cancer and Leukemia Group B study. Cancer Treat Rep 1984; 68:1305.

194. Dhingra HM, Umsawasdi T, Chiuten DF, et al. Spirogermanium (NSC 192-965) in advanced nonsmall-cell lung cancer. Proc Am Soc Clin Oncol 1985; 4:C761.

195. Evrard M, McGuire WP, Cobleigh M, et al. Phase 2 trial of spirogermanium advanced nonsmall-cell lung cancer. Proc Am Soc Clin Oncol 1985; 4:C720.

196. Harvey J, Bowers MW, Woolley PV et al. A phase 1 trial of oral spirogermanium. Proc Am Soc Clin Oncol 1984; 3:138.

197. Woolley PV, Priego V, Luc V, et al. A phase 1 trial of spirogermanium administered as a five-day continuous infusion. Proc Am Assoc Cancer Res 1983; 24:539.

References—Chapter 12

1. Karow M, Chirakawa S. The locus of action of 1-β-D-arabinofuranosyl cytosine in the cell cycle. Cancer Res 1970; 29:687–96.

2. Major PP, Egan EM, Beardsley GP, et al. Lethality of human myeloblasts correlated with the incorporation of arabinofuranosyl cytosine into DNA. Proc Natl Acad Sci USA 1981; 78:3235–39.

3. Wiley JS, Jones SP, Sawyer WH. Cytosine arabinoside transport by human leukemia cells. Eur J Cancer Clin Oncol 1983; 19:1067–71.

4. Wann SH, Huffman DH, Azarnoff DL, Hoogstraten B, Larsen WE. Pharmacokinetics of 1-β-D-arabinosylcytosine in humans. Cancer Res 1974; 34:392–97.

5. Chabner BA. Cytosine arabinoside. In: Chabner BA, ed. Pharmacologic principles of cancer treatment. Philadelphia: WB Saunders, 1982; 387–401.

6. Coleman CN, Stoller RG, Drake JC, et al. Deoxycytidine kinase: properties of the enzyme from human leukemic granulocytes. Blood 1975; 46:791–803.

7. Tattersall MNH, Ganeshagur UK, Hoffbrand AV. Mechanisms of resistance of human acute leukemia cells to cytosine arabinoside. Br J Haematol 1974; 27:39–46.

8. Iwagaki A, Nakamura T, Wakisake G. Studies on the mechanism of action of 1-β-D-arabinofuranosylcytosine as an inhibitor of DNA synthesis in human leukemic leukocytes. Cancer Res 1969; 29:2169–76.

9. Chu MY, Fisher GA. A proposed mechanism of action of 1-β-D-arabinofuranosylcytosine as an inhibitor of leukemic cells. Biochem Pharmacol 1962; 11:423–30.

10. Major PP, Egan EM, Beardsley GP, et al. Lethality of human myeloblasts correlated with the incorporation of arabinosylcytosine into DNA. Proc Natl Acad Sci USA 1981; 78:3235–39.

11. Major PP, Egan EM, Herrick P, Kufe DW. Instability of (ara-C) DNA under alkaline conditions. Biochem Pharmacol 1982; 31:861–66.

12. Atkinson MP, Deutscher M, Kornberg A, et al. Enzymatic synthesis of DNA termination of chain growth by a 2'-3'-dideoxyribonucleotide. Biochemistry 1969; 8:4897–4904.

13. Chu MY, Fisher GA. Comparative studies of leukemia cells sensitive and resistant to cytosine arabinoside. Biochem Pharmacol 1965; 14:333–41.

14. Dijkwel PA, Wanka F. Enhanced release of nascent single strands from DNA synthesized in the presence of arabinosyl cytosine. Biochim Biophys Acta 1978; 520:461–71.

15. Stewart CD, Burke PJ. Cytosine deaminase and the development of resistance to arabinosylcytosine. Nature 1971; 233:109–10.

16. Harris AL, Potter C, Bunch C, et al. Pharmacokinetics of cytosine arabinoside in patients with acute myeloid leukemia. Br J Clin Pharmacol 1979; 8:219–27.

17. Liversidge GG, Nishihata T, Higuchi T, Schaffer R, Cortese M. Simultaneous analysis of 1-β-D-arabinofuranosyl cytosine, 1-β-D-arabinofuranosyluracil and sodium silicylate in biological samples by high performance liquid chromatography. J Chromatog 1983; 276:375–79.

18. Skipper HE, Schabel FM Jr, Wilcox WS. Experimental evaluation of potential anticancer agents. XXI. Scheduling of arabinosyl cytosine to take advantage of its S-phase specificity against leukemia cells. Cancer Chemother Rep 1967; 51:125–41.

19. Frei E III, Bickers JN, Hewlett JS, et al. Dose schedule and antitumor studies of arabinosyl cytosine (NSC 63878). Cancer Res 1969; 29:1325–32.

20. Cottman CA, Freireich EJ, Pendleton O, et al. Adult acute leukemia studies utilizing cytarabine: early Southwest Oncology Group trials. Med Pediatr Oncol 1982; 1:173–83.

21. Kantarjian H, Barlogie B, Plunke HW, et al. High-dose cytosine arabinoside in non-Hodgkin's lymphoma. J Clin Oncol 1983; 1:689–94.

22. Ellison RR, Carey RW, Holland JF. Continuous infusion of arabinosyl cytosine in patients with neoplastic disease. Clin Pharmacol Therap 1967; 8:800–09.

23. Gale RP. Advances in the treatment of acute myelogenous leukemia. N Engl J Med 1979; 300:1189–99.

24. Ellison RR, Holland JF, Weil M, et al. Arabinosyl cytosine: a useful agent in the treatment of acute leukemia in adults. Blood 1968; 37:507–23.

25. Frei E, Bickers JN, Hewlett JS, et al. Dose schedule and antitumor studies of arabinosylcytosine. Cancer Res 1967; 29:1325–32.

26. Rai KR, Holland JF, Glidewell OJ, et al. Treatment of acute myelocytic leukemia: a study by Cancer and Leukemia Group B. Blood 1981; 58:1203–12.

27. Ho DHW, Frei E. Clinical pharmacology of 1-β-D-arabinofuranosylcytosine. Clin Pharmacol Therap 1971; 12:944–54.

28. Riva CM, Rustum YM, Priesler HD. Pharmacokinetics and cellular determinants of response to 1-β-D-arabinofuranosylcytosine. Semin Oncol 1985; 12:1–8.

29. Capizzi RL, Yang J, Rathmell JP, et al. Dose-related pharmacologic effects of high-dose ara-C and its self-potentiation. Semin Oncol 1985; 12:65–75.

30. Capizzi RL, Yang J, Cheng EC, et al. Alteration of the pharmacokinetics of high-dose ara-C by its metabolite, high ara-U, in patients with acute leukemia. J Clin Oncol 1983; 1:763–71.

31. Yang J, Cheng EH, Capizzi RL, et al. Effect of uracil arabinoside on metabolism and cytotoxicity of cytosine arabinoside in L5178Y leukemia. J Clin Invest 1985; 75:141–46.

32. Canten G, Brenne JK: High dose cytosine arabinoside for acute nonlymphocytic leukemia. Am J Hematol 1984; 16:59–64.

33. Early AP, Priesler HF, Higby DJ, et al. High-dose cytosine arabinoside: clinical response to therapy in acute leukemia. Med Pediatr Oncol Supp 1982; 1:239–41.

34. Hertig RH, Wolf SN, Lazarus HM, et al: High-dose cytosine arabinoside therapy for refractory leukemia. Blood 1983; 62:361–66.

35. Priesler HD, Early AP, Raza A, et al. Therapy for secondary acute leukemia with cytarabine. N Engl J Med 1983; 308:21–22.

36. Forman SJ, Nademance AP, O'Donnell MR, et al. High-dose cytosine arabinoside and daunomycin as primary therapy for adults with acute nonlymphoblastic leukemia: a pilot study. Semin Oncol 1985; 12:114–15.

37. Hines JD, Mazza MM, Oken MM. High-dose cytosine arabinoside and m-AMSA induction and consolidation in patients with previously untreated de novo acute nonlymphocytic leukemia: a phase 1 pilot study for the Eastern Cooperative Oncology Group. Semin Oncol 1985; 12:117–19.

38. Barnett MJ, Waxman JJ, Richards MA, et al. High dose cytosine arabinoside in the initial treatment of acute leukemia. Semin Oncol 1985; 12:133–38.

39. Capizzi RL, Powell BL, Cooper MR. Sequential high dose ara-C and asparaginase in the therapy of previously treated and untreated patients with acute leukemia. Semin Oncol 1985; 12:105–13.

40. Magee RJ, Schiffer CA, Peterson BA, et al. Intensive post-remission therapy in adults with acute nonlymphocytic leukemia with ara-C by continuous infusion or bolus administration: preliminary results of a CALGB phase 1 study. Semin Oncol 1985; 12:84–90.

41. Kufe DW, Spriggs DR. Biochemical and cellular pharmacology of cytosine arabinoside. Semin Oncol 1985; 12:34–48.

42. Keating MJ, Estey E, Iacoboni S, et al. Evaluation of clinical studies with high-dose cytosine arabinoside at the M. D. Anderson Hospital. Semin Oncol 1985; 12:98–104.

43. Plunkett W, Iacoboni S, Estey E, et al. Pharmacologically directed ara-C therapy for refractory

leukemia. Semin Oncol 1985; 12:20–30.

44. Plunkett W, Iacoboni S, Danhausen L, et al. Pharmacologically directed schedules of high-dose ara-C for relapsed acute leukemia. Proc Am Assoc Cancer Res 1984; 25:658.

45. Iacoboni S, Plunkett W, Danhausen L, et al. Clinical results of pharmacologically directed schedules of high-dose ara-C for relapsed acute leukemia. Proc Am Soc Clin Oncol 1984; 3:200.

46. Lotem J, Sachs L. Potential prescreening for therapeutic agents that induce differentiation in human leukemia cells. Int J Cancer 1980; 25:561–65.

47. Griffin J, Munroe D, Major P, Kufe D. Induction of differentiation of human myeloid leukemia cells by inhibitors of DNA synthesis. Exp Hematol 1982; 10:744–49.

48. Luise-DeLuca C, Mitchell T, Spriggs D, Kufe D. Induction of terminal differentiation in human K562 erythroleukemia cells by arabinofuranosylcytosine. J Clin Invest 1984; 74:821–28.

49. Craig R, Frankfurt O, Sakagami H, Takeda K, Bloch A. Macromolecular and cell cycle effects of human myeloblastic leukemia (ML-1) cells. Cancer Res 1984; 44:2421–27.

50. Spriggs D, Griffin J, Wiseb J, Kufe D. Clinical pharmacology of low-dose cytosine arabinoside. Blood 1985; 65:1087–89.

51. Moloney C, Rosenthal DS. Treatment of early acute nonlymphocytic leukemia with low-dose cytosine arabinoside. In: Modern trends in human leukemia, Vol. 4. Springer Biochem, 1981; 59–62.

52. Housset M, Daniel MT, Degos L. Small doses of ara-C in the treatment of acute myeloid leukemia: differentiation of myeloid leukemia cells. Brit J Haematol 1982; 51:125–29.

53. Wisch JS, Griffin JD, Kufe DW. Response of preleukemic syndromes to continuous infusion of low-dose cytarabine. N Engl J Med 1983; 309:1599–1602.

54. Griffin JD, Spriggs D, Wisch JS, Kufe DW. Treatment of preleukemic syndromes with continuous infusion of low-dose cytosine arabinoside. J Clin Oncol 1985; 3:982–91.

55. Tagawa M, Shibata J, Tomanaga M, et al. Low-dose arabinoside regimen induced a complete remission with normal karyotypes in a case with hypoplastic acute myeloid leukemia with No. 8 trisomy: in vitro and in vivo evidence for normal haematopoietic recovery. Brit J Haematol 1985; 60:449–55.

56. Beran M, Andersson BS, Ayyar RR, et al. Clinical response and mechanisms of action of low-dose cytosine arabinoside (ara-C) in myelodysplastic syndromes (MDS) and myelogenous leukemia (AML, CMML). Proc Am Assoc Clin Oncol 1985; 4:174.

57. Cheson BA, Jasperse DM, Simon R, Friedman MA. A critical appraisal of low-dose cytosine arabinoside in patients with acute nonlymphocitic leukemia and myelodysplastic syndromes. J Clin Oncol (in press).

58. Slevin ML, Piall EM, Aherne GW, et al. Effect of dose and schedule on pharmacokinetics of high-dose cytosine arabinoside in plasma and cerebrospinal fluid. J Clin Oncol 1983: 1:546–50.

59. Canellos GP, Sutcliffe SB, DeVita VT, Listen TA. Treatment of refractory splenomegaly in myeloproliferative disease by splenic artery infusion. Blood 1979; 53:1014–17.

60. Lukas G, Bundler SD, Greengard P. The route of absorption of intraperitoneally administered compounds. J Pharmacol Exp Therap 1971; 178:562–66.

61. King ME, Pfeifle CE, Howell SB. Intraperitoneal cytosine arabinoside therapy in ovarian cancer. J Clin Oncol 1984; 2:662–69.

62. Hamburger AW, Salmon SE, Kim MB, et al. Direct cloning of human ovarian cancer cells in a gas. Cancer Res 1979; 38:3438–44.

63. Markman M. The intracavitary administration of cytarabine to patients with nonhematologic malignancies: pharmacologic rationale and results of clinical trials. Semin Oncol 1985; 12:177–83.

64. Pfeifle CE, Howell SM, Markman M, et al. Totally implantable system for peritoneal access. J Clin Oncol 1984; 2:1277–80.

65. Markman M. Melphalan and cytarabine administered intraperitoneally as single agents and combination intraperitoneal chemotherapy with cisplatin and cytarabine. Semin Oncol 1985; 12:33–37.

References—Chapter 13

1. Bender RA. Vinca alkaloids and epipodophyllotoxins. In: Pinedo HM, ed. Cancer Chemotherapy 1979. New York: Elsevier, 1979; 93–106.

2. Root MA, Gerzon K, Dyke RW. A radioimmunoassay for vinblastine and vincristine. In: Federation of analytical chemistry and spectroscopy societies, abstract 183 (1975) 1254.

3. Sethi VS, Burton SS, Jackson DV. A sensitive radioimmunoassay for vincristine and vinblastine. Cancer Chemother Pharmacol 1980; 4:183–87.

4. Rahmani R, Barbet J, Cano JP. A ^{125}I-radiolabelled probe for vinblastine and vindestine radioimmunoassays: applications to measurements of vindesine plasma levels in man after intravenous injections and long-term infusions. Clin Chim Acta 1983; 129:51–69.

5. Ratain MJ, Holt JA, Sinkule JA, Vogelzang NJ. Modificaiton of the vinca alkaloid radioimmunoassay for improved sensitivity: application for measurement of serum concentrations during prolonged continuous vinblastine infusion (submitted for publication).

6. Owellen RJ, Root MA, Hains FO. Pharmacokinetics of vindesine and vincristine in humans. Cancer Res 1977; 37:2603–07.

7. Owellen RJ, Hartke CA, Harris FO. Pharmacokinetics and metabolism of vinblastine in humans. Cancer Res 1977; 37:2597–2602.

8. Nelson RL, Dyke RW, Root MA. Comparative pharmacokinetics of vindesine, vincristine and vinblastine in patients with cancer. Cancer Treat Rev 1980; 7 (suppl):17–24.

9. Jackson DV, Sethi VS, Long TR, Mass HB, Spurr CL. Pharmacokinetics of vindesine bolus and infusion. Cancer Chemother Pharmacol 1984; 13:114–19.

10. Rahmani R, Martin M, Faure R, Cano JP, Barbet J. Clinical pharmacokinetics of vindesine: repeated treatments by intravenous bolus injections. Eur J Cancer Clin Oncol 1984; 20:1409–17.

11. Ohnuma T, Norton L, Andrejczuk A, Holland JF. Pharmacokinetics of vindesine given as an intravenous bolus and 24-hour infusion in humans. Cancer Res 1985; 454:464–69.

12. Ratain MJ, Vogelzang NJ, Sinkule JA, Holt JA. Phase 1 pharmacokinetic (PK) and toxicity study of prolonged continuous infusion vinblastine (CIV) using infusion (INF) pumps. Proc Am Assoc Canc Res 1985; 26:162.

13. Hande K, Gay J, Gober J, Greco FA. Toxicity and pharmacology of bolus vindesine injection and prolonged vindesine infusion. Cancer Treat Rev 1980; 7 (suppl):25–30.

14. Jackson DV, Castle MC, Bender RA. Biliary excretion of (^{3}H)-vincristine in man. Clin Pharmacol Ther 1978; 24:101–07.

15. Dyke RW, Nelson RL. Phase 1 anti-cancer agents: vindesine (desacetyl vinblastine amide sulfate). Cancer Treat Rev 1977; 4:135–42.

16. Valdivieso M, Richman S, Burgess MA, Bodey GP, Freireich EJ. Initial clinical studies of vindesine. Cancer Treat Rep 1981; 65:873–75.

17. Frei E, Franzino A, Shnider BI, et al. Clinical studies of vinblastine. Cancer Chemother Rep 1961; 12:125–29.

18. Bruce WR, Meeker BE, Powers WE, Valeriote FA. Comparison of the dose — and time — survival curves for normal hematopoietic and lymphoma colony-forming cells exposed to vinblastine, vincristine, arabinosylcytosine, and amethopterin. J Natl Cancer Inst 1969; 42:1015–23.

19. Jusko WJ. A pharmacodynamic model for cell-cycle-specific chemotherapeutic agents. J Pharmacokin Biopharm 1973; 1:175–200.

20. Hill BT, Whelan RDH. Comparative effects of vincristine and vindesine on cell cycle kinetics in vitro. Cancer Treat Rev 1980; 7 (suppl):5–15.

21. Ludwig R, Alberts DS, Miller TP, Salmon SE. Evaluation of anticancer drug schedule dependency using an in vitro human tumor clonogenic assay. Cancer Chemother Pharmacol 1984; 12:135–41.

22. Matsushima Y, Kanzawa F, Hoshi A, et al. Time-schedule dependency of the inhibiting activity of various anticancer drugs in the clonogenic assay. Cancer Chemother Pharmacol 1985; 14:104–07.

23. Lengsfeld AM, Dietrich J, Schultz-Maures B. Accumulation and release of vinblastine and vincris-

tine by Hela cells: light microscopic, cinematographic, and biochemical study. Cancer Res 1982; 42:3798–3805.

24. Ferguson PJ, Phillips JR, Selner M, Cass CE. Differential activity of vincristine and vinblastine against cultured cells. Cancer Res 1984; 44:3307–12.

25. Owellen RJ, Donigan DW, Hartke CA, Harris FO. Correlation of biologic data with physicochemical properties among the vinca alkaloids and their congeners. Biochem Pharmacol 1977; 26:1213–19.

26. Ferguson PJ, Cass CE. The basis of differential toxicity of vincristine and vinblastine against HL-60/cl cells is rapid release of vinblastine. Proc Am Assoc Canc Res 1985; 26:236.

27. Gout PW, Noble RL, Bruchorsky N, Beer CT. Vinblastine and vincristine-growth-inhibitory effects correlate with their retention by cultured Nb 2 node lymphoma cells. Int J Cancer 1984; 34:245–48.

28. Yap HY, Blumenschein GR, Keating MJ, Hortobagyi GN, Tashima CK, Loo TL. Vinblastine given as a continuous 5-day infusion in the treatment of refractory advanced breast cancer. Cancer Treat Rep 1980; 64:279–83.

29. Young JA, Howell SB, Green MR. Pharmacokinetics and toxicity of 5-day continuous infusion of vinblastine. Cancer Chemother Pharmacol 1984; 12:43–45.

30. Zeffren J, Yagoda A, Kelsen D, Will R. Phase 1–2 trial of a 5-day continuous infusion of vinblastine sulfate. Anticancer Res 1984; 4:411–14.

31. Lokich JJ, Zipoli TE, Perri J, Bothe A. Protracted vinblastine infusion. Phase 1–2 study in malignant melanoma and other tumors. Am J Clin Oncol 1984; 7:551–53.

32. Lokich J, Bothe A, Fine N, Perri J. The delivery of cancer chemotherapy by constant venous infusion. Ambulatory management of venous access and portable pump. Cancer 1982; 50:2731–35.

33. Ensminger W, Niederhuber J, Dakhil S, Thrail J, Wheeler R. Totally implanted drug delivery system for hepatic arterial chemotherapy. Cancer Treat Rep 1981; 65:393–400.

34. Vogelzang NJ, Ruane MJ, Demeester TR. Phase 1 trial of implanted battery-powered, programmable drug delivery system for continuous doxorubicin administration. J Clin Oncol 1985; 3:407–14.

35. Lu K, Yap HY, Loo TL. Clinical pharmacokinetics of vinblastine by continuous intravenous infusion. Cancer Res 1983; 43:1405–08.

36. Chacon RD, Kotliar ML, Cavarva G, et al. Phase 2 study with vinblastine continuous infusion (Vb CI). Proc Am Soc Clin Oncol 1982; 1:33.

37. Tannock I, Erlichman C, Perrault D, Quirt I, King M. Failure of 5-day vinblastine in the treatment of patients with advanced refractory breast cancer. Cancer Treat Rep 1982; 66:1783–84.

38. Ingle JN, Ahmann DL, Gersther JG, Green SJ, O'Connell MJ, Kuols LK. Evaluation of vinblastine administered by 5-day continuous infusion in women with advanced breast cancer. Cancer Treat Rep 1984; 68:803–04.

39. Shah MK, Greech RH, Catalono RB, St. Mariek. Phase 2 study of vinblastine infusion in the treatment of refractory advanced breast cancer. Proc Am Soc Clin Oncol 1982; 1:73.

40. Yau JC, Yap YY, Buzdar AU, Hortobagyi GN, Body GP, Blumenschein GR. A comparative randomized trial of vinca alkaloids in patients with metastatic breast cancer. Cancer 1985; 55:337–40.

41. Paschold EH, Jackson DV. Spurr CL, et al. Continuous infusion of vincristine (VCR) and vinblastine (VLB) in refractory lymphoma: a phase 2 study. Proc Am Soc Clin Oncol 1982; 1:159.

42. Kavanagh JJ, Wharton JT, Rutledge FN. Continuous-infusion vinblastine for treatment of refractory epithelial carcinoma of the ovary: a phase 2 trial. Cancer Treat Rep 1984; 68:1417–18.

43. Kuebler JP, Hogan TF, Trump DL, Bryan GT. Phase 2 study of continuous 5-day vinblastine infusion in renal adenocarcinoma. Cancer Treat Rep 1984; 68:925–26.

44. Yap BS, Benjamin RS, Plager C, Burgess MA, Papadoupolos N, Bodey GP. A randomized study of continuous infusion vindesine versus vinblastine in adults with refractory sarcomas. Am J Clin Oncol 1983; 6:235–38.

45. Yap HY, Blumenschein GR, Hortobagyi GN, Buzdar AU, Schell FC, Bodey GP. Combination chemotherapy with continuous infusion vinblastine and peptichemio for patients with advanced metastatic breast cancer. Am J Clin Oncol 1982; 5:511–14.

46. Tannir N, Yap HY, Hortobagyi GH, Hug V, Buzdar AU, Blumenschein GR. Sequential continuous infusion with doxorubicin and vinblastine: an effective chemotherapy combination for patients with

advanced breast cancer previously treated with cyclophosphamide, methotrexate, 5-FU, vincristine, and prednisone. Cancer Treat Rep 1984; 68:1039–41.

47. Logothetis CJ, Samuels ML, Selig D, Swanson D, Johnson DE, von Eschenbach AC. Improved survival with cyclic chemotherapy for nonseminomatous germ cell tumors of the testis. J Clin Oncol 1985; 3:326–35.

48. Chong C, Logothetis C, Fristche H, Gietner A, Savaraj N, Samuels M. Peak vinblastine concentration as a monitor of nonhematologic toxicity in patients with testicular cancer. Proc Am Assoc Canc Res 1985; 26:173.

49. Ohnuma T, Greenspan EM, Holland JF. Initial clinical study with vindesine: tolerance to weekly I.V. bolus and 24-hour infusion. Cancer Treat Rep 1980; 64:25–30.

50. Gilby ED. A comparison of vindesine administration by bolus injection and by 24-hour infusion. Cancer Treat Rev 1980; 7 (suppl): 47–51.

51. Yap HY, Blumenschein GR, Bodey GP, Hortobagyi GN, Buzdar AU, DiStefano A. Vindesine in the treatment of refractory breast cancer: improvement in therapeutic index with continuous 5-day infusion. Cancer Treat Rep 1981; 65:775–79.

52. Bodey GP, Yap HY, Blumenschein GR, Savaraj N, Loo TL. Continuous infusion of vindesine in breast carcinoma. Clinical and pharmacology studies. In: Brade W, Nagel GA, Seeber S, eds. Proc International Vinca Alkaloid Symposium — Vindesine, Basel: S. Karger, 1981; 203–11.

53. Hansen PV, Brincker H. Vindesine in the treatment of metastatic breast cancer. Eur J Cancer Clin Oncol 1984; 20: 1221–25.

54. Gralla R, Raphael B, Golbey RB, Young CW. Phase 2 evaluation of vindesine in patients with nonsmall-cell carcinoma of the lung. Cancer Treat Rep 1979; 63:1343–46.

55. Bodey GP, Yap HY, Yap BS, Valdivieso M. Continuous infusion vindesine in solid tumors. Cancer Treat Rev 1980; 7 (suppl):39–45.

56. Bodey GP, Valdivieso M, Bedikian AY, Yap BS, Freireich EJ. Vindesine in the therapy of solid tumors. In: Proc International Vinca Alkaloid Symposium — Vindesine. 1981; 84–91.

57. Dirks HP, Drings P, Manke HG, Vollhaber HH. Continuous vindesine infusion therapy in cases of advanced nonsmall-cell bronchogenic carcinoma. In: Proc International Vinca Alkaloid Symposium — Vindesine. 1981; 344–49.

58. Magill GB, Sordillo P, Gralla R, Golbey RB. Phase 2 trials of DVA, AMSA and DCNU as single agents in adult sarcomas. Proc Am Soc Clin Oncol 1980; 21:362.

59. Popkin JD, Bromer RH, Vaughan CW, et al. Continuous vindesine infusion in advanced head and neck cancer. Am J Clin Oncol 1983; 6:301–04.

60. Mayol XF, Beltran J, Rubio-Bazan R, Rifa J, Rosell Costa R, Lopez JJ. Multicenter phase 2 trial with 5-day continuous infusion of vindesine in metastatic malignant melanoma. Cancer Treat Rep 1984; 68:1199–1200.

61. Wagstaff J, Anderson HA, Shiu W, Thatcher N. Phase 2 study of vindesine infusion in visceral metastatic malignant melanoma. Cancer Treat Rep 1983; 67:839–40.

62. Bayssas M, Gonreia J, Ribaud P, et al. Phase 2 trial with vindesine for regression induction in patients with leukemias and hematosarcomas. Cancer Chemother Pharmacol 1979; 2:247–55.

References—Chapter 14

1. Jackson DV Jr, Bender RA. The clinical pharmacology of the vinca alkaloids, epipodophyllotoxins, and maytansine. In: Pinedo, HM, ed. Clinical pharmacology of anti-neoplastic drugs. New York: Elsevier/North Holland Biomedical Press, 1978; 277–94.

2. Jackson DV Jr, Castle MC, Poplack DG, Bender RA. Pharmacokinetics of vincristine in the cerebrospinal fluid of subhuman primates. Cancer Res 1980; 40:722–24.

3. Jackson DV Jr, Sethi VS, Spurr CL, McWhorter JM. Pharmacokinetics of vincristine in the cerebrospinal fluid of humans. Cancer Res 1981; 41:1466–68.

4. Jackson DV Jr, Castle MC, Bender RA. Biliary excretion of [³H]-vincristine in man. Clin Pharmacol Ther 1978; 24:101–07.

5. Barringer M, Sterchi JM, Jackson DV Jr, Meredith J. Chronic biliary sampling via a subcutaneous system: a canine model. Lab Anim Sci 1982; 32:283–85.

6. Jackson DV Jr, Barringer ML, Sterchi JM, Rosenbaum DL, Sethi VS, Spurr CL. Prolonged biliary excretion of vincristine following intravenous injection. Clin Res 1982; 30:419A.

7. Jackson DV, Bender RA: Cytotoxic thresholds of vincristine in a murine and human leukemia cell line in vitro. Cancer Res 1979; 39:4346–49.

8. Jackson DV, Sethi VS, Spurr CL, et al. Pharmacokinetics of vincristine infusion. Cancer Treat Rep 1981; 65:1043–48.

9. Ferreira PPC. Vincristine infusion in advanced cancer. Proc Am Soc Clin Oncol 1976; 17:309.

10. Weber W, Nagel GA, Nagel-Studer E, Albrecht R. Vincristine infusion: A phase 1 study. Cancer Chemother Pharmacol 1979; 3:49–55.

11. Jackson DV, Sethi VS, Spurr CL, et al. Intravenous vincristine infusion: phase 1 trial. Cancer 1981; 48:2559–64.

12. Sethi VS, Burton SS, Jackson DV Jr. A sensitive radioimmunoassay for vincristine and vinblastine. Cancer Chemother Pharmacol 1980; 4:183–87.

13. Jackson DV Jr, Chauvenet AR, Callahan RD, Atkins JN, Trahey TF, Spurr CL. Phase 2 trial of vincristine infusion in acute leukemia. Cancer Chemother Pharmacol 1985; 14:26–29.

14. Jackson DV Jr, Spurr CL, Muss HB, et al. Vincristine infusion in refractory leukemia. Clin Res 1983; 31:409A.

15. Jackson DV Jr, Paschold EH, Spurr CL, et al. Treatment of advanced non-Hodgkin's lymphoma with vincristine infusion. Cancer 1984; 53:2601–06.

16. Hopkins JO, Jackson DV Jr, White DR, et al. Vincristine by continuous infusion in refractory breast cancer: a phase 2 study. Am J Clin Oncol 1983; 6:529–32.

17. Jackson DV, Hire EA, Rardin DA, Pope EK, Spurr CL. Phase 2 study of vincristine infusion in refractory small-cell carcinoma of the lung. Am J Clin Oncol (in press).

18. Jackson D, Spurr C, Richards F, et al. Vincristine infusion in refractory multiple myeloma. Proc Am Soc Clin Oncol 1985; 4:216.

19. Jobson V, Jackson D, Homesley H, et al. Treatment of recurrent gynecologic malignancies with prolonged intravenous vincristine (VCR) infusion. Proc Am Soc Clin Oncol 1983; 2:149.

20. Craig J, Jackson D, Powell B, et al. Continuous infusion vincristine (V) as a component of initial chemotherapy for stage 3-4 diffuse histiocytic lymphoma (DHL). Proc Am Assoc Cancer Res 1985; 26:182.

21. Jackson DV Jr, Muss HB, Richards F II et al. CCNU in combination chemotherapy for advanced histologically unfavorable non-Hodgkin's lymphoma. Cancer Chemother Pharmacol 1983; 11:191–95.

22. Jackson DV Jr, Richards F II, Spurr CL, et al. Hepatic intra-arterial infusion of vincristine. Cancer Chemother Pharmacol 1984; 13:120–22.

23. Jackson DV Jr, Wu WC, Spurr CL. Treatment of vincristine-induced ileus with sincalide, a cholecystokinin analog. Cancer Chemother Pharmacol 1982; 8:83–85.

24. Costa G, Hreshchyshyn MM, Holland JF. Initial clinical studies with vincristine. Cancer Chemother Rep 1962; 24:39–44.

25. Carbone PP, Bono V, Frei E III, Brindley CO. Clinical studies with vincristine. Blood 1963; 21:640–47.

26. Smart CR, Ottoman RE, Rochlin DB, Hornes J, Silva AR, Goepfert H. Clinical experience with vincristine (NSC-67574) in tumors of the central nervous system and other malignant diseases. Cancer Chemother Rep 1968; 52:733–41.

27. Holland JF, Scharlav C, Gailane S, et al. Vincristine treatment of advanced cancer: a cooperative study of 392 cases. Cancer Res 1973; 33:1258–64.

28. Bachmann P, Philip T, Biron P, et al. Perfusion intraveineuse continue de vincristine a forte dose. Lyon Medical 1983; 249:153–58.

29. Bodey GP, Yap HY, Blumenschein GR, Hortobagyi GN, Buzdar AV. A randomized comparative

study of vinblastine, vindesine and vincristine in patients with refractory metastatic breast cancer. Drugs Exptl Clin Res 1982; 8:559–63.

30. Martin J, Compston N. Vincristine sulphate in the treatment of lymphoma and leukemia. Lancet 1963; 2:1080–83.

31. Whitelaur DM, Cowan DH, Cassidy FR, Patterson TA. Clinical experience with vincristine. Cancer Chemother Rep 1963; 30:13–20.

32. Bohannon RA, Miller DG, Diamond HD. Vincristine in the treatment of lymphomas and leukemias. Cancer Res 1963; 23:613–21.

33. Schrek R. Cytotoxicity of vincristine to normal and leukemic cells. Amer J Clin Path 1974; 62:1–7.

34. Hreshchyshyn MM. Vincristine treatment of patients with carcinoma of the uterine cervix. Proc Am Assoc Cancer Res 1963; 4:29.

35. Reitemeier RJ, Moertel CG, Blackburn CM. Vincristine (NSC-67574) therapy of adult patients with solid tumors. Cancer Chemother Rep 1964; 34:21–23.

36. Korbitz BC, Davis HL Jr, Ramirez G, Ansfield FJ. Low doses of vincristine (NSC-67574) for malignant disease. Cancer Chemother Rep 1969; 53:249–54.

37. Rosenthal SM and Kaufman S. Vincristine neurotoxicity. Ann Intern Med 1974; 30:733–37.

38. Weiss HD, Walker MD, Wiernik PH. Neurotoxicity of commonly used antineoplastic agents. N Engl J Med 1974; 291:75–81.

39. Kaplan RS, Wiernik PH. Neurotoxicity of antineoplastic drugs. Sem Oncol 1982; 9:103–30.

40. Jackson DV Jr, Nichols AP, Bender RA. Interaction of albumin and vincristine with a human lymphoblastic leukemia cell line in vitro. Cancer Biochem Biophys 1980; 4:133–36.

41. Cruz J, Paschold E, Sterchi M, et al. Evaluation of a totally implantable system for venous access. Proc Am Soc Clin Oncol 1984; 3:101.

42. Jackson DV Jr, Barringer ML, Rosenbaum DL, et al. Continuous intravenous infusion of vinca alkaloid using a subcutaneously implanted pump in a canine model. Cancer Chemother Pharmacol 1983; 10:217–20.

43. Jackson DV, Sterchi JM, Morris DS, et al. Continuous intravenous infusion of vinca alkaloid using a subcutaneously implanted pump. Clin Res 1984; 32:417A.

44. Jackson DV Jr, Rosenbaum DL, Carlisle LH, Long TR, Wells HB, Spurr CL. Glutamic acid modification of vincristine toxicity. Cancer Biochem Biophys 1984; 7:245–52.

45. Jackson D Jr, Long T, Rosenbaum D, et al. Folinic acid modification of vincristine-induced toxicity. Proc Am Assoc Cancer Res 1983; 24:276.

46. Jackson D, Long T, Rich C, et al. Pyridoxine modification of vincristine toxicity. Proc Am Assoc Cancer Res 1984; 25:313.

47. Jackson DV, Long TR, Sethi VS, et al. Cholestyramine enhancement of vincristine excretion. Clin Res 1984; 32:417A.

48. Jackson DV Jr, Pope EK, Case LD, et al. Improved tolerance of vincristine by glutamic acid. J Neuro Oncol 1984; 2:219–22.

49. Jackson DV, Case LD, White DR, et al. Preliminary clinical trial of pyridoxine to reduce vincristine neurotoxicity. Clin Res 1984; 32:854A.

References—Chapter 15

1. Chien M, Grollman AP, Horwitz SB. Bleomycin-DNA interaction: fluorescence and proton magnetic resonance studies. Biochemistry 1977; 16:3641.

2. Dubrowiak JC, Greenaway FT, Sanbillo FS, et al. The iron complexes of bleomycin and tallysomycin. Biochem Biophys Res Commun 1979; 91:721.

3. Twentyman PR. Bleomycin's mode of action with particular reference to the cell cycle. Pharmacol Ther 1983; 23:417–41.

4. Drewinko B, Novak JK, Barranco SC. The response of human lymphoma cells in vitro to bleomycin and 1,3-bis(2-chloroethyl)-1-nitrosourea. Cancer Res 1972; 32:1206–08.

5. Barranco SC, Novak JK, Humphrey RM. Response of mammalian cells following treatment with bleomycin and 1,3-bis(2-chloroethyl)-1-nitrosourea during plateau phase. Cancer Res 1973; 33:691–94.

6. Barranco SC, Luce JK, Romsdahl MM, et al. Bleomycin as a possible synchronizing agent for human tumor cells in vivo. Cancer Res 1973; 33:882–87.

7. Kus MT and Hsu TC. Bleomycin causes release of nucleosomes from chromatin and chromosomes. Nature 1979; 271:83.

8. Umezawa H, Takeuchi T, Hori S, Sawa T, Ishizuka M. Studies on the mechanism of antitumor effect of bleomycin on squamous cell carcinoma. J Antibiot 1972; 25:409–20.

9. Crooke ST, Comis RL, Einhorn LH, et al. Effects of variations in renal function on the clinical pharmacology of bleomycin administered as an I.V. bolus. Cancer Treat Rep 1977; 61:1631–36.

10. Crooke ST, et al. Bleomycin serum pharmacokinetics as determined by radioimmunoassay and a microbiologic assay in a patient with compromised renal function. Cancer 1977; 39:1430–34.

11. Boughton A, Strong JE, Holoye PY, Bedrossian CWM. Clinical pharmacology of bleomycin folowing intravenous infusion as determined by radioimmunoassay. Cancer 1977; 40:2772–78.

12. Comis RL. Bleomycin pulmonary toxicity. In: Carter S, Crooke ST, Umezawa H, eds. Bleomycin: current status and new developments. New York: Academic Press, 1978; 279–91.

13. Peng YM, Alberts DS, Chen HSG, et al. Antitumor and plasma kinetics of bleomycin by continuous and intermittent administration. Br J Cancer 1980; 41:644–47.

14. Sikic BI, Collins JM, Mimnaugh EG, et al. Improved therapeutic index of bleomycin when administered by continuous infusion in mice. Cancer Treat Rep 1978; 62:2011–17.

15. Osieka R, Glatte P, Schmidt CG. Continuous infusion versus intermittent bolus injection of bleomycin in a human embryonal testicular cancer xenograft. Cancer Treat Rep 1984; 68:799–801.

16. Suzuki Y, Urano M, Ando K, et al. Repair of potentially lethal damage after single injection or continuous infusion of bleomycin. Gan 1978; 69:195–99.

17. Twentyman PR. Dose fractionation does not prevent repair of potentially lethal damage induced by bleomycin in vivo. Cancer Treat Rep 1976; 60:259–60.

18. Dorr RT, Fritz WL. Drug data sheets: bleomycin sulfate. In: Dorr RT, Fritz WL, eds. Cancer chemotherapy handbook. New York: Elsevier, 1980; 274–83.

19. Benvenuto JA, Anderson RW, Kerkof K, Smith RG, Loo TL. Stability and compatibility of antitumor agents in glass and plastic containers. Am J Hosp Pharm 1981; 38:1914–18.

20. Vogelzang NJ. Continuous infusion chemotherapy: a critical review. J Clin Oncol 1984; 2:1289–1304.

21. Carlson CW, and Sikic BI: Continuous infusion or bolus injection in cancer chemotherapy. Ann Intern Med 1983; 99:823–33.

22. Samuels ML, Johnson DE, Holoye PY. Continuous intravenous bleomycin (NSC-125066) therapy with vinblastine (NSC-49842) in stage 3 testicular neoplasia. Cancer Chemother Rep 1975; 59:563–70.

23. Samuels ML, Ianzotti VJ, Holoye PY, Howe CD. Stage 3 testicular cancer: complete response by substage to Velban plus continuous bleomycin infusion (VB-3). Proc Am Assoc Cancer Res 1977; 18:146.

24. Krakoff IH, Cvitkovic E, Currie V, et al. Clinical pharmacology and therapeutic studies of bleomycin given by continuous infusion. Cancer 1977; 40:2027–37.

25. Vugrin D, Herr HW, Whitmore WF, Sogani PC, Golbey RB. VAB-6 combination chemotherapy in disseminated cancer of the testis. Ann Intern Med 1981; 95:59–61.

26. Williams S., Einhorn L, Greco A, Birch R, and Irwin L. Disseminated germ cell tumors: a comparison of cisplatin plus bleomycin plus either vinblastine (PVB) or VP-16 (BEP). Proc Am Soc Clin Oncol 1985; 4:100 (abstract C-390).

27. Randolph VL, Vallejo A. Spiro RH, et al. Combination therapy of advanced head and neck cancer. Cancer 1978; 41:460–67.

28. Hong WK, Shapshay SM, Bhutani R, et al. Induction chemotherapy in advanced squamous head and neck carcinoma with high-dose cis-platinum and bleomycin infusion. Cancer 1979; 44:19–25.

29. Glick JH, Marcial V, Richter M, Velez-Garcia E. The adjuvant treatment of inoperable stage 3 and

4 epidermoid carcinoma of the head and neck with platinum and bleomycin infusions prior to definitive radiotherapy: an RTOG pilot study. Cancer 1980; 46:1919–24.

30. Cooper KR, and Hong WK. Prospective study of pulmonary toxicity of continuously infused bleomycin. Cancer Treat Rep 1981; 65:419–25.

31. Baker LH, Opipari MI, Wilson H, Bottomley R, Coltman CA Jr. Mitomycin-C, vincristine, and bleomycin therapy for advanced cervical cancer. Obstet Gynecol 1978; 52:146–50.

32. Yagoda A, Mukherji B, Young B, et al. Bleomycin, an antitumor antibiotic: clinical experience in 274 patients. Ann Intern Med 1972; 77:861–70.

33. Schein PS, DeVita VT Jr, Hubbard S, et al. Bleomycin, Adriamycin, cyclophosphamide, vincristine, and prednisone (BACOP) combination chemotherapy in the treatment of advanced diffuse histiocytic lymphoma. Ann Intern Med 1976; 85:417–22.

34. Skarin AT, Rosenthal DS, Moloney WC, Frei E. Combination chemotherapy of advanced non-Hodgkin's lymphoma with bleomycin, Adriamycin, cyclophosphamide, vincristine, and prednisone (BACOP). Blood 1977; 49:759–70.

35. Ginsberg SJ, Crooke ST, Bloomfield CD, et al. Cyclophosphamide, doxorubicin, vincristine, and low-dose continuous infusion bleomycin in non-Hodgkin's lymphoma: Cancer and Leukemia Group B study #7804. Cancer 1982; 49:1346–52.

36. Ginsberg S, Anderson J, Bloomfield L, et al. Therapy of advanced, intermediate grade lymphoma with cyclophosphamide, Adriamycin, vincristine and prednisone with or without bleomycin (CAVPB vs CAVP) followed by high-dose methotrexate or standard dose methotrexate (HMTX vs. LMTX): a randomized trial. Proc Am Soc Clin Oncol 1985; 4:202 (abstract C-786).

37. Hollister D, Silver RT, Gordon B, Coleman M. Continuous infusion vincristine and bleomycin with high-dose methotrexate for resistent non-Hodgkin's lymphoma. Cancer 1982; 50:1690–94.

38. Kolaric K, Marici Z, Dujmovic I. Bleomycin infusions combined with radiotherapy in the treatment of inoperable esophageal cancer. Tumori 1980; 66:615–21.

39. Nathanson L, Wittenberg BK. Pilot study of vinblastine and bleomycin combinations in the treatment of metastatic melanoma. Cancer Treat Rep 1980; 64:133–37.

40. Mabel JA, Merker PC, Sturgeon ML, Wodinsky I, Geran RI. Combination chemotherapy against B16 melanoma: bleomycin/vinblastine, bleomycin/cis-diamminedichloroplatinum, 5-fluorouracil/BCNU, and 5-fluorouracil/methyl-CCNU. Cancer 1978; 42:1711–19.

41. Nathanson L, Kaufman SD, Carey RW. Vinblastine, infusion bleomycin, and cis-dichlorodiammine-platinum chemotherapy in metastatic melanoma. Cancer 1981; 48:1290–94.

42. Anon. Vinblastine, bleomycin, and cis-platinum for the treatment of metastatic malignant melanoma. J Clin Oncol 1984; 2:131–34.

43. Luikart SD, Kennealey GT, Kirkwood JM. Randomized phase 3 trial of vinblastine, bleomycin, and cis-dichlorodiammine-platinum versus dacarbazine in malignant melanoma. J Clin Oncol 1984; 2:164–68.

44. Morantz RA. Intraneoplastic chemotherapy in the treatment of primary brain tumors. Presented at "A professional briefing-totally implantable pumps: intraspinal analgesia, CNS malignancies, Alzheimer's disease and other neurotransmitter disorders." Wild Dunes Resort, Isle of Palms, SC, Sep 19, 1984.

References—Chapter 16

1. Issell BF, Tihon C, Curry ME. Etoposide (VP16-213) and teniposide (VM26) comparative in vitro activities in human tumors. Cancer Chemother Pharmacol 1982; 7:113–15.

2. Loike JD, Horwitz SB. Effect of VP16-213 on the intracellular degradation of DNA in Hela cells. Biochem 1976; 15:5443–48.

3. Roberts D, Hilliard S, Peck C. Sedimentation of DNA from L1210 cells after treatment with 4'-

demethylepipodophyllotoxin -9-(4, 6-0-2-thenylidine-β-D-glucopyranoside) or 1-β-D-arabinofurano-sylcytosine or both drugs. Cancer Res 1980; 40:4225–31.

4. Wozniak AJ, Ross WE. DNA damage as a basis for 4′-demethylepipodophyllotoxin -9-(4, 6-0-ethylidine-β-D-glucopyranoside) (etoposide) cytotoxicity. Cancer Res 1983; 43:120–24.

5. Kalwinsky DK, Look AT, Ducore J, et al. Effects of the epipodophyllotoxin VP16-213 on cell cycle traverse, DNA synthesis, and DNA strand size in cultures of human leukemic lymphoblasts. Cancer Res 1983; 43:1592–97.

6. Long BH, Musial ST, Brattain MG. Comparison of cytotoxicity and DNA breakage activity of congeners of podophyllotoxin including VP16-213 and VM26: a quantitative structure activity relationship. Biochem 1984; 23:1182–88.

7. Long BH, Brattain MG. The activity of etoposide (VP16-213) and teniposide (VM-26) against human lung tumor cells in vitro: cytotoxicity and DNA breakage. In: Issell BF, Muggia FM, Carter SK, eds. Etoposide (VP-16): current status and new developments. New York: Academic Press, 1984; 63–86.

8. Chen GL, Yang L, Rowe TC, et al. Nonintercalative antitumor drugs interfere with the breakage-reunion reaction of mammalian DNA topoisomerase II. J Biol Chem 1984; 259:13560–66.

9. Minocha A, Long BH. Inhibition of the DNA catenation activity of type II topoisomerase by VP16-213 and VM-26. Biochem Biophys Res Commun 1984; 122:165–70.

10. Misra NC, Roberts D. Inhibition by 4′-demethyl-epipodophyllotoxin 9-(4,6-0-2-thenylidine-β-D-glucopyranoside) of human lymphoblast cultures in G_2 phase of the cell cycle. Cancer Res 1975; 35:99–105.

11. Krishan A, Paika K, Frei E III. Cytofluorometic studies on the action of podophyllotixin and epipodophyllotoxins (VM-26, VP16-213) on the cell cycle traverse of human lymphoblasts. J Cell Biol 1975; 66:521–30.

12. Creaven PJ, Allen LM. EPEG, a new antineoplastic epipodophyllotoxin. Clin Pharmacol Ther 1975; 18:221–26.

13. Allen LM, Creaven PJ. Comparison of the human pharmacokinetics of VM-26 and VP-16, two antineoplastic epipodophyllotixin glucopyranoside derivatives. Europ J Cancer 1975; 11:697–707.

14. Strife RJ, Jardine I. Analysis of the anticancer drugs VP16-213 and VM-26 and their metabolites by high-performance liquid chromatography. J Chromatogr 1980; 182:221.

15. Lawrie S, Dodson M, Arnold A, et al. Pharmacokinetics and bioavailability of VP16-213 in man. Cancer Chemother Pharmacol 1982; 7:236–37.

16. Farina P, Marzillo G, D'Incalci M. High-pressure liquid chromatography determination of 4′-demethyl-epipodophyllotoxin-9-(4,6-0-ethylidine-β-D-glucopyranoside) (VP-16-213) in human plasma. J Chromatogr 1981; 222:141–45.

17. Scalzo AJ, Comis R, Fitzpatrick A, et al. VP-16 pharmacokinetics in adults with cancer as determined by a new high-pressure liquid chromatography (HPLC) assay. Proc Am Soc Clin Oncol 1982; 1:129.

18. Snodgrass W, Walker L. Heideman R, et al. Kinetics of VP-16 epipodophyllotoxin in children with cancer. Proc Am Assoc Cancer Res, Am Soc Clin Oncol 1980; 21:333.

19. Evans WE, Sinkule JA, Crom WR, et al. Pharmacokinetics of teniposide (VM-26) and etoposide (VP16-213) in children with cancer. Cancer Chemother Pharmacol 1982; 7:147–50.

20. Aherne GW, Marks V. A radioimmunoassay for VP16-213 in plasma. Cancer Chemother Pharmacol 1982; 7:117–21.

21. Ho DHW, Kanellopoulos KA, Yap HY, et al. Clinical pharmacology of etoposide by radioimmunoassay. Pro Am Assoc Cancer Res 1983; 24:131.

22. Evans WE, Sinkule JA, Horvath A, et al. Clinical pharmacology of VM-26 (NSC 122819) and VP-16 (NSC 141540) in children with cancer. Proc Am Assoc Cancer Res, Am Soc Clin Oncol 1981; 22:174.

23. D'Incalci M, Farina P, Sessa C. Pharmacokinetics of VP16-213 given by different methods. Cancer Chemother Pharmacol 1982; 7:141–45.

24. Allen LM, Marks C, Creavan PJ. 4′-demethyl-epipodophyllic acid -9-(4,6-0-ethylidine- β-D-glucopyranoside), the major urinary metabolite of VP16-213 in man. Proc Am Assoc Cancer Res, Am Soc Clin Oncol 1976; 17:16.

25. Sinkule JA, Evans WE. High-pressure liquid chromatographic analysis of the semisynthetic epipodophyllotoxins teniposide and etoposide using electrochemical detection. J Pharm Sci 1984; 73:164–68.

26. Dow LW, Sinkule JA, Look AT, et al. Comparative cytotoxic and cytokinetic effects of the epipodophyllotoxins 4'-demethylepipodophyllotixin-9-(4,6-0-2-ethylidene-β-D-glucopyranoside) and 4' - demethylepipodophyllotoxin-9-(4,6-0-2-thenylidene-β-D-glucopyranoside) and their metabolites on human leukemic lymphoblasts. Cancer Res 1983; 43:5699–5706.

27. Pfeffer M, Scalzo AJ, Nardella PA, et al. The absolute oral bioavailability and pharmacokinetics of etoposide. In: Issell BF, Muggia FM, Carter SK, eds. Etoposide (VP-16): current status and new developments. New York: Academic Press, 1984; 127–140.

28. Hande KR, McKay CM, Wedlund PJ, et al. Clinical pharmacology of high dose VP16-213. Proc Am Assoc Cancer Res 1982; 23:131.

29. Creavan PJ, Allen LM. PTG, a new antineoplastic epipodophyllotoxin. Clin Pharmacol Ther 1975; 18:227.

30. Sinkule JA, Stewart CF, Crom WR, et al. Teniposide (VM26) disposition in children with leukemia. Cancer Res 1984; 44:1235–37.

31. Sessa C, D'Incalci M, Farina P, et al. Pharmacokinetics of VM26 after 60 minutes or 24 hours continuous infusion. Proc Am Assoc Cancer Res 1982; 23:128.

32. Rossi C, Zucchetti M, Sessa C, et al. Pharmacokinetic study of VM26 given as a prolonged IV infusion to ovarian cancer patients. Cancer Chemother Pharmacol 1984; 13:211–14.

33. Loike JD, Brewer CF, Sternlicht H, et al. Structure-activity study of the inhibition of microtubule assembly in vitro by podophyllotixin and its congeners. Cancer Res 1978; 38:2668–93.

34. Dombernowsky P, Nissen NI. Schedule dependency of the antileukemic activity of the podophyllotoxin-derivative VP16-213 (NSC-141540) in L1210 leukemia. Acta Path Microbiol Scan 1973; 81(A):715–24.

35. Venditti JM. Treatment schedule dependency of experimentally active antileukemic (L1210) drugs. Cancer Chemother Rep 1971; 2:35–59.

36. Broggini M, Colombo T, D'Incalci M. Activity and pharmacokinetics of teniposide in Lewis lung carcinoma-bearing mice. Cancer Treat Rep 1983; 67:555–59.

37. Radice PA, Bunn PA, Inde DC. Therapeutic trials with VP16-213 and VM26: active agents in small-cell lung cancer, non-Hodgkin's lymphomas, and other malignancies. Cancer Treat Rep 1979; 63:1231–39.

38. Cavalli F, Sonntag RW, Jungi F. VP16-213 monotherapy for remission induction of small-cell lung cancer: a randomized trial using three dosage schedules. Cancer Treat Rep 1978; 62:473–75.

39. Dorr RT, Fritz WL. Cancer chemotherapy handbook. New York: Elsevier Science, 1980; 420–21.

40. Bristol-Myers Pharmaceutical Research and Development. Pharmaceutical data on file. Syracuse, NY, May 1980.

41. U.S. Department of Health and Human Services, Public Health Service, National Institutes of Health. NCI investigational drugs pharmaceutical data, 1985.

42. Lokich JJ, Corkery J. Phase 1 study of VP16-213 (etoposide) administered as a continuous 5-day infusion. Cancer Treat Rep 1981; 65:887–89.

43. Aisner J, VanEcho DA, Whitacre M, et al. A phase 1 trial of continuous infusion VP16-213 (etoposide). Cancer Chemother Pharmacol 1982; 7:157–60.

44. Schell FC, Yap HY, Hortobagyi GN, et al. Phase 2 study of VP16-213 (etoposide) in refractory metastatic breast carcinoma. Cancer Chemother Pharmacol 1982; 7:223–25.

45. Steward WP, Thatcher N, Edmundson JM, et al. Etoposide infusions for treatment of metastatic lung cancer. Cancer Treat Rep 1984; 68:897–98.

46. Aisner J, Whitacre M, Van Echo DA, et al. Doxorubicin, cyclophosphamide, and etoposide (ACE) by bolus or continuous infusion for small-cell carcinoma of the lung (SCCL). Proc Am Soc Clin Oncol 1983; 2:196.

47. Creaven PJ. The clinical pharmacology of etoposide (VP-16) in adults. In: Issell BF, Muggia FM, Carter SK, eds. Etoposide (VP-16): current status and new developments. New York: Academic Press 1984; 103–115.

48. Evans WE, Sinkule JA, Hutson PR, et al. The clinical pharmacology of etoposide (VP16-213) in children with cancer. In: Issell BF, Muggia FM, Carter SK, eds. Etoposide (VP-16): current status and new developments. New York: Academic Press, 1984; 117–25.

References—Chapter 17

1. Tobias J, and Griffiths CT. Management of ovarian carcinoma. N Engl j Med 1976; 294:877–82.

2. Bedikian Ay, Bodey GP. Phase 1 study of cyclophosphamide (NSC 26271) by 72-hour continuous infusion. Am J Oncol (CCT) 1982; 6:365–68.

3. Solidoro A, Otero J, Vellejos C, et al. Intermittent continuous I.V. infusion of high-dose cyclophosphamide for reduction in acute lymphotropic leukemia. Cancer Treat Rep 1981; 65:213–18.

4. Lokich J, and Bothe A Jr. Phase 1 study of continuous infusion cyclophosphamide for protracted durations: a preliminary report. Cancer Drug Deliv 1984; 1(4):329–32.

5. Egorin MJ, Adman SR, Guttierrez PL. Plasma pharmacokinetics and tissue distribution of thiotepa in mice. Cancer Treat Rep 1984; 68(10):1265–68.

6. Kreis W, Budman DR, Vinciguerra V, et al. Phase 1 continuous infusion of triethylenethiophosphamide (thio-tepa) over 48 hrs. Proc AACR 1983; 552:140.

7. Tullis J. Triethylenephophoramide in the treatment of disseminated melanoma. JAMA. 1958; 166 (1):37–41.

8. Alberts DS, Peng Y, Fisher B. Minimal melphelan (LPAM) systemic avalability (SA): a potential cause for failure of adjuvant breast cancer therapy trials. Proc ASCO 1984; C-149:38.

9. Cumberlin R, DeMoss E, Lassus M, Friedman M. Isolation perfusion for malignant melanoma of the extremity: a review. J Clin Oncol 1985; 3(7):1022–31.

10. Buice RN, Niell HB, Sidhu P. Pharmacokinetics of mitomycin-C in non-oat cell carcinoma of the lung. Cancer Chemother Pharmacol 1984; 13:1–4.

11. Miller DC, Weiss RB, Issell BF. Mitomycin: ten years after approval for marketing. J Clin Oncol 1985; 3(2):276–86.

12. Lokich J, Perri J, Fine N, et al. Mitomycin-C: Phase 1 study of constant infusion ambulatory treatment schedule. Am J Clin Oncol: Cancer Clin Trials 1982; 5:443–47.

13. Loo TL, Luck JK, Sullivan MP, et al. Clinical pharmacological observations on 6-mercaptopurine and 6-methylthiopurine ribonucleoside. Clin Pharmacol Ther 1968; 9:180–94.

14. Zimm S, Ettinger LJ, Holcenberg JS, et al. Phase 1 and clinical pharmacological study of mercaptopurine administered as a prolonged intravenous infusion. Cancer Res 1985; 45:1869–73.

15. Beckloff GL, Lerner HJ, Frost D, et al. Hydroxurea (NSC-32065) in biologic fluids: dose-concentration relationship. Cancer Chemother Rep 1965; 48:57–58.

16. Ariel IM. Treatment of disseminated cancer by intravenous hydroxyurea and autogenous bone-marrow transplants: experience with 35 patients. J Surg Oncol 1975; 7:331–35.

17. Belt RJ, Haas CD, Kennedy J, et al. Studies of hydroxyurea administered by continuous infusion: toxicity, pharmacokinetics and cell-synchronization. Cancer 1980; 46:455–62.

18. Savlov ED, Hall TC, Oberfield RA. Intra-arterial therapy of melanoma with dimetheyl triazeno imidazole carboxamide (NSC-45388) Cancer 1971; 28 (5):1161–64.

19. Einhorn LH, McBride CM, Luce JK, Caoili E, Gottlieb JA. Intra-arterial infusion therapy with 5-(3,3-dimethyl-l-triazeno) imidazole-4-carboxamide (NSC 45388) for malignant melanoma. Cancer 1973; 32:749–55.

20. Casimir A, Kavanagh J, Liu F, et al. Phase 1 trial of intravenous procarbazine administered as a five-day continuous infusion: correlation with plasma levels of peridoxal phosphate. Proc Am Assoc Cancer Res 1983 (abstr); 24:144.

21. Seibert K, Golub G, Smiledge P, Scott J. Continuous streptozotocin infusion: a phase 1 study. Cancer Treat Rep 1979; 63 (11–12):2035–37.

22. Lokich JJ, Zipoli TE, Sonneborn H, Paul S, Phillips D. Streptozotocin for metastatic malignant melanoma. Amer J Clin Oncol 1985; 8:45–46.

23. Blumenreich MS, Woodcock TM, Richman SP, et al. A phase 1 trial of dactinomycin intravenous infusion in patients with advanced malignancies. Cancer 1985; 56:256–58.

24. Gutterman JU, Rosenblum MG, Rios A, Fritsche HA, Quesada JR. Pharmacokinetic study of partially pure y-interferon in cancer. Cancer Res 1984; 44:4164–71.

25. Miro J Jr., Kalwinsky D, Whisnant J, Weck P, Chesney C, Murphy S. Coagulopathy induced by continuous infusion of high doses of human lymphoblastoid interferon. Cancer Treat Rep 1985; 69(3):315–17.

References—Chapter 18

1. Legha S, Ajani JA, Bodey GP. Phase 1 study of spirogermanium given daily. J Clin Oncol 1983; 1:331–35.

2. Kavanagh JJ, Saul PB, Copeland LJ, Gershenson DM, Krakoff IH. Continuous-infusion spirogermanium for the treatment of refractory carcinoma of the ovary: a phase 2 trial. Cancer Treat Rep 1985; 69:139–40.

3. Woolley PV, Ahlgren JD, Byrne PJ, Priego VM, Schein PS. A phase 1 trial of spirogermanium administered on a continuous infusion schedule. Invest New Drugs 1984; 2:305–309.

4. Pinnamaneni K, Yap HY, Legha SS, Blemenschein GR, Bodey GP. Phase 2 study of spirogermanium in the treatment of metastatic breast cancer. Cancer Treat Rep 1984; 68:1197–98.

5. Warrell RP Jr., Coonley CJ, and Gee TS. Homoharringtonine: an effective new drug for remission induction in refractory nonlymphoblastic leukemia. J Clin Oncol 1985; 3:617–21.

6. Legha SS, Keating M, Picket S, Ajani JA, Ewer M, Bodey GP. Phase 1 clinical investigation of homoharringtonine. Cancer Treat Rep 1984; 68:1085–91.

7. Malamud SC, Ohnuma T, Coffey V, Paciucci PA, Wasserman LR, Holland JF. Phase 1 study of homoharringtonine (HHT) in 10 day schedule: 6 hr infusion daily vs. continuous infusion. Proc Ann Meet Am Assoc Cancer Res 1984; 25:179.

8. Neidhart JA, Young DC, Derocher D, Metz EN. Phase 1 trial of homoharringtonine. Cancer Treat Rep 1983; 67:801–04.

9. Connley CJ, Warrell RP Jr., Young CW. Phase 1 trial of homoharringtonine administered as a 5-day continuous infusion. Cancer Treat Rep 1983; 67:693–96.

10. Whitacre MY, Van Echo DA, Applefeld M, Wiernik PH, Aisner J. Phase I study of homoharringtonine (NSC 141-633). Proc Am Soc Clin Oncol 1983; 2C:129.

11. Smith CR, Mikolajczak KL, Powell RG. Harringtonine and related cephalotaxine esters. Med Chem 1980; 16:391–416.

12. Smith CR, Powell RG, Mikolajczak KL. The genus cephalotaxus: source of homoharringtonine and related anticancer alkaloids. Cancer Treat Rep 1976; 60:1157–70.

13. Lee EJ, Van Echo DA, Egorin MJ, Nayar B, Schulman P, Schiffer CA. A phase 1-2 study of continuous infusion diaziquone (AZQ) for refractory adult leukemia. Proc Am Soc Clin Oncol 1984; 3:195.

14. Lee EJ, Van Echo DA, Egorin MJ, Nayar MSB, Shulman P, Schiffer CA. Diaziquone given as continuous infusion is an active agent for relapsed adult acute nonlymphocytic leukemia. Blood 1985 (in press).

15. Neidhart JA, Derocher D, Grever MR, Kraut EH, Malspeis L. Phase 1 trial of teroxirone. Cancer Treat Rep 1984; 68:1115–19.

16. Ames MM, Kovach JS, Rubin J. Pharmacological characterization of teroxirone, a triepoxide antitumor agent, in rats, rabbits, and humans. Cancer Res 1984; 44:4151–56.

17. Atassi G, Dumont P, Fisher U, Ziedler M, Budnowski M. Preclinical evaluation of the antitumor activity of new epoxyde derivatives. Cancer Treat Rev, 1984; 11:99–110.

18. Rozencwig M, Crespeigne N, Nicaise C et al. Phase 1 trial of 1,2,4-triglycidylurazol (TGU, NSC 332488) with a daily × 5 schedule. Proc Ann Meet Am Assoc Cancer Res 1984; 25:201

19. Budnowski M. Preparation and properties of the diastereoisomeric 1,3,5-triglycidyl-5-triazinetriones. Agnew Chem 1968; 7:827–28.

20. Ames MM, Gretsch SK, DNA-DNA and DNA-protein crosslink formation by the experimental antitumor agent teroxirone (NSC-296934) in murine L1210 leukemia and human A204 rhabdomyosarcoma cell lines. Proc Ann Meet Am Assoc Cancer Res 1985; 26:211.

21. Attasi G, Spreafico F, Dumont P et al. Antitumor effect in mice of a new triepoxide derivative: alpha-1,3,5-triglycidyl-5-triazine-trione (NSC 296934). Eur J Cancer 1980; 16:1561–67.

22. Shoemaker DD, O'Dwyer PJ, Marsoni S, Plowman J, Davignon JP Davis RD. Spiromustine: a new agent entering clinical trials. Invest New Drugs 1983; 1:303–08.

23. Plowman J, Lakings DB, Owens ES, Adamson RH. Initial studies on the penetration of spirohydantoin mustard into the cerebrospinal fluid of dogs. Pharmacol 1977; 15:359–66.

24. Hilton J, Sessions RH, Walker MD. Cross-linking of DNA in rat brain tumor and bone marrow by spirohydantoin mustard (SHM). Proc Am Assoc Cancer Res 1977;18:112.

25. Kobayashi T, Blasberg RG, Patlak CS, Fenstermacher JD. Spirohydantoin mustard (NSC-172112) penetration of brain and systemic organs. Proc Am Assoc Cancer Res 1979; 20:104.

26. Flora KP, Cradock JC, Kelley JA. The hydrolysis of spirohydantoin mustard. J Pharmacol Sci 1982; 71:1206–11.

27. Sigman LM, Van Echo DA, Egorin MJ et al. Phase 1 trial of spiromustine (NSC 172112). Proc Ann Meet Am Soc Clin Oncol 1984; 3:31.

28. Simon S, McSherry JW, Krakoff IH, Stewart JA. Spiromustine (spirohydantoin mustard; NSC 172112) a phase 1 trial. Proc Ann Meet Am Soc Clin Oncol 1984; 3:29.

29. Brown T, Ettinger D, Rice A, Poremski C, Donehower R. A phase 1 clinical trial of spirohydantoin mustard (SHM). Proc Ann Meet Am Soc Clin Oncol 1984; 3:33.

30. Simon S, McSherry JW, Krakoff IH, Stewart JA. Spiromustine (spirohydantoin mustard; NSC 172112): a phase 1 trial. Proc Ann Meet Am Soc Clin Oncol 1984; 3:29.

31. Reuben RC, Rifkind RA, Marks PA. Murine erythroleukemia cells: induction of erythroid differentiation with hexamethylene bisacetamide. Fed Proc 1977; 36:886.

32. Reuben RC, Wife RL, Breslow R, Rifkind RA, Marks PA. Identification of a new group of potent inducers of differentiation in murine erythroleukemia cells. Proc Am Assoc Cancer Res 1976; 17:76.

33. Reuben RC, Wife RL, Breslow R, Rifkind RA, Marks PA. A new group of potent inducers of differentiation in murine erythroleukemia cells. Proc Natl Acad Sci USA 1976; 73:862–66.

34. Fibach E, Reuben RC, Rifkind RA, Marks PA. Effect of hexamethylene bisacetamide on the commitment to differentiation of murine erythroleukemia cells. Cancer Res 1977; 37:440–44.

35. Rabson AS, Stern R, Tralka TS, Costa J, Wilczek J. Hexamethylene bisacetamide induces morphologic changes and increased synthesis of procollagen in cell line from glioblastoma multiforme. Proc Natl Acad Sci USA 1977; 74:5060–64.

36. Palfrey C, Kimhi Y, Littauer UZ, Reuben RC, Marks PA. Induction of differentiation in mouse neuroblastoma cells by hexamethylene bisacetamide. Biochem Biophys Res Commun 1977; 76:937–42.

37. Reuben RC. Studies on the mechanism of action of hexamethylene bisacetamide, a potent inducer of erythroleukemia differentiation. Biochim Biophys Acta 1979; 588:310–21.

38. Paulin D, Perreau J, Jakob H, Jacob F, Yaniv M. Tropomyosin synthesis accompanies formation of actin filaments in embryonal carcinoma cells induced to differentiate by hexamethylene bisacetamide Proc Natl Acad Sci USA 1979; 1891–95.

39. Hughes EH, Schut HA, and Thorgeirsson SS. Effects of hexamethylene bisacetamide on alpha-fetoprotein, albumin, and transferrin production by two rat hepatoma cell lines. In Vitro 1982; 18:157–64.

40. Osborne HB, Bakke AC, Yu J. Effect of dexamethasone on hexamethylene bisacetamide-induced friend cell erythrodifferentiation. Cancer Res 1982; 42:513–18.

41. Kraut EH, Malspeis L, Balcerzak SP, Grever MR. Phase 1 clinical trial of pibenzimol (NSC 322921) Proc Am Soc Clin Oncol 1985; 4:36.

42. Calvert AH, Harland SJ, Newell DR, et al. Early clinical studies with cis-diammine-1,1-cyclobutane dicarboxylate platinum (II). Cancer Chemother Pharmacol 1982; 9:140–47.

43. Koeller JM, Earhart RH, Davis TE, Trump DL, Tormey DC. Phase 1 trial of carboplatin (NSC 241240) by bolus intravenous injection. Proc Am Assoc Cancer Res 1983; 24:643.

44. Lessus M. Ohnuma T, Leyvraz S, Holland JF. A phase 1 study of CBDCA (carboplatin). Proc Am Soc Clin Oncol 1983; 2:C-144.

45. Curt GA, Grygiel JJ, Corden BJ, Ozols RF, Weiss RB, Tell DT, et al. A phase 1 and pharmacokinetic study of diamminecyclobutane-dicarboxylatoplatinum (NSC 241240). Cancer Res 1983; 43:4470–73.

46. Rozencweig M, Nicaise C, Beer M, et al. Phase 1 study of carboplatin given on a five-day intravenous schedule. J Clin Oncol 1983; 1:621–26.

47. Joss RA, Goldhirsch A, Sessa C, Brunner KW, and Cavalli F. A phase 1 trial of cis-diammine-1,1-cyclobutane dicarboxylate platinum II (carboplatin, CBDCA, JM-8) with a single dose every five week-schedule. Invest New Drugs 1984; 2:297–304.

48. Van Echo DA, Egorin MJ, Whitacre MY, Olman EA, Aisner J. Phase 1 clinical and pharmacologic trial of carboplatin daily for five days. Cancer Treat Rep 1984; 68:1103–14.

49. Ohnuma T, Zimet AS, Coffey VA, Holland JF, Greenspan EM. Phase 1 trial of taxol in a 24-hr infusion schedule. Proc Ann Meet Am Assoc Cancer Res 1985; 26:167.

50. O'Connell JP, Kris MG, Gralla RJ, Wertheim MS, Young CM, Sykes, M. Phase 1 trial of taxol given as a three-hour infusion every three weeks. Proc Ann Meet Am Assoc Cancer Res 1985; 26:169.

51. Legha S, Tenney D, Dimery I, Krakoff I. A phase 1 study of taxol (NSC 125973). Proc Ann Meet Am Assoc Cancer Res 1985; 26:173.

52. Longnecker S, Donehower R, Grochow L, et al. Phase 1 and pharmacokinetic study of taxol in patients with advanced cancer. Proc Am Soc Clin Oncol 1983; 4:32.

53. Tutsch KD, Swaminathan S, Alberti D, et al. Phase 1 clinical trial with pharmacokinetic analysis of taxol (NSC 125973) given on a daily × 5 schedule. Proc Am Soc Clin Oncol 1985; 4:40.

54. Harvey J, Priego V, Binder R, Byrne P, Smith F, Woolley P. A phase 1 study of echinomycin (quinomycin A), NSC-526417 administered on an intermittent bolus schedule. Proc Ann Meet Am Soc Clin Oncol 1984; 3:35.

55. Haas C, Baker L, Leichman L, Decker D. Phase 1 evaluation of echinomycin administered on a weekly × 4 schedule. Proc Ann Meet Am Soc Clin Oncol 1984; 3:29.

56. Kuhn J, Von Hoff D, Schick M, et al. Phase 1 trial of echinomycin (NSC 526417). Proc Ann Meet Am Soc Clin Oncol 1984; 3:24.

57. Kuhn JG, Von Hoff DD, Clark GM, et al. Phase 1 evaluation of echinomycin (quinomycin A; NSC 526417). Proc Am Soc Clin Oncol 1983; 2:C-96.

58. Curt GA, Kelley JA, Fine RL, et al. A phase 1 and pharmacokinetic study of diahydroazacytidine (DHAC; NSC-264880). Proc Ann Meet Am Soc Clin Oncol 1984; 3:37.

59. Bjornson G, Stewart JA, McCormack JJ, Mathews LA, Ershler WB, Krakoff IH. Clinical and clinical pharmacologic study of dihydroazacytidine (DHAC). Proc Am Soc Clin Oncol 1983; 2:C-138.

60. McGovren JP, Nelson KG, Lassus M, Cradock JC, Plowman J, Christopher JP. Menogaril: a new anthracycline agent entering clinical trials. Invest New Drugs 1984; 2:359–67.

61. Zimet AS, Ohnuma T, Perlow L, Coffey VA, Holland JF, Goldsmith MA. A phase 1 trial of menogaril (7-CON-O-methylnogarol) in a daily 3 × schedule. Proc Ann Meet Am Assoc Cancer Res 1985; 26:167.

62. Sigman LM, Van Echo DA, Egorin MJ, Whitacre MY, and Aisner J. Menogaril (7-OMEN, NSC 269148) phase 1 study. Proc Ann Meet Am Assoc Cancer Res 1985; 26:170.

63. Long HJ, Powis G, Schutt AJ, Moertel CG, and Kovach JS. Menogaril by 72-hour continuous infusion: a phase 1 study with pharmacokinetics. Proc Am Soc Clin Oncol 1985; 4:28.

64. Dodion P, Sessa C, Gerard B, et al. Phase 1 trial of menogaril with a single-dose schedule. Proc Am Soc Clin Oncol 1986; 4:26.

65. Brown TD, Donehower RC, Grochow LB, Ettinger DS, Rice AP, Waalkes TP. A phase 1 study of menoril in patients with advanced cancer. Proc Am Soc Clin Oncol 1985; 4:32.

66. Durr A, Von Hoff D, Kuhn J, Kisner D. Phase 1 clinical trial of menogaril. Proc Am Soc Clin Oncol 1985; 4:39.

67. Cowan JD, Clark G, Von Hoff DD. Activity of mitoxantrone and bisantrene in a human tumor cloning system. EORTC Monogr Ser 1983; 12:39–46.

68. Dodion P, Bron D, Rozencweig M, et al. Differential sensitivity of normal marrow myeloid progenitor cells to mitoxantrone and bisantrene. EORTC Monogr Ser 1983; 12:29–38.

69. Callahan SK, Coltman CA Jr., Kitten C, Von Hoff DD. Tumor cloning assay: application and potential usefulness in lung cancer management. Cancer Treat Res 1983; 11:51–71.

70. Cowan JD, Von Hoff DD, Clark GM. Comparative cytotoxicity of Adriamycin, mitoxantrone and bisantrene as measured by a human tumor cloning system. Invest New Drugs 1983; 1:139–44.

71. Drewinko B, Yang LY, Barlogie B, Trujillo JM. Comparative cytotoxicity of bisantrene, mitoxantrone, amentantrone, dihydroxyanthracenedione, dihydroxyanthracenedione diacetate, and doxorubicin on human cells in vitro. Cancer Res 1983; 43:2648–53.

72. Yap B-S, Yap H-Y, Blumenschein GR, Bedikian AY, Pocelinko R, Bodey GP. Phase 1 clinical evaluation of 9,10-anthracenedicarboxyladehyde-bis (4,5-dihydro-1H-imidazol-2-YL)-hydrazone dihydrochloride (bisantrene). Cancer Treat Rep 1982; 66:1517–20.

73. Spiegel RJ, Blum RH, Levin M, et al. Phase 1 clinical trial of 9,10-anthracene dicarboxaldehyde (bisantrene) administered in a five-day schedule. Cancer Res 1982; 42:354–58.

74. Alberts DS, Mackel C, Pocelinko R, Salmon SE. Phase 1 clinical investigation of 9,10-anthracenedicarboxaldehyde bis (4,5-dihydro-1 H-imidazol-2-YL) hydrazone dihydrochloride with correlative in vitro human tumor clonogenic assay. Cancer Res 1982; 42:1170–75.

75. Powis G, Kovach JS. Disposition of bisantrene in humans and rabbits: evidence for intravascular deposition of drug as a cause of phlebitis. Cancer Res 1983; 43:925–29.

76. Kvols LK, Powis G, O'Connell MJ, Kovach JS. Phase 1 study of bisantrene (bis) administered at low concentration by 72-hour intravenous infusion. Proc Am Soc Clin Oncol 1983; 2:C-88.

77. Powell RG, Weisleder D, Smith CR. Antitumor alkaloids from cephalotaxus harringtonia: structure and activity. J Pharm Sci 1972; 61:1227–30.

78. Smith CR, Powell RG, Mikolajczak KL. The genus cephalotaxus: source of homoharringtonine and related anticancer alkaloids. Cancer Treat Rep 1976; 60:1157–70.

79. Smith CR, Mikolajczak KL, Powell RG. Harringtonine and related cephalotaxine esters. Med Chem 1980; 16:391–416.

80. Leukemia Coordination Group. Homoharringtonine and harringtonine in acute nonlymphocytic leukemia: clinical observations of 40 cases. Zhonghua Neike Zazhi 1978; 17:162–64.

81. Hematology Research Division. High remission induction (traditional sino-western hoap) regimen for acute nonlymphocytic leukemia. Chin Med J 1980; 93:565–68.

82. Douros J, Suffness M. New natural products under development at the national cancer institute. Recent Cancer Res 1981; 76:153–75.

83. Suffness M, Douros JD. Discovery of antitumor agents from natural sources. Trends Pharmacol Sci 1981; 2:307–310.

84. Clinical Brochure. Homoharringtonine (NSC-141633). Bethesda: Investigational Drug Branch, Cancer Therapy Evaluation Program, Division of Cancer Treatment, National Cancer Institute, Aug. 1982.

85. Legha SS, Keating M, Picket S, Ajani JA, Ewer M, Bodey GP. Phase 1 clinical investigation of homoharringtonine. Cancer Treat Rep 1984; 68:1085–91.

86. Malamud SC, Ohnuma T, Coffey V, Paciucci PA, Wasserman LR, Holland JF. Phase 1 study of homoharringtonine (HHT) in 10 day schedule: 6 hr infusion daily vs. continuous infusion. Proc Ann Meet Am Assoc Cancer Res 1984; 25:179.

87. Neidhart JA, Young DC, Derocher D, Metz EN. Phase 1 trial of homoharringtonine. Cancer Treat Rep 1983; 67:801–04.

88. Coonley Cj, Warrell RP Jr., Young CW. Phase 1 trial of homoharringtonine administered as a 5-day continuous infusion. Cancer Treat Rep 1983; 67:693–96.

89. Warrell RP Jr., Coonley CJ, Gee TS. Homoharringtonine: an effective new drug for remission induction in refractory nonlymphoblastic leukemia. J Clin Oncol 1985; 3:617–621.

90. Arlin Z, Gaddipati J, Mittelman A, et al. Phase 1-2 trial of homoharringtonine in acute myelogenous leukemia Proc Am Soc Clin Oncol 1985; 4:173.

91. Neidhart JA, Kraut E, Metz EN, Howenstine B. Phase 1 study of homoharringtonine administered by prolonged continuous infusion. Proc Am Soc Clin Oncol 1985; 4:49.

92. Driscoll JS, Hazard GF, Wood HB Jr., Goldin A. Structure-antitumor activity relationships among quinone derivatives. Cancer Chemother Rep Part 2 1974; 4:1–361.

93. Hartleib J. Untersuchungen uber das washstum von zwei tumoren des soliden yoshida-sarcoms der ratter beim gleichen tier sowie uber die reaktion verschieden grosser tumoren auf behandlung mit 2,3,5-trisathylenimonbenzochinon-(1,4). Z. Krebsforsch 1974; 81:1–6.

94. Mattern J, Wayss K, Volm M. Cytostaticawirkugen auf jurzzeit-(^{3}H-uridineinbau und gewebekulturen (zellzahl) menschilcher tumoren. Arch Gynaekol 1974; 216:273–79.

95. Nakao H, Arakawa M. Antileukemic agents. I. Some 2,5-disubstituted p-benzoquinones. Chem Pharm Bull (Tokyo),1972; 20:1962–67.

96. Nakao H, Arakawa M, Nakamura T, Fukushima M. Antileukemic agents. II. New 2,5-bis(1-aziridinyl)p-benzoquinone derivatives. Chem Pharm Bull (Tokyo) 1972; 20:1968–79.

97. Petersen S, Gauss W, Urbschat E. Synthese ein facher chinon-derivative mit fungiziden bakteriostatischem oder cytostatischen eigenschaften. Angew Chem Int Ed Engl 1955; 67:217–31.

98. Saito T, Ohira S, Wakui T, et al. Clinical experience with a new anticancer agent carbazilquinone (NSC 134679). Cancer Chemother Rep 1983; 57:447–57.

99. Chou F-T, Khan AH, Driscoll JS. Potential central nervous system antitumor agents aziridinylbenzoquinones, 2. J Med. Chem 1976; 19:1302–08.

100. Driscoll JS, Dudeck L, Congleton G, Geran RI. Potential CNS antitumor agents VI. Arizidinylbenzoquinones III. J Pharm Sci 1979; 68:185–88.

101. Khan AH, Driscoll JS. Potential central nervous system antitumor agents. Aziridinylbenzoquinones. J Med Chem 1976; 19:313–17.

102. Griffin JP, Newman RA, McCormack JJ, Krakoff IH. Clinical and clinical pharmacologic studies of aziridinylbenzoquinone. Cancer Treat Rep 1982; 66:1321–25.

103. Schilcher RB, Young JD, Leichman LP, Haas CD, Baker L. Phase 1 evaluation and pharmacokinetics of aziridinylbenzoquinone using a weekly intravenous schedule. Cancer Res 1983; 43:3907–11.

104. Schilsky RL, Kelley JA, Ihde DC, Howser DM, Cordes RS, Young RC. Phase 1 trial and pharmacokinetics of azirdinylbenzoquinone (AZQ) in humans. Cancer Res 1982; 42:1582–86.

105. Tan C, Hancock C, Miller L, Caparros B, Leyland-Jones B. Phase 1 study of aziridinylbenzoquinone (AZQ, NSC 182986) in children with cancer. Proc Am Assoc Cancer Res 1982; 22:120.

106. Taylor SA, Belt RJ, Haas CD, Hoogstraten B, Stephens RL. Phase 1 trial of carbamic acid (AZQ, NSC 182986). Proc Am Soc Clin Oncol 1981; 22:389.

107. Whitacre MY, Van Echo DA, Budman DR, Shulman P, Aisner J, Wiernik PH. A phase 1 trial of 5-day continuous infusion of aziridinyl benzoquinone (AZQ, NSC 182986). Proc Am Soc Clin Oncol 1982; 1:24.

108. Walters RS, Keating MJ, Bodey GP, McCredie KB, Freirich EJ. Phase 1-2 study of aziridinylbenzoquinone in actue leukemia. Proc Am Soc Clin Oncol 1982; 1:134.

109. Van Echo DA, Schulman P, Budman DR, Ferrari A, Wiernik PH. A phase 1 trial of aziridinylbenzoquinone (NSC 182986) in patients with previously treated acute leukemia. Am J Clin Oncol 1982; 5:405–10.

110. Aroney RS, Kaplan RS, Salcman M, Montgomery E, Wiernik PH. A phase 2 trial of AZQ (NSC 182986) in patients with recurrent primary or metastatic brain tumors. Proc Am Soc Clin Oncol 1982; 1:24.

111. Carey RW, Comis RL. Phase 2 evaluation of aziridinylbenzoquinone (AZQ) in the primary treatment of locally advanced or extensive nonsmall-cell lung cancer. Proc Am Soc Clin Oncol 1982; 1:55.

112. Case DC Jr., Hyes DM. Phase 2 study of aziridinylbenzoquinone in refractory lymphoma. Cancer Treat Rep 1983; 67:993–96.

113. Curt GA, Kelley J, Kufta CV, et al. Phase 2 and pharmacokinetic study of aziridinylbenzo-quinone 2,5-diaziridinyl -3,6-bis (carboethoxyamino) -1,4- benzoqauinone diaziquone, NSC 182986 in high-grade gliomas. Cancer Res 1983; 43:6102–05.

114. Feun LG, Savaraj N, Bedikian AY, et al. Phase 2 study of 2,5-diaziridinyl-3,6-biscarboethox-yamino-1,4-benzoquinone (AZQ, NSC 182986) in recurrent malignant gliomas. Proc Am Assoc Cancer Res 1982; 22:161.

115. Kamen BA, Holcenberg JS, Spiegel SE. Aziridinylbenzoquinone (AZQ) treatment of central nervous system leukemia. Cancer Treat Rep 1982; 66:2105–06.

116. Nichols WC, Kvols LK, Richardson RL, Benson RC. Phase 2 study of aziridinylbenzoquinone (AZQ) in advanced genitourinary (GU) cancer. Proc Am Soc Clin Oncol 1982; 1:117.

117. Neidhard JA, Erlichman C, Robert F, Velez-Garcia E, Bender JF, Grillo-Lopez J. Phase 2 trial of diaziquone in patients with colon cancer. Cancer Treat Rep 1985; 69:215–17.

118. Frytak S, Eagan RT, Creagan ET, Nichols WC. Phase 2 study of diaziquone in patients with advanced carcinoma of the lung. Cancer Treat Rep 1984; 68:1193–94.

119. Creagan ET, Long HJ, Kvols LK, Edmonson JH, O'Fallon JR. Phase 2 trial of diaziquone in advanced upper aerodigestive cancer. Cancer Treat Rep 1985; 69:141.

120. Shildt R, Stephens RL, Subramanian VP, et al. Phase 2 trial of diaziquone in advanced large bowel carcinoma in previously treated and untreated patients: A Southwest Oncology Group study. Cancer Treat Rep 1985; 69:709–10.

121. Creagan ET, Schutt AJ, Ahmann DL, Green SJ. Phase 2 study of aziridinyl-benzoquinone (AZQ) in disseminated malignant melanoma. Cancer Treat Rep 1982; 66:2089–90.

122. Host RH, Joss R, Pinedo H, et al. Phase 2 trial of diaziquone (AZQ) in advanced malignant melanoma. Eur J Cancer Clin Oncol 1983; 19:295–98.

123. Budman DR, Forastiere A, Perloff M, Perry M, Aisner J, Weinberg V, Wood W. Aziridinylben-zoquinone (AZQ) in advanced breast cancer: a Cancer and Leukemia Group B phase 2 trial. Cancer Treat Rep 1982; 66:1875–76.

124. Lund B, Bramwell B, Renard J, Hansen HH, and Dombernowsky P. Phase 2 trial of diaziquone in advanced ovarian carcinoma. European Organization for Research on Treatment of Cancer early clinical trials group. Cancer Treat Rep 1985; 69:339–40.

125. Hansen M, Gallmeier WM, Vermorken J, et al. Phase 2 trial of diaziquone in advanced renal adenocarcinoma. Cancer Treat Rep 1984; 68:1055–56.

126. Madajewicz S, Spaulding M, Bhimani S, et al. Phase 1–2 diaizquione chemotherapy in brain tumors. Cancer Treat Rep 1984; 68:913–14.

127. Aisner J, Fuks JZ, Van Echo DA, et al. Phase 2 study of aziridynlbenzoquinone (AZQ) in patients with refractory small-cell carcinoma of lung. Proc Am Soc Clin Oncol 1982; 1:148.

128. Vinciguerra V, Anderson K, McIntyre OR. Diaziquone for resistant multiple myeloma. Cancer and leukemia group B. Cancer Treat Rep 1985; 69:331–32.

129. Handa K, Sato S. Generation of free radicals of quinone group containing anticancer chemicals in NADPH-microsome system as evidenced by initiation of sulfite oxidation. Gann 1975; 66:43–47.

130. Bachur NR, Gordon SL, Gee MV. A general mechanism for microsomal activation of quinone anticancer agents to free radicals. Cancer Res 1978; 38:1745–50.

131. Egorin MJ, Fox BM, Spiegel JF, Gutierrez PL, Friedman RD, Bachur NR. Cellular pharmacol-ogy in murine and human leukemic cell lines of diaziquone (NSC 182986). Cancer Res 1985; 45:992–99.

132. Spiegel JF, Egorin MJ, Collins JM, Lerner BD, Bachur NR. The murine disposition and pharma-cokinetics of the antineoplastic agent, diaziquone (NSC 182986). Drug Metab Dispos 1983; 11:41–46.

References—Chapter 19

1. Sullivan RD, Young CW, Miller E, Glastein N, Clarkson B, Burchenal JH. The clinical effects of the continuous administration of fluorinated pyrimidines (5-fluorouracil and 5-fluoro-2'-deoxyuridine. Cancer Treat Res 1960; 8:77–83.

2. Lokich JJ, Bothe A, Fine N, Perri J. Phase 2 study of protracted venous infusion of 5-fluorouracil. Cancer 1981; 48:2565–68.

3. Lokich JJ, Moore C. Chemotherapy associated palmar-plantar erythrodysesthesia syndrome. Ann Intern Med 1984; 101:789–800.

4. Vogelzang NJ, Bosl GJ, Johnson K, Kennedy BJ. Raynaud's phenomenon: a common toxicity after combination chemotherapy for testicular cancer. Ann Intern Med 1981; 95:228–92.

5. Vogelzang NJ, Bosl GJ, Johnson K, Kennedy BJ. Raynaud's phenomenon: common toxicity after combination chemotherapy for testicular cancer. Ann Intern Med 1981; 95:288–92.

6. DeConti RC, Kaplan SR, Papak RJ, Calabresi P. Continuous intravenous infusion of 5-fluoro-2'-deoxyuridine in the treatment of solid tumors. Cancer 1973; 894–98.

7. Sullivan RD, Miller E. The clinical effects of prolonged intravenous infusion of 5-fluoro-2'-deoxyuridine. Cancer Res 1965; 25:1025–30.

8. Lokich JJ, Sonneborn H, Paul S, Zipoli T. Phase 1 study of continuous venous infusion of floxuridine (5-FUDR) chemotherapy. Cancer Treat Rep 1983; 791–93.

9. Kelvin FM, Gramm HF, Gluck WL, Lokich JJ. Radiologic manifestations of small bowel toxicity due to floxuridine therapy. Am J Radiol 1986; 146:39–43.

10. Legha SS, Benjamin RS, Makay B, et al. Reduction of doxorubicin cardiotoxicity by prolonged continuous intravenous infusion. Ann Intern Med 1982; 96:133–39.

11. Garnick MB, Weiss GR, Steele GD, et al. Clinical evaluation of long-term continuous-infusion doxorubicin. Cancer Treat Rep 1983; 67:133–42.

12. Vogelzane NJ, Ruane M, DeMeester TR. Phase 1 trial of an implanted battery-powered, programmable drug delivery system for continuous doxorubicin administration. J Clin Oncol 1985; 3(3):407–14.

13. Lokich JJ, Bothe A, Zipoli T, et al. Constant infusion schedule for adriamycin: a phase 1–2 clinical trial of a 30-day schedule by ambulatory pump delivery system. J Clin Oncol 1983; 1(1):24–28.

14. Lokich JJ, Perri J, Fine N, Bothe A. Mitomycin C: phase 1 study of a constant infusion ambulatory treatment schedule. Am J Clin Oncol cancer trials 1982; 5:443–47.

15. Lokich JJ. Phase 1–2 study of cis-diamminedichloroplatinum (II) administered by constant 5-day infusion. Cancer Treat Rep 1980; 64:905–908.

16. Salem P, Jadboury K, Khalil M, et al. Cis-diammine-dichloroplatinum by 5-day continuous infusion—toxicity pattern. Proc Am Assoc Cancer Res and ASCO 1979; 20:84.

17. Lokich JJ, Zipoli TE. Phase 1 study of protracted infusion of cisplatin. Cancer Drug Deliv 1984; 1(3):247–50.

18. Sullivan R, Miller E, Zurek W, et al. Re-evaluation of methotrexate as an acute cancer. Cancer Chemother Rep 1968; 52:655.

19. Campbell MA, Perrier DG, Dorr RT, Alberts DS, Finley PR. Methotrexate: bioavailability and pharmacokinetics. Cancer Treat Rep 1985; 69(7–8): 833–38.

20. Goldin A, Venditti JM, Humphreys SR, Mantel N. Modification of treatment schedules in the management of advanced mouse leukemia with amethopterin. J Natl Cancer Inst 1956; 17:203–12.

21. Lokich JJ, Curt G. A phase 1 and pharmacology study of continuous infusion low dose methotrexate. Cancer 1985; 56:2391–94.

22. Zeffren J, Yagoda A, Kelsen D, Winn R. Phase 1 trial of a 4-day infusion of vinblastine (VLB). Proc Am Assoc Cancer Res and ASCO 1980; 21:178.

23. Lokich JJ, Zipoli TE, Perri J, Bothe A. Protracted vinblastine infusion phase 1–2 study in malignant melanoma and other tumors. Am J Clin Oncol (CCT) 1984; 7:551–53.

24. Bedikian AY, Bodey CP. Phase 1 study of cyclophosphamide (NSC 26271) by 72-hour continuous intravenous infusion. Am J Clin Oncol (CCT) 1983; 6:365–68.

25. Solidoro A, Otero J, Vellejos C, et al. Intermittent continuous I.V. infusion of high-dose cyclophosphamide for remission induction to acute lymphocytic leukemia. Cancer Treat Rep 1981; 65(3–4):213–18.

26. Lokich JJ, Bothe A. Phase 1 study of continuous infusion cyclophosphamide for protracted durations. Cancer Drug Deliv 1984; 4:329–32.

27. Lokich JJ, Becker B. Subclavian vein thrombosis in patients treated with infusion chemotherapy for advanced malignancy. Cancer 1983; 52:1586–89.

28. Rich TA, Lokich JJ, Chaffey JT. A pilot study of protracted venous infusion of 5-fluorouracil and concomitant radiation therapy. J Clin Oncol 1985; 3:402–06.

References—Chapter 20

1. Silverberg E. Lancer Statistics 1982. Cancer 1982; 32:15–31.

2. Al-Sarraf M. Chemotherapy Strategies in squamous carcinoma of the head and neck. CRC Critical Rev in Oncol/Hematol 1984; 1(4):323–55.

3. Merino OR, Lindberg RD, Fletcher GH. An analysis of distant metatases from squamous cell carcinoma of the upper respiratory and digestive tracts. Cancer 1977; 40:145–51.

4. Carter S. The chemotherapy of head and neck cancer. Sem Oncol 1978; 4:413–24.

5. Amer MH, Al-Sarraf M, et al. Factors that effect response to chemotherapy and survival of patients with adenoid head and neck cancer. Cancer 1979; 43:2202–06.

6. Cachin Y. Adjuvant chemotherapy in head and neck carcinoma. Clin Otolaryngol 1982; 7:121–32.

7. Grunberg SM. Future directions in the chemotherapy of head and neck cancer. Am J Oncol (CCT) 1985; 8:51–54.

8. Oster MW. Chemotherapy before radiotherapy and/or surgery for equally advanced squamous cell carcinomas of the head and neck. Arch Otolaryngol 1981; 107:297–99.

9. Hong WK, Bromer R. Current concepts: chemotherapy in head and neck cancer. New Engl J Med 1983; 308:75–79.

10. Schuller DE, Wilson HE, Smith RE, Batley F, James AD. Prospective reductive chemotherapy for locally advanced carcinoma of the oral cavity, oropharynx and hypopharynx. Cancer 1983; 51:15–19.

11. Tarpley JL, Chretien PB, Alexander JC, Joyce RC, Block JB, Ketcham A, Ketcham AS. High-dose methotrexate as a preoperative adjuvant in the treatment of epidermoid carcinoma of the head and neck: a feasibility study and clinical trial. Am J Surg 1975; 130:481–86.

12. Leone LA, Albala MM, Rege VB. Treatment of carcinoma of the head and neck with intravenous methotrexate. Cancer 1968; 21:820–37.

13. Bertino JR, Boston B, Capizzi RL. The role of chemotherapy in the management of cancer of the head and neck: a review. Cancer 1975; 36:752–57.

14. Amer MH, Izbicki RM, Vaitkevicius VK, Al-Sarraf M. Combination chemotherapy with cis-diamminedichloroplatium, oncovin and bleomycin (COB) in advanced head and neck cancer: phase 2. Cancer 1980; 45:217.

15. Kish JA, Weaver A, Jacobs J, et al. Cisplatin and 5-fluorouracil infusion in patients with recurrent and disseminated epidermoid cancer of the head and neck. Cancer 1984; 53:1819–24.

16. DeConti RC, Schoenfeld D. A randomized prospective comparison of intermittent methotrexate, methotrexate with leucovorin and/or methotrexate combination head and neck cancer. Cancer 1981; 48:1061.

17. Drelichman A, Cummings G, Al-Sarraf M. A randomized trial of the combination of cis-platinum, oncovin and bleomycin (COB) vs. methotrexate in patients with advanced squamous cancer of the head and neck. Cancer 1983; 53:399–403.

18. Capizzi RL, DeConti RC, Marsh JC, Bertino JR. Methotrexate therapy of head and neck cancer: improvement in therapeutic index by the use of leucovorin rescue. Cancer Res 1970; 30:1782.

19. Kirkwood JM, Canellos GP, Ervin TJ, et al. Increased therapeutic index using moderate dose methotrexate-leucovorin in patients with advanced squamous carcinoma of the head and neck: a safe new effective regimen. Cancer 1981; 47:2414.

20. Al-Sarraf M. The cost and clinical value of combination of cis-platinum, oncovin and bleomycin (COB) vs. methotrexate in patients with advanced head and neck epidermoid cancer. Proc ASCO 1980; 21:354.

21. Witter RE. Combination chemotherapy of head and neck cancer in the United States — recent research. Cancer Res 1981; 76:276 – 89.

22. Haas CD, Coltman CA Jr, Gottlieb JA, et al. Phase 2 evaluation of bleomycin, a Southwest Oncology Group study. Cancer 1976; 38:8 – 12.

23. Hong WK, Schaefer S, Issell B, et al. A prospective randomized trial of methotrexate vs. cis-platinum in the treatment of recurrent squamous cell carcinomas of the head and neck (abst.). Proc ASCO 1982; 1:202.

24. Grose EW, Lehane D, Dixon DO, et al. A comparison of methotrexate and cis-platinum for patients with advanced squamous cell carcinomas of the head and neck region. Cancer (in press).

25. Wittes RE, Cvitkovic E, Shah J, Gerold RP, Strong EW. Cis-dichlorodiaminineplatinum (II) in the treatment of epidermoid carcinoma of the head and neck. Cancer Treat Rep 1977; 61:359 – 66.

26. Sako K, Razack MS, Koclnius I. Chemotherapy for advanced and recurrent squamous cell carcinoma of the head and neck with high and low dose cis-diamminedichloroplatinum. Am J Surg 1978; 136:529 – 33.

27. Rozencweig M, Slavic M, Muggia FM, Carter SK. Overview of early and investigational chemotherapeutic agents in solid tumors. Med Pediatr Oncol 1976; 2:417.

28. Rozencweig M, VonHoff DD, Muggia FM. Investigation chemotherapeutic agents in head and neck cancer. Sem Oncol 1977; 4:425.

29. Wittes RE. Chemotherapy of head and neck cancer. Otolaryngol Clin N Am 1980; 13:515.

30. Papaioannou AN. Preoperative chemotherapy for operable solid tumors. Eur J Cancer 1981; 17:263 – 69.

31. Randolph VL, Vallajo A, Spiro RH, et al. Combination therapy of advanced head and neck cancer. Induction of remissions with diamminedichloroplatinum (II), bleomycin and radiation therapy. Cancer 1978; 41:460.

32. Kloss R, Oster M, Blitzer A, et al. Cis-platinum and bleomycin for previously untreated equally advanced squamous cell carcinoma of the head and neck. Proc ASCO 1981; 22:535.

33. Glick JH, Marcial V, Richter M, et al. The adjuvant treatment of inoperable stage 3 and 4 epidermoid carcinoma of the head and neck with platinum and bleomycin infusion prior to definitive radiotherapy: An RTOG pilot study. Cancer 1980; 46:1919.

34. Al-Sarraf M, Amer MH, Vaishampayan G, et al. A multidisciplinary therapeutic approach for advanced previously untreated epidermoid cancer of the head and neck: preliminary report. Int J Radiation Oncol Biol Phys 1979; 5:1421.

35. Wittes R, Heller K, Randolph V, et al. Cis-dichlorodiammineplatinum (II) based chemotherapy as initial treatment of advanced head and neck cancer. Cancer Treat Rep 1979; 63:1533.

36. Hong WK, Shapshay SM. Treatment of previously untreated stage 3 and 4 squamous cell carcinoma of the head and neck. Otolaryngol Clin N Am 1980; 13:521.

37. Al-Sarraf M, Drelichman A, Jacobs J, et al. Adjuvant chemotherapy with cis-platinum, oncovin and bleomycin followed by surgery and/or radiotherapy in patients with advanced previously untreated head and neck cancer, In: Final report in adjuvant therapy of cancer III. Jones SE, Salmon SE, eds. New York: Grune and Stratton, 1981.

38. Spaulding MB, Klotch D, Grillo J, et al. Adjuvant chemotherapy in the treatment of advanced tumors of the head and neck. Am J Surg 1980; 140:538.

39. Brown AW, Blom J, Butler WM, et al. Combination chemotherapy with vinblastine, bleomycin and cis-diamminedichloroplatinum (II) in squamous cell carcinoma of the head and neck. Cancer 1980; 45:2830.

40. Elias EG, Chretien PB, Monnard E, et al. Chemotherapy prior to local therapy in advanced

squamous cell carcinoma of the head and neck. Preliminary assessment of an intensive drug regimen. Cancer 1979; 43:1025.

41. Hong WK, Shapsay SM, Bhutani R, et al. Induction chemotherapy in advanced squamous head and neck carcinoma with high-dose cis-platinum and bleomycin infusion. Cancer 1979; 44:19.

42. Schuller DE, King GW, Smith RE, et al. Combination therapy protocol for stage 3 or 4 carcinoma of the oral cavity, oropharynx and hypopharynx. Laryngoscope 1980; 90:1263.

43. Weaver A, Fleming S, Kish J, et al. Cis-platinum and 5-fluorouracil as induction therapy for advanced head and neck cancer. Am J Surg 1982; 144:445.

44. Schwert R, Jacobs JR, Crissman J, Kinzie J, et al. Improved survival in patients with advanced head and neck cancer achieving complete clinical response to induction chemotherapy. Proc ASCO 1983; 24:159.

45. Al-Kourainy K, Crissman J, Ensley J, et al. Achievement of superior survival of histologically negative vs histologically positive clinically complete responders to cisplatinum (CACP) combinations in patients with locally advanced head and neck cancer. Proc AACR 1985; 26:164.

46. Snow JB, Gelber RD, Kramer S, et al. Comparison of preoperative and postoperative radiation therapy for patients with carcinoma of the head and neck. Acta Otolaryngeal 1981; 91:611 – 26.

47. Vogl SE, Lerner H, Kaplan BH, Coughlin C, et al. Failure of effective initial chemotherapy to modify the course of stage 4 (MO) squamous cancer of the head and neck. Cancer 1982; 50:840 – 44.

48. Goffinet DR, Bagshaw MA. Clinical use of radiation sensitizing agents. Cancer Treat Rev 1974; 1:15 – 26.

49. Clifford P, O'Connor AD, Druden-Smith J, et al. Synchronous multiple drug chemotherapy and radiotherapy for advanced (stage 3 and 4) squamous carcinoma of the head and neck. Antibiot Chemother 1978; 24:60 – 72.

50. O'Connor D, Clifford P, Edwards WG, Dalley VM, et al. Long-term results of VBM and radiotherapy in advanced head and neck cancer. Int J Radiat Oncol Biol Phy 1982; 8:1525 – 31.

51. Borgelt BB, Davis LW. Combination chemotherapy and irradiation for head and neck cancer: a review. Cancer Clin Trials 1978; 1:49 – 59.

52. Glick JH, Fazekas JT, Davis LW, et al. Combination chemotherapy-radiotherapy for advanced inoperable head and neck cancer: a RTOG pilot study. Cancer Clin Trials 1979; 2:129 – 36.

53. Chabner B, ed. Pharmacologic principles of cancer treatment. Philadelphia: WB Saunders Co., 1982.

54. Skipper HE, et al. Experimental evaluation of potential anticancer agents XIII: on the critical and kinetic association with "curability" of experimental leukemia. Cancer Chemother Rep 1964; 35:1 – 111.

55. Skipper HE, et al. Implications of biomedical, cytokinetic, pharmacologic, and toxicologic relationship in the design of optimal therapeutic schedules. Cancer Chemother Rep 1970; 54:431.

56. Skipper HE. Leukocyte kinetics in leukemia and lymphoma. In: Leukemia-lymphoma. Chicago: Year Book Medical Publishers, 1970.

57. Clarkson BD, Fried J. Changing concepts of treatment in acute leukemia. Med Clin N Am 1971; 55:561 – 600.

58. Ziegler JL, Morrow RH, Foss L, et al. Treatment of burritis tumor with cyclophosphamide. Cancer 1970; 26:474 – 84.

59. Goldin A, Venditti JM, Humphreys SB, et al. Modification of treatment schedules in the management of advanced mouse leukemia with amethopterin. J Natl Cancer Inst 1956; 17:203 – 12.

60. Sikic BI, Collins JM, Humphreys SB, et al. Improved therapeutic index of bleomycin when administered by continuous infusion in mice. Cancer Treat Rep 1978; 62:2022 – 7.

61. Krakoff IH, Cvitkovic E, Currie V, Yeh S, LaMonte C. Clinical pharmacologic and therapeutic studies of bleomycin given by continuous infusion. Cancer 1977; 40:2027 – 37.

62. Seifert P, Baker LH, Reed ML, Vaitkevicius VK. Comparison of continuously infused 5-fluorouracil with bolus injection in treatment of patients with colorectal adenocarcinoma. Cancer 1975; 36:123 – 8.

63. Legha SS, Benjamin RS, MacKay B, et al. Reduction of doxorubicin cardiotoxicity by prolonged continuous intravenous infusion. Ann Intern Med 1982; 96:133 – 9.

64. Carlson RW, Sific BI. Continuous infusion or bolus injection in cancer chemotherapy. Ann Intern Med 1983; 99:823 – 33.

65. Crooke ST, Bradner WT. Bleomycin – a review. J Med 1976; 7:333 – 428.

66. Page YM, Alberts DS, Chen HSG, et al. Anti-tumor activity and plasma kinetics of bleomycin by continuous and intermittent administration. Br J Cancer 1980; 41:641 – 7.

67. Cooper KR, Hong WK. Prospective study of the pulmonary toxicity of continuous infused bleomycin. Cancer Treat Rep 1981; 65:419 – 25.

68. Lennon HM. Reduction of 5-fluorouracil toxicity in man with retention of anti-cancer effects by prolonged intravenous administration in 5% dextrose. Cancer Chemother Rep 1981; 65:419 – 25.

69. Lokich J, Bothe A Jr., Fine N, et al. Phase 1 study of protracted venous infusion of 5-fluorouracil. Cancer 1981; 48:2565 – 8.

70. Fraile RJ, Baker LH, Buroker TR, Horwitz J, Vaitkevicius VK. Pharmacokinetics of 5-fluorouracil administered orally, by rapid intravenous and by slow infusion. Cancer Res 1980; 40:2223 – 28.

71. Kish J, Ensley J, Weaver A, et al. Superior response rate with 96 hour 5-fluorouracil infusion vs 5-FU bolus combined with cis-platinum in a randomized trial for recurrent and advanced squamous head and neck cancer. Proc ASCO 1984; 3:179.

72. Drewinko B, Brown BW, Gottlieb JA. The effect of cis-diamminedichloroplatinum (II) on cultured human lymphoma cells and its therapeutic implications. Cancer Res 1973; 33:3091 – 5.

73. Moray RE, Strauss MJ. Effects of pulse and continuous intravenous infusion of cis-diamminedichloroplatinum on L1210 leukemia in vitro. Cancer Res 1981; 41 (12 pt. 1):4993 – 6.

74. Jacobs C, Bertino JR, Goffinet DR, et al. 24-hour infusion of cis-platinum in head and neck cancers. Cancer 1978; 42:2135 – 40.

75. Bazzino JM, Prasad V, Koriech OM. Avoidance of renal toxicity by 24-hour infusion of cisplatin. Cancer Treat Rep 1981; 65:351 – 2.

76. Leichman CG, Corbett T, Leichman L. Improved treatment results in murine colon tumors treated with infusion 5-FU vs standard bolus schedule. Proc ASCO 1985; 355:1402.

77. Rooney M, Stanley R, Weaver A, et al. Superior results in complete response rate and overall survival in patients with advanced head and neck cancer treated with 3 courses of 120-hour 5-FU infusion + cis-platinum. Proc ASCO 1983; 2:159.

78. Hill BT, Price LA, MacRae K. Importance of primary site in assessing 6-year survival data in advanced epidermoid head and neck cancer treated with initial combination chemotherapy without cis-platin. Proc ASCO 1984; 3:178.

79. Ervin TJ, Weichselbaum RR, Fabian RL, et al. Advanced squamous carcinoma of the head and neck: a preliminary report of neoadjuvant chemotherapy with cis-platin, bleomycin, and methotrexate. Arch Otolaryngeal 1984; 110:241 – 45.

80. Ensley JF, Jacobs JR, Weaver A, et al. Correlation between response to cis-platinum-combination chemotherapy and subsequent radiotherapy in previously untreated patients with advanced squamous cell cancers of the head and neck. Cancer 1984; 54:811 – 14.

81. Jacobs C, Meyers F, Hendrickson C, et al. A randomized phase 3 study of cisplatin with or without methotrexate for recurrent squamous cell carcinoma of the head and neck. A NCOG study. Cancer 1983; 52:1563 – 69.

82. Creagen ET, O'Fallon JR, Woods JE, et al. Cis-diamminedichloroplatinum (II) administered by 24-hour infusion in the treatment of patients with advanced upper aerodigestive cancer. Cancer 1983; 51:2020 – 23.

83. Lokich JJ. Phase 1 study of cis-diamminedichloroplatinum (II) administered as a constant 5-day infusion. Cancer Treat Rep 1980; 64:905 – 08.

84. Tapazoglou E, Kish J, Ensley J, Al-Sarraf M. The activity of a single agent 5-fluorouracil infusion in advanced and recurrent head and neck cancer. Cancer 1986; 57:1105 – 09.

85. Kish J, Tapazoglou E, Ensley J, Al-Sarraf M. Activity of 96-hour to 120-hour 5-fluorouracil infusion in advanced and recurrent head and neck cancer. Proc ASCO 1985; C – 667.

86. Costanzi JJ, Loukas D, Gagliano RG, et al. Intravenous bleomycin infusion as a potential synchronizing agent in human disseminated malignancies: a preliminary report. Cancer 1976; 38:1503–06.

87. Ervin TJ, Weichselbaum R, Miller D, et al. Treatment of advanced squamous cell carcinoma of the head and neck with cisplatin, bleomycin, and methotrexate (PBM). Cancer Treat Rep 1981; 65:787–91.

88. Amrein PC, Fingert H, Weitzman SA. Cisplatin-vincristine-bleomycin therapy in squamous cell carcinoma of the head and neck. J Clin Oncol 1983; 1, 7 (July):421–27.

89. Plasse TF, Ohnuma T, Brooks S, et al. Bleomycin infusion followed by cyclophosphamide, methotrexate and 5-fluorouracil in advanced squamous carcinoma of the head and neck. Cancer 1984; 53:841–43.

90. Gonzalez MF, Valdivieso JG, Sartiano GP. Five-drug combination chemotherapy for advanced or recurrent head and neck neoplasms. Proc ASCO 1982.

91. Carey RZ, Grace WR, Sarg MJ. Treatment of advanced head and neck cancer in a pilot study with cytoxan, methotrexate, 5-FU, bleomycin and cis-platinum. Proc ASCO 1982.

92. Kish J, Drelichman A, Jacobs J, et al. Clinical trial of cis-platinum and 5-FU infusion as initial treatment for advanced squamous carcinoma of the head and neck. Cancer Treat Rep 1982; 66:471–74.

93. Kish JA, Drelichman A, Weaver A, et al. Cis-platinum and 5-FU infusion chemotherapy in advanced recurrent cancer of the head and neck. Proc ASCO 1984.

94. Rowland KM, Taylors SG, O'Donnell MR, et al. Cisplatin/5-FU infusion chemotherapy in advanced recurrent cancer of the head and neck. Proc ASCO 1984.

95. Fosser VP, Paccaguella A, Venturelli E, et al. Cisplatin + 5-FU 120-hour infusion in patients with recurrent and disseminated head and neck cancer. Proc ASCO 1985.

96. Amrein P, Weitzman S. 24-Hour infusion cisplatin and 5-day infusion 5-fluorouracil in squamous cell carcinoma of the head and neck. Proc ASCO 1985; C–519.

97. Spaulding MB, DeLos Santos R, Samani S, et al. Infusion 5-FU/Velban: a nontoxic combination active in head and neck cancer. Proc ASCO 1982; C–772.

98. Weaver A, et al. Combined modality therapy for advanced head and neck cancer. Am J Surg 1980; 140:549–52.

99. Spaulding MB, Kahn A, DeLos Santos R, et al. Adjuvant chemotherapy in advanced head and neck cancer: an update. Am J Surg 1982; 144:432–36.

100. Tannock I, Cummings B, Sorrenti V. The ENT group: combination chemotherapy used prior to radiation therapy for locally advanced squamous cell carcinoma of the head and neck. Cancer Treat Rep 1982; 66:1421–24.

101. Weaver A, Fleming S, Ensley J, et al. Superior clinical response and survival rates with initial bolus of cisplatin and 120-hour infusion of 5-fluorouracil before definitive therapy for locally advanced head and neck cancer. Am J Surg 1984; 148:525–29.

102. Popkin J, Bromer R, Byrne R, et al. Seven day continuous bleomycin induction chemotherapy in advanced squamous cell carcinoma of the head and neck. Proc ASCO 1982; C–777.

103. Spaulding MG, DeLos Santos R, Klotch D, et al. Induction chemotherapy in head and neck cancer: superiority of a bleomycin-containing regimen. Proc ASCO 1982; 3:187.

104. Laccourrey H, Brasnu D, Lacau St. Guily J, et al. High response rate after induction chemotherapy in stage 3 head and neck cancer. Proc ASCO 1984; 3:187.

105. Baker SR, Makuch RW, Wolf T. Preoperative cisplatin and bleomycin therapy in head and neck squamous carcinoma – prognostic factors for tumor response. Arch Otolaryngol 1981; 107:683–89.

106. Israel L, Aguilera J, Soudant J, et al. Bleomycin and cis-platinum with or without mitocycin-C in 110 previously untreated patients with head and neck cancer. Am J Clin Oncol (CCT) 1983; 5:305–11.

107. Jacobs C, Wolf GT, Makuch RW, et al. Adjuvant chemotherapy for head and neck squamous carcinomas. Proc ASCO 1984; 3:182.

108. Spaulding MB, Kahn A, Sundquist N, et al. Preoperative chemotherapy for hypopharyngeal carcinoma. Laryngoscope 1983; 93:346–49.

109. Decker DA, Drelichman A, Jacobs J, et al. Adjuvant chemotherapy with high-dose bolus cis-diamminedichloroplatinum (II) and 120-hour infusion 5-FU in stage 3 and 4 squamous cell carcinoma of the head and neck. Proc ASCO 1982; 1:195.

110. Rooney M, Kish JA, Jacobs J, et al. Improved complete response rate and survival in advanced head and neck cancer after three-course induction therapy with 120-hour 5-FU infusion and cisplatin. Cancer 1985; 55:1123–28.

111. Ensley J, Kish JA, Jacobs J, et al. Survival advantages observed in complete responders when achieved with chemotherapy alone versus comparable response requiring chemotherapy and radiotherapy in patients with advanced squamous cell cancer of the head and neck. Cancer—Baltimore (July 22–27) 1984; 109.

112. Jacobs JR, Kinzie J, Al-Sarraf M, et al. Combination of cis-platinum and 5-FU infusion before surgery in patients with resectable head and neck cancer. Proc ASCO 1984; 3:180.

113. Ensley J, Kish JA, Jacobs J, et al. The use of a 5-course alternating combination chemotherapy induction regimen in advanced squamous cell cancer of the head and neck. Proc ASCO 1985; 4:143.

114. Greenberg B, Ahmann F, Garewel H, et al. Neoadjuvant therapy for advanced head and neck cancer with allopurinol modulated high-dose 5-FU and cis-platinum. Proc ASCO 1985; 4:146.

115. Al-Sarraf M, Drelichman A, Peppard S, et al. Adjuvant cis-platinum and 5-fluorouracil 96-hour infusion in previously untreated epidermoid cancers of the head and neck. Proc ASCO 1981; 22:428.

116. Al-Sarraf M, Kish J, Ensley J, et al. Induction cis-platinum and 5-fluourouracil infusion before surgery and/or radiotherapy in patients with locally advanced head and neck cancer: progress report. Proc AACR 1984; 25:196.

References—Chapter 21

1. Powers WE, Tolmach LV. Preoperative radiation therapy: biological basis and experimental investigation. Nature 1964; 201:172–204.

2. Vaitkevicius VK, Brennan MJ, Beckett VL, et al. Clinical evaluation of cancer chemotherapy with 5-fluorouracil. Cancer 1961; 14:131–52.

3. Seifert P, Baker LH, Reed ML, et al. Comparison of continuously infused 5-fluorouracil with bolus injection in treatment of patients with colorectal adenocarcinoma. Cancer 1975; 36(1):123–28.

4. Fraile RJ, Baker LH, Buroker TR, et al. Pharmacokinetics of 5-fluorouracil administered orally, by rapid intravenous and by slow infusion. Cancer Res 1980; 40:2223–28.

5. Byfield JE, Barone RM, Mendelsohn J, et al. Infusional 5-fluorouracil and x-ray therapy for nonresectable esophageal cancer. Cancer 1980; 45:703–08.

6. Quan SHQ, Deddish MR, Stearns MW. The effect of preoperative roentgen therapy upon the 10 and 15 year results of the surgical treatment of cancer of the rectum. Surg Gynecol Obstet 1960; 111:507–08.

7. Leichman LP, Won J, et al. Pre-operative radiation therapy causing downstaging of adenocarcinoma of the rectum: preliminary results. Proc Mich St Med Soc 1981.

8. Nigro ND, Vaitkevicius VK, Considine B. Combined therapy for cancer of the anal canal: a preliminary report. Dis Colon Rectum 1974; 17:354–56.

9. Stearns MW Jr., ed. Cancer of the anal canal. Curr Probl Cancer IV No 12. Chicago: Year Book Medical Publishers Inc., 1980.

10. Leichman LP, Nigro ND, Vaitkevicius VK, et al. Cancer of the anal canal: model for preoperative adjuvant combined modality therapy. Am J Med 1985; 78:211–15.

11. Byfield JE, Barone RM, Sharp TR, Fraukel SS. Conservative managmeent without alkylating agents of squamous cell anal cancer using clinical 5FU alone and x-ray therapy. Cancer Treat Rep 1983; 67:709–12.

12. Michaelson RA, Magill GB, Quan SH, et al. Preoperative chemotherapy and radiation therapy in the management of anal epidermoid carcinoma. Cancer 1983; 51:390–95.

13. Cummings BJ, Rider WD, Harwood AR, et al. Combined radical radiation therapy and chemotherapy for primary squamous cell carcinoma of the anal canal. Cancer Treat Rep 1982; 66:489–92.

14. John M, Flam M, Wittlinger P, Padmanabhan A, Podolsky W, Ager-Mowry P. Clinical exposure with synchronous radiation and chemotherapy in advanced squamous cell carcinoma. Proc ASCO 1985; 4:78.

15. Tiver KW, Langlands AO. Synchronous chemotherapy and radiotherapy for carcinoma of the anal canal—an alternative to abdominoperineal resection. Aust NZJ Surg 1984; 54:101—08.

16. Franklin R, Steiger Z, Vaishampayan G, et al. Combined modality therapy for esophageal squamous cell carcinoma. Cancer 1983; 51:1062—71.

17. Panettiere F, Leichman L, O'Bryan R, et al. Cisdiamminedichloride platinum (II) an effect agent in the treatment of epidermoid carcinoma of the esophagus. Cancer Clin Trials 1981; 4:29—31.

18. Leichman L, Steiger Z, Seydel HG, et al. Preoperative chemotherapy and radiation therapy for patients iwth cancer of the esophagus: a potentially curative approach. J Clin Oncol 1984; 2:75—79.

19. Carey R, Choi NC, Hilgenberg AD. Preoperative chemotherapy (5-FU/DDP) as initial component in multimodality treatment program for esophageal cancer. Proc ASCO 1985; 4:78.

20. Engstrom P, Coia L, Paul A. Nonsurgical management of stage 1 and 2 esophageal cancer. Proc ASCO 1985; 4:91.

21. Coia LR, Engstrom PF, Paul A, et al. A pilot study of combined radiotherapy and chemotherapy for esophageal carcinoma. Am J Clin Oncol 1984; 7:653—59.

22. Lokich J, Chaffey J, Rich T. Protracted infusion 5-FU with sequential radiation for esophageal cancer. Proc NE Cancer Soc Sept 1984.

23. Trillet V, Moutbarbou X, de Laroche G, Lambert R, Gerard JP. combination 5-fluorouracil and cisplatin prior to laser and radiotherapy in 47 patients with resectable esophageal cancer. Proc First Int Conf Neoadjuvant Ther Nov 1985.

24. Abitbol A, Straus MJ, Franklin G, Billet D, Sullivan P, Moran RE. Infusional chemotherapy and cyclic radiation therapy in inoperable esophageal and gastric cardia carcinoma. Am J Clin Oncol 1983; 6:195—201.

25. Hellerstein S, Rosen S, Kies M, et al. Diamminedichloro platinum and 5-FU combined chemotherapy of epidermoid esophageal cancer. Proc ASCO 1983; 2:127.

26. Coonley CJ, Bains M, Hilaris B, Chapman R, Kelsen DP. Cisplatin and bleomycin in the treatment of esophageal carcinoma. Cancer 1984; 54:2351—55.

27. Bosset J, Horteloup P, Bontemas P, et al. A phase 2 trial of bleomycin and cisplatin in advanced esophagus carcinoma (abstr). Proc 13th Int Cancer Cong 1982; 13:41.

28. Kelson D, Coonley C, Hilaris B, et al. Cisplatin, vindesine, bleomycin combination chemotherapy of loco-regional and advanced esophageal carcinoma. Am J Med 1983; 75:639—52.

29. Forestiere A, Patel H, Hawkins J, et al. Cisplatin, bleomycin, and VP16-213 in combination for epidermoid carcinoma for epidermoid carcinoma of the esophagus. Proc ASCO 1983; 2:123.

30. Hermann R, Schlag P, Manegold C, Buhr C, Herfartdz C, Schettler G. Preoperative chemotherapy in esophageal cancer. Results of a phase 2 pilot study. Proc First Int Symp Neoadjuvant Ther (Paris) (abstr 64) Nov 1985; 30.

31. Marontz A, Schmilovich A, Sautos J, Muro A, Block J, Hunis A, Chacou R. Combined therapy of inoperable locally advanced carcinoma of the esophagus. First Int Symp Neoadjuvant Ther (Paris) (abstr 66) Nov. 1985; 30.

32. Kelsen D, et al. Chemotherapy for cancer of the esophagus. Sem Oncol 1984; 11:159—68.

33. Resbeut M, Prise-Fleury EL, Ben-Hassel M, et al. Squamous cell carcinoma of the esophagus. Treatment by combined vincristine-methotrexate plus folinic acid rescue and cisplatin before radiotherapy. Cancer 1985; 56:1246—50.

34. Advani SH, Saikia TK, Swaroop S, et al. Anterior chemotherapy in esophageal cancer. Cancer 1985; 56:1502—06.

35. Gisselbrecht C, Calvo F, Mignot L, et al. Fluorouracil (F), adriamycin (A), and cisplatin (P) (FAP): combination chemotherapy of advanced esophageal carcinoma. Cancer 1983; 52:974—77.

36. Leichman L, Steiger Z, Seydel HG, Vaitkevicius VK. Combined preoperative chemotherapy and radiation therapy for cancer of the esophagus. Wayne State University Southwest Oncology Group and Radiation Therapy Oncology Group Exp Sem Oncol 1984; 11:178—85.

References—Chapter 22

1. Ansfield F, Klotz J, Nealon T, et al. A phase 3 study comparing the clinical utility of four regimens of 5-fluorouracil. A preliminary report. Cancer 1977; 39:34—40.

2. Douglass HOJ, Lavin PT, Woll J, Conroy JF, Carbone P. Chemotherapy of advanced measurable colon and rectal carcinoma with oral 5-fluorouracil, alone or in combination with cyclophosphamide or 6-thioguanine, with intravenous 5-fluorouracil or beta-2'-deoxythioguanosine or with oral 3(4-methyl-cyclohexyl)-1(2-chloroethyl)-1-nitrosurea: A phase 2-3 study of the Eastern Cooperative Oncology Group (EST:4273). Cancer 1978; 42:2538—45.

3. Presant CA, Denes AE, Liu C, Bartolucci AA. Prospective randomized reappraisal of 5-fluorouracil in metastatic colorectal carcinoma. A comparative trial with 6-thioguanine. Cancer 1984; 53:2610—14.

4. Windschitl H, Scott M, Schutt A, et al. Randomized phase 2 studies in advanced colorectal carcinoma: a North Central Cancer Treatment Group study. Cancer Treat Rep 1983; 67(11):1001—08.

5. Moertel CG, Schutt AJ, Hahn RG, Reutmeir RJ. Therapy of advanced colorectal cancer with a combination of 5-FU, methyl CCNU, and vincristine. J Natl Cancer Inst 1975; 54:69—72.

6. Lokich JJ, Skarin AT, Mayer RJ, Henderson IC, Blum R, Frei E III. lack of effectiveness of combined 5-fluorouracil and methyl CCNU in advanced colorectal cancer. Cancer 1977; 40:2792—96.

7. Engstrom PF, MacIntyre JM, Mittlean A, Klassen DJ. Chemotherapy of advanced colorectal carcinoma: fluorouracil alone vs two drug combinations using fluorouracil, hydroxyurea, semustine, dacarbazine, rozoxane, and mitomycin. Am J Clin Oncol 1984; 7:313—18.

8. Boroker T, Moertel C, Flemming T, et al. A randomized comparison of 5-FU-containing drug combinations with 5-FU alone in advanced colorectal carcinoma. Proc ASCO 1984; 3:138.

9. Madajewicz S, Petrelli N, Rustum YM, et al. Phase 1-2 trial of high-dose calcium leucovorin and 5-fluorouracil in advanced colorectal cancer. Cancer Res 1984; 44(10):4667—69.

10. Ajani JA, Kanojia MD, Bedikian AY, Korinek JK, Stein SH, Espinoza EG, Bodey GP. Sequential methotrexate and 5-flourouracil in the primary treatment of metastatic colorectal carcinoma. Am J Clin Oncol (CCT) 1985; 8:69—71.

11. Herrmann R, Spehn J, Beyer J, et al. Sequential methotrexate and 5-fluorouracil: improved response rate in metastatic colorectal cancer. J Clin Oncol 1984; 2(6):591—94.

12. Beck TM, Curtis PW, Woodard DA, Hart NE, Smith CE. Treatment of metastatic colorectal carcinoma with 5-FU, mitomycin, vincristine, and methotrexate. Cancer Treat Rep 1984; 68(4):647—50.

13. Einhorn LH, Williams SD, Loehrer PJ. Combination chemotherapy with platinum (P) plus 5-FU in metastatic colorectal carcinoma (abstr). Proc Ann Meet Am Soc Clin Oncol 1984; 3:133.

14. Reitemeier RJ, Moertel CG. Comparison of rapid and slow intravenous administration of 5-florouracil in treating patients with advanced carcinoma of the large intestine. Cancer Chemother Rep 1962; 25:87—89.

15. Moertel CG, Schutt AJ, Reitemeier RJ, Hahn RG. A comparison of 5-fluorouracil administered by slow infusion and rapid injection. Cancer Res 1972; 32:2717—19.

16. Seifert P, Baker LH, Reed ML, et al. Comparison of continuously infused 5-fluorouracil with bolus injection in treatment of patients with colorectal adenocarcinoma. Cancer 1975; 36:123—28.

17. Kish J, Ensley J, Weaver A, Jacobs J, Cummings G, Al-Sarraf M. Superior response rate with 96-hour 5-fluorouracil (5-FU) infusion vs 5-FU bolus combined with cis-platinum (CACP) in a randomized trial for recurrent and advanced squamous head and neck cancer, (HNG) ASCO Abstr 1984; C—695.

18. Hartman HA, Kessinger A, Lemon HM, Foley JF. Five-day continuous infusion of 5-fluorouracil for advanced colorectal, gastric, and pancreatic adenocarcinoma. J Surg Oncol 1979; 11:227—38.

19. Shah A, MacDonald W, Goldie J, Gudauskas G, Briesebois B. 5-FU infusion in advanced colorectal cancer: a comparison of three dose schedules. Cancer Treat Rep 1985; 69(7—8):739—42.

20. Lokich JJ, Bothe A, Fine N, Perri J. Phase 1 study of protracted venous infusion of 5-fluorouracil. Cancer 1981; 48:2565—68.

21. Shepard KV, Faintuch J, Bitnan JD, Sweet DL, Robin E, Levin B. Treatment of metastatic colorectal cancer with cisplatin and 5-FU. Cancer Treat Rep 1985; 69(1):123−24.

22. Benedetto P, Davila E, Solomon J. Chronic continuous systemic infusion of 5-fluorouracil (CCI-5-FU) in the treatment of metastatic colorectal carcinoma (CRC). Proc ASCO 1984; C−556.

23. Ausman R, Caballero G, Quebbeman E, Hansen R. Response of metastatic colorectal adenocarcinomas to long-term continuous ambulatory intravenous infusion (CAII) of 5-fluorouracil (5-FU). Proc ASCO 1985; 4:C−336.

24. Belt RJ, Davidner ML, Myron MC, Barrett S. Continuous low-dose 5-fluorouracil (5-FU) for adenocarcinoma: confirmation of activity. Proc ASCO 1985; 4:349.

25. Leichman L, Leichman CG, Kinzie J, Weaver D, Evans L. Long-term low-dose 5-fluorouracil (5-FU) in advanced measurable colon cancer: no correlation between toxicity and efficacy. Proc ASCO 1985; 4:C−333.

26. Faintuch J, Shepard KV, O'Laughlin K, Beschorner J, Gaynor E, Levin B. Toxicity of continuous infusion of 5-FU. Proc ASCO 1985; 4:C−357.

27. Buroker T, Kim PN, Heilbrun L, Vaitkevicius VK. 5-FU infusion with mitomycin-C vs 5-FU infusion with methyl CCNU in the treatment of advanced colon cancer. A phase 3 study. ASCO Abstr 1977; C−18.

28. Shepard KV, Faintuch J, Bitran JD, Sweet DL, Robin E, Levin B. Treatment of metastatic colorectal carcinoma with cisplatin and 5-FU. Cancer Treat Rep 1985; 69(1):123−24.

29. Einhorn L. Personal communications.

30. Budd GT, Bukowski R, Fleming T, McCracken P. A randomized comparison of 2 dose-schedules of 5-fluorouracil (5-FU) and folinic acid (FA) for the treatment of metastatic colorectal cancer. Proc ASCO 1985; 4:C−318.

31. Lokich JJ, Phillips D, Greene R, et al. 5-fluorouracil and methotrexate administered simultaneously as a continuous infusion: a phase 1 study. Cancer 1985; 56:2395−98.

32. Lynch G, Kemeny N, Chun H, Martin D, Young C. Phase 1 evaluation and pharmacokinetic study of weekly I.V. thymidine and 5-FU in patients with advanced colorectal carcinoma. Cancer Treat Rep 1985; 69(2):179−84.

33. Vogel S, Presaut CA, Ratkin GA, Klahr C. Phase 1 study of thymidine plus 5-fluorouracil infusions in advanced colorectal carcinoma. Cancer Treat Rep 1979; 63:1−5.

34. O'Connell MJ, Moertel CG, Rubin J, Hahn RG, Kvols LK, Schutt AJ. Clinical trials of sequential N phosphoneacetyl-1-aspartate, thymidine, and 5-fluorouracil in advanced colorectal carcinoma. J Clin Oncol 1984; 2(10):1133−38.

35. Howell SB, Wung WE, Taetle R, Hussain F, Romine JS. Modulation of 5-fluorouracil toxicity by allopurinol in man. Cancer 1981; 48:1281−89.

36. Reitemeier RJ, Moertel CG, Hahn RG. Comparison of 5-fluorouracil (NSC-19893) and 2'-deoxy-5-fluorouridine (NSC-27640) in treatment of patients with advanced adenocarcinoma of colon or rectum. Cancer Chemother Rep 1965; 44:39−43.

37. Ansfield FJ, Curreri AR. Further clinical comparison between 5-fluorouracil (5-FU) and 5-fluoro-2'-deoxyuridine (5-FUDR). Cancer Chemother Rep 1963; 32:101−05.

38. Sullivan RD, Miller E. The clinical effects of prolonged intravenous infusion of 5-fluoro-2'-deoxyuridine. Cancer Res 1965; 25:1025−30.

39. Moertel CG, Reitemeier RJ, Hahn RG. A controlled comparison of 5-fluoro-2'-deoxyuridine therapy administered by rapid intravenous injection and by continuous intravenous infusion. Cancer Res 1967; 27:549−52.

40. Ansfield FJ, Schroeder JM, Curreri AR. A preliminary comparison of 5-fluoro-2'-deoxyuridine administered by rapid daily intravenous injections and by slow continuous infusion. Cancer Chemother Rep 1962; 16:389−90.

41. Lokich JJ, Sonneborn H, Paul S, Zipoli T. Phase 1 study of continuous venous infusion of floxuridine (5-FUDR) chemotherapy. Cancer Treat Rep 1983; 67:791−93.

42. DeConti RC, Kaplan SR, Papak RJ, Calabresi P. Continuous intravenous infusion of 5-fluoro-2'-deoxyuridine in the treatment of solid tumors. Cancer 1973; 32:894−98.

43. Kemeny N, Daly J, Oderman P, Chun H, Petroni G, Geller N. Randomized study of intrahepatic vs. systemic infusion of fluorodeoxyridine in patients with liver metastases from colorectal carcinoma. ASCO Abstr 1984; C−551.

44. Staff R, Friedman M, Lewis B, et al. Current status of NCOG randomized trial of continuous intra-arterial (IA) versus intravenous (IV) floxuridine (FUDR) in patients with colorectal carcinoma metastatic to the liver. ASCO Abstr 1984; C−577.

45. Bedikian AY, Karlin D, Stroehlein J, Bodey GP, Korinek J. A comparative study of oral tegafur and intravenous 5-fluorouracil in patients with metastatic colorectal cancer. Am J Clin Oncol 1983; 6:181−86.

46. Abele R, Alberto P, Kaplan S, et al. Phase 2 study of doxifluridine in advanced colorectal adenocarcinoma. J Clin Oncol 1983; 1(12):750−54.

47. Livingston R, Carter SK. Single agents in cancer chemotherapy. New York: IFI/Plenum, 1970.

48. Moertel C, Reitemeier R, Hahn R. Evaluation of hydroxyurea by parenteral infusion. Cancer Chemother Rep 1965; 49:27.

49. Regelson W, Holland J, Frei E, et al. Comparative clinical toxicity of 6 mercaptopurine (6MP) and 6MP ribonucleoside. Cancer Chemother Rep 1964; 36:41.

50. Moore G, Brass I, Ausman R. Effects of mercaptopurine in 290 patients with advanced cancer. Cancer Chemother Rep 1968; 52:655.

51. Sullivan R, Miller E, Zurek W, et al. Re-evaluation of methotrexate as an anticancer drug. Surg Gyn Obst 1967; 125:819.

52. Frank W, Osterberg AE. Mitomycin C − an evaluation of the Japanese reports. Cancer Chemother Rep 1960; 9:114.

53. Miller E, Sullivan RD, Chryssochoos T. The clinical effects of mitomycin-C by continuous intravenous administration. Cancer Chemother Rep 1962; 21:129.

54. Holdener EE, Hansen HH, Host H, et al. Phase 2 trial of 4-epidadriamycin in advanced colorectal cancer. ASCO Abstr 1983; C−451.

55. Moertel C, Childs DS, Reitemeier R. Combined 5-fluorouracil and supervoltage radiation therapy of locally unresectable gastrointestinal cancer. Lancet 1969; 2:865−67.

56. Lokich JJ, The Gastrointestinal Tumor Study Group. Comparative therapeutic trial of radiation with or without chemotherapy in pancreatic carcinoma. Int J Rad Oncol Biol Physics 1979; 5:1643−47.

57. Rich TA, Lokich JJ, Chaffey JT. A pilot study of protracted venous infusion of 5-fluorouracil and concomitant radiation therapy. J Clin Oncol 1985; 3:402−06.

58. Cochran M, Gyves J, Han I, Wollner I, Walker S, Ensminger W. Combination chemo-radiation therapy for extrahepatic biliary tract obstruction due to metastatic GI cancer. Proc ASCO 1985; 4:C−317.

References—Chapter 23

1. Moertel CG. The stomach. In: Hollard JF, Frei E III, eds. Cancer medicine. Philadelphia: Lea & Febiger, 1982; 1767.

2. Falkson G. Halogenated pyrimidines as radiopotentiators in the treatment of stomach cancer. In: Paoletti R, Vertua R, eds. Progress in biochemical pharmacology − Vol I. Basel and New York: S Karger, 1964.

3. Falkson G, Sandison AG, Jacobs EL, Fichardt T. Combined telecobalt and 5-fluorouracil therapy in cancer of the stomach. S Afr Med J 1963; 36:712−17.

4. Moertel CG, Childs DS Jr, Reitemeier RJ, Colby MY Jr, Holbrooke MA. Combined 5-fluorouracil and supervoltage radation therapy of locally unresectable gastrointestinal cancer. Lancet 1969; 2:865-67.

5. Kovach JS, Moertel CG, Schutt AJ. A controlled study of combined 1,3-bis(2-chloroethyl)-1-nitrosourea and 5-fluorouracil therapy for advanced gastric and pancreatic cancer. Cancer 1974; 33:563.

6. Moertel CG, Mittelman JA, Bakermeier RF, Engstrom P, Hanely J. Sequential and combination chemotherapy of advanced gastric cancer. Cancer 1976; 38:678.

7. Comis RL, Carter SK. Integration of chemotherapy into combined modality treatment of solid tumors. III: Gastric Cancer. Cancer Treat Rev 1974; 1:221.

8. Moertel CG. Chemotherapy of gastrointestinal cancer. Clin Gastroenterol 1976; 5:777.

9. Moertel CG, Lavin PT. Phase 2-3 chemotherapy studies in advanced gastric cancer. Cancer Treat Rep 1979; 63:1863.

10. Gastrointestinal Tumor Study Group. Phase 2-3 chemotherapy studies in advanced gastric cancer. Cancer Treat Rep 1979; 63:1871.

11. Kolaric K, Potrebica V, Cervek J. Phase 2 clinical trial of 4'epidoxórubicin in metastatic solid tumors. J Cancer Res Clin Oncol 1983; 106:148—52.

12. Robustelli Della Cuna G, Ganzina F, Tramarin R, Pavesi L. Phase 2 evaluation of 4'epidoxorubicin in advanced solid tumors. 12th Int Cong Chemother, Florence, Italy; 1982; 75.

13. Holdener EE, ten Bokkel WH, Hansen HH, et al. Phase 2 trial of 4'-deoxydoxorubicin (4'-deoxyDX) in advanced gastrointestinal cancer. Proc Am Soc Clin Oncol 1984; 3:139.

14. Bedikian AY, Stroehlein J, Korinek J, Karlin D, Valdirieso M, Bodey GP. Phase 2 evaluation of dihydroxyanthracenedione (DHAD, NSC 301739) in patients with upper gastrointestinal tumors: a preliminary report. Am J Clin Oncol 1983; 6:473—76.

15. Leichman L, MacDonald B, Dindogru A, Samson M. Platinum: a clinically active drug in advanced adenocarcinoma of the stomach. Proc Am Assoc Clin Res 1982; 23:110.

16. Ajani J, Kantarjian H, Kanojia M, Karlin D. Phase 2 trial of cis-platinum in advanced upper gastrointestinal cancer. Proc Am Soc Clin Oncol 1984; 3:147.

17. Gailani S, Holland JF, Falkson G, Leone L, Burningham R, Larsen V. Comparison of treatment of metastatic gastrointestinal cancer with 5-fluorouracil (5-FU) to a combination of 5-FU with cytosine arabinoside. Cancer 1972; 29:1308—13.

18. Falkson G, van Eden EB, Sandison AG. A controlled clinical trial of fluorouracil plus imidazole carboxamide dimethyl triazeno plus vincristine plus bis-chloroethyl nitrosourea plus radiotherapy in stomach cancer. Med Pediatr Oncol 1976; 2:111—17.

19. MacDonald JS, Wooolley PV, Symthe T, Ueno W, Hoth D, Schein PS. 5-fluorouracil, Adriamycin, and mitomycin-C (FAM) combination chemotherapy in the treatment of advanced gastric cancer. Cancer 1979; 44:42—47.

20. MacDonald JS, Schein PS, Woolley PV, et al. 5-fluorouracil, mitomycin-C, and Adriamycin (FAM): a new combination chemotherapy program for advanced gastric carcinoma. Ann Intern Med 1980; 93:533.

21. Bitran JD, Desser RK, Kozloff MF, Billings AA, Shapiro CM. Treatment of metastatic pancreatic and gastric adenocarcinomas with 5-fluorouracil, Adriamycin, and mitomycin-C (FAM). Cancer Treat Rep 1979; 63:2049—51.

22. Haim N, Cohen Y, Honizman J, Robinson E. Treatment of advanced gastric carcinoma with 5-fluorouracil, Adriamycin and mitomycin-C (FAM). Cancer Chemother Pharmacol 1982; 8:277—80.

23. Beretta G, Fraschini P, Labianca R, Luponini G. The value of FAM polychemotherapy in advanced gastric carcinoma. Proc ASCO 1982; 1:C-400.

24. Biran H, Sulkes A. A possible dose response relationship in "FAM" chemotherapy for advanced gastric cancer. Proc Am Soc Clin Oncol 1984; 3:132.

25. Haim N, Epelbaum R, Cohen Y, Robinson E. Further studies on the treatment of advanced gastric cancer by 5-fluorouracil, Adriamycin (doxorubicin), and mitomycin-C (modified FAM). Cancer 1984; 54:1999—2002.

26. Gastrointestinal Tumor Study Group. A comparative clinical assessment of combination chemotherapy in the management of advanced gastric cancer. Cancer 1982; 49:1362—66.

27. Douglass HO, Lavin PT, Goudsmit A, Klassen DJ. Phase 2-3 evaluation of combinations of

methyl-CCNU, mitomycin-C, Adriamycin and 5-fluorouracil in advanced measurable gastric cancer. Proc Am Soc Clin Oncol 1983; 2:121.

28. Gastrointestinal Tumor Study Group. Randomized study of combination chemotherapy in unresectable gastric cancer. Cancer 1984; 53:13 – 17.

29. Panettiere FJ, Haas C, McDonald B, et al. Drug combination in the treatment of gastric adenocarcinoma: a randomized Southwest Oncology Group study. J Clin Oncol 1984; 2:420 – 24.

30. Cullinan S, Moertel C, Fleming T, Everson L, Krook J, Schutt A. A randomized comparison of 5-FU alone (F), 5-FU + Adriamycin (FA) and 5-FU + Adriamycin + mitomycin-C (FAM) in gastric and pancreatic cancer. Proc Am Soc Clin Oncol 1984; 3:137.

31. Woolley P, Smith F, Estevez R, et al. A phase 2 trial of 5-FU, Adriamycin, and cisplatin (FAP) in advanced gastric cancer. Proc Am Assoc Cancer Res 1981; 22:455.

32. Wagner DJM, Burghouts JMM, van Dam FE, et al. A phase 2 trial of 5-fluorouracil, Adriamycin and cisplatin (FAP) in advanced gastric cancer. Proc Am Soc Clin Oncol 1983; 2:115.

33. Moertel C, Fleming T, O'Connell M, Schutt A, Rubin J. A phase 2 trial of combined intensive course 5-fluorouracil, Adriamycin and cisplatin in advanced gastric and pancreatic carcinoma. Proc Am Soc Clin Oncol 1984; 3:137.

34. Bruckner HW, Stablein DM. Single arm trials of triazinate, cisplatin, and methotrexate combinations in advanced gastric cancer. Proc Am Soc Clin Oncol 1984; 3:144.

35. Vogl S, Engstrom PF. Cisplatin, doxorubicin, and 5-fluorouracil in combination for advanced gastric cancer. Cancer Treat Rep 1984; 68:1273 – 79.

36. Haas C, Oishi N, McDonald B, Coltman C, O'Bryan R. Southwest Oncology Group phase 2-3 gastric cancer study: 5-fluorouracil, Adriamycin and mitomycin-C + vincristine (FAM versus V-FAM) compared to chlorozotocin (CZT), m-AMSA, and dihydroxyanthracenedione (DHAD) with unimpressive differences. Clinical trials: gastrointestinal tract. Proc Am Soc Clin Oncol 1983; 2:122.

37. Beretta G, Fraschini P, Ravaioli A, Amadori D, Luporini G. FA/FAMB polychemotherapy for advanced carcinoma of the stomach (ACS): a randomized study. Clinical trials: gastrointestinal tract. Proc Am Soc Clin Oncol 1983; 2:131.

38. Carter SK, Comis RL. Adenocarcinoma of the pancreas, prognostic variables, and criteria of response. In: Staquet MJ, ed. Cancer therapy: prognostic factors and criteria of response. New York: Raven Press, 1975; 237.

39. Douglass HO Jr, Lavin PT, Moertel CG. Nitrosoureas: useful agents for treatment of advanced gastrointestinal cancer. Cancer Treat Rep 1976; 60:769.

40. Broder LE, Carter SK. Streptozotocin: clinical brochure. Bethesda: Thereapy Evaluation Program, National Cancer Institute, 1971.

41. Dupriest RW, Hintington M, Massey WH, Wiess AJ, Wilson WL, Fletcher WS. Streptozotocin therapy in 22 cancer patients. Cancer 1974; 35:358 – 67.

42. Stolinsky DC, Sadoff L, Braunwald J, Bateman JR. Streptozotocin in the treatment of cancer: phase 2 study. Cancer 1972; 30:61 – 67.

43. Schein PS, Lavin PT, Moertel CG, et al. Randomized phase 2 clinical trial of Adriamycin, methotrexate and actinomycin-D, in advanced measurable pancreatic carcinoma. A Gastrointestinal Tumor Study Group report. Cancer 1978; 42:19 – 22.

44. Nicoletto O, Vinante O, Cartei G. Clinical activity of 4'-epi-doxorubicin in advanced pancreatic adenocarcinoma (abstr). EORTC Symp on treatment of advanced gastrointestinal cancer. Padova 23, 1983.

45. Hochster H, Green M, Speyer J, Blum R, Wernz J, Muggia F. Activity of 4'-epidoxorubicin (EPIDX) in hepatoma (HEP) and pancreatic cancer (PANC). Proc Am Soc Clin Oncol 1984; 3:147.

46. Horton J, Gelbert RD, Engstrom P, et al. Trials of single-agent and combiantion chemotherapy for advanced cancer of the pancreas. Cancer Treat Rep 1981; 65:65 – 68.

47. Loehrer PJ, Williams SD, Einhorn LH, Estes NC. A phase 1-2 trial of ifosfamide (IFOS) and N-acetylcysteine (NAC) in advanced pancreatic cancer (PC). Proc Am Soc Clin Oncol 1984; 3:149.

48. Lokich J, Chawla PL, Brooks J, Frei E III. Chemotherapy in pancreatic carcinoma: 5-fluorouracil (5-FU) and 1,3 Bis-(2 chlorethyl)-1-nitrosourea (BCNU). Ann Surg 1974; 179(4):450 – 53.

49. Wiggans G, Woolley PV, MacDonald JS, Smythe T, Ueno W, Schein PS. Phase 2 trial of strepto-zotocin, mitomycin-C and 5-fluorouracil (SMF) in the treatment of advanced pancreatic cancer. Cancer 1978; 41:387 – 95.

50. Bukoski RM, Abderhalten RT, Hewlett JS. Phase 2 trial of streptozotocin, mitomycin-C and 5-fluorouracil in adenocarcinoma of the pancreas. Cancer Clin Trials 1980; 3:321.

51. Bitran JD, Desser RK, Kozloff MF, Billings AA, Shapiro CM. Treatment of metastatic pancreatic and gastric adenocarcinoma with 5-fluorouracil, Adriamycin and mitomycin-C (FAM). Cancer Treat Rep 1979; 63:2049 – 51.

52. Smith FP, Hoth DF, Levin BL. 5-fluorouracil, Adriamycin and mitomycin-C (FAM) chemother-apy for advanced adenocarcinoma of the pancreas. Cancer 1980; 46:2014.

53. Sternberg CN, Magill GB, Sordillo PP, Cheng E. Preliminary trial of MIFA III (mitomycin-C, 5-fluorouracil and Adriamycin) in adenocarcinoma of the pancreas. Clinical trials: gastrointestinal tract. Proc Am Soc Clin Oncol 1982; 1:99.

54. Smith FP, Stablein DM, Schein PS. Phase 2 combination chemotherapy trials in advanced measur-able pancratic cancer. Proc Am Soc Clin Oncol 1984; 3:151.

55. Oster MW, Theologides A, Cooper MR, et al. Fluorouracil (F) + Adriamycin (A) + mitomycin (M) (FAM) versus fluorouracil (F) + streptozotocin (S) + mitomycin (M) (FSM) in advanced pancreatic cancer. Proc Am Soc Clin Oncol 1982; 1:90.

56. Bukowski RM, Schacter LP, Groppe CW. Phase 2 trial of 5-fluorouracil, Adriamycin, mitomycin-C and streptozotocin (FAM-S) in pancreatic carcinoma. Cancer 1982; 50:197.

57. Smith FP, Priego V, Lokey L, et al. Phase 2 evaluation of hexamethylmelamine + FAM (HEXA - FAM) in advanced measurable pancreatic cancer (PC). Proc Am Soc Clin Oncol 1983; 2:126.

58. Smith FP, Rustgi VK, Schertz G, Woolley PV, Schein PS. Phase 2 study of 5-FU, doxorubicin and mitomycin (FAM) and chlorozotocin in advanced measurable pancreatic cancer. Cancer Treat Rep 1982; 66(12):2095 – 96.

59. Gisselbrecht C, Smith FP, Woolley PV, et al. Phase 2 trial of FAP (5-fluorouracil, Adriamycin and cisdiammin dichloroplatinum) chemotherapy for advanced measurable pancreatic cancer (PC) and adeno-carcinoma of unknown origin (AUO). Proc Am Soc Clin Oncol 1981; 22:454.

60. Falkson G. The management of tumours of the liver and biliary tract. In: Carter SK, Gladstein E, Livingston RB, eds. Principles of cancer treatment. New York: McGraw Hill, 1982; 426 – 433.

61. Haskell CM. Cancer of the liver. In: Haskell CM, ed. Cancer treatment. Philadelphia: WB Saun-ders, 1980; 319 – 570.

62. Cambareri RJ, Smith FP, Kales A, Warren R, Woolley PV, Schein PS. 5-fluorouracil, Adriamycin and mitomycin-C in cholangiocarcinoma. Proc Am Soc Clin Oncol 1980; 21:419.

63. Harvey JH, Smith FP, Schein PS. 5-fluorouracil, mitomycin, and doxorubicin (FAM) in carci-noma of the biliary tract. J Clin Oncol 1984; 2(11).

64. Falkson G, MacIntyre JM, Moertel CG. Eastern Cooperative Oncology Group experience with chemotherapy for inoperable gallbladder and bile duct cancer. Cancer 1984; 54:965 – 69.

65. Sullivan RD, Young CW, Miller E, Gladstein E, Clarkson B, Burchenal JH. The clinical effects of the continuous administration of fluorinated pyrimidines (5-fluorouracil and 5-fluoro-2'-deoxyuridine). Cancer Treat Res 1960; 8:77 – 83.

66. Reitemeier RJ, Moertel CG. Comparison of rapid and slow intravenous administration of 5-fluorouracil in treating patients with advanced carcinoma of the large intestine. Cancer Chemother Rep 1962; 25:87 – 89.

67. Seifert P, Baker LH, Reed ML, Vaitkevicius VK. Comparison of continuously infused 5-fluorouracil with bolus injection in treatment of patients with colorectal adenocarcinoma. Cancer 1975; 36:123 – 28.

68. Grillo-Lopez AZ, Velez-Garcia E, Elliott A. Survival of patients with advanced gastrointestinal cancer treated with 5-fluorouracil (5-FU) Proc Am Soc Clin Oncol, 1977.

69. Nixon DW, Vogler WR, Jacobs J, Heffner LT, Winton EF, Garrett PR. Phase 1 study of 5-FU — methyl CCNU — methotrexate with leucovorin in advanced adenocarcinoma. Proc Am Cancer Res 1978; 19:326.

70. Hartman HA Jr, Kessinger A, Lemon HM, Foley JF. Five-day continuous infusion of 5-fluorouracil for advanced colorectal, gastric, and pancreatic adenocarcinoma. J Surg Oncol 1979; 11:227 — 38.

71. Krauss S, Sonoda T, Solomon A. Treatment of advanced gastrointestinal cancer with 5-fluorouracil and mitomycin-C. Cancer 1979; 43:1598 — 1603.

72. Lokich JJ. Protracted ambulatory venous infusion of chemotherapeutic agents (meeting). Strategies for clinical cancer 22 — 24, 1980.

73. Lokich JJ, Bothe A, Fine N, et al. Phase 1 study of protracted venous infusion of 5-fluorouracil. Cancer 1981; 48:2565 — 68.

74. Lokich JJ, Philips D, Perri J, et al. Cancer chemotherapy via ambulatory infusion pump. Am J Clin Oncol (CCT) 1983; 6:355 — 63.

75. Vaughn CB, Brady P, Chinn BJ, Daversa GC, Parzuchowski JS. Combination chemotherapy in advanced gastrointestinal malignancy. Oncology 1980; 37:57 — 61.

76. Bruckner HW, Storch JA, Brown JC, Goldberg J, Chamberlin K. Phase 2 trial of combination chemotherapy for pancreatic cancer with 5-fluorouracil, mitomycin-C and hexamethylmelamine. Oncology 1983; 40:165 — 69.

77. Cazap E. Phase 2 study of bleomycin (BL) by 5-day continuous intravenous infusion (5-CII) in advanced adenocarcinoma (AA). Proc Am Soc Clin Oncol 1984; 3:45.

78. Bukowski RM, Vaughn CB, Hampton J, Stuckey WJ. Anguidine in gastrointestinal malignancies: SWOG phase 2 study (meeting abstr). Proc Am Assoc Cancer Res 1980; 21:352.

79. Falkson G, Lombaard CM, McDonald TPS. the Treatment of advanced cancer with intra-arterial triethyleneglycol diglycidyl ether. S Afr Cancer Bull 1964; 8:3 — 17.

80. Geddes EW, Falkson G. Malignant hepatoma in the Bantu. Cancer 1970; 25:1271 — 78.

81. Freckman HA. Arterial infusion chemotherapy. In: Badellino F, ed. 4th int symp on locoregional treatment of tumors — III. Saint Vincent: Pan Med 17:277 — 79.

82. Davis HL Jr, Ramirez G, Ansfield FJ. Adenocarcinomas of stomach, pancreas, liver and biliary tracts (survival of 328 patients treated with fluoropyrimidine therapy). Cancer 1974; 33:193 — 97.

83. Yoshikawa, K. Ten years experience with intra-aortic infusion chemotherapy for gastrointestinal malignant tumors. Proc in Oncol 1981; 11(2):351.

84. Theodor A, Livingston RB, Bukowski RM, Weick JK, Hewlett JS. Intermittent regional infusion of chemotherapy for pancreatic adenocarcinoma. Am J Clin Oncol (CCT) 1982; 5:555 — 58.

85. Marlow Lord Smith, Gazet JC. Intra-arterial chemotherapy for patients with inoperable carcinoma of the pancreas. Ann R Coll Surg Eng 1980; 62:208 — 12.

86. Vogelzang NJ. Continuous infusion chemotherapy: a critical review. J Clin Oncol 1984; 2:1289 — 1304.

87. Lokich JJ, Becker B. Subclavian vein thrombosis in patients treated with infusion chemotherapy for advanced malignancy. Cancer 1983; 52:1586 — 89.

88. Clouse ME, Ahmed R, Ryan RB, et al. Complications of long-term transbrachial hepatic arterial infusion chemotherapy. Am J Roentgenol 1977; 129:799 — 803.

89. Anderson JR, Cain KC, Gelber RD, Gelman RS. Analysis and interpretation of the comparison of survival by treatment outcome variables in cancer clinical trials. Cancer Treat Symp (in press).

References—Chapter 24

1. Vogelzang NJ. Continuous infusion chemotherapy: a critical review. J Clin Oncol 1984; 2:1289 — 1304.

2. Legha SS, Benjamin RS, Mackay B, et al. Adriamycin therapy by continuous intravenous infusion in patients with metastatic breast cancer. Cancer 1982; 9:1762−66.

3. Tannir Z, Yap HY, Hortobagyi GH, Hug V, Buzdar AU, Blumenschein GR. Sequential continuous infusion with doxorubicin and vinblastine: an effective chemotherapy combination for patients with advanced breast cancer previously treated with cyclophosphamide, methotrexate, 5-FU, vincristine and prednisone. Cancer Treat Rep 1984; 68:1039−41.

4. Bitran JD, Desser RK, Kozloff MF, Shapiro CM, Robin E, Billings AA. Continuous infusion Adriamycin and Velban chemotherapy in refractory, stage 4 adenocarcinoma of the breast. Proc Am Soc Clin Oncol (Abstr C381) 1983; 2:98.

5. Legha SS, Benjamin RS., Mackay B, et al. Reduction of doxorubicin cardiotoxicity by prolonged continuous intravenous infusion. Ann Intern Med 1982; 96:133−39.

6. Legha SS, Benjamin R, Ewer M, et al. Reduction of Adriamycin cardiotoxicity by continuous IV infusion: the effect of duration of infusion on cardiotoxicity. Proc Am Assoc Cancer Res (Abstr 499) 1982; 23:127.

7. Hortobagyi G, Frye D, Blumenschein G, et al. FAC with Adriamycin by continuous infusion for treatment of advanced breast cancer. Proc Am Soc Clin Oncol (Abstr C408) 1983; 2:105.

8. Legha S, Benjamin R, Mackay B, et al. Reutilization of Adriamycin in previously treated patients. Proc Am Soc Clin Oncol (Abstr C792) 1981; 22:534.

9. Yap HY, Blumenschein GR, Keating MJ, Hortobagyi GN, Tashima CK, Loo TL. Vinblastine given as a continuous 5-day infusion in the treatment of refractory advanced breast cancer. Cancer Treat Rep 1980; 64:279−83.

10. Ingle JN, Ahmann DL, Gerstner JG, Green SJ, O'Connell MJ, Kvols LK. Evaluation of vinblastine administered by 5-day continuous infusion in women with advanced breast cancer. Cancer Treat Rep 1984; 68:803−04.

11. Fraschini G, Yap HY, Barnes BC, Buzdar AU, Hortobagyi GN, Blumenschein GR. Continuous five-day infusion of vinblastine for refractory metastatic breast cancer. Proc Am Soc Clin Oncol (Abstr C302) 1982; 1:78.

12. Yap HY, Blumenschein GR, Bodey GP, Hortobagyi GN, Buzdar AU, DiStefano A. Vindesine in the treatment of refractory breast cancer: improvement in therapeutic index with continous 5-day infusion. Cancer Treat Rep 1981; 65:775−79.

13. Fleishman GB, Yap HY, Bodey GP, Chuang VP, Blumenschein GR. Comparability in therapeutic index with continuous 5-day infusion and 5-day bolus vindesine in the treatment of refractory breast cancer. Proc Am Soc Clin Oncol (Abstr C316) 1982; 1:82.

14. Yau JC, Yap HW, Buzdar AU, Hortobagyi GN, Bodey GP, Blumenschein GR. A comparative randomized trial of vinca alkaloids in patients with metastatic breast carcinoma. Cancer 1985; 55:337−40.

15. Bedikian AY, Bodey GP. Phase 1 study of cyclophosphamide (NSC 26271) by 72-hour continuous intravenous infusion. Am J Clin Oncol 1983; 6:365−68.

16. Yap HY, Valdivieso M, Blumenschein G, Hortobagyi G, Bedikian A. A phase 1-2 study of continuous 5-day infusion mitomycin-C. Am J Clin Oncol 1983; 6:109−12.

17. Seifert P, Baker LH, Reed ML, Vaitkevicius VK. Comparison of continuously infused 5-fluorouracil with bolus injection in treatment of patients with colorectal adenocarcinoma. Cancer 1975; 36:123−28.

18. Malik R, Blumenschein GR, Legha SS, et al. A randomized trial of high-dose 5-fluorouracil, doxorubicin and cyclophosphamide vs. conventional FAC regimen in metastatic breast cancer. Proc Am Soc Clin Oncol (Abstr C303) 1982; 1:79.

19. Schell FC, Yap HY, Hortobagyi GN, Issell B, Esparza L. Phase 2 study of VP16-213 (etoposide) in refractory metastatic breast carcinoma. Cancer Chemother Pharmacol 1982; 7:223−25.

20. Forastiere AA, Hakes TB, Wittes JT, Wittes RE. Cisplatin in the treatment of metastatic breast carcinoma. Am J Clin Oncol 1982; 5:243−47.

21. Yap HY, Salem P, Hortobagyi GN, et al. Phase 2 study of cis-dichlorodiammineplatinum (II) in advanced breast cancer. Cancer Treat Rep 1978; 62:405−08.

References—Chapter 25

1. Vogelzang NJ. Continuous infusion chemotherapy: a critical review. J Clin Oncol 1984; 2:1289–1304.

2. Lokich JJ, Perri J, Bothe A Jr., et al. Ambulatory pump infusion chemotherapy: clinical trials of 5 agents, 125 patients. Proc Am Assoc. Cancer Res (abstr. 518) 1982; 23:132.

3. Gregoriadis G. Targeting of drugs: implications in medicine. Lancet 1981; 2:241–46.

4. Gabizon A, Dagan A, Goren D. Barenholz Y, Fuks Z. Liposomes as in vivo carriers of Adriamycin: reduced cardiac uptake and antitumor activity in mice. Cancer Res 1982; 42:4734–39.

5. Ross DD, Joneckis CC, Schiffer CA. Effects of verapamil on in vitro intracellular accumulation and retention of daunorubicin in marrow cell blasts from patients with acute nonlymphoblastic leukemia (ANLL). Proc Am Soc Clin Oncol (abstr. C171) 1985; 4:45.

6. Gau TC, Natale RB, Ensminger W, Gyves J, Niederhuber J. A prospective double-blind test of the capacity of the human tumor cloning assay (HTCA) to predict the in vivo sensitivity of hepatic tumors treated with single agents administered by continuous arterial infusion with a totally implantable pump. Proc Am Soc Clin Oncol (abstr. C479) 1983; 2:123.

7. Ferreira PPC. Vincristine infusion in advanced cancer. Proc Am Soc Clin Oncol (abstr C289) 1976; 17:309.

8. Jackson DV Jr., Sethi VS, Spurr CL, et al. Pharmacokinetics of vincristine infusion. Cancer Treat Rep 1981; 65:1043–48.

9. Jackson DV, Sethi VS, Spurr CL, et al. Intravenous vincristine infusion: phase 1 trial. Cancer 1981; 48:2559–64.

10. Weber W, Nagel GA, Nagel-Studer E, Albrecht R. Vincristine infusion: a phase 1 study. Cancer Chemother Pharmacol 1979; 3:49–55.

11. Jackson D, Spurr C, Richards F, et al. Vincristine infusion in refractory multiple myeloma. Proc Am Soc Clin Oncol (abstr C839) 1985; 4:216.

12. Jackson DV, Paschold EH, Spurr CL, et al. Treatment of advanced non-Hodgkin's lymphoma with vincristine infusion. Cancer 1984; 53:2601–06.

13. Paschold EH, Jackson DV Jr., Spurr CL, et al. Continuous infusion of vincristine (VCR) and vinblastine (VLB) in refractory lymphoma: a phase 2 study. Proc Am Soc Clin Oncol (abstr C618) 1982; 1:159.

14. Lu K, Yap H-Y, Loo TL. Clinical pharmacokinetics of vinblastine by continuous infusion. Cancer Res 1983; 43:1404–08.

15. Yap H-Y, Blumenschein GR, Keating MJ, Hortobagyi GN, Tashima CK, Loo TL. Vinblastine given as a continuous five-day infusion in the treatment of refractory-advanced breast cancer. Cancer Treat Rep 1980; 64:279–83.

16. Zeffren J, Yagoda A, Kelson G. Phase 1 trial of a 5-day infusion of vinblastine. Proc Am Assoc Cancer Res 1980; 21:1978.

17. Lokich JJ, Zipoli TE, Perri J, Bothe A Jr. Protracted vinblastine infusion. Phase 1–2 study in malignant melanoma and other tumors. Am J Clin Oncol 1984; 7:551–53.

18. Yap H-Y, Blumenschein GR, Bodey GP, Hortobagyi GN, Buzdar AU, DiStefano A. Vindesine in the treatment of refractory breast cancer: improvement in therapeutic index with continuous five-day infusion. Cancer Treat Rep 1981; 65:775–79.

19. Fleishman GB, Yap HY, Bodey GP, Chuang VP, Blumenchein GR. Comparability in therapeutic index with continuous 5-day infusion and 5-day bolus vindesine in the treatment of refractory breast cancer. Cancer Treat Rep 1981; 65:775–79.

20. Maraninchi D, Gastaut JA, Tubiana N, Carcassonne Y. Etude de la vindesine en perfusion de 5 jours dans le traitment de leucemies et lymphomes. Bull Cancer 1981; 68:338–42.

21. Lokich JJ, Corkery J. A phase 1 study of VP-16-213 (etoposide) administered as a continuous five-day infusion. Cancer Treat Rep 1981; 65:887–89.

22. Aisner J, Van Echo DA, Whitacre M, Wiernik PH. A phase 1 trial of continuous infusion VP-16-213 (etoposide). Cancer Chemother Pharmacol 1982; 7:157–60.

23. Ho DHW, Kanellopoulos KA, Yap H-Y et al. Clinical pharmacology of etoposide by radioimmunoassay. Proc Am Assoc Cancer Res (abstr 519) 1983; 24:131.

24. Sessa C, D'Incalci M, Farina P, Rossi C, Cavalli F, Mangioni C, Garattini S. Pharmacokinetics of VM 26 after 60 minutes or 24 hours continuous infusion. Proc Am Assoc Cancer Res (abstr 502) 1982; 23:128.

25. Riggs CE Jr., Tipping SJ, Angelou JE, Bachur NR, Wiernik PH. Human pharmacokinetics of continuous infusion Adriamycin (ADR). Proc Am Soc Clin Oncol (abstr C126) 1983; 2:32.

26. Legha SS, Benjamin RS, MacKay B, et al. Reduction of doxorubicin cardiotoxicity by prolonged continuous intravenous infusion. Ann Intern Med 1982; 96:133–39.

27. Weiss AJ, Manthel RW. Experience with the use of doxorubicin in combination with other anti-cancer agents using a weekly schedule with particular reference to lack of toxicity. Cancer 1977; 40:2046–52.

28. Lokich J, Bothe A Jr., Zipoli T, et al. Constant infusion schedule for Adriamycin: a phase 1–2 clinical trial of a 30–day schedule by ambulatory pump delivery system. J Clin Oncol 1983; 1:24–28.

29. Torti FM, Bristow MR, Howes AE, et al. Reduced cardiotoxicity of doxorubicin delivered on a weekly schedule. Ann Intern Med 1983; 99:745–49.

30. Chlebowski RT, Paroly WJ, Pugh RP, et al. Doxorubicin given as a weekly schedule without a loading course: clinically effective with reduced incidence of cardiotoxicity. Cancer Treat Rep 1980; 64:47–51.

31. Green MD, Speyer JS, Blum R, Wernz J, Muggia FM. The effect of six-hour infusions of doxorubicin (ADR) on anthracycline cardiotoxicity. Proc Am Soc Clin Oncol (abstr C100) 1983; 2:26.

32. Lokich JJ, Perri J. Protracted venous infusion of Adriamycin by portable infusion pump. Proc Am Soc Clin Oncol (abstr C85) 1982; 1:21.

33. Garnick MB, Weiss GR, Steele GD Jr., et al. Clinical evaluation of long-term continuous infusion doxorubicin. Cancer Treat Rep 1983; 67:133–43.

34. Legha SS, Benjamin RS, MacKay B, et al. Doxorubicin therapy by continuous intravenous infusion in patients with metastatic breast cancer. Cancer 1982; 49:1762–66.

35. Legha SS, Benjamin R, Ewer M, et al. Reduction of Adriamycin cardiotoxicity by continuous I.V. infusion: the effect of duration of infusion on cardiotoxicity. Proc Am Assoc Cancer Res (abstr 499) 1982; 23:127.

36. Straus MJ, Moran RE. Comparison of toxicity and antitumor effect of pulse and continuous infusion schedule of Adriamycin in CDF₁ mice. Proc Am Assoc Cancer Res (abstr 694) 1982; 23:177.

37. Drewinko B, Novak JK, Barranco SC. The response of human lymphoma cells in vitro to bleomycin and 1, 3 bis (2-chlorethyl)-1-nitrosourea. Cancer Res 1972; 32:1206–08.

38. Haas CD, Coltman CA, Gottlieb JA, et al. Phase 2 evaluation of bleomycin. Cancer 1976; 38:8–12.

39. Krakoff IH, Cvitkovic E, Currie V, Yeh S, LaMonte C. Clinical pharmacology and therapeutic studies of bleomycin given by continuous infusion. Cancer 1977; 40:2027–37.

40. Sikic BI, Collins JM, Mimnaugh EG, Gram TE. Improved therapeutic index of bleomycin when administered by continuous infusion in mice. Cancer Treat Rep 1978; 62:2011–17.

41. Cooper KR, Hong WK. Prospective study of the pulmonary toxicity of continuously infused bleomycin. Cancer Treat Rep 1981; 65:419–25.

42. Seibert K, Golub G, Smiledge P, Nystrom JS. Continuous streptozotocin infusion: a phase 1 study. Cancer Treat Rep 1979; 63:2035–37.

43. Solidoro A, Otero J, Vallejos C, et al. Intermittent continuous I.V. infusion of high-dose cyclophosphamide for remission induction in acute lymphocytic leukemia. Cancer Treat Rep 1981; 65:213–18.

44. Steuber CP, Pernbach DJ, Starling KA. High-dose cyclophosphamide (NSC 26271) therapy in childhood acute leukemia. Cancer Chemother Rep 1974; 58:417–19.

45. Kreis W, Budman DR, Vinciguerra V, et al. Phase 1 continuous infusion of triethylenethiophosphamide (thio-tepa) over 48 hours. Proc Am Assoc Cancer Res (abstr 552) 1983; 24:140.

46. Richardson VJ, Ryman BE. Effect of liposomally trapped antitumor drugs on a drug-resistant mouse lymphoma in vivo. Br J Cancer 1982; 45:552.

47. Skipper H, Schabel F, Wilcox W. Experimental evaluation of potential anticancer agents. XXI scheduling of arabino-sylcytosine to take advantage of its S-phase specificity against leukemia cells. Cancer Chemother Rep 1967; 51:125–65.

48. Kantarjian H, Barlogie B, Plunkett W, et al. High-dose cytosine arabinoside in non-Hodgkin's lymphoma. J Clin Oncol 1983; 1:689–94.

49. Capizzi, RL, Yang J-L, Cheng E, et al. Alteration of the pharmacokinetics of high-dose ara-C by its metabolite, high ara-U, in patients with acute leukemia. J Clin Oncol 1983; 1:763-71.

50. Slevin ML, Piall EM, Aherne GW, et al. Effect of dose and schedule on pharmacokinetics of high-dose cytosine arabinoside in plasma and cerebrospinal fluid. J Clin Oncol 1983; 1:546–51.

51. Wisch JS, Griffin JD, Kufe DW. Response of preleukemic syndromes to continuous infusion of low-dose cytarbine. N Engl J Med 1983; 309:1599–1602.

52. Kufe DW, Griffin JD, Spriggs DR. Cellular and clinical pharmacology of low-dose ara-C. Sem Oncol 12 (suppl 3) 1985; 200–07.

53. Kreis W, Budman DR, Chan K, et al. Pharmacokinetics of continuous infusion of low-dose cytosine arabinoside (ara-C) in eleven patients. Proc Am Soc Clin Oncol (abstr 150) 1985; 4:40.

54. Sachs L. The differentiation of myeloid leukemia cells: new possibilities for therapy. Br J Haematol 1978; 40:509–17.

55. Griffin J, Munroe D, Major P, Kufe D. Induction of differentiation of human myeloid leukemia cells by inhibitors of DNA synthesis. Exp Hematol 1982; 10:774–81.

56. Castaigne S, Daniel MT, Tilly H, Herait P, Degos L. Does treatment with ara-C in low dosage cause differentiation of leukemic cells? Blood 1983; 62:85–86.

57. Beran M, Andersson BS, Ayyar R, et al. Clinical response and mechanisms of action of low-dose cytosine arabinoside (ara-C) in myelodysplastic syndromes (MDS) and myelogenous leukemia. Proc Am Soc Clin Oncol (abstr C678) 1985; 4:174.

58. Schiff RD, Mertelsmann R, Andreeff M, et al. Low-dose cytarabine (LD ara-C) in RAEB in tansformation (RAEBIT) and poor risk leukemias. Proc Am Soc Clin Oncol (abstr C643) 1985; 4:165.

59. Harousseau JL, Castaigne S, Milpied N, Marty M, Degos L. Treatment of acute nonlymphoblastic leukemia in elderly patients. Lancet II 1984; 288.

60. Degos L, Castaigne S, Tilly H, Sigaux F, Daniel MT. Treatment of leukemia with low-dose ara-C: a study of 160 cases. Sem Oncol 1985; 12:196–99.

61. Desforges JF. Cytarabine: low-dose, high-dose, no dose. N Engl J Med. 1983; 309:1637–39.

62. Preisler H, Royer G, eds. Cytosar-U: therapeutic new dimensions. Sem Oncol (Suppl 3) 1985; 12:1–236.

63. Plunkett W, Liliemark JO. Evidence that accumulation of ara-CTP by leukemic cells is saturated during high dose ara-C infusion: suggestion for increased efficiency of drug administration. Proc Am Soc Clin Oncol (abstr C192) 1985; 4:50.

64. Spriggs DR, Robbins G, Takvorian T, Kufe DW. Continuous infusion of high-dose 1-B-D-arabinofurnasylcytosine: a phase 1 and pharmacological study. Cancer Res 1985; 45:3932–36.

65. Jones GR, Ettinger LJ. Continuous infusion of high-dose cytosine arabinoside (HDARAC) for treatment of childhood acute leukemia and non-Hodgkin's lymphoma in relapse. Blood 1984; 64 (Suppl 1) 166a (abstr 574).

66. Jones G. Ettinger LJ. Continuous infusion of high-dose cytosine arabinoside for treatment of childhood acute leukemia and non-Hodgkin's lymphoma in relapse. Sem Oncol 1985; 12 (Suppl 3), 150–54.

67. Ochs JJ, Look AT, Sinkule J, et al. Continuous infusion high-dose cytosine arabinoside (ara-C) in refractory pediatric leukemia. Proc Am Assoc Cancer Res (abstr 629) 1983; 24:159.

68. Iacoboni S, Plunkett W, Keating M, McCredie K, Frieireich E. Pharmacologic direction of continuous infusion high dose ara-C (CIHDAC) for refractory acute leukemia (RAL) and chronic myelogenous leukemia blast crisis (CML-BC). Proc Am Soc Clin Oncol (abstr C674) 1985; 4:173.

69. Blumenreich MS, Woodcock TM, Andreef M, et al. Effect of very high dose thymidine infusion on leukemia and lymphoma patients. Cancer Res 1984; 44:2203–07.

70. Zittoun R, Marie JP, Zittoun J, Marquet J, Haanen C. Modulation of cytosine arabinoside (Ara-C) and high-dose Ara-C in acute leukemia. Sem Oncol (Suppl 3) 1985; 139–143.

71. Moran RE, Straus MJ. Cytokinetic analysis of L1210 leukemia after continuous infusion of hydroxyurea in vivo. Cancer Res 1979; 39:1616–22.

72. Moran RE, Straus MJ. Synchronization of L1210 leukemia with hydroxyurea infusion and the effect of subsequent pulse dose chemotherapy. Cancer Treat Rep 1980; 64:81–86.

73. Belt RJ, Haas CD, Kennedy J, Taylor S. Studies of hydroxyurea administered by continuous infusion: toxicity, pharmacokinetics, and cell synchronization. Cancer 1980; 46:455–62.

74. Posner MR, Belliveau JF, Ferrari L, et al. Clinical and pharmacokinetic study of five-day continuous infusion cis-platinum. Proc Am Soc Clin Oncol (abstr 145) 1985; 4:38.

75. Salem P, Hall SW, Benjamin RS, et al. Clinical phase 1–2 study of cis-dichlorodiammineplatinum (II) given by continuous IV infusion. Cancer Treat Rep 1978; 62:1553–55.

76. Moran RE, Straus MJ. Effects of pulse and continuous intravenous infusion of cis-diamminedichloroplatinum on L1210 leukemia in vitro. Cancer Res 1981; 41:4993–96.

77. Bedikian AY, Valdivieso M, Bodey GP. Phase 1 clinical studies with gallium nitrate. Cancer Treat Rep 1978; 62:1449–1553.

78. Kelson DP, Alcock N, Yen S, Brown J, Young CW. Pharmacokinetics of gallium nitrate in man. Cancer 1980; 46:2009–13.

79. Warrell RP, Coonley CJ, Straus DJ, Young CW. Treatment of patients with advanced malignant lymphoma using gallium nitrate administered as a seven-day continuous infusion. Cancer 1983; 51:1982–87.

80. Casimir MT, Miller A, Ewer MS, et al. Phase 1 clinical study of 24-hour continuous infusion (CI) aclacinomycin (ACLA) with cardiac and pharmacologic monitoring. Proc Am Soc Clin Oncol (abstr C90) 1982; 1:23.

81. Ehninger G, Proksch B, Heinzel G, Woodward D. Pharmacokinetics and metabolism of mitoxantrone in man. Proc Am Soc Clin Oncol (abstr C105) 1985; 4:28.

82. Gams R, Keller J, Case D, et al. Mitoxantrone in refractory lymphoma. Proc Soc Clin Oncol (abstr C821) 1985; 4:210.

83. Legha SS, Ajani JA, Bodey GP. Phase 1 study of spirogermanium given daily. J Clin Oncol 1983; 1:331–36.

84. Woolley P, Priego V, van Luc, Bollenbacher B, Schein P. A phase 1 trial of spirogermanium administered as a five-day continuous infusion. Proc Am Assoc Cancer Res (abstr 539) 1983; 24:136.

85. Coonley CJ, Warrell RP Jr., Young CW. Phase 1 trial of homoharringtonine administered as a 5-day continuous infusion. Proc Am Assoc Cancer Res (abstr 537) 1983; 24:136.

86. Neidhart JA, Kraut E, Metz EN, Howenstein B. Phase 1 study of homoharringtonine (HH) administered by prolonged continuous infusion. Proc Am Soc Clin Oncol (abstr C188) 1985; 4:49.

87. Boyd AW, Sullivan JR. Leukemic cell differentiation in vivo and in vitro: arrest of proliferation parallels the differentiation induced by the antileukemic drug harringtonine. Blood 1984; 63:384–92.

88. Lee EJ, van Echo DA, Egorin MJ, Mayar B, Schulman P, Schiffer CA. A phase 1–2 study of continuous infusion diaziquone (AZQ) for refractory adult leukemia. Proc Am Soc Clin Oncol (abstr 759) 1984; 3:195.

89. Whitacre MY, van Echo DA, Budman DR, Schulman P, Aisner J, Wiernik PH. A phase 1 trial of 5-day continuous infusion aziridinylenzoquinone (AZQ, NSC 182986) Proc Am Soc Clin Oncol (abstr C94) 1982; 1:24.

90. Sinkule JA, Murphy SB, Evans WE, Rivera G. Pharmacodynamics of continuous infusion 2'-Deoxycoformycin (dCF) in refractory acute lymphoblastic leukemia (ALL). Proc Am Assoc Cancer Res (abstr 535) 1983; 24:135.

91. Klein HO, Wickramanayake PD, Christian E, Coerper C. Therapeutic effects of single-push or fractionated injection or continuous infusion of oxazaphosphorines (cyclophosphamide, ifosfamide, ASTA Z7557). Cancer 1984; 54:1193–1203.

92. Bodner AJ, Ting RC, Gallo RC. Induction of differentiation of human promyelocytic leukemia cells HL-60 by nucleoside and methotrexate. J Natl Cancer Inst 1981; 67:1025.

93. Christman JK, Mendelsohn N, Herzog D, Schneiderman V. Effect of 5-azacytidine on differentiation and DNA methylation in human promyelocytic leukemia cell (HL-60). Cancer Res 1983; 43: 763–70.

94. Pinto A, Attadia V, Fusco A, Ferrara F, Spada OA, DiFiore PP. 5-AZA-2'-deoxycytidine induces terminal differentiation of leukemic blasts from patients with acute myeloid leukemias. Blood 1984; 64:922–29.

95. Coleman M, Boyd DB, Berhhardt B, Gerstein G, Silver RT, Pasmantier R, Knope S. COPBLAM III: combination chemotherapy for diffuse large cell lymphoma (LCL) with cyclophosphamide (c), infusional oncovin (0), prednisone (P), infusional bleomycin (BL), Adriamycin (A), and matulane (M). Proc Am Soc Clin Oncol (abstr C964) 1984; 3:246.

96. Hollister D Jr., Silver RT, Gordon B, Coleman M. Continuous infusion vinblastine and bleomycin with high dose methotrexate for resistant non-Hodgkin's lymphoma. Cancer 1982; 50:1690–94.

97. Kaplon M, Jackson DV, Spurr CL, et al. VP-16-213 ± vincristine (VCR) infusion in refractory non-Hodgkin's lymphoma (NHL). Proc Am Soc Clin Oncol (abstr 789) 1985; 4:202.

98. Barlogie B, Smith L, Alexanian R. Effective treatment of advanced multiple myeloma refractory to alkylating agents. N Engl J Med 1984; 310:1353–56.

99. Lewis JP, Meyers F, Armstrong O, Tanaka L. Continuous infusion daunomycin (DNM) in remission induction of acute nonlymphoblastic leukemia (ANLL). Blood (abstr 725) 1983; 62 (Suppl 1):205.

100. Kalwinsky D, Crom W, Mirro J, Evans W, Fridland A, Dahl G. Combined continuous infusions of etoposide (VP-16) and cytarabine (ara-C) in childhood acute myelogenous leukemia (AML) clinical and pharmacologic effects. Proc Am Soc Clin Oncol (abstr C608) 1985; 4:156.

101. Price LA, Hill BT. Reduced toxicity of etoposide (VP16-213) alone and in combination chemotherapy using 24-hour approach: a feasibility study. Proc Am Soc Clin Oncol (abstr C770) 1985; 4:198.

102. Ginsberg SJ, Crooke ST, Bloomfield CD, et al. Cyclophosphamide, doxorubicin, vincristine and low-dose continuous infusion bleomycin in non-Hodgkin's lymphoma. Cancer 1982; 49:1346–52.

103. Ginsberg S, Anderson J, Bloomfield C, et al. Therapy for advanced intermediate grade lymphoma with cyclophosphamide, Adriamycin, vincristine and prednisone with or without bleomycin (CAVPB vs CAVP) followed by high-dose methotrexate or standard dose methotrexate (HMTX vs LMTX): a randomized trial. Proc Am Soc Clin Oncol (abstr C786) 1985; 4:202.

104. Williams SF, Gaynor E, Watson S, Ultmanon JE. Management of advanced, resistant Hodgkin's disease (HD) and non-Hodgkin's lymphoma (NHL) with a noncross-resistant drug program: cisplatinum (P), VP-16 (E), bleomycin (B), lomustine (CCNU), or cormustine (BCNU) and methotrexate (MTX) with leucovorum (L). A phase 2 study. Proc Am Soc Clin Oncol (abstr 797) 1985; 4:204.

105. Guthrie TH. Continuous infusion cyclophosphamide, cytosine arabinoside, vincristine, and prednisone (HIC-OAP) is an effective, well tolerated therapy for refractory adult acute leukemia (RAAL). Blood 1984; 64:(Suppl 1) 165a.

106. Fiere D, Campos L, Coiffier B, et al. Intensive timed chemotherapy for 51 acute myeloid leukemia patients with poor prognosis. Sem Oncol 12 (suppl 3) 1985; 12:130–32.

107. Gisselbrecht C, Lepage E, Fermand JP, et al. Diffuse non-Hodgkin's lymphoma (NHL): treatment by intensive induction. Proc Am Soc Clin Oncol (abstr C782) 1985; 4:201.

108. Hainsworth JD, Wolff SN, Stein RS, Greer JP, Collins RD, Greco FA. Treatment of very poor prognosis lymphoid neoplasms with mega COMLA/CHOP, a high-dose modification of the COMLA protocol: preliminary results. Proc Am Soc Clin Oncol (abstr C769) 1985; 4:197.

109. Amadori S, Guglielmi C, Anselmo AP, Cimino G, Papa G, Mandelli F. F-MACHOP: a new intensive chemotherapy program for diffuse aggressive lymphoma. Proc Am Soc Clin Oncol (abstr 772) 1985; 4:198.

References—Chapter 26

1. Cano JP, Israel L, Catalin J. Clinical pharmacokinetics of Cis-DDP in patients after 5-6 days fractionated administration by infusion (20 mg/m^2/day). Communication to 12th Int Cong Chemother. Florence, 1981.

2. Einhorn LH, Donohue J. Cis-diammino dichloro platinum, vinblastine and bleomycin chemotherapy in disseminated testicular cancer. Ann Intern Med 1977; 27:293-98.

3. Haas CD, Coltman CA, Gottlieb JA, et al. Phase 2 evaluation of bleomycin. Cancer 1976; 38:8-12.

4. Okuyama S, Mishina H. Consecutive therapy of cancer aimed at perpetuation of repairable damage: a hypothesis unifying radiotherapy and chemotherapy. J Clin Hematol Oncol 1980; 10:83-93.

5. Einhorn LH, Donohue J. Combination chemotherapy in disseminated testicular cancer. The Indiana University experience. Sem Oncol 1979; 6:87-93.

6. Israel L, Aguilera J, Soudant J, Penot JC, Breau JL, Morere JF. Bleomycin and cisplatinum with or without mitomycin-C in 110 previously untreated patients with head and neck cancer. Am J Clin Oncol 1983; 6:305-11.

7. Cooper KR, Hong WK. Prospective study of the pulmonary toxicity of continuously infused bleomycin. Cancer Treat Rep 1981; 65:419-25.

8. Sikic B, Collins JM, Mimnaugh EG, Gram TE. Improved therapeutic index of bleomycin when administered by continuous infusion in mice. Cancer Treat Rep 1978; 62:2011-17.

9. Peng YM, Albert DS, Chen HSG, Mason N, Hoon TE. Antitumor activity and plasmakinetics of bleomycin by continuous and intermittent administration. Br J Cancer 1980; 41:644-51.

10. Breau JL, Israel L, Pochmalicki G, Spaulding C. Efficacité de la méthylprednisolone dans la prévention des vomissements dus aux chimiothérapies par sels de platine dans un essai randomisé. Nouv Presse Méd 1983; 12:2058.

11. Israel L, Breau JL, Baudelot J, et al. Plasma exchange as a means of decreasing bleomycin induced pulmonary toxicity. Bull Cancer (in press).

12. Longeval E, Klastersky J. Combination chemotherapy with cisplatin and etoposide in thrombopenic squamous cell carcinoma and adenocarcinoma. A study by the EORTC Lung Cancer Working Party (Belgium). Cancer 1982; 50:2751-56.

13. Pedersen AG, Hansen HH. Etoposide (VP-16) in the treatment of lung cancer. Cancer Treat Rev 1983; 10:245-54.

14. Gralla JR, Casper ES, Kelsen DP, et al. Cisplatin and vindesine combination chemotherapy for advanced carcinoma of the lung: a randomized trial investigating two dosage schedules. Ann Intern Med 1981; 95:414-20.

15. Elliott JA, Ahmedzai S, Stevenson RD, Durward AJ, Calman KC. Vindesine and cisplatin combination chemotherapy composed with vindesine as a single agent in the management of nonsmall-cell lung cancer: a randomized study. Eur J Clin Oncol 1984; 20:1025-32.

16. Niederle J, Shutte N, Roer N, Seeber S, Schmidt CG (1983). Inoperable large-cell carcinoma of the lung. Treatment with vindesine (VDS) and cisplatin (DDP). Proc AACR (abstr 606) 1983.

17. Briancon S, Thisse JY, Feintrenie X, Barral D, Lamaze R, Lamy P. Vindesine in stage 3 nonsmall-cell carcinoma of the lung: a randomized trial combination with either cyclophosphamide or cisplatin. Proc 13th Int Cong Chemother, Vienna SE 12.1.15 Part 248 1983; 63-68.

18. Longeval E, Klastersky J. Combination chemotherapy with cisplatin and etoposide in bronchogenic squamous cell carcinoma and adenocarcinoma. A study by the EORTC Lung Cancer Working Party (Belgium). Cancer 1982; 50:2751-56.

19. Klastersky J, Sculier JP, Nicaise C, et al. Combination chemotherapy with cisplatin, etoposide and vindesine in nonsmall-cell lung carcinoma. A clinical trial of the EORTC Lung Cancer Working Party. Cancer Treat Rep 1983; 67:727-30.

20. Miller TW. Treatment of advanced nonsmall-cell lung cancer (NSLC) with mitomycin-C plus

cisplatin plus vindesine (MiPE): comparisons to other mitomycin-C plus vinca-containing combinations (for the Southwest Oncology Group). Proc. ASCO (Abstr C898) 1984.

21. Rafkin HS. Etude de la survie des tumeurs bronchiques classées T3 opérées à l'exclusion des carcinomes anaplasiques à petites cellules. Thèse de doctorat en médecine, Université Paris VII. Faculté de médecine Xavier Bichat. Paris: Editions de la Faculté de Médecine Xavier Bichat, 1984.

22. Livingston RB, Carter SK. Single agents in cancer chemotherapy. New York: Plenum, 1970.

23. Kish J, Ensley J, Weaver A, Jacobs J, Cummings G, Al-Sarraf M. Superior response rate with 96 hour 5-fluorouracil (5-FU) infusion vs 5-FU bolus combined with cis-platinum (CACP) in a randomized trial for recurrent and advanced squamous head and neck cancer. ASCO abstr C695, 1984.

24. Weiden PL, Einstein AB, Rudolph RH. Cisplatin and 5-FU infusion chemotherapy for nonsmall-cell lung cancer (meeting abstr). Proc Annu Meet Am Soc Clin Oncol 1984; 3:215.

25. Trybula M, Taylor SG, Bonomi P, et al. Preoperative simultaneous cisplatin/5-fluorouracil and radiotherapy in clinical stage 3 nonsmall-cell bronchogenic carcinoma. ASCO abstr C873 1984.

26. Byfield JE, Stanton W, Sharp TR, Frankel SS, Koziol J. Phase 1–2 study of 120-hour infused 5-FU and split-course radiation therapy in localized nonsmall-cell lung cancer. Cancer Treat Rep 1983; 67(10):933–36.

27. Matelski HW, Lokich JJ, Huberman MS, et al. Adriamycin, cyclophosphamide, and etoposide (VP-16-213) in extensive-stage small-cell lung cancer. Am J Clin Oncol 1984; 729–32.

28. O'Donnell JF, Maurer LH, Forcier RJ, LeMarbre PA, Quinn BM, Stern R. Intensive cytosine arabinoside therapy in small-cell carcinoma of the lung. Am J Clin Oncol 1984; 7:415–18.

29. Huberman M, Lokich JJ, Greene R, et al. Vinblastine plus cis-platin in advanced nonsmall-cell lung cancer: lack of advantage for vinblastine infusion schedule. Cancer Treat Rep 1986; 70:287–89.

References—Chapter 27

1. Samuels ML, Holoye PY, Johnson DE. Bleomycin combination chemotherapy for metastatic testicular carcinoma. Cancer Bulletin 1973; 25(3):53–5.

2. Samuels ML, Johnson DE, Holoye PY. Continuous intravenous bleomycin (NSC-125066) therapy with vinblastine (NSC-49842) in stage 3 testicular neoplasia. Cancer Chemo Rep 1975; 59(3):563–70.

3. Samuels ML, Lanzotti VJ, Boyle PY, Smith TL, Johnson DE. Combination chemotherapy in germinal cell tumors. Cancer Treat Rev 1976; 3:185–204.

4. Bauer KA, Skarin AT, Balikian JP, Garnick MB, Rosenthal DS, Canellos GP. Pulmonary complications associated with combination chemotherapy programs containing bleomycin. Am J Med 1983; 74:557–63.

5. Logothetis CJ, Samuels ML, Selig D, et al. Cyclic chemotherapy with Cytoxan, Adriamycin and cisplatinum (CISCA) and VB-bleomycin (VB$_{IV}$) in advanced germ cell tumors: results in 100 patients. Am J Med (in press).

6. Sikic BI, Collins JM, Mimnaugh EG, et al. Improved therapeutic index of bleomycin when administered by continuous infusion in mice. Cancer Treat Rep 1978; 62:2011–17.

7. Goldinger PL, Schweizer O. The hazards of anesthesia and surgery in bleomycin-treated patients. Semin Oncol 1970; 6:121–24.

8. Logothetis CJ, Samuels ML. Surgery in the management of stage 3 germinal cell tumors: observations of the M. D. Anderson Hospital experience, 1971–79. Cancer Treat Rev 1984; 11:27–37.

9. Samuels ML, Johnson DE, Holoye PY, Lanzotti VJ. Large-dose bleomycin therapy and pulmonary toxicity: a possible role of prior radiotherapy. JAMA 1976; 235(11):1117–20.

10. Samuels ML, Howe CD. Vinblastine sulfate in the treatment of germinal tumors of the testis. In: Diagnosis and management of cancer—specific sites. Oncology 1970; 4:335–41.

11. Samuels ML, Johnson DE, Bracken RB. Adjuvant chemotherapy in metastatic testicular neoplasia: results with vinblastine-bleomycin. The University of Texas M. D. Anderson Hospital and Tumor Institute. In: Johnson DE, Samuels ML, eds. Cancer of the genitourinary tract. Raven Press, 1979; 173-79.

12. Einhorn LH, Williams SD. Chemotherapy of disseminated testicular cancer: a random prospective study. Cancer 1980; 46:1339-44.

13. Stoter G, Vendrik CPJ, Struyvenberg A, et al. Five-year survival of patients with disseminated nonseminomatous testicular cancer treated with cisplatin, vinblastine, and bleomycin. Cancer 1984; 54:1521-24.

14. Peckham MJ, Barrett A, McElwain TJ, Hendry WF. Combined management of malignant teratoma of the testis. Lancet 1979; 2:267-70.

15. Logothetis CJ, Samuels ML, Selig DE, et al. Chemotherapy of extragonadal germ cell tumors. J Clin Oncol 1985; 3(3):316-25.

16. Newlands ES, Rustin GJS, Begent RHJ, Parker D, Bagshawe KD. Further advances in the management of malignant teratomas of the testis and other sites. Lancet 1983; 1:948-51.

17. Fitzharris BM, Kaye SB, Saverymuttu S, et al. VP16-213 as a single agent in advanced testicular tumors. Eur J Cancer 1980; 16:1193-97.

18. Peckham Mj, Barrett A, Liew KH, et al. The treatment of metastatic germ-cell testicular tumors with bleomycin, etoposide and cis-platin (BEP). Br J Cancer 1983; 47:613-19.

19. Williams S, Einhorn L, Greco A, Birch R, Irwin L. Disseminated germ cell tumors: a comparison of cisplatin plus bleomycin plus either vinblastine (PVB) or VP-16 (BEP). Am Soc Clin Oncol (abstr C390) 1985; 100.

20. Stoter G, Vendrik CPJ, Struyvenberg A, et al. Five-year survival of patients with disseminated nonseminomatous testicular cancer treated with cisplatin, vinblastine, and bleomycin. Cancer 1984; 54:1521-24.

21. Bosl GJ, Geller N, Cirrincinone C, Scher H, Whitmore W, Golbey R. A multivariate analysis of prognostic variables in patients with metastatic germ cell tumors of the testis (GCT). Cancer Res 1983; 43:3403.

22. Chong CDK, Logothetis CJ, Fritsche H, Gietner A, Savaraj N, Samuels ML. Peak vinblastine concentration as a monitor of nonhematologic toxicity in patients with testicular cancer. Am Assoc Cancer Res (abstr 685) 1985; 173.

23. Dexeus F, Logothetis CJ, Samuels ML, Hossan E, von Eschenbach AC. Continuous infusion of vinblastine for advanced hormone-refractory prostate cancer. Cancer Treat Rep 1985; 69:885-86.

24. Logothetis CJ, Samuel M, von Eschenbach A, et al. Doxorubicin, mitomycin-C and 5-fluorouracil (DFMO) in the treatment of metastatic hormonal refractory adenocarcinoma of the prostate: with a note on the staging of metastatic prostate cancer. J Clin Oncol 1983; 1(6):368-79.

25. Samuels ML, Moran ME, Johnson DE, Bracken RB. CISCA combination chemotherapy for metastatic carcinoma of the bladder. The University of Texas M. D. Anderson Hospital and Tumor Institute. In: Johnson DE, Samuels ML, eds. Cancer of the genitourinary tract. Raven Press, 1979; 101–06.

26. Sternberg J, Bracken RB, Handel PB, Johnson DE. Combination chemotherapy (CISCA) for advanced urinary tract carcinoma. JAMA 1977; 238:2282–87.

27. Logothetis CJ, Samuels ML, Ogden S, et al. CISCA chemotherapy for patients with locally advanced urothelial tumors with or without nodal metastases. J Urol 1985; 134:460.

28. Sternberg CN, Yagoda A, Scher HI, et al. M-VAC: update of methotrexate (MTX), vinblastine (VLB), Adriamycin (ADM), and cisplatin (DDP) for urothelial tract cancer. Am Soc Clin Oncol (abstr C409) 1985; 105.

29. Stoter G, Fossa SD, Klein JGM, et al. Combination chemotherapy with cisplatin (DDP) and methotrexate (MTX) in advanced bladder cancer. Am Soc Clin Oncol (abstr C413) 1985; 106.

References—Chapter 28

1. Silverberg E. Cancer statistics, CA 1985; 35:19–35.

2. Miller AB, Hoogstraten B, Staquet M, et al. Reporting results of cancer treatment. Cancer 1981; 47:207–14.

3. Beecham JB, Helmkamp BF, Rubin P. Tumors of the female reproductive organs. In: Rubin P, ed. Clinical oncology: a multidisciplinary approach. New York: American Cancer Society, 1983; 428–81.

4. Shackney SE, McCormack GW, Cuchural GJ Jr. Growth rate patterns of solid tumors and their relation to responsiveness to therapy. Ann Intern Med 1978; 89:107–21.

5. Charbit A, Malaise EP, Tubiana M. Relation between the pathological nature and growth rate of human tumors. Eur J Cancer 1971; 7:307–25.

6. Averette HE, Weinstein GD, Ford JH Jr., et al. Cell kinetics and programmed chemotherapy for gynecologic cancer. Am J Obstet Gynecol 1976; 124:912–23.

7. Bonomi PD, Yordan EL Jr. Chemotherapy of cervical carcinoma. In: Deepe G, ed. Chemotherapy of gynecologic cancer. New York: Alan R. Liss, 1984; 103–24.

8. Salem P, Khalyl K, Jabboury K, et al. Cis-diamminedichloroplatinum (II) by 5-day continous infusion: a new dose schedule with minimal toxicity. Cancer 1984; 53:837–40.

9. Thigpen JT, Blessing J, Lewis G. A randomized trial of bolus cisplatin versus 24-hour infusion in advanced carcinoma of the cervix. Gynecologic Oncology Group (personal communication).

10. Rozencweig M, Nicaise C, Beer M, et al. Phase 1 study of carboplatin given on a five-day intravenous schedule. J Clin Oncol 1983; 1:621–26.

11. Jobson V, Jackson D, Homesley H, et al. Treatment of recurrent gynecologic malignancies with prolonged intravenous vincristine (VCR) infusion. Proc ASCO 1983; 2:149.

12. Hakes T, Nikrui M, Magill G, et al. Cervix cancer: treatment with combination vincristine and high doses of methotrexate. Cancer 1979; 43:459–64.

13. Forney JP, Morrow CP, DiSaia PH, et al. Seven-drug polychemotherapy in the treatment of advanced and recurrent squamous carcinoma of the female genital tract. Am J Obstet Gynecol 1974; 123:748–52.

14. O'Quinn AG, Barranco SC, Costanz JJ. Tumor cell kinetics-directed chemotherapy for advanced squamous carcinoma of the cervix. Gynecol Oncol 1984; 18:135–44.

15. Wade JL, Richman CM, Senekjian E, et al. Objective response in advanced carcinoma of the cervix using cis-platinum and infusion 5-fluorouracil (5-FU) chemotherapy. Proc ASCO 1984; 3:172.

16. Sorbe B, Frankendal B. Bleomycin-Adriamycin-cisplatin combination chemotherapy in the treatment of primary advanced and recurrent cervical carcinoma. Obstet Gynecol 1984; 63:167–70.

17. Lele SB, Piver MS, Barlow JJ. Cyclophosphamide, Adriamycin, and platinum chemotherapy in treatment of advanced and recurrent cervical carcinoma. Gynecol Oncol 1983; 15:15–18.

18. Yordan E, Graham J, Reddy S, et al. Treatment of advanced pelvic malignancies with simultaneous cisplatin, 5-FU, and radiation therapy (personal communication).

19. Thomas G, Dembo A, Beale F, et al. Concurrent radiation, mitomycin C and 5-fluorouracil in poor prognosis carcinoma of cervix: preliminary results of a phase 1-2 study. Int J Radiat Oncol Biol Phys 1984; 10:1785–90.

20. Kalra J, Cortes E, Chen S, et al. Effective multimodality treatment for advanced epidermoid carcinoma of the female genital tract. Proc ASCO 1983; 2:152.

21. Nakajima Y, Miyamoto T, Tanabe M, et al. Enhancement of mammalian cell killing by 5-fluorouracil in combination with x-rays. Cancer Res 1979; 39:3763–67.

22. Ochoa M Jr., Beattie EJ, Tamimi H, et al. Carcinoma of the cervix: treatment with continuous intravenous bleomycin. Clin bull 1976; 6:159–62.

23. Krakoff IH, Cvitkovic E, Currie V, et al. Clinical pharmacologic and therapeutic studies of bleomycin given by continuous infusion. Cancer 1977; 40:2027–37.

24. Baker LH, Opipari MI, Wilson H, et al. Mitomycin C, vincristine, and bleomycin therapy for advanced cervical cancer. Obstet Gynecol 1977; 52:146–50.

25. Hannigan EV, Dillard EA Jr., Van Dinh T. Bleomycin, vincristine, and methotrexate with citrovorum factor rescue in the treatment of advanced squamous cell carcinoma of the cervix. Gynecol Oncol 1984; 19:57−59.

26. Alberts DS, Martimbeau PW, Surwit EA, et al. Mitomycin-C, bleomycin, vincristine, and cis-platinum in the treatment of advanced, recurrent squamous cell carcinoma of the cervix. Cancer Clin Trials 1981; 4:313−16.

27. Surwit EA, Alberts DS, Aristizbal S, et al. Treatment of primary and recurrent advanced squamous cell cancer of the cervix with mitomycin-C + vincristine + bleomycin (MOB) plus cisplatin (PLAT). Proc ASCO 1983; 2:153.

28. Rosenthal CJ, Khumpateea N, Boyce J, et al. Effective chemotherapy for advanced carcinoma of the cervix with bleomycin, cisplatin, vincristine, and methotrexate. Cancer 1983; 52:2025−30.

29. Israel L, Aguitera J, Breau J-L. Traitement des cancers épidermoides par bleomycine et platine en administration continue prolongée. La Nouvelle Presse Médicale, 1981; 10:1817−24.

30. Daghestani AN, Hakes TB, Lynch G, et al. Cervix carcinoma: treatment with combination cisplatin and bleomycin. Gynecol Oncol 1983; 16:334−39.

31. Hakes T, Wertheim M, Daghestani A, et al. Adjuvant chemotherapy for poor risk stage IB/IIA cervix carcinoma patients−a pilot study with cisplatin/bleomycin. Proc ASCO 1984; 3:171.

32. Bauer K, Knapp R, Bloomer W, et al. Cis-DDP, bleomycin, MTX-LCV (PBM) chemotherapy in advanced, previously untreated carcinoma of the cervix (CaC). Proc ASCO 1984; 3:169.

33. Cromer JK, Bateman JC, Berry N, et al. Use of intra-arterial nitrogen mustard therapy in the treatment of cervical and vaginal cancer. Am J Obstet Gynecol 1952; 63:538−48.

34. Boiman RE, Holzaepfel JH, Barnes AC. Intra-arterial nitrogen mustard in advanced pelvic malignancies. Am J Obstet Gynecol 1956; 72:1319−25.

35. Krakoff IH, Sullivan RD. Intra-arterial nitrogen mustard in the treatment of pelvic cancer. Ann Intern Med 1958; 48:839−50.

36. Boutselis JG, Ullery JC, Page W. Palliation chemotherapy of pelvic carcinoma by systemic, perfusion, and infusion modalities. Ohio St Med J 1971; 67:721−25.

37. Parker RT, Shingleton WW. Chemotherapy in genital cancer: systemic therapy and regional perfusion. Am J Obstet Gynecol 1962; 83:981−1003.

38. Trussell RR, Mitford-Barberton GD. Carcinoma of the cervix treated with continuous intra-arterial methotrexate and intermittent intramuscular leucovorin. Lancet 1961; 1:971−72.

39. Laufe LE, Blockstein RS, Parsi FZ, et al. Infusion through inferior gluteal artery for pelvic cancer. Obstet Gynecol 1966; 28:650−59.

40. Carlson JA Jr., Freedman RS, Wallace S, et al. Intra-arterial cis-platinum in the management of squamous cell carcinoma of the uterine cervix. Gynecol Oncol 1981; 12:92−98.

41. Bateman Jr, Hazen JG, Stolinsky DC, et al. Advanced carcinoma of the cervix treated by intra-arterial methotrexate. Am J Obstet Gynecol 1966; 96:181−87.

42. Fallappa P, Trodella L, et al. Advanced carcinoma of the cervix treated by continuous pelvic arterial infusion with cytostatics and radiation therapy. Eur J Radiol 1982; 2:307−09.

43. Oberfield RA. Intra-arterial infusion in tumors of the pelvis. Recent Results Cancer Res 1983; 86:15−25.

44. Kim EE, Bledin AG, Kavanagh J, et al. Chemotherapy of cervical carcinoma: use of Tc-99m-MAA infusion to predict drug distribution. Radiology 1984; 150:677−81.

45. Cavanagh D, Hovadhana P, Comas MR. Regional chemotherapy−a comparison of pelvic perfusion and intra-arterial infusion in patients with advanced gynecologic cancer. Am J Obstet Gynecol 1975; 123:435−41.

46. Calvo DB III, Patt YZ, Wallace S, et al. Phase 1-2 trial of percutaneous intra-arterial cis-diamminedichloro platinum (II) for regionally confined malignancy. Cancer 1980; 45:1278−83.

47. Mahaley MS Jr., Woodhall B. The effect of anticancer agents on nervous tissue. Cancer Chemother Rep 1962; 16:543−44.

48. Morrow CP, DiSaia PH, Mangan CF. Continuous pelvic arterial infusion with bleomycin for

squamous carcinoma of the cervix recurrent after irradiation therapy. Cancer Treat Rep 1977; 61:1403–05.

49. Kraybill WG, Harrison M, Sasaki T, et al. Regional intra-arterial infusion of Adriamycin in the treatment of cancer. Surg Gynecol Obstet 1977; 144:335–38.

50. Lifshitz S, Railsback LD, Buchsbaum HJ. Intra-arterial pelvic infusion chemotherapy in advanced gynecologic cancer. Obstet Gynecol 1978; 52:476–80.

51. Swenerton KD, Evers JA, White GW, et al. Intermittent pelvic infusion with vincristine, bleomycin, and mitomycin-C for advanced recurrent carcinoma of the cervix. Cancer Treat Rep 1979; 63:1379–81.

52. Smith JP, Randall GE, Castro JR, et al. Hypogastric artery infusion and radiation therapy for advanced squamous cell carcinoma of the cervix. Am J Roentgenol Radium Ther Nuc Med 1972; 114:110–15.

53. Kavanagh J, Wallace S, Delcios L, et al. Induction intra-arterial chemotherapy for advanced squamous cell carcinoma of the cervix. Clinical trials. Proc ASCO 1983; 2:154.

54. Douple EB, Richmond RC. A review of the interactions between platinum coordination complexes and ionizing radiation: implications for cancer therapy. In: Prestayko AW, Crooke ST, Carter SK, eds. Cisplatin: current status and new developments. New York: Academic Press, 1980; 125–148.

55. Collins JM. Pharmacologic rationale for regional drug delivery. J Clin Oncol 1984; 2:498–504.

56. Bruckner HW. Chemotherapy: the common epithelial ovarian carcinomas. In: Deppe G, ed. Chemotherapy of gynecologic cancer. New York: Alan R. Liss, 1984; 151–94.

57. Lokich JJ. Phase 1 study of cis-diamminedichloroplatinum (II) administered as a constant 5-day infusion. Cancer Treat Rep 1980; 64:905–08.

58. Kavanagh JJ, Wharton JT, Rutledge FN. Continuous-infusion vinblastine for treatment of refractory epithelial carcinoma of the ovary: a phase 2 trial. Cancer Treat Rep 1984; 68:1417–18.

59. Shah MK, St. Marie K, Catalano RB, et al. Phase 2 study of 5-day infusion of vinblastine in patients with advanced ovarian carcinoma. Cancer Treat Rep 1985; 69:229–30.

60. Papac RJ, Calabresi P. Infusion of floxuridine in the treatment of solid tumors. JAMA 1966; 197:79–83.

61. Legha SS, Ajani JA, Bodey GP. Phase 1 study of spirogermanium given daily. J Clin Oncol 1983; 1:331–35.

62. Lokich J, Perri J, Fine N, et al. Mitomycin-C: phase 1 study of a constant infusion ambulatory treatment schedule. Am J Clin Oncol 1982; 5:443–47.

63. Izibicki RM, Baker LH, Samson MK, et al. 5-FU infusion and cyclophosphamide in the treatment of advanced ovarian cancer. Cancer Treat Rep 1977; 61:1573–75.

64. Vriesdendorp R, Aalders JG, Sleijfer DT, et al. Effective high-dose chemotherapy with autologous bone marrow infusion in resistant ovarian cancer. Gynecol Oncol 1984; 17:271–76.

65. Drapkin R, Stanton G, Nealy R, et al. Sequential methotrexate, Velban, and cis-diamminedichloroplatinum in advanced ovarian cancer refractory to initial chemotherapy. Proc ASCO 1984; 3:175.

66. Deppe G, Cohen CJ, Bruckner HW. Treatment of advanced endometrial adenocarcinoma with cis-dichlorodiammine platinum (II) after intensive prior therapy. Gynecol Oncol 1980; 10:51–54.

67. Aisner J, Van Echo DA, Whitacre M, et al. A phase 1 trial of continuous infusion VP-16-213 (etoposide). Cancer Chemother Pharmacol 1982; 7:157–60.

68. Deppe G. Chemotherapy of endometrial cancer. In: Deppe G, ed. Chemotherapy of gynecologic cancer. New York: Alan R. Liss, 1984; 139–50.

69. Slayton RE. Management of germ cell and stromal tumors of the ovary. Semin Oncol 1984; 11:299–313.

70. Carlson RW, Sikic BI, Turbow MM, et al. Cisplatin, vinblastine, and bleomycin (PVB) therapy for ovarian germ cell cancer. Proc ASCO 1983; 2:156.

71. Decker A, Drelichman A, Jacobs J, et al. Adjuvant chemotherapy with cis-diamminodichloroplatinum II and 120-hour infusion 5-fluorouracil in stage 3 and 4 squamous cell carcinoma of the head and neck. Cancer 1983; 51:1353–55.

72. Leichman L, Steiger Z, Seydel HG, et al. Preoperative chemotherapy and radiation therapy for patients with cancer of the esophagus. J Clin Oncol 1984; 2:75–79.

73. Cummings B, Keane T, Thomas G, et al. Results and toxicity of the treatment of anal canal carcinoma by radiation therapy or radiation therapy and chemotherapy. Cancer 1984; 54:2062–68.

References—Chapter 29

1. Bramwell VHC, Mouridron HT, Malder JH, et al. Carminomycin versus Adriamycin in advanced soft tissue sarcoma. Eur J Cancer Clin Oncol 1983; 19:1097.

2. Gottleib JA, Baker LH, O'Bryan RM, et al. Adriamycin used alone in combination for soft tissue and bony sarcomas. Cancer Chemother Rep 1975; 6(3):271–82.

3. Subramanian S, Wiltshaw E. Chemotherapy of sarcoma. A comparison of three regimens. Lancet 1978; 683–86.

4. Rosenberg SA, Suit HD, Baker LH, Rosen G. Sarcomas of the soft tissue and bone. In: Cancer—principles and practice of oncology. Devita VT Jr., Hellman S, Rosenberg SA, eds. Philadelphia: JB Lippincott 1982; 1036–93.

5. Stuart-Harris RC, Harper PG, Parsons CA, et al. High-dose alkylation therapy using ifosfamide infusion with mesna in the treatment of adult soft tissue sarcoma. Cancer Chemother Pharmacol 1983; 11:69.

6. Burkett H. Ifosfamide: European perspective. Sem Oncol (Suppl. 1) 1983; 9:28.

7. Cortes EP, Holland JF, Wang JJ, et al. Adriamycin (NSC-123127) in 87 patients with osteosarcoma. Cancer Chemother Rep 1975; 6:305–13.

8. Pratt CB, Champion JE, Senzer N, et al. Treatment of unresectable or metastatic osteosarcoma with cisplatin and cisplatin-doxorubicin. Cancer 1985; 56:1930–33.

9. Ochs JJ, Freeman AI, Douglass HO Jr., et al. Cis-dichlorodiammineplatinum (II) in advanced osteogenic sarcoma. Cancer Treat Rep 1978; 62:239–45.

10. Rosen G, Nirenberg A, Caparros B. Evaluation of high dose methotrexate (HDMTX) with citrovorum factor rescue (CER) single agent chemotherapy in osteogenic sarcoma (OSA). Proc AACR 1980; March:177.

11. Rosen G, Caparros B,, Huvos AG, et al. Preoperative chemotherapy for osteogenic sarcoma: selection of postoperative adjuvant chemotherapy based on the response of the primary tumor to preoperative chemotherapy. Cancer 1982; 49:1221–30.

12. Eilber FR, Grant T, Morton DL. Adjuvant therapy for osteosarcoma: preoperative and postoperative treatment. Cancer Treat Rep 1978; 62:213–16.

13. Eilber FR, Morton DL, Eckardt J, Grant T, Weisenburger T. Limb salvage for skeletal and soft tissue sarcomas. Cancer 1984; 53:2579–84.

14. Azzarelli A, Quaglinolo V, Audiso RA, Boufouti G, Audreola S, Gemari L. Intra-arterial Adriamycin followed by surgery for limb sarcomas: preliminary report. Eur J Cancer Clin Oncol 1983; 19:885–90.

15. Jaffe N, Bowman R, Wang Y, et al. Chemotherapy for primary osteosarcoma by intra-arterial infusion: review of the literature and comparison of results achieved by the intravenous route. Cancer Bull 1984; 36:37–41.

16. Campbell TN, Howell SB, Pfeifle CE, Wung WE, Bookstein J. Clinical pharmacokinetics of intra-arterial cisplatin in humans. J Clin Oncol 1983; 1:755–62.

17. Jaffe N, Knapp J, Chuang VP, et al. Osteosarcoma: intra-arterial treatment of primary tumor with cisplatin. Cancer 1983; 51:402.

18. Benjamin RS, Chawla SP, Murray JP, et al. Response to preoperative chemotherapy of osteosarcoma improves disease-free survival and the chances of limb salvage. Proc AACR 1985; 26:174.

19. Jaffe N, Prudich J, Knapp J, et al. Treatment of primary osteosarcoma with intra-arterial and intravenous high-dose methotrexate. J Clin Oncol 1983; 1:428.

20. Akahoshi Y, Takeuchi S, Chen S, et al. The results of surgical treatment combined with intra-arterial infusion of anticancer agents in osteosarcoma. J Clin Orthop 1976; 120:102 – 09.

21. Legha SS, Benjamin RS, MacKay B, et al. Role of Adriamycin in breast cancer and sarcomas. In: Anthracycline antibiotics in cancer therapy. Muggia FM, Young CW, Carter SK, eds. Marinus Nijhoff Publishers, 1982; 432 – 44.

22. Lokich JJ, Bothe A, Gaj E, Rich T. Protracted systemic infusion of doxorubicin: studies in 83 patients with advanced malignancy. Cancer Treat Symp 1984; 3:85 – 89.

23. Gasparini M, Rouesse J, Van Oosterom A, et al. Phase 2 study of cisplatin in advanced osteogenic sarcoma. Cancer Treat Rep 1985; 69:211 – 13.

24. Gasparini M, Fossati B, Rottali L, Grairi C, Azzarelli A. Remission induction by chemotherapy (VCR, HDMTX, CDDP) in osteosarcoma. Proc ASCO 1983; 2:239.

25. Yap BS, Benjamin RS, Plager C, Burgess MA, Papdoupolos N, Bodey GP. A randomized study of continuous infusion vindesine versus vinblastine in adults with refractory sarcomas. Am J Clin Oncol 1983; 6:235 – 38.

26. Rosenberg SA. Prospective randomized trials demonstrating the efficacy of adjuvant chemotherapy in adult patients with soft tissue sarcomas. Cancer Treat Rep 1984; 68:1067 – 78.

27. Rosen G, Nirenberg A. Chemotherapy for primary osteogenic sarcoma: ten year evolution, and current status of preoperative chemotherapy. Adjuvant Ther Cancer 1984; IV:593 – 629.

28. Posner MR, Belliveau JF, Ferrari L, et al. Clinical and pharmacokinetic study of 5-day continuous infusion cis-platinum. Proc ASCO 1985; 4:C – 145.

29. Rosenthal CJ, Park HS, Choi K, Bhutiani I, Rotman M. Effective therapy for advanced localized soft tissue sarcomas (STS): Adriamycin (ADR) by continuous infusion (CI) and concomitant radiation therapy (RT). Proc ASCO 1985; 4:C – 565.

30. Bonadonna G, Santoro A. Bone and soft tissue sarcoma. In: Cancer chemotherapy annual 6. Pinedo HM, Chabner BA, eds. Elsevier Science Publishers B.V., 1984; 25:436 – 49.

References—Chapter 30

1. Costanza ME, Nathanson L, Schoenfeld D, et al. Results with methyl-CCNU and DTIC in metastatic melanoma. Cancer 1977; 40:1010 – 15.

2. Constanzi JJ. DTIC (NSC-45388) studies in the Southwest Oncology Group. Cancer Treat Rep 1976; 60:189 – 92.

3. Einhorn LH, Burgess MA, Vellejos C, et al. Prognostic correlations and response to treatment in advanced metastatic melanoma. Cancer Res 1974; 34:1995 – 2004.

4. Nathanson L, Wolter K, Horton J, et al. Characteristics of prognosis and response to an imidazole carboxamide in malignant melanoma. Clin Pharmacol Ther 1971; 12:955 – 62.

5. Luco JK. Chemotherapy of malignant melanoma. Cancer 1972; 30:1604 – 16.

6. Ramirez G, Wilson W, Grage T, et al. Phase 2 evaluation of 1, 3-bis (2-chloroethyl-1-nitrosourea)(BCNU; NSC-409962) in patients with solid tumors. Cancer Chemother Rep 1972; 56:787 – 90.

7. Pugh R, Jacobs E, et al. CCNU versus CCNU: vincristine in disseminated melanoma. Proc 11th Int Cancer Cong Florence, Italy, 1974; 540 – 55.

8. Lokich JJ, Zipoli TE, Sonneborn H, Paul S, Philips D. Streptozotocin for metastatic malignant melanoma. Am J Clin Oncol 1985; 8:45 – 46.

9. Hall SW, Benjamin RS, Lewinski U, et al. Actinomycin D, levamisole chemoimmunotherapy of refractory malignant melanoma. Cancer 1979; 43:1195 – 1200.

10. Chary KK, Higby DJ, Henderson ES, et al. Phase 1 study of high dose cis-dichlorodiammineplatinum (II) with forced diuresis. Cancer Treat Rep 1977; 61:367 – 70.

11. Maral J, Jacquillat CL, Weil M, Auclerc G, Sellami M, Banzet P. Chemotherapy of metastatic

malignant melanoma by cis. platyl (CDDP), Adriamycin (ADR), VP-16 and continuous infusion of 5-fluorouracil (5-FU) and bleomycin (Bleo). Proc ASCO 1985; 4:C593.

12. Cumberlin R, De Moss E, Lassus M, Friedman M. Isolation perfusion for malignant melanoma of the extremity: a review. J Clin Oncol 1985; 3(7):1022−31.

13. Stewart DJ, Wallace S, Feun L, et al. A phase 1 study of intracarotid artery infusion of cis-diamminedichloroplatinum (II) in patients with recurrent malignant intracerebral tumors. Cancer Res 1982; 42:2059−62.

14. Yamada K, Bremer AM, West CR, Ghoorha J, Park HY, Takita H. Intra-arterial BCNU therapy in the treatment of metastatic brain tumor from lung carcinoma. Cancer 1979; 44:2000−07.

15. Lokich JJ, Bothe A, Yanes L, Moore C. Continuous infusion with an ambulatory pump. 13th Int Cong Chemother Vienna, 1983.

16. Lokich JJ, Zipoli T, Moore C, Sonneborn H, Paul S, Greene R. Doxorubicin/vinblastine and doxorubicin/cyclophosphamide combination chemotherapy by continuous infusion. (in press).

17. Moertel CG, Hanley JA, Johnson LA. Streptozotocin alone compared with streptozotocin plus fluorouracil in the treatment of advanced islet-cell carcinoma. N Engl J Med 1980; 303(21):1189−94.

18. Kossinger A, Foley FJ, Lemon HG. Use of DTIC (dacarbazine) in the malignant carcinoid syndrome. Cancer Treat Rep 1977; 61:101.

19. Broder L, Carter S. Pancreatic islet cell carcinoma; clinical features of 52 patients. Ann Intern Med 1973; 79:101−07.

20. Harris AL. Chemotherapy for carcinoid syndrome: review. Cancer Chemother Pharmacol 1981; 5:133−38.

21. Moertel CG. Treatment of the carcinoid tumor and the malignant carcinoid: review article. J Clin Oncol 1983; 1(11):727−40.

22. Legha SS, Valdiviesco M, Nelson RS, Benjamin RS, Bodey GP. Chemotherapy for metastatic carcinoid tumors: experiences with 32 patients and a review of the literature. Cancer Treat Rep 1977; 61:1699−1703.

23. Sridhar KS, Holland JF, Brown JC, Cohen JM, Ohnuma T. Doxorubicin plus cisplatin in the treatment of apudomas. Cancer 1985; 55:2634−37.

24. Oberg K, Funs K, Alm G, et al. Effects of leukocyte interferon on clinical symptoms and hormone levels in patients with mid-gut carcinoid tumor. N Engl J Med 1983; 309:129−32.

25. Giaccone G, Musella R, Bertetto O, Donadio M, Calciati A. Cisplatin-containing chemotherapy in the treatment of invasive thymoma: report of five cases. Cancer Treat Rep 1985; 69(6):695−97.

26. Fornasiero A, Daniele O, Sperandio P, et al. Chemotherapy of invasive metastatic thymoma: report of 11 cases. Cancer Treat Rep 1984; 68(10):1205−10.

References—Chapter 31

1. Probert JC, Thompson RW, Bagshaw MA. Patterns of spread of distant metastases in head and neck cancer. Cancer 1974; 33:127−33.

2. Million RR, Cassisi NJ, Wittes RE. Cancer in the head and neck. In: Cancer: principles & practices of oncology. DeVita VT, Hellman S, Rosenberg SA, eds. Philadelphia: JB Lippincott. 1982; 301−95.

3. Parlavecchio G. Sul lavaggio antisettico interstizaile dei tessut dolla vie arteriosa. Policlinico (sez. Prat.) 1899; 6:667−74.

4. Ransohoff JL. Terminal arterial anesthesia. Ann Surg 1910; 51:453−56.

5. Hirsch HL, Myerson A, Halloran RD. Intracarotid route in the treatment of general paresis. N Engl J Med 1925; 192:713−17.

6. Klopp CT, Alfordd TC, Bateman J, Berry GN, Winship T. Fractionated intra-arterial cancer chemotherapy with methyl bis amine hydrochloride: a preliminary report. Ann Surg 1950; 132:811−32.

7. Sullivan RD, Miller E, Chryssochoos T, Watkins E Jr. The clinical effects of the continuous

intravenous and intra-arterial infusion of cancer chemotherapeutic compounds. Cancer Chemother Rep 1962; 16:449–510.

8. Clarkson B, Lawrence W Jr. Perfusion and infusion techniques in cancer chemotherapy. J Clin North Amer 1961; 45:689–710.

9. Sullivan RD, Miller E, Sikes MP. Antimetabolite-metabolite combination cancer chemotherapy: effects of intra-arterial methotrexate-intramuscular citrovorum factor therapy in human cancer. Cancer 1959; 12:1248–62.

10. Yollick BL, Corgill DA. Regional chemotherapy of head and neck tumors by intra-arterial infusion techniques. Tex State J Med 1963; 59:423–28.

11. Acquarelli M, Feder R, Gordon H. Continuous intra-arterial infusion of methotrexate for recurrent squamous cell carcinoma of head and neck. Am Surg 1964; 80:423–30.

12. Hayes DM, Wilkins FB, Meredith JH. Regional arterial infusion for localized malignancies. Arch Surg 1964; 88:1070–76.

13. Jesse R, Villarreal R, Leftayf V, et al. Intra-arterial infusion for head and neck cancers. Arch Surg 1964; 88:618–27.

14. Espiner H, Westbury G. Continuous chemotherapy by intra-arterial infusion. Acta Un Int Contra Cancrum 1964; 20:475–77.

15. Beahrs OH, Caldarola VT, Harrison EG. Treatment of cancer of the head and neck by chemotherapy. JAMA 1964; 189:765.

16. Baker RR, Gaertner RA. Regional arterial infusion of antimetabolites. J Surg Res 1965; 5:132–36.

17. Burn JI, Johnston ID, Davies AJ, et al. Cancer chemotherapy in continuous intra-arterial infusion of methotrexate. Br J Surg 1966; 53:329–36.

18. Gorgun B, Watne AL. Infusion chemotherapy in head and neck tumors. Arch Surg 1966; 92:951–57.

19. Tindel S. Intra-arterial chemotherapy in recurrent neoplasms. JAMA 1967; 200(11):913–17.

20. Couture J. Intra-arterial infusion therapy for oral cancer. Cancer J Surg 1968; 11:420–23.

21. Watkins E, Sullivan RD. Cancer chemotherapy by prolonged arterial infusion. Surg Gynec Obst 1964; 118(1):3–19.

22. Carter SK. The chemotherapy of head and neck cancer. Semin Oncol 1977; 4:413–24.

23. Hong WK, Bromer R. Chemotherapy in head and neck cancer. N Engl J Med 1983; 308:75–79.

24. Johnson RO, Kisken WA, Curreri AR. A report upon arterial infusion with 5-fluorouracil in 100 patients. Surg Gynec Obstet 1965; 120:530.

25. Freckman HA. Result in 169 patients with cancer of the head and neck treated by intra-arterial infusion therapy. Am J Surg 1972; 124:501–09.

26. Szabo G, Kovacs A. Possibilities of enhancing the effectiveness of intra-arterial chemotherapy. Int J Oral Surg 1980; 9:33–44.

27. Burkhardt A, Holtje WJ. Effects of intra-arterial bleomycin therapy in squamous cell carcinoma of the oral cavity: biopsy and autopsy examination. J Maxillofac Surg 3:217–30.

28. Richard JM, Sancho H. Intra-arterial chemotherapy of head and neck tumors: statistical study of 129 cases treated at the Institute Gustave Roussy. Biomedicine 1973; 18:429–35.

29. Inuyama Y. In: Carter SK, Crooke ST, Umeazwa, eds. Bleomycin: current status and new developments. New York: Academic Press, 1978; 267.

30. Matras H, Burke K, Watzek G, Kuhbock J, Potzi P, Dimopoulus J. Concept of cytostatic therapy in advanced cancers of the head and neck. J Maxillofac Surg 1979; 7:150–54.

31. Ziekle-Temme BC, Stevens KR Jr., Everts EC, Moseley HS, Ireland KM. Combined intra-arterial chemotherapy radiation therapy and surgery for advanced squamous cell carcinoma of the head and neck. Cancer 1980; 45:1527–32.

32. Bitter KJ. Pharmacokinetic behavior of bleomycin-cobalt-57 with special regard to intra-arterial perfusion of the maxillofacial region. J Maxillofac Surg 1976; 4:226–31.

33. Wittes RE, Cvitkovic E, Shah J, Gerold FP, Strong EW. Cisdichlorodiammineplatinum (II) in the treatment of epidermoid carcinoma of the head and neck. Cancer Treat Rep 1977; 61:359–66.

34. Stephens R, Coltman C, Rossof A, et al. Cisdichlorodiammineplatinum (II) in adult patients: Southwest Oncology Group studies. Cancer Treat Rep 1979; 63:1609−10.

35. Madajewica S, Kanter P, West C, et al. Plasma, spinal fluid and organ distribution of cisplatinum (DDP) following intravenous (IV) and intracarotid (IC) infusion. Proc Amer Assoc Cancer Res and ASCO 1981; 22:176.

36. Lehane DE, Sessions R, Johnson P, et al. Intra-arterial cisplatinum administration for advanced squamous cell carcinoma of the head and neck region. Int Head and Neck Oncol Res Conf, Rosslyn, VA (abstr 2.11) Sept 1980.

37. Donegan WL, Harris P. Regional chemotherapy with combined drugs in cancer of the head and neck. Cancer 1976; 38:1479−83.

38. Curioni C, Quado G. Clinical trial of intra-arterial polychemotherapy in the treatment of carcinoma of the oral cavity. J Maxillofac Surg 1978; 6:207−16.

39. Szabo G, Kovacs A. Intra-arterial chemotherapy of head and neck tumors. Acta Chir Acad Sci Hung 1979; 20:49−55.

40. Muggia FM, Wolf GT. Intra-arterial chemotherapy of head and neck cancer: worth another look? Cancer Clin Trials 1980; 3:375−79.

41. Andreasson L, Bjorklunk A, Landberg T, Mattson W, Merke C. Combination chemotherapy of advanced malignant head and neck tumors by means of regional intra-arterial infusions and systemic treatment. Int Head and Neck Oncol Res Conf, Rosslyn, VA, (abstr 2.10) Sept 1980.

42. Bier J. Intra-arterial chemotherapy in head and neck cancer: clinical and experimental experience of the DOSAK. Rev Sudam Oncol (Argent) 1979; 3:35−40.

43. Reese AB, Hyman GA, Herriam DR Jr., Forrest AW, Kliegerman MM. Treatment of retinoblastoma by radiation and triethylenemelamine. AMA Arch Ophth 1955; 53:503−13.

44. Bolman RE, Holzaepfel JH, Barnes AC. Intra-arterial nitrogen mustard in advanced pelvic malignancies. Am J Obst Gynecol 1956; 72: 1319−25.

45. Jesse R. Combined intra-arterial infusion in radiotherapy for treatment of advanced cancer of the head and neck. Front Radiat Ther Oncol 1969; 4:126−31.

46. Demard F, Colonna d'Istria J, Jausseran M, Vallicioni J, Gaillot M, Schneider M. Intra-arterial sequential chemotherapy in head and neck tumors. Med Oncol Abstr 4th Annu Meet Med Oncol Soc and Bi-Annu Meet Immunol and Immunother Group, Nice, France, Dec 2-4, 1978. New York: Springer-Verlag, 1978; 29.

47. Danko J, Satko I, Durkovsky J. Combined regional chemotherapy and radiation therapy in the treatment of epidermoid carcinoma of the oro-facial region. Neoplasma 1979; 26(3):345−50.

48. Molinari R. Experience with intra-arterial chemotherapy prior to surgery or radiotherapy for advanced cancer of the oral cavity. Rev Sudam Oncol (Argent) 1979; 3:18−25.

49. Cruz AB Jr., McInnis WD, Aust JB. Triple drug intra-arterial infusion combined with x-ray therapy and surgery for head and neck cancer. Am J Surg 1974; 128:573−79.

50. Auersperg M, Furlan L, Marolt F, Jereb B. intra-arterial chemotherapy and radiotherapy in locally advanced cancer of the oral cavity and oropharynx. Int J Radiat Oncol Biol Phys 1978; 4:273−77.

51. Hervi, Perrino A, Valente V. Protracted intra-arterial chemotherapy with sequential courses of antimitotics and radiotherapy in the treatment of extended head and neck. Tumori 1968; 54:199−219.

52. Bagshaw M, Doggett RLS. A clinical study of chemical radiosensitization. Front Rad Ther Oncol 1969; 4:164−73.

53. Rooney M, Kish J, Jacobs J, Kinzie J, et al. Improved complete response rate and survival in advanced head and neck cancer after three-course induction therapy with 120-hour 5-FU infusion and cisplatin. Cancer 1985; 55:1123−28.

54. Baker SR, Wheeler RH, Medvec BR. Innovative regional therapy for head and neck cancer. Arch Otolaryngol 1982; 108:703−08.

55. Frei E III, Canellos GP. Dose: a critical factor in cancer chemotherapy. Am J Med 1980; 69:583−94.

56. Bruce WR, Meeker BE, Powers WE, Valeriote FA. Comparison of the dose- and time-survival

curves for normal hematopoietic and lymphoma colony-forming cells exposed to vinblastine, vincristine, arabinosylcytosine and amethopterin. J Natl Cancer Inst 1969; 42:1015–23.

57. Mellett LB. Considerations in design of optimal therapeutic schedules. In: Pharmacology and the future of man. Proc 5th Int Cong Pharmacol, San Francisco, Vol. 3. Basal: Karger, 1973; 332–53.

58. Pinedo HM, Chabner BA. Role of drug concentration, duration of exposure and endogenous metabolites in determining methotrexate cytotoxicity. Cancer Treat Rep 1977; 61:708–15.

59. Chabner BA, Young RC. Threshhold methotrexate concentration for in vivo inhibition of DNA synthesis in normal and tumorous target tissues. J Clin Invest 1973; 52:1804–11.

60. Bruce WR, Meeder BE, Valeriote FA. Comparison of the sensitivity of normal hematopoietic and transplanted lymphoma colony-forming cells to chemotherapeutic agents administered in vivo. J Natl Cancer Inst 1966; 37:233–45.

61. Young RC, Rosenoff SA, Myers CE, Btereton H, Chabner BA. Alterations in DNA synthesis induced by chemotherapeutic agents in vivo: potential applications to clinical treatment schedules. In: Growth kinetics and biochemical regulation of normal and malignant cells. Drewinko B, Humphrey RM, eds. Baltimore: Williams & Wilkins Co., 1977; 787–809.

62. Skipper HE, Schabd FM. Quantitative and cytokinetic studies in experimental tumor systems. In: Cancer medicine. Holland JF, Frei E III, eds. Philadelphia: Lea and Febiger, 1982; 663–85.

63. Blum RH, Frei E III, Holland JF. Principles of dose, schedule and combination chemotherapy. In: Cancer medicine. Holland JF, Frei E III, eds. Philadelphia: Lea and Febiger, 1982; 730–52.

64. Jusko WJ. A pharmacodynamic model for cell-cycle-specific chemotherapeutic agents. J Pharmacokin Biopharm 1973; 1:175–200.

65. Collins JM, Dedrick RL. Pharmacokinetics of anticancer drugs. In: Pharmacologic principles of cancer treatment. Chaber B, ed. Philadelphia: W.B. Saunders Co., 1982; 77–99.

66. Fensmacher J, Gazendam J. Intra-arterial infusions of drugs and hyperosomotic solutions as ways of enhancing CNA chemotherapy. Cancer Treat Rep 1981; 65(Suppl 2):27–38.

67. Levin VA, Landahl HD, Patlak CS. Drug delivery to CNS tumors. Cancer Treat Rep 1981; 65(Suppl 2):19–26.

68. Chen HG, Gross JF. Intra-arterial infusion of anticancer drugs: theoretic aspects of drug delivery and review of responses. Cancer Treat Rep 1980; 64:31–40.

69. Eckman WW, Pallak CS, Fenstermacher JD. A critical evaluation of the principles governing the advantages of intra-arterial infusions. J Pharmacokin Biopharm 1974; 2:257–85.

70. Wheeler RH, Zeissman HA, Medvec BR, et al. Tumor blood flow and systemic shunting in patients receiving intra-arterial chemotherapy for head and neck cancer. Cancer Res 1986; 46:4200-04.

71. Baker SR, Wheeler RH. Long-term intra-arterial chemotherapy infusion of ambulatory head and neck cancer patients. J Surg Oncol 1982; 21:125–31.

72. Mattesson J, Appelgren L, Bertil H, Peterson HI. Tumor vessel innervation and influence of vasoactive drugs on tumor blood flow. In: CRC tumor blood circulation. Peterson HI, ed. Boca Raton, FL: CRC Press, Inc., 1979.

73. Billing L, Lindgren AGH. Die patologishe-anatomische unterlage der geschwulstarteriographie. Eine untersuchung der arteriellen gefässe des hypernephroms und des magenkarzinoma. Acta Radiol 1944; 25:625.

74. Lagergren C, Lindbom A, Söderberg G. Vascularization of fibromatous and fibrosarcomatous tumors. Histopathologic, microangiographic and angiographic studies. Acta Radiol 1960; 53:1.

75. Forastiere AA, Ziessman HA, Wheeler RH, et al. The use of a vasoconstrictor to improve tumor blood flow in intra-arterial chemotherapy: preliminary report. Nuc Med Commun 1985; 6:777–86.

76. Goldman HL, Bilbao MK, Rosch J, Dotter CT. Complications of indwelling chemotherapy catheters. Cancer 1975; 36:1883–90.

77. Helsper JT, DeMoss EV. Regional intra-arterial infusion of 5-fluorouracil for cancer. Surgery 1964; 56:340–48.

78. Hanna DC, Gaisford JC, Goldwyn RM. Intra-arterial nitrogen mustard for control of pain in head and neck cancer. Am J Surg 1963; 106:783–85.

79. Watkins E Jr., Sullivan RD. Cancer chemotherapy by prolonged arterial infusion. SGO 1964; 118(1):3 – 19.

80. Zimmerman HA, Rand JH III. A pressure pump for administering intra-arterial or intravenous fluids. J Lab Clin Med 1950; 35:993 – 94.

81. Pegg DE, Trotman RE, Pierce NH. Apparatus for continuous infusion chemotherapy. Br Med J 1963; 1:207 – 08.

82. Addison BA, Jennings ER. A simplified technique for cancer infusion chemotherapy. J Med Assoc Ga 1963; 52:203 – 04.

83. McDonald IR. An assisted infusion apparatus. Med J Aust 1963; 50(1):661 – 62.

84. Donaldson RC, Paletta FX. An improved method of direct cannulation of the carotid artery for infusion. Am J Surg 1963; 106:712 – 15.

85. Herter FT, Markowitz AM, Feind CR. Cancer chemotherapy by continuous intra-arterial infusion of antimetabolites. Am J Surg 1963; 105:628 – 39.

86. Kisken WA, Johnson RO, Curreri AR. A technique of continuous intra-arterial infusion. Cancer Chemother Rep 1962; 24:27 – 28.

87. Watkins E Jr. Chronometric infusor – an apparatus for protracted ambulatory infusion therapy. N Engl J Med 1963; 269:850 – 51.

88. Burn JI, Gains E. The chemofusor: a new apparatus for maintaining continuous intra-arterial infusion chemotherapy. Br J Surg 1973; 60(5):375 – 77.

89. Rutherford WI. M.D. Anderson: treating cancer on an outpatient basis. Tex Hosp 1980; 36:10 – 12.

90. Blackshear PJ, Dorman FD, Blackshear PL Jr., Varco RL, Buchwald H. A permanently implantable self-recycling low-flow constant rate multipurpose infusion pump of simple design. Surg Forum 1970; 21:137.

91. Blackshear PJ, Dorman FD, Blackshear PL Jr., Varco RL, Buchwald H. The design and initial testing of an implantable infusion pump. SGO 1972; 134:51 – 56.

92. Blackshear PJ, Rohde TD, Varco RL, Buchwald H. One year of continuous heparinization in the dog using a totally implantable infusion pump. SGO 1975; 141:176 – 86.

93. Rohde TD, Blackshear PJ, Varco RL, Buchwald H. Chronic heparin anticoagulant in dogs by continuous infusion with a totally implantable pump. Trans Am Soc Artif Intern Organs 1975; 21:510 – 14.

94. Rohde TD, Blackshear PJ, Varco RL, Buchwald H. Protracted parenteral drug infusion in ambulatory subjects using an implantable infusion pump. Trans Am Soc Artif Intern Organs 1977; 23:13 – 16.

95. Baker SR, Wheeler RH, Medvec BR. Surgical aspects of intra-arterial therapy of outpatients with head and neck cancer. Otolaryngol Head Neck Surg 1985; 93:192-99.

96. Wheeler RH, Baker SR, Medvec BM. Single agent and combination drug regional chemotherapy for head and neck cancer using an implantable infusion pump. Cancer 1984; 54:1504 – 12.

97. Duff JK, Sullivan RD, Miller E, Ulm AH, Charlson BC, Clifford P. Antimetabolite-metabolite cancer chemotherapy using continuous intra-arterial methotrexate with intermittent intramuscular citovorum factor method of therapy. Cancer 1961; 14:744 – 52.

98. Ramsden CH, Duff JK. Continuous arterial infusion of head and neck tumors, improvements in technique by retrograde temporal artery catherterization. Cancer 1963; 16:133 – 35.

99. Engeset A, Brennhovd I, Stovner J. Intra-arterial infusions in cancer chemotherapy, a technique for testing drug distribution. Lancet 1962; 1:1382 – 83.

100. Rapoport A, Sobrinho J de A, Serson D, Nunes JE De O. The value of ^{131}I-labeled albumin macroaggregate in the localization of intra-arterial chemotherapy for the treatment of advanced cancer of the head and neck. Tumori 1974; 60:355 – 59.

101. Kaplan WD, Ensminger WD, Come SE, et al. Radionuclide angiography to predict patient response to hepatic artery chemotherapy. Cancer Treat Rep 1980; 64(12):1217 – 22.

102. Baker SR, Wheeler RH, Ziessman H, Medvec BR, Thrall JH, Keyes JW. Radionuclide localization of intra-arterial infusion in head and neck cancer. Cancer Drug Del 1984; 1:145 – 56.

References—Chapter 32

1. Pickren JW, Tsukada Y, Lane WW. Liver metastasis: analysis of autopsy data. In: Weiss L, Gilbert H, eds. Liver metastasis. Boston: G.K. Hall Medical Publishers, 1982; 2–18.

2. Lee Y-T. Regional management of liver metastases. I and II. Cancer Invest 1983; 1:237–57, 321–32.

3. Abrams HL, Spiro R, Goldstein N. Metastases in carcinoma: analysis of 1,000 autopsied cases. Cancer 1950; 3:74–85.

4. Welch JP, Donaldson GA. The clinical correlation of an autopsy study of recurrent colorectal cancer. Ann Surg 1979; 189:496–502.

5. Cady B, Monson DO, Swinton NW. Survival of patients after colonic resection for carcinoma with simultaneous liver metastasis. Surg Gyn Obstet 1970; 131:697–700.

6. Foster JH. Survival after liver resection for secondary tumors. Am J Surg 1978; 135:389–94.

7. Fortner JG, Pahnke LD. A new method for long-term intra-hepatic chemotherapy. Surg Gynecol Obstet 1976; 143:979–80.

8. Hagemeister FB Jr., Buzdar AU, Luna MA, et al. Causes of death in breast cancer: a clinicopathologic study. Cancer 1980; 46:162–67.

9. Viadana E, Cotter R, Pickren JW, et al. An autopsy study of metastatic sites of breast cancer. Cancer Res 1973; 33:179–81.

10. Jaffee BM, Donegan WL, Watson F, et al. Factors influencing survival in patients with untreated hepatic metastases. Surg Gynecol Obstet 1968; 127:1-11.

11. Wanebo JH, Semoglou C, Attiyeh F, et al. Surgicial management of patients with primary operable colorectal cancer and synchronous liver metastases. Am J Surg 1978; 135:81–85.

12. Wagner JS, Adson MA, Van Heerden JA, et al. The natural history of hepatic metastases from colorectal cancer: a comparison with resective treatment. Ann Surg 1984; 199:502–08.

13. Lahr CJ, Soong SJ, Cloud G, et al. A multifactorial analysis of prognostic factors in patients with liver metastases from colorectal carcinoma. J Clin Oncol 1983; 1:720–26.

14. Biefman HR, Byron RL, Miller ER, et al. Effects of intra-arterial administration of nitrogen mustard. Am J Med 1950; 8:535.

15. Klopp CT, Bateman J, Berry N, et al. Fractionated regional cancer chemotherapy. Cancer Res 1950; 10:229.

16. Sullivan RD, Miller E, Sikes MP. Antimetabolite-metabolite combination cancer chemotherapy. Cancer 1959; 12:1248–61.

17. Clarkson B, Lawrence W. Perfusion and infusion techniques in cancer chemotherapy. Med Clin N Am 1961; 45:689.

18. Niederhuber JE, Ensminger WD. Surgical considerations in the management of hepatic neoplasia. Semin Oncol 1983; 10:135–47.

19. Karakousis CP, Douglass HO, Holyoke ED. Technique of infusion chemotherapy, ligation of the hepatic artery and dearterialization in malignant lesions of the liver. Surg Gynecol Obstet 1979; 149:403–07.

20. Chuang VP, Wallace S. Current status of transcatheter management of neoplasms. Cardiovasc Intervent Radiol 1980; 3:256–65.

21. Daly JM, Kemeny N, Oderman P, et al. Long-term hepatic arterial infusion chemotherapy: anatomic considerations, operative technique, and treatment morbidity. Arch Surg 1984; 119:936–41.

22. Rosenberg HD, Wile AG, Aufrichtig D, et al. Hepatic artery-biliary fistula: an unusual complication of infusion therapy. Gastrointest Radiol 1983; 8:37–40.

23. Hohn D, Melnick J, Stagg R, et al. Biliary sclerosis in patients receiving hepatic arterial infusion of floxuride. J Clin Oncol 1985; 3:98–102.

24. Kemeny N, Daly J, Oderman P, et al. Hepatic artery pump infusion: toxicity and results in patients with metastatic colorectal carcinoma. J Clin Oncol 1984; 2:595–600.

25. Weidner N, Smith JG, LaVanway JM. Peptic ulceration with marked epithelial atypia following

hepatic arterial infusion chemotherapy: a lesion initially misinterpreted as carcinoma. Am J Surg Pathol 1983; 7:261–68.

26. Yang PJ, Thrall JH, Ensminger WD, et al. Perfusion scintigraphy (Tc-99m MAA) during surgery for placement of chemotherapy catheter in hepatic artery: concise communication. J Nucl Med 1982; 23:1066–69.

27. Bledin AG, Kim EE, Chuang VP, et al. Changes of arterial blood flow patterns during infusion chemotherapy, as monitored by intra-arterially injected technetium 99m macroaggregated albumin. Br J Radiol 1984; 57:197–203.

28. Ziessman HA, Thrall JH, Yang PJ, et al. Hepatic arterial perfusion scintigraphy with Tc-99m-MAA: use of a totally implanted drug delivery system. Radiology 1984; 152:167–72.

29. Bledin AG, Kim EE, Haynie TP. Technetium Tc 99m-macroaggregated albumin angiography and perfusion, intra-arterial chemotherapy for neoplasms. JAMA 1983; 250:941–43.

30. Kaplan WD, Come SE, Takvorian RW, et al. Pulmonary uptake of technetium 99m macroaggregated albumin: a predictor of gastrointestinal toxicity during hepatic artery perfusion. J Clin Oncol 1984; 2:1266–69.

31. Wallace S, Charnsangavej C, Carrasco CH, et al. Percutaneous transcatheter infusion and infarction in the treatment of human cancer: part 1. In: Hickey RC, ed. Current problems in cancer. 1984; 8:17; 1–62.

32. Ensminger WD, Rosowsky A, Raso V, et al. A clinical-pharmacological evaluation of hepatic arterial infusions of 5-fluoro-2-deoxyuridine and 5-fluorouracil. Cancer Res 1978; 38:3784–92.

33. Stagg RJ, Lewis BJ, Friedman MA, et al. Hepatic arterial chemotherapy for colorectal cancer metastatic to the liver. Ann Intern Med 1984; 100:736–43.

34. Huberman MS. Comparison of systemic chemotherapy with hepatic arterial infusion in metastatic colorectal carcinoma. Semin Oncol 1983; 10:238–48.

35. Patt YZ, Chuang VP, Wallace S, et al. The palliative role of hepatic arterial infusion and arterial occlusion in colorectal carcinoma metastatic to the liver. Lancet 1981; 1:349–50.

36. Cady B, Oberfield RA. Regional infusion chemotherapy of hepatic metastases from carcinoma of the colon. Am J Surg 1974; 127:220–27.

37. Tylen U, Dahl E, Fredlung P. Angiography after temporary inhibition of blood flow followed by intra-arterial 5-FU infusion in the treatment of liver metastases. Acta Radiol Diag 1981; 22:15–23.

38. Mittal R, Kowal C, Starzl T, et al. Accuracy of computerized tomography in determining hepatic tumor size in patients receiving liver transplatation or resection. J Clin Oncol 1984; 2:637–42.

39. Miller DL, Vermess M, Doppman JL, et al. CT of the liver and spleen with EOE-13: review of 225 examinations. AJR 1984; 143:235–43.

40. Labell JJ, Lucas RJ, Eisenstein B, et al. Hepatic artery catheterization for chemotherapy. Arch Surg 1968; 96:683–93.

41. Davis HL, Ramirez G, Ansfield FJ. Adenocarcinomas of stomach, pancreas, liver and biliary tracts. Cancer 1974; 33:193–97.

42. Petrek JA, Minton JP. Treatment of hepatic metastases by percutaneous hepatic arterial infusion. Cancer 1979; 43:2182–88.

43. Ansfield FJ, Ramirez G, Skibba JL, et al. Intrahepatic arterial infusion with 5-fluorouracil. Cancer 1971; 28:1147–51.

44. Ansfield FJ, Ramirez G. The clinical results of 5-fluorouracil intrahepatic arterial infusion in 528 patients with metastatic cancer to the liver. Prog Clin Cancer 1978; 7:201–06.

45. Reed ML, Vaitkevicius VK, Al-Sarraf M, et al. The practicality of chronic hepatic artery infusion therapy of primary and metastatic hepatic malignancies: ten-year results of 124 patients in a prospective protocol. Cancer 1981; 47:402–09.

46. Brennan MJ, Talley RW, Drake EH, et al. 5-fluorouracil treatment of liver metastases by continuous hepatic artery infusion via Cournand catheter. Ann Surg 1963; 158:405–19.

47. Freckman HA. Chemotherapy for metastatic colorectal liver carcinoma by intra-aortic infusion. Cancer 1971; 28:1152–60.

48. Fortuny IE, Theologides A, Kennedy BJ. Hepatic arterial infusion for liver metastases from colon

cancer: comparison of mitomycin-C (NSC-26980) and 5-fluorouracil (MSC-19893). Cancer Chemother Rep 1975; 59:401−04.

49. Oberfield RA, McCaffrey JA, Polio J, et al. Prolonged and continuous percutaneous intra-arterial hepatic infusion chemotherapy in advanced metastatic liver adenocarcinoma from colorectal primary. Cancer 1979; 44:414−23.

50. Douglass CC. Improved survival in liver metastases from colorectal carcinoma following periodic arterial infusions with mitomycin-C, 5-fluorouracil, Adriamycin, Velban, and vincristine. Proc Am Soc Clin Oncol 1979; 20:431.

51. Grage TB, Vassilopoulos PP, Shingleton WW, et al. Results of a prospective randomized study of hepatic artery infusion with 5-fluorouracil versus intravenous 5-fluorouracil in patients with hepatic metastases from colorectal cancer: a Central Oncology Group study. Surgery 1979; 86:550−55.

52. Grage TB, Shingleton WW, Jubert AV, et al. Results of a prospective randomized study of hepatic artery infusion with 5-fluorouracil vs. intravenous 5-fluorouracil in patients with hepatic metastases from colorectal cancer: a Central Oncology Group study (COG 7032). Front Gastrointest Res 1979; 5:116−29.

53. Bedikian AY, Chen TT, Malahy M-A, et al. Prognostic factors influencing survival of patients with advanced colorectal cancer: hepatic-artery infusion versus systemic intravenous chemotherapy for liver metastases. J Clin Oncol 1984; 2:174−80.

54. Fortner JG, Silva JS, Cox EB, et al. Multivariate analysis of a personal series of 247 patients with liver metastases from colorectal cancer. II. Treatment by intrahepatic chemotherapy. Ann Surg 1984; 199:317−24.

55. Rochlin DB, Smart CR. An evaluation of 51 patients with hepatic artery infusion. Surg Gynecol Obstet 1966; 123:535−38.

56. Ariel IM, Pack GT. Treatment of inoperable cancer of the liver by intra-arterial radioactive isotopes and chemotherapy. Cancer 1967; 20:793−804.

57. Massey WH, Fletcher WS, Judkins MP, et al. Hepatic artery infusion for metastatic malignancy using percutaneous placed catheters. Am J Surg 1971; 121:160−64.

58. Tandon RN, Bunnell IL, Copper RG. The treatment of metastatic carcinoma of the liver by the percutaneous selective hepatic artery infusion of 5-fluorouracil. Surgery 1973; 73:118−21.

59. Kraybill WG, Harrison M, Sasaki T, et al. Regional intra-arterial infusion of Adriamycin in the treatment of cancer. Surg Gynecol Obstet 1977; 144:335−38.

60. Misra NC, Jaiswal MSD, Singh RV, et al. Intrahepatic arterial infusion of combination of mitomycin-C and 5-fluorouracil in treatment of primary and metastatic liver carcinoma. Cancer 1977; 39:1425−29.

61. Robison EW. Metastatic liver disease: treatment by hepatic artery infusion. Rocky Mt Med J 1979; 76:185−86.

62. Helsper JT, Lance JS, Hall TC. Transfemoral hepatic artery infusion for metastatic carcinoma. J Surg Oncol 1981; 18:173−81.

63. Peetz M, Swanson J, Moseley HS, et al. Endocrine ablation and hepatic artery infusion in the treatment of metastases to the liver from carcinoma of the breast. Surg Gynecol Obstet 1982; 155:395−400.

64. Burrows JH, Talley RW, Drake EL, et al. Infusion of fluorinated pyrimidines into hepatic artery for treatment of metastatic carcinoma of the liver. Cancer 1967; 20:1886−92.

65. Donegan WL, Harris HS. Metastatic colorectal carcinoma: response to hepatic infusion. Mo Med 1970; 67:163−68.

66. Watkins E, Khazei AM, Nahra KS. Surgical basis for arterial infusion chemotherapy of disseminated carcinoma of the liver. Surg Gynecol Obstet 1970; 130:581−605.

67. Stehlin JS, Hafstrom L, Greeff PJ. Experience with infusion and resection in cancer of the liver. Surg Gynecol Obstet 1974; 138:855−63.

68. Ansfield FJ, Ramirez G, Davis HL, et al. Further clinical studies with intrahepatic arterial infusion with 5-fluorouracil. Cancer 1975; 36:2413−17.

69. Pettavel J, Morgenthaler F. Protracted arterial chemotherapy of liver tumors: an experience of 107 cases over a 12-year period. Prog Clin Cancer 1978; 7:217−33.

70. Sundqvist K, Hafstrom LO, Jonsson PE, et al. Treatment of liver cancer with regional intra-arterial 5-FU infusion. Am J Surg 1978; 136:328–31.

71. Patt YZ, Wallace S, Hersh EM, et al. Hepatic arterial infusion of corynebacterium parvum and chemotherapy. Surg Gynecol Obstet 1978; 147:897–902.

72. Calvo DB, Patt YZ, Wallace S, et al. Phase 1-2 trial of percutaneous intra-arterial cisdiamminedichloro-platinum (II) for regionally confined malignancy. Cancer 1980; 45:1278–83.

73. Storm FK, Kaiser LR, Goodnight JE, et al. Thermochemotherapy for melanoma metastases in liver. Cancer 1982; 49:1243–48.

74. Kondi ES, Gallitano AL, Evjy JT, et al. Prolonged survival in patients with hepatic malignant melanoma treated by intra-arterial bleomycin and later oral hydroxyurea. Am J Surg 1974; 128:85–87.

75. Gyves JW, Ensminger WD. Metastatic colorectal cancer–regional chemotherapy. Curr Concepts Oncol 1984; 6:9–18.

76. Patt YZ, Mavligit GM, Chuang VP, et al. Percutaneous hepatic arterial infusion (HAI) of mytomycin-C and floxuridine (FUDR): an effective treatment for metastatic colorectal carcinoma in the liver. Cancer 1980; 46:261–65.

77. Patt YZ, Chuang VP, Wallace S, et al. Hepatic arterial chemotherapy and occlusion for palliation of primary hepatocellular and unknown primary neoplasms in the liver. Cancer 1983; 51:1359–63.

78. Falk RE, Greig P, Makowka L, et al. Intermittent percutaneous infusion into the hepatic artery of cytotoxic drugs for hepatic tumors. Can J Surg 1982; 25:47–50.

79. Tilchen E, Patt YZ, McBride CM, et al. Sequence of regional chemotherapy and surgery. Arch Surg 1981; 116:959–60.

80. Hodgson WJB, Mittelman A, Ahmed T, et al. Combined intra-hepatic chemotherapy and surgical debulking for metastatic adenocarcinoma of the colon to the liver. Proc ASCO March 1984; 141.

81. Kano T, Kumashiro R, Abe Y, et al. Combination of hepatic arterial infusion and systemic chemotherapy for gastric cancer with synchronous hepatic metastases. Jpn J Surg 1984; 14:23–29.

82. Shigemasa K, Kawaguchi H, Kishimoto H, et al. Therapeutic significance of noncurative gastrectomy for gastric cancer with liver metastasis. Am J Surg 1980; 140:356–59.

83. Lee Y-TN. Hepatography with oily contrast medium injected via the portal vein system. Surgery 1968; 63:948–53.

84. Konno T, Maeda H, Iwai K, et al. Selective targeting of anticancer drug and simultaneous image enhancement in solid tumors by arterially administered lipid contrast medium. Cancer 1984; 54:2367–74.

85. Madding GF, Kennedy PA. Hepatic artery ligation. Surg Clinic N Am 1972; 52:719–28.

86. Markowitz J. The hepatic artery. Surg Gynecol Obstet 1952; 95:644–46.

87. Nilsson LAV. Therapeutic hepatic artery ligation in patients with secondary liver tumors. Rev Surg Sept–Oct 1966; 374–76.

88. Madding GF, Kennedy PA, Sogemeier E. Hepatic artery ligation for metastatic tumor in the liver. Am J Surg 1970; 120:94–96.

89. Benmark S, Ericsson M, Lunderquist A, et al. Temporary liver dearterialization in patients with metastatic carcinoid disease. World J Surg 1982; 6:46–53.

90. Berjian RA, Douglass HO, Nava HR, et al. The role of hepatic artery ligation and dearterialization with infusion chemotherapy in advanced malignancies in the liver. J Surg Oncol 1980; 14:379–87.

91. Murray-Lyon IM, Dawson JL, Parsons VA, et al. Treatment of secondary hepatic tumours by ligation of hepatic artery and infusion of cytotoxic drugs. Lancet 1970; 2:172–75.

92. Koudahl G, Funding J. Hepatic artery ligation in primary and secondary hepatic cancer. Acta Chir Scand 1972; 138:289–91.

93. Zike WL, Safaie-Shirazi S, Gulesserian HP, et al. Hepatic artery ligation and cytotoxic infusion in treatment of liver neoplasms. Arch Surg 1975; 110:641–43.

94. Cuschieri A, Swain C. Hepatic artery ligation and prolonged cytotoxic therapy in advanced primary and secondary liver tumours. Proc Soc Med 1975; 68:678–80.

95. Sparks FC, Mosher MB, Hallauer WC, et al. Hepatic artery ligation and postoperative chemotherapy for hepatic metastases: clinical and pathophysiological results. Cancer 1975; 35:1074–82.

96. Ramming KP, Sparks FC, Eilber FR, et al. Hepatic artery ligation and 5-fluorouracil infusion for metastatic colon carcinoma and primary hepatoma. Am J Surg 1976; 132:236−42.

97. Almersjo O, Bengmark S, Hafstrom L, et al. Results of liver dearterialization combined with regional infusion of 5-fluorouracil for liver cancer. Acta Chir Scand 1976; 142:131−38.

98. Nagasue N, Inokuchi K, Kobayashi M, et al. Hepatic dearterialization for nonresectable primary and secondary tumors of the liver. Cancer 1976; 38:2593−2603.

99. Lee Y-TN. Hepatic artery ligation and infusion chemotherapy for malignancy of the liver. J Am Med Women's Assoc 1979; 34:21−39.

100. Evans JT. Hepatic artery ligation in hepatic metastases from colon and rectal malignancies. Dis Colon Rectum 1979; 22:370−71.

101. Smith R. Tumours of the liver (Bradshaw Lect 1977). Ann R Coll Surg Engl 1979; 61:87−99.

102. Fortner JG, Papachristou DN. Surgery of liver tumors. Int Adv Surg Oncol 1979; 2:251−57.

103. Taylor I. Studies on the treatment and prevention of colorectal liver metastases. Ann R Coll Surg Engl 1981; 63:270−76.

104. Taylor I: Cytotoxic perfusion for colorectal liver metastases. Br J Surg 1978; 65:109−14.

105. Petrelli NJ, Barcewica PA, Evans JT, et al. Hepatic artery ligation for liver metastasis in colorectal carcinoma. Cancer 1984; 53:1347−53.

106. Laufman LR, Nims Ta, Guy JT, et al. Hepatic artery ligation and portal vein infusion for liver metastases from colon cancer. J Clin Oncol 1984; 2:1382−89.

107. Almersjo O, Bengmark S, Hafstrom L. Liver resection for cancer. Acta Chir Scand 1976; 142:139−44.

108. Lee Y-TN. Liver function tests after ligation of hepatic artery. J Surg Oncol 1978; 10:305−20.

109. El-Domeiri AA, Mojab K. Intermittent occlusion of the hepatic artery and infusion chemotherapy for carcinoma of the liver. Am J Surg 1978; 135:771−75.

110. El-Domeiri AA. Treatment of hepatic metastases in cancer of the colon and rectum: a preliminary report. Cancer 1980; 45:2245−48.

111. Karakousis CP, Kanter PM, Lopez R, et al. Modes of regional chemotherapy. J Surg Res 1979; 26:134−41.

112. Bengmark S, Fredlund PE. Temporary dearterialization combined with intra-arterial infusion of oncolytic drugs in the treatment of liver tumors. Prog Clin Cancer 1978; 7:207−16.

113. Dahl EP, Fredlund PE, Tylen U, et al. Transient hepatic dearterialization followed by regional intra-arterial 5-fluorouracil infusion as treatment for liver tumors. Ann Surg 1981; 193:82−88.

114. Lise M, Cagol PP, Nitti D, et al. Temporary occlusion of the hepatic artery plus infusion and systemic chemotherapy for inoperable cancer of the liver. Int Surg 1980; 65:315−23.

115. Aronsen KF, Hellekant C, Holmberg J, et al. Controlled blocking of hepatic artery flow with enzymatically degradable microspheres combined with oncolytic drugs. Eur Surg Res 1979; 11:99−106.

116. Ensminger WD, Thompson M, Come S, et al. Hepatic arterial BCNU: a pilot clinical-pharmacologic study in patients with liver tumors. Cancer Treat Rep 1978; 62:1509−12.

117. Dakhil S, Ensminger W, Cho K, et al. Improved regional selectivity of hepatic arterial BCNU with degradable microspheres. Cancer 1982; 50:631−35.

118. Lien WM, Ackerman NB. The blood supply of experimental liver metastases. II. A microcirculatory study of normal vessels of the liver with the use of perfused silicone rubber. Surgery 1970; 68:334−40.

119. Almersjo O, Gustavsson B, Hafstrom L. Results of regional portal infusions of 5-fluorouracil in patients with primary and secondary liver cancer. Ann Chir Gynaecol 1976; 65:27−32.

120. Chuang VP, Wallace S, Soo C-S, et al. Therapeutic Ivalon embolization of hepatic tumors. AJR 1982; 138:289−94.

121. Clouse ME, Lee RG, Duszlak RJ, et al. Peripheral hepatic artery embolization for primary and secondary hepatic neoplasms. Radiology 1983; 147:407−11.

122. Michaels NA. Blood supply and anatomy of the upper abdominal organs. Philadelphia: JB Lippincott Co., 1965.

123. Soo C-S, Chuang VP, Wallace S, et al. Treatment of hepatic neoplasm through extrahepatic collaterals. Radiology 1983; 147:45 – 49.

124. Chuang VP, Wallace S. Interventional approaches to hepatic tumor treatment. Semin Roentgenol 1983; 18:127 – 35.

125. Blumgart LH, Allison DJ. Resection and embolization in the management of secondary hepatic tumors. World J Surg 1982; 6:32 – 45.

126. Wallace S, Charnsangavej C, Carrasco H, et al. Infusion-embolization. Cancer 1984; 54:2751 – 65.

127. Patt YZ, Peters RE, Chuang VP, et al. Effective retreatment of patients with colorectal cancer and liver metastases. Am J Med 1983; 75:237 – 40.

128. Allison DJ, Modlin IM, Kenkins WJ. Treatment of carcinoid liver metastases by hepatic-artery embolization. Lancet 1977; 2:1323 – 25.

129. Martensson H, Nobin A, Bengmark S, et al. Embolization of the liver in the management of metastatic carcinoid tumors. J Surg Oncol 1984; 27:152 – 58.

130. Carrasco CH, Chuang VP, Wallace S. Apudomas metastatic to the liver: treatment by hepatic artery embolization. Radiology 1983; 149:79 – 83.

131. Chuang VP, Wallace S. Arterial infusion and occlusion in cancer patients. Semin Roentgenol 1981; 16:13 – 25.

132. Shermeta DW, Golladay ES, White RI. Preoperative occlusion of the hepatic artery with isobutyl 2-cyanoacrylate for resection of the "unresectable" hepatic tumor. Surgery 1978; 83:319 – 22.

133. Kato T, Nemoto R, Mori H, et al. Arterial chemoembolization with mitomycin-C microcapsules in the treatment of primary or secondary carcinoma of the kidney, liver, bone and intrapelvic organs. Cancer 1981; 48:674 – 80.

134. Balch CM, Urist MM, McGregor ML. Continuous regional chemotherapy for metastatic colorectal cancer using a totally implantable infusion pump. Am J Surg 1983; 145:285 – 90.

135. Balch CM, Urist MM, Soong S-J, et al. A prospective phase 2 clinical trial of continuous FUDR regional chemotherapy for colorectal metastases to the liver using a totally implantable drug infusion pump. Ann Surg 1983; 198:567 – 73.

136. Niederhuber JE, Ensminger W, Gyves J, et al. Regional chemotherapy of colorectal cancer metastatic to the liver. Cancer 1984; 53:1336 – 43.

References—Chapter 33

1. Lien WM, Ackerman NB. The blood supply of experimental liver metastases. II: a microcirculatory study of the normal and tumor vessels of the liver with the use of perfused silicone rubber. Surgery 1970; 68:334–40.

2. Breedis C, Young G. The blood supply of neoplasms in the liver. Am J Pathol 1954; 30:969–85.

3. Lee M. Regional management of liver metastases I. Cancer Invest 1983; 1 (3):237–57.

4. Blackshear PJ, Dorman FD, Blackshear PL Jr, et al. The design and initial testing of an implantable infusion pump. Surg Gynecol Obstet 1972; 134:51–56.

5. Rohde TD, Blackshear PJ, Varco RL, et al. One year of heparin anticoagulation: an ambulatory subject using a totally implantable infusion pump. Minn Med 1977; 60:719–22.

6. Buchwald H, Grage TB, Vassilopoulos PP, et al. Intra-arterial infusion chemotherapy for hepatic carcinoma using a totally implantable infusion pump. Cancer 1980; 45:866–69.

7. Barone RM, Byfield JE, Goldfarb PB, et al. Intra-arterial chemotherapy using an implantable infusion pump and liver irradiation for the treatment of hepatic metastases. Cancer 1982; 50:850–62.

8. Cohen AM, Kaufman SD, Wood WC, et al. Regional hepatic chemotherapy using an implantable drug infusion pump. Am J Surg 1983; 145:529–33.

9. Weiss GR, Garnick MB, Osteen RT, et al. Long-term hepatic arterial infusion of 5-fluorodeoxyuridine for liver metastases using an implantable infusion pump. J Clin Oncol 1983; 1:337–44.

10. Balch CM, Urist MM, Soong S, et al. A prospective phase 2 clinical trial of continuous FUDR regional chemotherapy for colorectal metastases to the liver using a totally implantable drug infusion pump. Ann Surg 1983; 198:567–73.

11. Niederhuber JE, Ensminger W, Gyves J. Regional chemotherapy of colorectal cancer metastatic to the liver. Cancer 1984; 53:1336–43.

12. Kemeny N, Daly J, Oderman P, et al. Hepatic artery pump infusion: toxicity and results in patients with metastatic colorectal carcinoma. J Clin Oncol 1984; 2(6):595–600.

13. Shepard KV, Levin B, Karl RC, et al. Therapy for metastatic colorectal cancer with hepatic artery infusion chemotherapy using a subcutaneous implanted pump. J Clin Oncol 1985; 3(2):161–69.

14. Buroker T, Samson M, Correa J, et al. Hepatic artery infusion of 5-FUDR after prior systemic 5-fluorouracil. Cancer Treat Rep 1976; 60:1277–79.

15. Lahr C, Soong S–J, Cloud G, et al. A multifactorial analysis of prognostic factors in patients with liver metastases from colorectal carcinoma. J Clin Oncol 1983; 1(11):720–26.

16. Wagner JS, Adson MA, VanHeerden JA, et al. The natural history of hepatic metastases from colorectal cancer: a comparison with resective treatment. Ann Surg 1984; 199:502–08.

17. Niederhuber JE, Ensminger WD. Surgical considerations in the management of hepatic neoplasia. Semin Oncol 1983; 10:135–47.

18. Cohen AM, Greenfield A, Wood WC, et al. Treatment of hepatic metastases by transaxillary hepatic artery chemotherapy using an implanted drug pump. Cancer 1983; 51:2013–19.

19. Hohn D, Melnick J, Stagg R, et al. Biliary sclerosis in patients receiving hepatic arterial infusions of floxuridine. J Clin Oncol 1985; 3(1): 98–102.

20. Kemeny MM, Goldberg DA, Browning SN, et al. Complications with continuous hepatic artery chemotherapy via an implantable pump. Proc ASCO 1984; 3:151.

21. Grage TB, Vassilopoulos PP, Shingleton WW, et al. Results of a prospective randomized study of hepatic artery infusion with 5-fluorouracil versus intravenous 5-fluorouracil in patients with hepatic metastases from colorectal cancer: a Central Oncology Group study. Surgery 1979; 86:550–55.

22. Lokich JJ. Hepatic artery chemotherapy: the relative importance of direct organ distribution vs. the constant infusion schedule. Am J Clin Oncol (CCT) 1984; 7:125–28.

23. Proceedings from 3rd Saddlebrook Conf: ongoing clinical trials using a totally implantable drug delivery system. Feb 1985. Spons by Intermedics Infusaid, Inc., Norwood, MA.

References—Chapter 34

1. Al-Sarraf M, Go TS, Kithier K, Vaitkevicius VK. Primary liver cancer: a review of the clinical features, blood groups, serum enzymes, therapy, and survival of 65 cases. Cancer 1974; 33:574–82.

2. Baker LH, Saiki JH, Jones SE, et al. Adriamycin and 5-fluorouracil in the treatment of advanced hepatoma: a Southwest Oncology Group study. Cancer Treat Rep 1977; 61:1595–97.

3. Balch CM, Urist MD, McGregor ML. Continuous regional chemotherapy for metastatic colorectal cancer using a totally implantable infusion pump: a feasibility study in 50 patients. Am J Surg 1983; 145:285–90.

4. Balch CM, Urist MM, Soong S-J, McGregor ML. A prospective phase 2 clinical trial of continuous FUDR regional chemotherapy for colorectal metastases to the liver using a totally implantable drug infusion pump. Ann Surg 1983; 198:567.

5. Bern MM, McDermott W, Cady B, et al. Intra-arterial hepatic infusion and intravenous Adriamycin for treatment of hepatocellular carcinoma: a clinical and pharmacology report. Cancer 1978; 42:399–405.

6. Bland KI, Knutson CO, Max MH. Hepatic arterial infusion chemotherapy for cancer of the liver. J Surg Oncol 1980; 13:253.

7. Cady B, Oberfield RA. Arterial infusion chemotherapy of hepatoma. Surg Gynecol Obstet 1974; 138:381.

8. Choi TK, Lee NW, Wong J. Chemotherapy for advanced hepatocellular carcinoma. Cancer 1984; 53:401–05.

9. Cohen AM, Greenfield A, Wood WC, et al. Treatment of hepatic metastases by transaxillary hepatic artery chemotherapy using an implanted drug pump. Cancer 1983; 51:2013–19.

10. El-Domeiri AA, Mojab K. Intermittent occlusion of the hepatic artery and infusion chemotherapy for carcinoma of the liver. Am J Surg 1978; 135:763.

11. Falkson G, Moertel CG, Lavin P, Pretorius FJ, Carbone PP. Chemotherapy studies in primary liver cancer. A prospective randomized clinical trial. Cancer 1978; 42:2149–56.

12. Farhi DC, Shikes RH, Murari PJ, Silverberg SG. Hepatocellular carcinoma in young people. Cancer 1983; 52:1516–25.

13. Garnick MB, Ensminger W, Israel M. A clinical-pharmacological evaulation of hepatic arterial infusion of Adriamycin. Cancer Res 1979; 39:4105–10.

14. Johnson PJ, Williams R, Thomas H, Sherlock S, Murray-Lyon IM. Induction of remission in hepatocellular carcinoma with doxorubicin. Lancet 1978; 1:1006–09.

15. Lack EE, Neave C, Vawter GF. Hepatocullular carcinoma: review of 32 cases in childhood and adolescence. Cancer 1983; 52:1510–15.

16. Lee YT. Systemic and regional treatment of primary carcinoma of the liver. Cancer Treat Rev 1977; 4:195–212.

17. Legha SS, Benjamin RS, Mackay B, et al. Reduction of doxorubicin cardiotoxicity by prolonged continuous intravenous infusion. Ann Int Med 1982; 96:133.

18. Melia WM, Johnson PJ, Williams R. Induction of remission in hepatocellular carcinoma. Cancer 1983; 51:206–10.

19. Morstyn G, Ihde DC, Eddy JL, Bunn PA, Cohen MH, Minna JD. Combination chemotherapy of hepatocellular carcinoma with doxorubicin and streptozotocin. Am J Clin Oncol 1983; 6:547–51.

20. Patt YZ, Charnsangavej C, Soski M. Hepatic arterial infusion of floxuridine, Adriamycin, and mitomycin-C for primary liver neoplasms. In: Bottino JC, Opfell R, Muggia F, eds. Therapy of neoplasms confined to the liver and biliary tract. New York: Martinus Nijhoff Publishers (in press).

21. Patt YZ, Chuang VP, Wallace S, Benjamin RS, Fuqua R, Mavligit GM. Hepatic arterial chemotherapy and occlusion for palliation of primary hepatocellular and unknown primary neoplasms in the liver. Cancer 1983; 51:1359–63.

22. Sack J, Urist MM, Balch CM, Aldrete JS. Hepatocellular carcinoma: characteristics and current management Ala J Med Sci 1983; 20:182–85.

23. Stehlin JS, Hafstrom L, Greeff PJ. Experience with infusion and resection in cancer of the liver. Surg Gynecol Obstet 1974; 138:855.

24. Urist MM and Balch CM. Intra-arterial chemotherapy for hepatoma using Adriamycin administered via an implantable constant infusion pump. Proc ASCO 1984; 3:148.

25. Vogel CL, Bayley AC, Brooker RJ, Anthony PP, Ziegler JL. A phase 2 study of Adriamycin (NSC 123127) in patients with hepatocellular carcinoma from Zambia and the United States. Cancer 1977; 39:1923–29.

References—Chapter 35

1. Wright RD. The blood supply of newly developed epithelial tissue in the liver. J Pathol Bacteriol 1937; 45:405–14.

2. Bierman HR, Byron RL, Kelley KH, Grady A. Studies on the blood supply of tumors in man. III. Vascular patterns of the liver by hepatic arteriography in vivo. J Nat Cancer Inst 1951; 12:107–17.

3. Suzuki T, Sarumaru S, Kawabe K, Honjo I. Study of vascularity of tumors of the liver. Surg Gynecol Obstet 1972; 134:27–34.

4. Kim DK, Watson RC, Pahnke LD, Fortner JG. Tumor vascularity as a prognostic factor for hepatic tumors. Ann Surg 1977; 185:31–34.

5. Nilsson LAV, Zettergren L. Blood supply and vascular pattern of induced primary hepatic carcinoma in rats. A microangiographic and histologic investigation. Acta Pathol Microbiol Scand 1967; 71:179–86.

6. Breedis C, Young G. The blood supply of neoplasms in the liver. Am J Pathol 1954; 30:969–77.

7. Burgener FA, Violante MR. Comparison of hepatic VX2-carcinomas after intra-arterial, intraportal and intraparenchymal tumor cell injection. An angiographic and computed tomographic study in the rabbit. Invest Radiol 1979; 14:410–14.

8. Honjo I, Matsumura H. Vascular distribution of hepatic tumors. Experimental study. Rev Int Hepatol 1979; 15:681–90.

9. Ackerman NB. The blood supply of experimental liver metastases. IV. Changes in vascularity with increasing tumor growth. Surgery 1974; 75:589–596.

10. Kido C. Hepatic angiography of experimental transplantable tumor. Invest Radiol 1970; 5:341–47.

11. Ackerman NB. Experimental studies on the circulatory dynamics of intrahepatic tumor blood supply. Cancer 1972; 29:435–39.

12. Ackerman NB, Lien WM, Kondi ES, Silverman NA. The blood supply of experimental liver metastases I. The distribution of hepatic artery and portal vein blood to "small" and "large" tumors. Surgery 1969; 66:1067–72.

13. Sundqvist K, Hafström L, Persson B. Measurements of total and regional tumor blood flow and organ blood flow using ^{99}Tcm labeled microspheres. An experimental study in rats. Eur Surg Res 1978; 10:433–43.

14. Hafström LO, Persson B, Sundqvist K. Blood flow in experimental liver tumors. Effect of vasoactive drugs. Acta Chir Scand 1980; 146:149–53.

15. Plengvanit U, Suwanik R, Chearani O, et al. Regional hepatic blood flow studied by intrahepatic injection of ^{133} xenon in normals and in patients with primary carcinoma of the liver, with particular reference to the effect of hepatic artery ligation. Aust NZ J Med 1972; 1:44–48.

16. Taylor I, Bennett R, Sherriff S. The blood supply of colorectal liver metastases. Br J Cancer 1979; 39:749–56.

17. Graham RR, Connell D. Accidental ligature of the hepatic artery. Report of a case, with a review of the cases in the literature. Br J Surg 1933; 20:566–578.

18. Markowitz J, Rappaport A, Scott AC. The function of the hepatic artery in the dog. Am J Dig Dis 1949; 16:344–48.

19. Pettersson H. Arterial collaterals in intrahepatic arterial occlusion. Acta Radiol (Diagn) 1975; 16:401–06.

20. Tygstrup N, Winkler K, Mellemgaard K, Andreassen M. Determination of the hepatic arterial blood flow and oxygen supply in man by clamping the hepatic artery during surgery. J Clin Invest 1962; 41:447–54.

21. Lindell B, Aronsen KF, Rothman U, Sjögren HO. The circulation in liver tissue and experimental liver metastases before and after embolization of the liver artery. Res Exp Med 1977; 171:63–70.

22. Ternberg JL, Butcher HR. Blood-flow relation between hepatic artery and portal vein. Science 1965; 150:1030–31.

23. Hasselgren PO, Almersjö O, Gustavsson B, Seeman T. Liver circulation and oxygen metabolism during short time ligation of the hepatic artery in the dog. Acta Chir Scand 1979; 145:471–77.

24. Hanson KM, Johnson PC. Local control of hepatic arterial and portal venous flow in the dog. Am J Physiol 1966; 211:712–20.

25. Kock NG, Hahnloser P, Roding B, Schenk WG. Interaction between portal venous and hepatic arterial blood flow: an experimental study in the dog. Surgery 1972; 72:414–19.

26. Gelin L-E, Lewis DH, Nilsson L. Liver blood flow in man during abdominal surgery. I. Description of a method utilizing intrahepatic injections of radioactive xenon (133 Xe). Normal values and effect of temporary occlusion. Acta Hepatosplenol 1968; 15:13–20.

27. Horvath SM, Farrand EA, Larsen R. Effect of hepatic arterial ligation on hepatic blood flow and related metabolic function. Arch Surg 1957; 74:565–70.

28. Lien WM, Ackerman NB. The blood supply of experimental liver metastases. II. A microcircula-

28. Lien WM, Ackerman NB. The blood supply of experimental liver metastases. II. A microcirculatory study of the normal and tumor vessels of the liver with the use of perfused silicone rubber. Surgery 1970; 68:334–40.

29. Rienhoff WF, Woods AC. Ligation of hepatic and splenic arteries in treatment of cirrhosis with ascitis. JAMA 1953; 152:687–90.

30. Nilsson LAV, Rudenstam CM, Zettergren L. Vascularization of liver tumours and the effect of hepatic artery ligature. 4th Europ Conf Microcirculation, Cambridge 1966. New York: Karger Basel 1967; Bibl Anat 9:425–31.

31. Bengmark S, Rosengren K. Angiographic study of the collateral circulation to the liver after ligation of the hepatic artery in man. Am J Surg 1970; 119:620–24.

32. Bengmark S, Fredlund P, Hafström LD, Vang J. Present experiences with hepatic dearterialization in liver neoplasm. Prog Surg 1974; 13:141–66.

33. Bengmark S, Börjesson B, Hafström L, Olsson A. A two-stage liver resection combined with long-term intraportal 5-FU infusion. Rev Surg 1971; 28:456–58.

34. Fortner JG, Pahnke LD. A new method for long-term intrahepatic chemotherapy. Surg Gynecol Obstet 1976; 143:979–80.

35. Nagasue N, Inokuchi K, Kobayashi M. Hepatic dearterialization for nonresectable primary and secondary tumors of the liver. Cancer 1976; 38:2593–2603.

36. Laufman LR, Nims TA, Guy JT, Guy JF, Courter S. Hepatic artery ligation and portal vein infusion for liver metastases from colon cancer. J Clin Oncol 1984; 2:1382–89.

37. Taylor I. Cytotoxic perfusion for colorectal liver metastases. Br J Surg 1978; 65:109–14.

References—Chapter 36

1. Aronson HA, Flanigan S, Mark JED. Chemotherapy of malignant brain tumors using regional perfusion: I. technic and patient selection. Ann Surg 1963; 157:394–99.

2. Beck DO, Hochberg FH. The rationale for pre-irradiation chemotherapy in the treatment of malignant gliomas. J Neurosurg 1985; 63:994–95.

3. Blasberg R. Brain Tumor Research Symp, Asheville NC, Oct. 1985.

4. Bonstelle, CT, et al. Intracarotid chemotherapy of glioblastoma after induced blood-brain barrier disruption. AJNR 1983; 4:810–12.

5. Cascino TL, Byrne TN, Deck MD, Posner JB. Intra-arterial BCNU in the treatment of metastatic brain tumors. J Neurooncol 1983; 1(3):211–18.

6. Crafts DC, Levin VA, Nielsen SA. Intracarotid BCNU (NCS-409962): a toxicity study in six rhesus monkeys. Cancer Treat Rep 1976; 60(5):541–45.

7. Debrun GM, Davis KR, Hochberg FH. Superselective injection of BCNU through a latex calibrated-leak balloon. AJNR 1983; 4(3):399–400.

8. Dedrick RL, Oldfield EH, Collins JM. Arterial drug infusion with extracorporeal removal. I. Theoretic basis with particular reference to the brain. Cancer Treat Rep 1984; 68(2):373–80.

9. DeWys WD, Fowler EH. Report of vasculitis and blindness after intracarotid injection of 1,3-bis(2-chloroethyl)-1-nitrosourea (BCNU: NSC-409962) in dogs. Cancer Chemother Rep 1973; 57:33–40.

10. Edland RW, Javid M, Ansfield FJ. Glioblastoma multiforme: an analysis of the results of postoperative radiotherapy alone versus radiotherapy and concomitant 5-fluorouracil (a prospective randomized study of 32 cases). Am J Roentgenol 1971; 111:337–42.

11. Egorin MJ, Bellis EH, Salcman M, Collins JM, Spiegel JF, Bachur NR. The pharmacology of diaziquone given in intravenous or intracarotid infusion to normal and intracranial tumor-bearing puppies. J Neurosurg 1984; 60:1005–13.

12. Ensminger WD. Wild Dunes Symp, Sept. 1984.

13. Epenelos AA, Courtenay-Luck N, Pickering D, et al. Antibody guided irradiation of brain glioma

by arterial infusion of radioactive monoclonal antibody against epidermal growth factor receptor and blood group A antigen. Br Med J 1985; 290:1463–66.

14. Fenstermacher JD, Cowles AL. Theoretic limitation of intracarotid infusions in brain tumor chemotherapy. Cancer Treat Rep 1977; 61(4):519–26.

15. Fenstermacher J, Gazendam J. Intra-arterial infusions of drugs and hyperosmotic solutions as ways of enhancing CNS chemotherapy. Cancer Treat Rep 1981; 65(2):27–37.

16. Feun LG, Wallace S, Stewart DJ, et al. Intracarotid infusion of cis-diamminedichloroplatinum in the treatment of recurrent malignant brain tumors. Cancer 1984; 54(5):794–99.

17. Feun LG, Stewart DJ, Maor M, Leavens M, Savaraj N, et al. A pilot study of cis-diamminedichloroplatinum and radiation therapy in patients with high grade astrocytomas. J Neurooncol 1983; 1(2):109–13.

18. French JD, West PM, von Amerongen FK, et al. Effects of intracarotid administration of nitrogen mustard on normal brain and brain tumors. J Neurosurg 1952; 9:378–89.

19. Gebarski SS, Greenberg HS, Gabrielsen TO, Vine AK. Orbital angiographic changes after intra-carotid BCNU chemotherapy. AJNR 1984; 5:55–58.

20. Greenberg HS, Ensminger WD, Seeser JF, et al. Intra-arterial BCNU chemotherapy for the treatment of malignant gliomas of the central nervous system: a preliminary report. Cancer Treat Rep 1981; 65(9–10):803–10.

21. Greenberg HS, Ensminger WD, Chandler WF, et al. Intra-arterial BCNU chemotherapy for treatment of malignant gliomas of the central nervous system. J Neurosurg 1984; 61:423–29.

22. Grimson BS, Mahaley MS Jr, Dubey HD, Dudka L. Ophthalmic and central nervous system complications following intracarotid BCNU (carmustine). J Clin Neuroophthalmol 1981; 1:262–64.

23. Hatiboglu I, Owens G. Results of intermittent prolonged infusion of nitrogen mustard into the carotid artery in twelve patients with cerebral gliomas. Surg Forum 1961; 12:396–99.

24. Hidemitsu N, Groothuis D, Blasberg RG. The effect of graded hypertonic intracarotid infusions on drug delivery to experimental RG-2 gliomas. Neurology 1984; 34:1571–81.

25. Hochberg FH, Pruitt A. Assumptions in the radiotherapy of glioblastoma. Neurology 1980; 30:907–11.

26. Hochberg FH, Pruitt A, Beck DO, Debrun G, Davis K. The rationale and methodology for intra-arterial chemotherapy with BCNU as treatment for glioblastoma. J Neurosurg (in press).

27. Johnson D, Parkinson D, Wolpert S, Kasdon, DL. Intracarotid chemotherapy with 1,3-bis(2 chlorethyl)-1-nitrosourea (BCNU) in D5W in the treatment of malignant glioma (submitted for publication).

28. Kapp J, Vance R, Parker JL, Smith RR. Limitations of high dose intra-arterial 1,3-bis (2-chloroethyl)-1-nitrosourea (BCNU) chemotherapy for malignant gliomas. Neurosurgery 1982; 10:715–19.

29. Kapp JP, Vance R. Treatment of recurrent brain tumors with intra-arterial cis-platinum and BCNU. J Miss State Med Assoc 1984; 25(1):1–6.

30. Kapp JP, Parker JL, Tucker EM. Supraophthalmic carotid infusion for brain chemotherapy: experience with a new single-lumen catheter and maneuverable tip. J Neurosurg 1985; 62:823–25.

31. Klopp CT, Bateman J, Berry GN, et al. Fractionated regional cancer chemotherapy. Cancer Res 1950; 10:229.

32. Layton PB, Greenberg HS, Stetson PL, Ensminger WD, Gyves JW. BCNU solubility and toxicity in the treatment of malignant astrocytomas. J Neurosurg 1984; 60:1134–37.

33. Levin VA, Jabra PM, Freeman-Dove M. Pharmacokinetics of intracarotid artery 14C-BCNU in the squirrel monkey. J Neurosurg 1978; 48:587–93.

34. Madajewicz S, West CR, Avellanosa AM, et al. Phase 2 study intra-arterial 1,3-bis(2-chloroethyl)-1 nitrosourea (BCNU) therapy for metastatic brain tumors (MET). ASCO Abstr Mar. 1980.

35. Madajewicz S, West CR, Park HC, et al. Phase 2 Study—intra-arterial BCNU therapy for metastatic brain tumors. Cancer 1981; 47:653–57.

36. Mealey J Jr. Treatment of malignant cerebral astrocytomas by intra-arterial infusion of vinblastine. Cancer 1970; 26:360–67.

37. Miller DF, Bay JW, Lederman RJ, et al. Ocular and orbital toxicity following intracarotid injection of BCNU (carmustine) and cisplatinum for malignant gliomas. Ophthalmology 1985; 92:402–06.

38. Neuwalt EA, Hill SA, Frnekel EP, et al. Osmotic blood-brain barrier disruption: pharmacodynamic studies in dogs and a clinical phase 1 trial in patients with malignant brain tumors. Cancer Treat Rep 1981; 65(2):39–43.

39. Owens G, Javid R, Tallon M, Stepanian G, Belmusto L. Arterial infusion chemotherapy of primary gliomas. JAMA 1963; 186:802–03.

40. Oldfield EH, Dedrick RL, Yeager RL, et al. Reduced systemic drug exposure by combining intra-arterial chemotherapy with hemoperfusion of regional venous drainage. J Neurosurg 1980; 63:726–32.

41. Perese DM, Day CE, Chardack WM. Chemotherapy of brain tumors by intra-arterial infusion. J Neurosurg 1962; 19:215.

42. Phillips TW, Chandler WF, Kindt GW, et al. New implantable continuous administration and bolus dose intracarotid drug delivery system for the treatment of malignant gliomas. Neurosurgery 1982; 11(2):213–18.

43. Ross RL, Kapp JP, Hochberg F, Krull IS, Xiang-Dong Ding BS, Selavka C. Solvent systems for intracarotid 1,3-bis(2-chloroethyl)-1-nitrosourea (BCNU) infusion. Neurosurgery 1983; 12:512–14.

44. Saki N, Kondo H, Shikinami A, et al. Post-operative treatment for malignant intracranial tumors — especially concerning intermittent intracarotid administration of Adriamycin. No-Shinkei-Geka 1984; 12(3):237–43.

45. Salazar OM, Rubin P, Feldstein ML, et al. High dose radiation therapy in the treatment of malignant glioma: final report. Int J Rad Oncol Biol Phys 1979; 5:1733–40.

46. Stewart DJ, Wallace S, Feun L, Leavens M, et al. A phase 1 study of intracarotid artery infusion of cis-diamminedichloroplatinum (II) in patients with recurrent malignant intracerebral tumors. Cancer Res 1982; 42(5):2059–62.

47. Stewart DJ, O'Bryan RM, Al-Sarraf M, Costanzi JJ, Dishi N. Phase 2 study of cisplatin in recurrent astrocytomas in adults: a Southwest Oncology Group study. J Neurooncol 1983; 1(2):145–47.

48. Stewart DJ, Grahavoc Z, Benoit B, et al. Intracarotid chemotherapy with a combination of 1,3-bis(2-chloroethyl)-1-nitrosourea (BCNU), cis-diamminedichloroplatinum (cis-platin), and 4'-0-demethyl-1-0-(4,6-0-2-thenylidene-beta-D-slucopyranosyl) epipodophyllotoxin (VM-26) in the treatment of primary and metastatic brain tumors. Neurosurgery 1984; 15(6):828–33.

49. Walker MD, Green SB, Byar DP, et al. Randomized comparisons of radiotherapy and nitrosoureas for the treatment of malignant glioma after surgery. N Engl J Med 1980; 303:1323–29.

50. Walker MD, Alexander E Jr, Hunt WE, et al. Evaluation of BCNU and/or radiotherapy in the treatment of naplastic gliomas: a cooperative clinical trial. J Neurosurg 1978; 49:333–43.

51. West CR, Yamada K, Karakousis CP, Takita H. Intra-arterial BCNU infusion for intracerebral metastases from malignant melanoma and lung cancer. ASCO Abstr 1979.

52. West CR, Avellanosa Am, Barua NR, Patel A, Hong CI. Intra-arterial 1,3-bis(2-chloroethyl)-1-nitrosourea (BCNU) and systemic chemotherapy for malignant gliomas: a follow-up study. Neurosurgery 1983; 13(4):420–6.

53. Wilson CB. Chemotherapy of brain tumors by continuous arterial infusion. Surg Forum 1962; 13:423–25.

54. Wilson CB. Chemotherapy of brain tumors by continuous arterial infusion. Surgery 1964; 55:640–53.

55. Yamada K, Bremer AM, West CR, Ghoorah J, Park HC, Takita H. Intra-arterial BCNU therapy in the treatment of metastatic brain tumor from lung carcinoma: a preliminary report. Cancer 1979; 44(6):2000–07.

56. Yamashita J, Handa H, Tokuriki Y, et al. Intra-arterial ACNU therapy for malignant brain tumors: experimental studies and preliminary clinical results. J Neurosurg 1983; 59(3):424–30.

57. Yumitori K, Handa H, Teraura T, Yamashita J. Treatment of malignant brain tumours with ACNU and phenobarbital: continuous infusion of ACNU into internal carotid artery and systemic administration of phenobarbital. Acta Neurochir (Wien) 1984; 70(304):155–268.

58. Zielke-Temme BC, Stevens KR Jr, Everts ED, Moseley HS, Ireland KM. Combined intra-arterial

chemotherapy, radiation therapy, and surgery for advanced squamous-cell carcinoma of the head and neck. Cancer 1980; 45(7):1527–32.

References—Chapter 37

1. Almersjo OE, Gustavsson BG, Regardh C-G, Wahlen P. Pharmacokinetic studies of 5-fluorouracil after oral and intravenous administration in man. Acta Pharmacol et Toxicol 1980; 46:329–36.

2. Ansfield FJ, Klotz J, Nealon T. A phase 3 study comparing the clinical utility of four regimens of 5-fluorouracil. Cancer 1977; 39:34–40.

3. Ardalan B, Cooney D, MacDonald JS. Physiological and pharmacological determinants of sensitivity and resistance to 5-fluorouracil in lower animals and man. Adv Pharmacol Chemother 1980; 17:289–320.

4. Bagshaw MA. Possible role of potentiators in radiation therapy. Am J Roentgenol 1961; 85:822–33.

5. Barone RM, Byfield JE, Goldfarb PB, et al. Intra-arterial chemotherapy using an implantable infusion pump and liver irradiation for the treatment of hepatic metastases. Cancer 1982; 50:850–62.

6. Bellamy AS, Hill BT. Interactions between clinically effective antitumor drugs and radiation in experimental systems. Biochim Biophys Acta 1984; 738:125–66.

7. Byfield JE. The combined use of drugs and radiation in the treatment of liver metastases. In: Herfarth C, Schlag P, eds. Therapeutic strategies in primary and metastatic liver cancer. Heidelberg: Springer Verlag (in press).

8. Byfield JE, Barone RM, Frankel SS, Sharp TR. Treatment with combined intra-arterial 5-FUDR infusion and whole liver radiation for colon carcinoma metastatic to the liver. Am J Clin Oncol 1984; 7:319–25.

9. Byfield JE, Barone RM, Mendelsohn J, et al. Infusional 5-fluorouracil and x-ray therapy for non-resectable esophageal carcinoma. Cancer 1979; 22:376–82.

10. Byfield JE, Barone RM, Sharp TR, Frankel SS. Conservative management of squamous anal cancer by cyclical 5-fluorouracil infusion alone and x-ray therapy. Cancer Treat Rep 1983; 67:709–12.

11. Byfield JE, Calabro-Jones P, Klisak I, Kulhanian F. Pharmacologic requirements for obtaining sensitization of human tumors cells in vitro to combined 5-fluorouracil or ftorafur and x-rays. Int J Radiat Oncol Biol Phys 1982; 8:1923–33.

12. Byfield JE, Frankel SS, Hornbeck CL, Sharp TR, Callipari F. Phase 1 and 2 trial of cyclical 72-hour infused 5-fluorouracil and hyperfractionated radiation in man. Int J Radiat Oncol Biol Phys (in press).

13. Byfield JE, Frankel SS, Hornbeck CL, Sharp TR, Floyd RA, Callipari F. Phase 1 and pharmacologic study of 72-hour infused 5-fluorouracil. Am J Clin Oncol (in press).

14. Byfield JE, Sharp TR, Hornbeck CL, Frankel SS, Floyd RA, Griffiths JJ. Phase 1 study of oral ftorafur and x-ray therapy in advanced gastro-intestinal cancer. Int J Radiat Oncol Biol Phys 1985; 11:597–602.

15. Byfield JE, Sharp TR, Tang S, Frankel SS, Callipari F. Phase 1 and 2 trial of cyclical 5-day infused 5-fluorouracil and coincident radiation in advanced cancer of the head and neck. J Clin Oncol 1984; 2:406–13.

16. Calabro-Jones PM, Byfield JE, Ward JF, Sharp TR. Time-dose relationships for 5-fluorouracil cytotoxicity against human epithelial cancer cells in vitro. Cancer Res 1982; 42:4413–20.

17. Collins JM, Dedrick RL, King FG, Speyer JL, Myers CE. Nonlinear pharmacokinetic models for 5-fluorouracil in man: intravenous and intraperitoneal routes. Clin Pharmacol Ther 1980; 28:235–46.

18. Cummings BJ, Byfield JE. Anal cancer. In: Withers HR, Peters LJ, eds. Innovations in radiation oncology research. Heidelberg: Springer-Verlag (in press).

19. Duschinsky R, Pleven E, Heidelberger C. The synthesis of 5-fluoropyrimidines. J Am Chem Soc 1957; 79:4559–60.

20. Floyd RA, Hornbeck CL, Byfield JE, Griffiths JC, Frankel SS. Clearance of continuously infused

5-fluorouracil in adults having lung or gastro-intestinal carcinoma with or without hepatic metastatses. Drug Intell Clin Pharm 1982; 16:665–67.

21. Gastrointestinal Tumor Study Group. A comparison of combination chemotherapy and combined modality therapy for locally advanced gastric cancer. Cancer 1982; 49:1771–77.

22. Hahn SS, Kim J-A, Constable WC. Concomitant chemotherapy and radiotherapy for advanced squamous cell carcinoma of head and neck. Int J Radiat Oncol Biol Phys 1984; 10: (suppl 2) 191.

23. Heidelberger C. Fluorinated pyrimidines and their nucleosides. In: Sartorelli AC, Johns DG, eds. Antineoplastic and immuno-suppressive agents, vol. 2. New York: Springer Verlag, 1975; 193–231.

24. Ingraham HO, Tseng BY, Goulian M. Nucleotide levels and incorporation of 5-fluorouracil and uracil into DNA of cells treated with fluorodeoxyuridine. Molec Pharmacol 1982; 21:211–16.

25. Keane TJ, Harwood AR, Beale et al. A pilot study of mitomycin-C and 5-fluorouracil infusion combined with split course radiation therapy for advanced carcinomas of the larynx and hypopharynx (in preparation).

26. Keane TJ, Harwood AR, Rider WD, Cummings BJ, Thomas GM. Concomitant radiation and chemotherapy for squamous cell carcinoma (SCC) esophagus. Int J Radiat Oncol Biol Phys 1984; 10 (suppl 2):89 (abstr).

27. Kinsella TJ, Russo A, Mitchell JB, et al. A phase 1 study of intravenous iododeoxyuridine as a clinical radiosensitizer (submitted for publication).

28. Kinsella TJ, Mitchell JB, Russo A, Morstyn G, Glatstein E. The use of halogenated thymidine analogues as clinical radiosensitizers: rationale, current status, and future prospects: non-hypoxic cell sensitizers. Int J Radiat Oncol Biol Phys 1984; 10:1399–1406.

29. Kinsella TJ, Russo A, Mitchell JB, et al. A phase 1 study of intermittent intravenous BUDR with conventional radiation. Int J Radiat Oncol Biol Phys 1984; 10:69–76.

30. Klecker RW, Jenkins JF, Kinsella TJ, Fine RL, Strong JM, Collins JM. Clinical pharmacology of 5-iodo-2'-deoxyuridine and 5-iodouracil and endogenous pyrimidine modulation (submitted for publication).

31. Leichman L, Steiger Z, Seydel HG, et al. Preoperative chemotherapy and radiation therapy for patients with cancer of the esophagus: a potentially curative approach. J Clin Oncol 1984; 2:75–79.

32. Lokich JJ, Bothe A Jr, Fine N, Perri J. Phase 1 study of protracted venous infusion of 5-fluorouracil. Cancer 1981; 48:2565–68.

33. Looney W, Schaffer JG, Trefil JS, Kovacs CJ, Hopkins HA. Solid tumor model for the assessment of different treatment modalities: IV. The combined effects of radiation and 5-fluorouracil. Br J Cancer 1976; 34:254–61.

34. McCracken JD, Weatherall TJ, Oishi N, Janaki L, Boyer C. Adjuvant intrahepatic chemotherapy with mitomycin and 5-FU combined with hepatic irradiation in high-risk patients with carcinoma of the colon: a Southwest Oncology Group phase 2 pilot study. Cancer Chemother Rep 1985; 69:129–31.

35. Moertel CG, Childs DS, Reitemeier RJ, Colby MY, Holbrook MA. Combined 5-fluorouracil and supervoltage radiation therapy of locally unresectable gastrointestinal cancer. Lancet 1969; 2:865–67.

36. Mukherjee KL, Boohar J, Wentland D, Ansfield FJ, Heidelberger C. Studies of fluoropyrimidines. XVI. Metabolism of 5-fluorouracil-C-14 and 5-fluoro-2'-deoxyuridine in cancer patients. Cancer Res 1963; 23:49–66.

37. Myers, CE. The pharmacology of the fluoropyrimidines. Pharmacol Rev 1981; 33:1–15.

38. Nigro ND, Vaitkevicius VK, and Considine B. Combined therapy for cancer of the anal canal: a preliminary report. Dis Colon Rectum 1974; 17:354–56.

39. Phuphanich S, Levin EM, Levin VA. Phase 1 study of intravenous bromodeoxyuridine used concomitantly with radiation therapy in patients with primary malignant brain tumors. Int J Radiat Oncol Biol Phys 1984; 10:1769–72.

40. Prusoff WH, Goz B. Halogenated pyrimidine deoxyribonucleosides. In: Sartorelli AC, Johns DG, eds. Antineoplastic and immunosuppressive agents, vol. 2. New York: Springer-Verlag, 1975; 272–347.

41. Russo A, Gianni L, Kinsella TJ, et al. Pharmacological evaluation of intravenous delivery of 5-bromodeoxyuridine to patients with brain tumors. Cancer Res 1984; 44:1702–05.

42. Showell JL, Murthy AK, Hutchinson LD, Caldarelli DE, Taylor SS. Synchronous radiation

therapy and cis-platin-5-FU chemotherapy in advanced head and neck cancer. Proc 2nd Eur Conf Clin Oncol (abstr) 1983; 162.

43. Siefert P, Baker LH, Reed ML, Vaitkevicius VK. Comparison of continuously infused 5-fluorouracil with bolus injection treatment of patients with colorectal adenocarcinomas. Cancer 1975; 36:123–28.

44. Sischy B, Qazi R, Hinson EJ. A pilot study of concurrent radiation, mitomycin-C, and 5-FU in marginally operable carcinomas of the rectum. Int J Radiat Oncol Biol Phys 1984; 10 (suppl 2):91 (abstr).

45. Steiger Z, Franklin R, Wilson RF, et al. Complete eradication of squamous cell carcinoma of the esophagus with combined chemotherapy and radiotherapy. Am Surg 1981; 95–98.

46. Szybalski W. X-ray sensitization by halopyrimidines. Cancer Chemother Rep 1974; 58:539–57.

47. Thomas G, Dembo A, Beale F, et al. Concurrent radiation, mitomycin-C, and 5-fluorouracil in poor prognosis carcinoma of cervix: preliminary results of a phase 1–2 study. Int J Radiat Oncol Biol Phys 1984; 10:1785–90.

48. Thomlinson RH, Gray LH. The histological structure of some human cancers and the possible implications for radiotherapy. Br J Cancer 1955; 9:539–49.

49. Vietti T, Eggerding F, Valeriote F. Combined effect of x-radiation and 5-fluorouracil on survival of transplanted leukemic cells. J Nat Cancer Inst 1971; 47:865–70.

50. Zimbrick JF, Ward JF, Myers LS Jr. Studies on the chemical basis of cellular radiosensitization by 5-bromouracil substitution of DNA. I. Pulse and steady-state radiolysis of 5-bromouracil and thymine. Int J Radiat Biol 1969; 16:502–23.

51. ——, II. Pulse and steady-state radiolysis of bromouracil substituted and unsubstituted DNA. Int J Radiat Biol 1969; 16:525–34.

References—Chapter 38

1. Weisberger AS, Levine B, Storaasli JP. Use of nitrogen mustard in treatment of serous effusions of neoplastic origin. JAMA 1955; 159:1704–07.

2. Green TH. Hemisulfer mustard in the palliation of patients with metastatic ovarian carcinoma. Obstet Gynecol 1959; 13:383–93.

3. Kottmeier HL. Treatment of ovarian cancer with thio-tepa. Clin Obstet Gynecol 1968; 11:447–48.

4. Suhrland LG, Weisberger AS. Intracavitary 5-fluorouracil in malignant effusions. Arch Intern Med 1965; 116:431–33.

5. Cunningham TJ, Olson KB, Horton J, et al. A clinical trial of intravenous and intracavitary bleomycin. Cancer 1972; 29:1413–19.

6. Paladine W, Cunningham TJ, Sponzo R, Donavan M, Olson K, Horton J. Intracavitary bleomycin in the management of malignant effusions. Cancer 1976; 38:1903–08.

7. Bitran JD, Brown C, Desser RK, Kozloff MF, Shapira C, Billings AA. Intracavitary bleomycin for the control of malignant effusions. J Surg Oncol 1981; 16:273–77.

8. Ostrowski MJ, Halsall GM. Intracavitary bleomycin in the management of malignant effusions: a multicenter study. Cancer Treat Rep 1982; 66:1903–07.

9. Kefford RF, Woods RL, Fox RM, Tattersall MHN. Intracavitary Adriamycin, nitrogen mustard and tetracycline in the control of malignant effusions: a randomized study. Med J Aust 1980; 2:447–48.

10. Anderson CB, Philpott GW, Ferguson TB. The treatment of malignant pleural effusions. Cancer 1974; 33:916–22.

11. Fracchia AA, Knapper WH, Carey JT, Farrow JH. Intrapleural chemotherapy for effusion from metastatic breast carcinoma. Cancer 1970; 26:626–29.

12. Ariel IM, Oropeza R, Pack GT. Intracavitary administration of radioactive isotopes in the control of effusions due to cancer: results in 267 patients. Cancer 1966; 19:1096–1102.

13. Izbicki R, Weyhing BT, Baker L, Caoili EM, Vaitkevicius VK. Pleural effusion in cancer patients:

a prospective study of pleural drainage with the addition of radioactive phosphorous to the pleural space vs. pleural drainage alone. Cancer 1975; 36:1511-18.

14. Osborne MP, Copeland BE. Intracavitary administration of radioactive colloidal gold (Au[198]) for the treatment of malignant effusions: a report of thirty-one cases and an appraisal of results. N Engl J Med 1956; 255:1122-27.

15. Dedrick RL, Myers CE, Bungay PM, DeVita VT Jr. Pharmacokinetic rationale for peritoneal drug administration in the treatment of ovarian cancer. Cancer Treat Rep 1978; 62:1-9.

16. Collins JM. Pharmacokinetic rationale for regional drug delivery. J Clin Oncol 1984; 2:498-504.

17. Kraft AR, Tompkins RK, Jesseph JE. Peritoneal electrolyte absorption: analysis of portal, systemic venous and lymphatic transport. Surgery 1968; 64:148-53.

18. Lukas G, Brindle SD, Greengard P. The route of absorption of intraperitoneally administered compounds. J Pharmacol Exp Ther 1971; 178:562-66.

19. Lockhard RD, Hamilton GF, Fyfe FW. Anatomy of the human body. Philadelphia: JB Lippincott Co., 1960.

20. Romanes GB, ed. Cunningham's textbook of anatomy. London: Oxford University, 1964.

21. Leak LV, Rahil K. Permeability of the diaphragmatic mesothelium: the ultrastructural basis for "stomata." Am J Anat 1978; 151:577-94.

22. Bollman JL, Cain JC, Grindlay JH. Techniques for the collection of lymph from liver, small intestine, or thoracic duct of the rat. J Lab Clin Med 1948; 33:1349-52.

23. Reininger EJ, Saperstein LA. Effect of digestion on distribution of blood flow in the rat. Science 1957; 126:1176.

24. Torres IJ, Litterst CL, Guarino AM. Transport of model compounds across the peritoneal membrane in the rat. Pharmacology 1978; 17:330-40.

25. Speyer JL, Sugarbaker PH, Collins JM, Dedrick RL, Klecker RW, Myers CE. Portal levels and hepatic clearance of 5-fluorouracil after intraperitoneal administration in humans. Cancer Res 1981; 41:1916-22.

26. Litterst CL, Torres IJ, Arnold S, et al. Absorption of antineoplastic drugs following large-volume IP administration to rats. Cancer Treat Rep 1982; 66:147-55.

27. Dedrick RL, Flessner MF, Collins JM, Schultz JS. Is the peritoneum a membrane? Am Soc Artificial Int Organs 1982; 5:1-8.

28. Nolph KD, Popovich RP, Ghods AJ, Twardowski Z. Determinants of low clearances of small solutes during peritoneal dialysis. Kidney Int 1978; 13:117-123.

29. Nolph KD. Short dialysis, middle molecules, and uremia. Ann Intern Med 1977; 86:93-97.

30. Maher JF. Principles of dialysis and dialysis of drugs. Am J Med 1977; 62:475-81.

31. Nolph KD. Peritoneal clearances. J Lab Clin Med 1979; 94:519-25.

32. Maher JF. Peritoneal transport rates: mechanism, limitations and methods for augmentation. Kidney Int 1980; 18:117-20.

33. Tully TE, Goldberg ME, Loken MK. The use of ^{99}Tc-sulfur colloid to assess the distribution of ^{32}P chromic phosphate. J Nucl Med 1974; 15:190-91.

34. Taylor A, Baily NA, Halpern SE, Ashburn WL. Loculation as a contraindication to intracavitary ^{32}P chromic phosphate therapy. J Nucl Med 1975; 16:318-19.

35. Vider M, Deland FM, Maruyama Y. Loculation as a contraindication to intracavitary ^{32}P chronic phosphate therapy. J Nucl Med 1976; 17:150-51.

36. Rosenshein N, Blake D, McIntyre PA, et al. The effect of volume on the distribution of substances instilled into the peritoneal cavity. Gynecol Oncol 1978; 6:106-10.

37. Dunnick NR, Jones RB, Doppmen JL, Speyer J, Myers CE. Intraperitoneal contrast infusion for assessment of intraperitoneal fluid dynamics. AJR 1979; 133:221-23.

38. Howell SB, Pfeifle CE, Wung WE, et al. Intraperitoneal cisplatin with systemic thiosulfate protection. Ann Intern Med 1982; 97:845-51.

39. Levin VA, Patlak CS, Landahn MD. Heuristic modelling of drug delivery to malignant brain tumors. J Pharmacokinet Biopharm 1980; 8:257-96.

40. West GW, Weichselbau R, Little JB. Limited penetration of methotrexate into human osteosar-

coma spheroids as a proposed model for solid tumor resistance to adjuvant chemotherapy. Cancer Res 1980; 40:3665−68.

41. Durand RE. Flow cytometry studies of intracellular Adriamycin in multicell spheroids in vitro. Cancer Res 1981; 41:495−98.

42. Schwartz HS. A fluorometric assay for daunomycin and Adriamycin in animal tissues. Biochem Med 1973; 7:396−404.

43. Donelli MG, Martini A, Colombo T, Bossi A, Garattini S. Heart levels of Adriamycin in normal and tumor-bearing mice. Eur J Cancer 1976; 12:913−23.

44. Ozols RF, Locker GY, Doroshow JH, Grotzinger KR, Myers CE, Young RC. Pharmacokinetics of Adriamycin and tissue penetration in murine ovarian cancer. Cancer Res 1979; 39:3209−14.

45. Ozols RF, Grotzinger KR, Fisher RI, Myers CE, Young RC. Kinetic characterization and response to chemotherapy in a transplantable murine ovarian cancer. Cancer Res 1979; 39:3202−08.

46. Ozols RF, Locker GY, Doroshow JH, et al. Chemotherapy for murine ovarian cancer: a rationale for IP therapy with Adriamycin. Cancer Treat Rep 1979; 63:269−73.

47. Fenstermacher JD, Patlak CS, Blasberg RG. Transport of material between brain extracellular fluid, brain cells and blood. Fed Proc 1974; 33:2070−74.

48. Blasberg RG, Patlak C, Fenstermacher JD. Intrathecal chemotherapy: brain tissue profiles after ventriculocisternal perfusion. J Pharmacol Exp Ther 1975; 195:73−83.

49. Blasberg RG, Patlak C, Shapiro WR. Distribution of methotrexate in the cerebrospinal fluid and brain after intraventricular administration. Cancer Treat Rep 1977; 61:633-41.

50. Collins JM, Dedrick RL, King FG, Speyer JL, Myers CE. Non-linear pharmacokinetic models for 5-fluorouracil in man: intravenous and intraperitoneal routes. Clin Pharmacol Ther 1980; 28:235−46.

51. Collins JM, Dedrick RL, Flessner MF, Guarino AM. Concentration-dependent disappearance of fluorouracil from peritoneal fluid in the rat: experimental observations and distributed modeling. J Pharm Sci 1982; 71:735−38.

52. Howell SB, Chu BCF, Wung WE, Metha BM, Mendelsohn J. Long-duration intracavitary infusion of methotrexate with systemic leucovorin protection in patients with malignant effusions. J Clin Invest 1981; 67:1161−70.

53. Jones RB, Collins JM, Myers CE, et al. High-volume intraperitoneal chemotherapy with methotrexate in patients with cancer. Cancer Res 1981; 41:55−59.

54. Howell SB, Pfeifle CE, Wung WE, Olshen RA. Intraperitoneal cisplatin with systemic thiosulfate protection. Cancer Res 1983; 43:1426−31.

55. Speyer JL, Collins JM, Dedrick RL, et al. Phase 1 pharmacologic studies of 5-fluorouracil administered intraperitoneally. Cancer Res 1980; 567−72.

56. Markman M, Howell SB, Lucas WE, Pfeifle CE, Green MR. Combination intraperitoneal chemotherapy with cisplatin, cytarabine, and doxorubicin for refractory ovarian carcinoma and other malignancies principally confined to the peritoneal cavity. J Clin Oncol 1984; 2:1321−26.

57. Markman M, Howell SB, Pfeifle CE, Lucas WE, Green MR. Intraperitoneal chemotherapy with high dose cisplatin and cytarabine in patients with refractory ovarian carcinoma and other malignancies confined to the abdominal cavity. Proc Am Soc Clin Oncol 1984; 3:165.

58. Pfeifle CE, Howell SB, Markman M. Intracavitary cisplatin chemotherapy for mesothelioma. Cancer Treat Rep 1985; 69:205.

59. Deserga GS, Holtz GD. Cause and prevention of postsurgical pelvic adhesions. In: Osotsky HS, ed. Advances in clinical obstetrics and gynecology. Baltimore: Williams and Wilkins Co., 1982; 277−89.

60. Stangel JJ, Nisbet JD, Settles H. formation and prevention of postoperative abdominal adhesions. J Repro Med 1984; 29:143−56.

61. Alberts DS, Chen HSG, Change SY, Peng YM. The disposition of intraperitoneal bleomycin, melphalan, and vinblastine in cancer patients. Recent Results Cancer Res 1980; 74:293−99.

62. Litterst CL, Collins JM, Lowe MC, Arnold ST, Powell DM, Guarino AM. Local and systemic toxicity resulting from large-volume IP administration of doxorubicin in the rat. Cancer Treat Rep 1982; 66:157−61.

63. Ozols RF, Young RC, Speyer JL, et al. Phase 1 and pharmacological studies of Adriamycin administered intraperitoneally to patients with ovarian cancer. Cancer Res 1982; 42:4265−69.

64. Gloor HJ, Nichols WK, Sorkin MI, et al. Peritoneal access and related complications in continuous ambulatory peritoneal dialysis. Am J Med 1983; 74:593−98.

65. Rubin J, Rogers WA, Taylor HM, et al. Peritonitis during continuous ambulatory dialysis. Ann Intern Med 1980; 92:7−13.

66. Krothapalli RK, Senekjian HO, Ayus JC. Efficacy of intravenous vancomycin in the treatment of gram-positive peritonitis in long-term peritoneal dialysis. Am J Med 1983; 75:345−48.

67. Knight KR, Polak A, Crump J, Maskell R. Laboratory diagnosis and oral treatment of CAPD peritonitis. Lancet 1982; 2:1301−04.

68. Glasson P, Favre H. Treatment of peritonitis in continuous ambulatory peritoneal dialysis patients with co-trimaxazole. Nephron 1984; 36:65−67.

69. Nolph KD, Sorkin M. Diagnosis and treatment of peritonitis. In: Montcrief JW, Popovich RP, eds. CAPD update. New York: Masson Publishing USA, Inc., 1981; 265−72.

70. Low DE, Vas SI, Oreopoulos DG, et al. Randomized clinical trial of cephalexin in CAPD. Lancet 1980; 2:753−54.

71. Vas I. Microbiologic aspects of chronic ambulatory peritoneal dialysis. Kindey Int 1983; 23:83−92.

72. Kaplan RA, Markman M, Lucas WE, Pfeifle CE, Howell SB. Infectious peritonitis in patients receiving intraperitoneal chemotherapy. Am J Med 1985; 78:49−53.

73. Myers C. The use of intraperitoneal chemotherapy in the treatment of ovarian cancer. Semin Oncol 1984; 11:275−84.

74. Jenkins J, Sugarbaker PH, Gianola FJ, Myers CE. Technical considerations in the use of intraperitoneal chemotherapy administered by Tenckhoff catheter. Surg Gynecol Obstet 1982; 154:858−64.

75. Lucas WE. Surgical principles of intraperitoneal access and therapy. In: Howell SB, ed. Intra-arterial and intracavitary chemotherapy. Boston: Martinus Nijhoff (in press), 1985.

76. Pfeifle CE, Howell SB, Markman M, Lucas WE. Totally implantable system for peritoneal access. J Clin Oncol 1984; 2:1277−80.

77. Jones RB, Myers CE, Guarino AM, Dedrick RL, Hubbard SM, DeVita VT. High volume intraperitoneal chemotherapy ("belly bath") for ovarian cancer. Cancer Chemother Pharmacol 1978; 1:161−66.

78. Speyer JL, Myers CE. The use of peritoneal dialysis for delivery of chemotherapy to intraperitoneal malignancies. Recent Results Cancer Res 1980; 74:264−69.

79. Clarkson B. Relationship between cell type, glucose concentration, and response to treatment in neoplastic effusions. Cancer 1964; 17:914−28.

80. Clarkson B, O'Connor A, Winston L, Hutchison D. The physiologic disposition of 5-fluorouracil and 5-fluoro-2'-deoxyuridine in man. Clin Pharmacol Ther 1964; 5:581−610.

81. Niederhuber JE, Ensmigner WE. Surgical considerations in the management of hepatic neoplasia. Semin Oncol 1983; 10:135−47.

82. Demicheli R, Jirillo A, Bonciarelli G, et al. Pharmacological data and technical feasibility of intraperitoneal 5-fluorouracil administration. Tumori 1982; 68:437−41.

83. Gyves JW, Ensminger WD, Stetson P, et al. Constant intraperitoneal 5-fluorouracil infusion through a totally implanted system. Clin Pharmacol Ther 1984; 35:83−89.

84. Ozols RF, Myers CE, Young RC. Intraperitoneal chemotherapy (editorial). Ann Intern Med 1984; 101:118−20.

85. Roboz J, Jacobs AJ, Holland JF, Deppe G, Cohen CJ. Intraperitoneal infusion of doxorubicin in the treatment of gynecoloigc carcinomas. Med Pediatr Oncol 1981; 9:245−50.

86. Tobias JS, Griffiths CT. Management of ovarian carcinoma: current concepts and future prospects. N Engl J Med 1976; 294:877−82.

87. Casper ES, Kelsen DP, Alcock NW, Lewis JL. IP cisplatin in patients with malignant ascites: pharmacokinetic evaluation and comparison with the IV route. Cancer Treat Rep 1983; 67:235−38.

88. Pretorius RG, Hacker NF, Berek JS, et al. Pharmacokinetics of IP cisplatin in refractory ovarian carcinoma. Cancer Treat Rep 1983; 67:1085−92.

89. Howell SB, Taetle R. Effect of sodium thiosulfate on cis-dichlorodiammineplatinum (II) toxicity and antitumor activity in L1210 leukemia. Cancer Treat Rep 1980; 64:611−16.

90. Iwamoto Y, Kawano T, Uozumi J, Aoki K, Baba T. "Two-route chemotherapy" using high-dose IP cisplatin and IV sodium thiosulfate, its antidote, for peritoneally disseminated cancer in mice. Cancer Treat Rep 1984; 68:1367−73.

91. Belt RJ, Himmelstein KJ, Patton TF, Bannister SJ, Sternson LA, Repta AJ. Pharmacokinetics of nonprotein-bound platinum species following administration of cis-dichlorodiammineplatinum (II). Cancer Treat Rep 1979; 63:1515−21.

92. Pfeifle CE, Howell SB, Felthouse RD, Woliver TBS, Markman M. High-dose cisplatin with sodium thiosulfate. J Clin Oncol 1985; 3:237.

93. Shea M, Koziol JA, Howell SB. Kinetics of sodium thiosulfate, a cisplatin neutralizer. Clin Pharmacol Ther 1984; 35:419−25.

94. Antman KH, Blum RH, Greenberger JS, Flowerdew G, Skarin AT, Canellos GP. Multimodality therapy for malignant mesothelioma based on a study of natural history. Am J Med 1980; 68:356−62.

95. Aisner J, Wiernik PH. Chemotherapy in the treatment of malignant mesothelioma. Semin Oncol 1981; 8:335−43.

96. Ho DH, Frei E III. Clinical pharmacology of 1-beta-D-arabinofuranosyl cytosine. Clin Pharmacol Ther 1971; 12:944−54.

97. Van Prooijen R, Van der Kleijn E, Haanen C. Pharmacokinetics of cytosine arabinoside in acute myeloid leukemia. Clin Pharmacol Ther 1977; 21:744−50.

98. Wasserman TH, Comis RL, Goldsmith M, et al. Tabular analysis of the clinical chemotherapy of solid tumors. Cancer Chemother Rep 1975; 6:399−419.

99. Bodey GP, Freireich EJ, Monto RW, Hewlett JS. Cytosine arabinoside (NSC-63878) therapy for acute leukemia in adults. Cancer Chemother Rep 1969; 53:59−66.

100. Ellison RR, Holland JF, Weil M, et al. Arabinosyl cytosine: a useful agent in the treatment of acute leukemia in adults. Blood 1968; 32:507−23.

101. King ME, Pfeifle CE, Howell SB. Intraperitoneal cytosine arabinoside in ovarian carcinoma. J Clin Oncol 1984; 2:662−69.

102. Holcenberg J, Anderson T, Ritch P, et al. Intraperitoneal chemotherapy with melphalan plus glutaminase. Cancer Res 1983; 43:1381−88.

103. Howell SB, Pfeifle CE, Olshen RA. Intraperitoneal chemotherapy with melphalan. Ann Intern Med 1984; 101:14−18.

104. Vistica DT, Von Hoff DD, Torain B. Uptake of melphalan by human ovarian carcinoma cells and its relationship to the amino acid content of ascitic fluid. Cancer Treat Rep 1981; 65:157−61.

105. Gyves J, Ensminger W, Niederhuber J, et al. Phase 1 study of intraperitoneal 5-day continuous 5-FU infusion and bolus mitomycin-C. Proc Am Soc Clin Oncol 1982; 1:15.

106. Adams SC, Patt YZ, Rosenblum MG. Pharmacokinetics of mitomycin-C following intraperitoneal administration of mitomycin-C and floxuridine for peritoneal carcinomatosis. Proc Am Assoc Cancer Res 1984; 25:361.

107. Allen LM, Tejada F, Okonmah AD, Nordquist S. Combination chemotherapy of the epipodophyllotoxin derivatives, teniposide and etoposide: a pharmacodynamic rationale? Cancer Chemother Pharmacol 1982; 7:151−56.

108. Stahelin H. Delayed toxocity of epipodophyllotoxin derivatives (VM-26 and VP-16-213), due to a local effect. Eur J Cancer 1976; 12:925−31.

109. Panasci LC, Skalski V, St-Germain J, Lazarus P, Shinder M, Margolese R. Pharmacology and toxicity of IP streptozotocin in ovarian cancer: a case report. Cancer Treat Rep 1982; 66:1595−96.

110. Spratt JS, Adcock RA, Sherrill W, Travathen S. Hyperthermic peritoneal perfusion system in canines. Cancer Res 1980; 40:253−55.

111. Spratt JS, Adcock RA, Muskovin M, Sherill W, McKeown J. Clinical delivery system for intraperitoneal hyperthermic chemotherapy. Cancer Res 1980; 40:256−60.

112. Gianni L, Jenkins JF, Greene RF, Lichter AS, Myers CE, Collins JM. Pharmacokinetics of the hypoxic radiosensitizers misonidazole and demethylmisonidazole after intraperitoneal administration in humans. Cancer Res 1983; 43:913—16.

113. Stratford IJ, Adams GE, Horsman MR, et al. The interaction of misonidazole with radiation, chemotherapeutic agents, or heat: a preliminary report. Cancer Clin Trials 1980; 3:231—36.

114. Goldie JH, Coldman AJ. A mathematical model for relating the drug sensitivity of tumors to their spontaneous mutation rate. Cancer Treat Rep 1979; 63:1727—33.

115. Goldie JH, Coldman AJ, Gudauskas GA. Rationale for the use of alternating noncross-resistant chemotherapy. Cancer Treat Rep 1982; 66:439—49.

116. Drewinko B, Green C, Loo TL. Combination chemotherapy in vitro with cis-dichlorodiammineplatinum (II). Cancer Treat Rep 1976; 60:1619—25.

117. Bergerat J-P, Green C, Drewinko B. Combination chemotherapy in vitro. IV. Response of human colon carcinoma cells to combinations using cis-diamminodichloroplatinum. Cancer Biochem Biophys 1979; 3:173—80.

118. Bergerat J-P, Drewinko B, Corry P, Barlogie B, Ho DH. Synergistic lethal effect of cis-dichlorodiammineplatinum and 1-beta-D-arabinofuranosylcystosine. Cancer Res 1981; 41:25—30.

119. Einhorn LH, Donohue J. Cis-diamminedichloroplatinum, vinblastine, and bleomycin combination chemotherapy in disseminated testicular cancer. Ann Intern Med 1977; 87:293—98.

120. Stoter G, Vendrik CPJ, Struyvenberg A, et al. Combination chemotherapy with cis-diamminedichloro-platinum, vinblastine, and bleomycin in advanced testicular non-seminoma. Lancet 1979; 1:941—45.

121. Mascharak PK, Sugiura Y, Kuwahara J, Suzuki T, Lippard SJ. Alteration and activation of sequence-specific cleavage of DNA by bleomycin in the presence of the antitumor drug cis-diamminedichloroplatinum (II). Proc Natl Acad Sci 1983; 80:6795—98.

122. Alberts DS, Chen HSG, Mayersohn M, Perrier D, Moon TE, Gross JF. Bleomycin pharmacokinetics in man. II. Intracavitary administration. Cancer Chemother Pharmacol 1979; 2:127—32.

123. Alberts DS, Slamon SE, Chen HSG, et al. In-vitro clonogenic assay for predicting response of ovarian cancer to chemotherapy. Lancet 1980; 2:340—42.

124. Blackledge G, Lawton F, Buckley H, Crowther D. Phase 2 evaluation of bleomycin in patients with advanced epithelial ovarian cancer. Cancer Treat Rep 1984; 68:549—50.

125. Canetta R, Hilgard P, Florentine S, Bedogni P, Lenaz L. Current development of podophyllotoxins. Cancer Chemother Pharmacol 1982; 7:93—98.

126. Schabel FM, Trader MW, Laster WR, Corbett TH, Griswold DP. Cis-dichloro-diammineplatinum (II): combination chemotherapy and cross-resistance studies with tumors of mice. Cancer Treat Rep 1979; 63:1459—73.

127. Williams SD, Einhorn LH. Etoposide salvage therapy for refractory germ cell tumors: an update. Cancer Treat Rev 1982; 9(suppl A):67—71.

128. Evans WK, Osoba D, Feld R, et al. Etoposide (VP-16) and cisplatin: an effective treatment for relapse in small-cell lung cancer. J Clin Oncol 1985; 3:65—71.

129. Williams CJ, Stevenson KE, Buchanan RB, Whitehouse JMA. Advanced ovarian carcinoma: pilot study of cis-dichlorodiamminplatinum (II) in combination with Adriamycin and cyclophosphamide in previously untreated patients and as a single agent in previously treated patients. Cancer Treat Rep 1979; 63:1745—53.

130. Williams CJ, Mead B, Arnold A, Green J, Buchanan R, Whitehouse M. Chemotherapy of advanced ovarian carcinoma: initial experience using a platinum-based combiantion. Cancer 1982; 49:1778—83.

131. Cohen CJ, Goldberg JD, Holland JF, et al. Improved therapy with cisplatin regimens for patients with ovarian carcinoma (FIGO stages 3 and 4) as measured by surgical end-staging (second-look) operation. Am J Obstet Gynecol 1983; 145:955—67.

132. Myers CE, Collins JM. Pharmacology of intraperitoneal chemotherapy. Cancer Invest 1983; 1:395—407.

133. Markman M, Howell SB, Green MR. Combination intercavitary chemotherapy for malignant pleural disease. Cancer Drug Delivery 1984; 1:333 – 36.

134. Markman M, Howell SB. Intrapericardial instillation of cisplatin in a patient with a large malignant effusion. Cancer Drug Delivery 1985; 2(pt.1):49-52.

References—Chapter 39

1. Abelson HT. Methotrexate and central nervous system toxicity. Cancer Treat Rep 1978; 62(12):1999.

2. Abelson HT, Kufe DW, Skarin AT, Major P, et al. Treatment of central nervous system tumors with methotrexate. Cancer Treat Rep 1981; 65(Supp.1):137-40.

3. Aisner J, Aisner SC, Ostrow S, Govindan S, Mummert K, Wiernik P. Meningeal carcinomatosis from small cell carcinoma of the lung consequence of improved survival. Acta Cytologica 1979; 292-96.

4. Alberts MC, Terrence CF. Hearing loss in carcinomatous meningitis. J Laryngol Otol 1978; 92:233.

5. Altrocchi PA, Reinhardt PH, Eckman PB. Blindness and meningeal carcinomatosis. Arch Ophthal 1972; 88:508.

6. Amer MH, Al-Sarraf M, Baker LH, Vaitkevicius VK. Malignant melanoma and central nervous system metastases: incidence, diagnosis, treatment and survival. Cancer 1978; 42:660-68.

7. Ballentine P. Intraventricular lithium infusion and potential applications in psychiatry. In: A professional briefing – totally implantable pumps: intraspinal analgesia, CNS malignancies, Alzheimer's disease and other neurotransmitter disorders. Invitat Conf Sept. 1984; 113-36.

8. Blasberg RG, Patlak C, Fenstermacher JD. Intrathecal chemotherapy: brain tissue profiles after ventriculocisternal perfusion. J Pharmacol Exp Ther 1975; 195:75-83.

9. Blasberg RG, Patlak CS, Shapiro WR. Distribution of methotrexate in the cerebrospinal fluid and brain after intraventricular administration. Cancer Treat Rep 1977; 61:633-41.

10. Bleyer WA. Current status of intrathecal chemotherapy for human meningeal neoplasms. Natl Cancer Inst Mono 1977; 46:171-8.

11. Bleyer WA, Poplack DG, Simon RM, et al. 'Concentration × time' methotrexate via a subcutaneous reservoir: a less toxic regimen for intraventricular chemotherapy of central nervous system neoplasms. Blood 1978; 51:835.

12. Bleyer WA, Drake JC, Chabner BA. Neurotoxicity and elevated cerebrospinal fluid methotrexate concentration in meningeal leukemia. N Engl J Med 1973; 289:770-73.

13. Breuer AC, Blank NK, Schoene WC. Multifocal pontine lesions in cancer patients treated with chemotherapy and CNS radiotherapy. Cancer 1978; 41:2112-20.

14. Chabner BA, Young RC. Threshold methotrexate concentration for in vivo inhibition of DNA synthesis in normal and tumorous target tissues. J Clin Invest 1973; 52:1804-11.

15. Cobb CA, French BN, Smith KA. Intrathecal morphine for pelvic and sacral pain caused by cancer. Surg Neurol 1984; 22:63-68.

16. Dakhil S, Ensminger W, Kindt G, et al. Implanted system for intraventricular drug infusion in central nervous system tumors. Cancer Treat Rep 1981; 65:401-11.

17. Ensminger WD, Frei E. The prevention of methotrexate toxicity by thymidine infusions in humans. Cancer Res 1977; 37:1857-63.

18. Enzmann DR, Krikorian J, Yorke C, Hayward R. Computed tomography in leptomeningeal spread of tumor. J Comput Assist Tomogr 1978; 2:448-55.

19. Erickson DL, Blacklock JB, Michaelson M, Sperling KB, Lo JN. Control of spasticity by implantable continuous flow morphine pump. Neurosurgery 1985; 16:215-17.

20. Foley KM. Kinetics of intraspinal opiates and update on their acute and chronic use. In: A professional briefing – totally implantable pumps: intraspinal analgesia, CNS malignancies, Alzheimer's disease and other neurotransmitter disorders. Invitat Conf, Sept. 1984; 55-58.

21. Grossman SA, Trump DL, Chen DCP, Thompson G, Camargo EE. Cerebrospinal fluid flow abnormalities in patients with neoplastic meningitis: an evaluation using [111]Indium-DTPA ventriculography. JAMA 1982; 73:641.

22. Gutin PH, Weiss HD, Wiernik PH, Walker MD. Intrathecal N. N', N"— triethylenethiophosphoramide [thio-tepa (NSC 6396)] in the treatment of malignant meningeal disease: phase 1-2 study. Cancer 1976; 38:1471-75.

23. Harbaugh RE. Intracranial bethanechol infusion in patients with Alzheimer's disease. In: A professional briefing—totally implantable pumps: intraspinal analgesia, CNS malignancies, Alzheimer's disease and other neurotransmitter disorders. Invitat Conf Sept. 1984; 91-103.

24. Jackson DV, Richards F, Cooper MR, Ferree C, et al. Prophylactic cranial irradiation in small cell carcinoma of the lung: a randomized study. JAMA 1977; 237:2730-33.

25. Katz JL, Valsamis MP, Jampel RS. Ocular signs in diffuse carcinomatous meningitis. J Ophthal 1961; 52:681-90.

26. Kim KS, Ho SU, Weinberg PE, Lee C. Spinal leptomeningeal infiltration by systemic cancer: myelographic features. AJR 1982; 130:361-65.

27. Little JR, Dale AJD, Okazaki H. Meningeal carcinomatosis. Arch Neurol 1974; 30:138-43.

28. Maguire LC, Corder MP, Wiesenfeld M. Monitoring central nervous system methotrexate levels via subcutaneous reservoir sources of errors in sampling and their avoidance. Cancer Clin Trials 1980; 3:337-40.

29. Mehta BM, Glass JP, Shapiro WR. Serum and cerebrospinal fluid distribution of 5-methyltetrahydrofolate after intravenous calcium leucovorin and intra-Ommaya methotrexate administration in patients with meningeal carcinomatosis. Cancer Res 1983; 43:435-38.

30. Munsat TL. Intrathecal TRH in motor neuron diseases. In: A professional briefing—totally implantable pumps: intraspinal analgesia, CNS malignancies, Alzheimer's disease and other neurotransmitter disorders. Invitat Conf Sept. 1984; 85.

31. Nurchi G. Use of intraventricular and intrathecal morphine in intractable pain associated with cancer. Neurosurgery 1984; 15:801-03.

32. Olson ME, Chernik NL, Posner JB. Infiltration of the leptomeninges by systemic cancer. Arch Neurol 1974; 30:122-37.

33. Price RA, Jamieson PA. The central nervous system in childhood leukemia. II. Subacute leukoencephalopathy. Cancer 1975; 35:306-18.

34. Price RA, Birdwell DA. The central nervous system in childhood leukemia. III. Mineralizing microangiopathy and dystrophic calcification. Cancer 1978; 42:717-28.

35. Rosen ST, Aisner J, Makuch RW, et al. Carcinomatous leptomeningitis in small cell lung cancer: a clinicopathologic review of the National Cancer Institute experience. Medicine 1982; 61(1):45-53.

36. Rubinstein LJ, Herman MM, Long TF, Wilbur JR. Disseminated necrotizing leukoencephalopathy: a complication of treated central nervous system leukemia and lymphoma. Cancer 1975; 35:291-305.

37. Rubenstein MK. Cranial mononeuropathy as the first sign of intracranial metastases. Ann Intern Med 1969; 70:49-54.

38. Schold SC, Wasserstrom WR, Fleisher M, Schwartz MK, Posner JB. Cerebrospinal fluid biochemical markers of central nervous system metastases. Ann Neurol 1980; 8:597-604.

39. Schousboe A. Glial GABA uptake inhibitors and epilepsy. In: A professional briefing—totally implantable pumps: intraspinal analgesia, CNS malignancies, Alzheimer's disease and other neurotransmitter disorders. Invitat Conf Sept. 1984; 117-33.

40. Sondak V, Deckers PJ, Feller JH, Mozden PJ. Leptomeningeal spread of breast cancer: report of case and review of the literature. Cancer 1981; 48:395-99.

41. Shapiro WR, Young DF, Mehta BM. Methotrexate: distribution in cerebrospinal fluid after intravenous, ventricular and lumbar injections. N Engl J Med 1975; 293:161-66.

42. Shapiro WR, Allen J, Horten B. Chronic methotrexate toxicity to the central nervous system. Clin Bull 1980; 10:49.

43. Susac JO, Smith JL, Powell JO. Carcinomatous optic neuropathy. Am J Ophthalmol 1973; 76(5):672–79.

44. Sullivan MP, Vietti TJ, Haggard ME, et al. Remission maintenance therapy for meningeal leukemia: intrathecal methotrexate vs intravenous bis-nitrosourea. Blood 1971; 38:680–87.

45. Theodore WH, Gendelman S. Meningeal carcinomatosis. Arch Neurol 1981; 38:696–99.

46. Wasserstrom WR, Glass P, Posner JB. Diagnosis and treatment of leptomeningeal metastases from solid tumors: experience with 90 patients. Cancer 1982; 49:759–72.

47. Yap HY, Yap BS, Tashima CK, DiStefano A, Glumenschein GR. Meningeal carcinomatosis in breast cancer. Cancer 1978; 42:283–86.

48. Yap HY, Yap BS, Rasmussen SH, Levens ME, Hortobagyi GN, Blumenschein GR. Treatment for meningeal carcinomatosis in breast cancer. Cancer 1982; 49:219–22.

49. Zimm S, Collins JM, Curt GA, O'Neill D, Poplack DG. Cerebrospinal fluid pharmacokinetics of intraventricular and intravenous aziridinylbenzoquinone. Cancer Res 1984; 44:1698–1701.

50. Zimm S, Collins JM, Miser J, Chatterji D, Poplack DG. Cytosine arabinoside cerebrospinal fluid kinetics. Clin Pharmacol Ther 1984; 35(6):826–30.

References—Chapter 40

1. CA—A cancer journal for clinicians. 1985; 35:1.

2. Gilbert HA, Logan JL, Kagan AR, et al. The natural history of papillary transitional cell carcinoma of the bladder and its treatment in an unselected population on the basis of histologic grading. J Urol 1978; 119:448–92.

3. Williams JL, Hammond JC, Saunders N. T-1 bladder tumors. Br J Urol 1977; 49:663–668.

4. Heney N, Ahmed S, Flanagan MJ, et al. Superficial bladder cancer: progression and recurrence. J Urol 1983; 130:1083–86.

5. Lerman IL, Hutter RVP, Whitmore WF Jr. Papilloma of the urinary bladder. Cancer 1970; 25:333–42.

6. Melicow MM. Tumors of the urinary bladder: a clinicopathological analysis of over 2500 species and biopsies. J Urol 1955; 74:498.

7. Sontag JM. Experimental identification of genitourinary carcinogens. Urol Clin N Am 1980; 7:803.

8. Morrison AS, Cole T. Epidemiology of bladder cancer. Urol Clin N Am 1976; 3:13.

9. Morrison AJ, Buring JE, Verhoek WG, et al. An international study of smoking and bladder cancer. J Urol 1984; 131:650–54.

10. Hultergren N, Lagengren C, Ljungqvist A. Carcinoma of the renal pelvis in papillary necrosis. Acta Clin Scand 1965; 130:314.

11. Brand KG. Schistosomiasis-cancer: etiological considerations. A review. Acta Trop (Basel) 1979; 36:203.

12. Utz DC, Hanash KA, Farrow G. The plight of the patient with carcinoma in situ of the bladder. J Urol 1970; 103:160.

13. Baker R, Maxted W. Tumors of the renal pelvis, ureter and urinary bladder. In: Kendall AR, Karafin L, eds. Urology. New York: Harper and Row, 1983.

14. Farrow GM, et al. Clinical observations on 69 cases of in situ carcinoma of the urinary bladder. Cancer Res 1977; 37:2794–98.

15. Rife CC, Farrow GM, Utz DC. Urinary cytology of transitional cell neoplasms. Urol Clin North Am 1979; 6:599–612.

16. Devonec M, Darzynkiewicz Z, Kostyrka-Claps ML, et al. Flow cytometry of low-stage bladder tumors. Cancer 1982; 48:109–18.

17. Devonec M, Darzynkiewicz A, Whitmore WF, et al. Flow cytometry for followup examinations of conservatively treated low-stage bladder tumors. J Urol 1981; 126:166–170.

18. Klein FA, Herr HW, Sogani PC, et al. Detection and followup of carcinoma of the urinary bladder by flow cytometry. Cancer 1982; 50:389–95.

19. Schade ROK, Swinney J. The association of urothelial atypism with neoplasia: its importance in treatment and prognosis. J Urol 1973; 109:619.

20. Eisenberg RB, Roth RB, Schweinsberg MH. Bladder tumors and associated proliferative musocal lesions. J Urol 1960; 84:544.

21. Soloway MS, Murphy W, Rao MK, Cox C. Serial multiple site biopsies in patients with bladder cancer. J Urol 1978; 120:57.

22. Murphy WM, Najy GK, Rao MK, et al. Normal urothelium in patients with bladder cancer. Cancer 1979; 44:1050.

23. Cooper TP, Wheelis RF, Correa RJ Jr, et al. Random mucosal biopsies in the evaluation of patients with carcinoma of the bladder. J Urol 1977; 117:46.

24. Heney MM, Daly J, Prout GR Jr. Biopsy of apparently normal urothelium in patients with bladder cancer. J Urol 1978; 120:559.

25. Whitmore WF Jr. Management of bladder cancer. Curr Prob Cancer 1979; 4:1–48.

26. McDonald DR, Thorson T. Clinical implications of transplantability of induced bladder tumors to intact transitional epithelium in dogs. J Urol 1956; 75:690–694.

27. Wallace AC, Hershfield ES. The experimental implantation of tumor cells in the urinary tract. Br J Cancer 1958; 12:622–30.

28. Weldon TE, Soloway MS. Susceptibility of urothelium to neoplastic cellular implantation. Urology 1975; 5:824–827.

29. Soloway MS, Masters S. Implantation of transitional tumor cells on the cauterized murine urothelial surface. Proc Am Assoc Cancer Res 1979; 20:256.

30. Franksson C. Tumors of the urinary bladder: a pathological and clinical study of 434 cases. Acta Chir Scand 1950; (suppl) 515:1–203.

31. Kiefer JH. Bladder tumor recurrence in the urethra: a warning. J Urol 1953; 60:652–656.

32. Hinman F Jr. Recurrence of bladder tumors by surgical implantation. J Urol 1956; 75:695–696.

33. Boyd PJR, Burnand KG. Site of bladder tumor recurrence. Lancet 1974; 1:1290–1292.

34. Page BH, Levison VB, Curwen MP. The site of recurrence of noninfiltrating bladder tumor. Br J Urol 1978; 50:237–242.

35. Hollands FG. The results of diathermy treatment of villous papilloma of the bladder. Br J Urol 1950; 22:342–375.

36. Van der Werf-Messing B. Carcinoma of the bladder treated by suprapubic radium implants. Eur J Cancer 1969; 5:277–285.

37. Greene LF and Yalowitz PA. The advisability of concomitant transurethral excision of vesical neoplasm and prostatic hyperplasia. J Urol 1972; 107:445.

38. Falor WH, Ward RM. Fifty-three month persistence of ring chromosome in noninvasive bladder carcinoma. Acta Cytol 1976; 20:270.

39. Sandberg AA. Chromosome markers and progression in bladder cancer. Cancer Res 1977; 37:2950.

40. Melicow MM. Histological study of vesical urothelium intervening between gross neoplasms in total cystectomy. J Urol 1952; 68:261–79.

41. Cooper PH, Waisman J, Johnston WH, et al. Severe atypia of transitional epithelium and carcinoma of the urinary bladder. Cancer 1973; 31:1055–60.

42. Koss LG, Tiamson EM, Robbins MA. Mapping cancerous and precancerous bladder changes. A study of the urothelium in ten surgically removed bladders. JAMA 1974; 227:281–86.

43. Farrow GM, Utz DC, Rife CC. Morphological and clinical observations of patients with early bladder cancer treated with total cystectomy. Cancer Res 1976; 36:2495–2501.

44. Soto EA, Friedell GH, Tiltman AJ. Bladder cancer as seen in giant histologic sections. Cancer 1977; 39:447–455.

45. Jacobs JB, Masayuki A, Cohen SM, Friedell GH. A long-term study of reversible and progressive

urinary bladder cancer lesions in rats fed N-4-(5-Nitro-2-furyl)-2-thiazolyl formamide. Cancer Res 1977; 37:2817–21.

46. Greene LF, Hanash KA, Farrow GM. Benign papilloma or papillary carcinoma of the bladder? J Urol 1973; 110:205–07.

47. England HR, Paris AMI, Blandy JP. The correlation of T-1 bladder tumor history with prognosis and followup requirements. Br J Urol 1981; 53:593–97.

48. Lutzeyer W, Rubben H, Dahm H. Prognostic parameters in superficial bladder cancer: an analysis of 315 cases. J Urol 1982; 127:250–52.

49. O'Flynn JD, Smith JM, Hanson JS. Transurethral resection for assessment and treatment of vesical neoplasms. Eur Urol 1975; 1:38–40.

50. Barnes RW, Hadley HL, et al. Survival following transurethral resection of bladder carcinoma. Cancer Res 1977; 37:2895–97.

51. Heney NM, Nocks BN, Daly JJ, et al. Ta and T1 bladder cancer: location, recurrence and progression. Br J Urol 1982; 54:152–57.

52. Dalesio O, Schulman CC, Sylvester R, et al. Prognostic factors in superficial bladder tumors. A study of the European Organization for Research on Treatment of Cancer: Genitourinary Tract Cancer Cooperative Group. J Urol 1983; 129:730–33.

53. Koss LG. Tumors of the urinary bladder. AFIP Fascicle, 2nd series, Fascicle II 62–69.

54. Utz DC, Hanash KA, Farrow GM. The plight of the patient with carcinoma in situ of the bladder. J Urol 1970; 103:160.

55. Farrow GM, Utz DC, Rife CC, Greene LF. Clinical observations on sixty-nine cases of in situ carcinoma of the urinary bladder. Cancer Res 1977; 37:2794–98.

56. Riddle PR, Chisholm GD, Trott PA. Flat carcinoma in situ of the bladder. Br J Urol 1975; 47:829–33.

57. Prout GR Jr, Griffin PP, Daly JJ, Heney NM. Carcinoma in situ of the urinary bladder with and without associated vesical neoplasms. Cancer 1983; 52:524–32.

58. Melamed MR, Voutso NG, Grabstald H. Natural history and clinical behavior of in situ carcinoma of the human urinary bladder. Cancer 1964; 17:1533–45.

59. Althausen AF, Prout GR Jr, Daly JJ. Noninvasive papillary carcinoma of the bladder associated with carcinoma in situ. J Urol 1976; 116:575–80.

60. Sadoughi N, Johnson RA, Ezdinli EZ, et al. Intravesical bleomycin in treatment of carcinoma of the bladder. JAMA 1973; 226:465.

61. Smith TH, McCollum CN. Intravesical bleomycin in bladder cancer. JAMA 1976; 235:906.

62. Bracken RB, Johnson DE, Rodriguez L, et al. Treatment of multiple superficial tumors of the bladder with intravesical bleomycin. Urology 1977; 9:161.

63. Pavone-Macaluso M. Chemotherapy of vesical and prostatic tumors. Br J Urol 1971; 43:701.

64. Esquivel EL Jr, Mackenzie AR, Whitmore WF Jr. Treatment of bladder tumors by instillation of thio-tepa, actinomycin-D or 5-fluorouracil. Invest Urol 1964; 2:381.

65. Blumenreich MS, Needles B, Yagoda A, et al. Intravesical cisplatin for superficial bladder tumors. Cancer 1982; 50:863.

66. Dennis LJ, Viggiano G, Oosterlink W, et al. Phase 3 chemotherapy with thio-tepa, Adriamycin and cisplatinum for recurrent superficial bladder tumors (abstr 287). J Urol 1985; 133(4).

67. Riddle PR. The management of superficial bladder tumors with intravesical Epodyl. Br J Urol 1973; 45:84.

68. Kurth KH, Schroder FH, Tunn U, et al. Adjuvant chemotherapy of superficial transitional cell bladder carcinoma: preliminary results of a European Organization for Research on Treatment of Cancer randomized trial comparing doxorubicin hydrochloride, ethoglucid and transurethral resection alone. J Urol 1984; 132:258–62.

69. Jones HC, Swinney J. Thio-tepa in the treatment of tumors of the bladder. Lancet 1961; 2:615–18.

70. Veenema RJ, Dean AL Jr, Roberts M, et al. Bladder carcinoma treated by direct instillation of thio-tepa. J Urol 1962; 88:60–63.

71. Abbassian A, Wallace DM. Intracavitary chemotherapy of diffuse, noninfiltrating papillary carcinoma of the bladder. J Urol 1966; 96:461–65.

72. Veenema RJ, Dean AL Jr, Uson AC, et al. Thio-tepa bladder instillations: therapy and prophylaxis for superficial bladder tumors. J Urol 1969; 101:711–15.

73. Edsmyr R, Boman J. Instillation of thio-tepa (Tifosyl) in vesical papillomatosis. Acta Radiol 1970; 9:395–400.

74. Koontz WW Jr, Prout GR Jr, Smith W, et al. The use of intravesical thio-tepa in the management of noninvasive carcinoma of the bladder. J Urol 1981; 125:307–12

75. Heney NM, Koontz WK, Bartin B, et al. A comparative study of intravesical thio-tepa and mitomycin-C in patients with superficial bladder carcinoma (abstr 286). J Urol 1985; 130(4) Part II.

76. Pavone-Macaluso M, Gebbia N, Biondo F, et al. Permeability of the bladder mucosa to thio-tepa, Adriamycin and daunomycin in men and rabbits. Urol Res 1976; 4:9–13.

77. Hollister D Jr, Coleman M. Hematologic effects of intravesicular thio-tepa therapy for bladder carcinoma. JAMA 1980; 244:2065–67.

78. Bruce BW, Edgcomb JH. Pancytopenia and generalized sepsis following treatment of cancer of the bladder with instillations of triethylene thiophosphoramide. J Urol 1967; 97:482.

79. Soloway MS, Ford KS. Thio-tepa induced myelosuppression: review of 670 bladder instillations. J Urol 1983; 130:889–91.

80. Burnand KG, Boyd PJR, Mayo ME, et al. Single dose intravesical thio-tepa as an adjuvant to cystodiathermy in the treatment of transitional cell carcinoma. Br J Urol 1976; 48:55–59.

81. Gavrell GJ, Lewis RW, Meehan WL, et al. Intravesical thio-tepa in the immediate postoperative period in patients with recurrent transitional cell carcinoma of the bladder. J Urol 1978; 120:410–411.

82. England HR, Flynn JT, Paris AMI, Blandy JP. Early multiple dose adjuvant thio-tepa in a control of multiple and rapid T1 tumor neogenesis. Br J Urol 1981; 53:588–92.

83. Prout GR Jr, Kopp J. Resume of selected studies of the National Bladder Cancer Collaborative Group A and new protocols. In: Progress in clinical and biological research. Alan R. Liss, Inc. 1984; Vol. 162B:397–427.

84. Wescott JW. The prophylactic use of thio-tepa in transitional cell carcinoma of the bladder. J Urol 1966; 96:913–918.

85. Byar D, Blackard C. Comparisons of placebo, pyridoxine and topical thio-tepa in preventing recurrence of stage 1 bladder cancer. Urology 1977; 10:556–61.

86. Schulman CC, Robinson M, Denis L, et al. Prophylactic chemotherapy of superficial transitional cell bladder carcinoma: An EORTC randomized trial comparing thio-tepa, and epipodophyllotoxin (VM-26) and TUR alone. Eur Urol 1982; 8:207–212.

87. Prout GR, Koontz WW Jr, Coombs LJ, et al. Long-term fate of 90 patients with superficial bladder cancer randomly assigned to receive or not to receive thio-tepa. J Urol 1983; 130:677–680.

88. Fluchter FH, Harzmann R, Dichler KH. Local mitomycin-C therapy of transitional cell carcinoma of the bladder serum resorption study and clinical results. In: Ogawa M, Rozencweig M, Staquet MJ, eds. Mitomycin-C: Current impact on cancer chemotherapy. Amsterdam: Excerpta Medica, 1982; 143–152.

89. DeWall JG, Kurth KH, vanOosterom AT, et al. Plasma levels of mitomycin-C during its intravesical instillation. Am Urolog Assoc 1984; 131 (part II): 139A.

90. Wajsman Z, Dhafir RA, Pfeffer M, et al. Studies of mitomycin-C absorption after intravesical treatment of superficial bladder tumors. J Urol 1984; 132:30–33.

91. Mishina T, Oda K, Murata S, et al. Mitomycin-C bladder instillation therapy for bladder tumors. J Urol 1975; 114:217–19.

92. Mishina T, Watanabe H. Mitomycin-C bladder instillation therapy for bladder tumors. In: Carter SK, Crooke ST, eds. Mitomycin-C: Current status and new developments. New York: Academic Press, Inc., 1979; 193–203.

93. Harrison GSM, Green DF, Newling DWW, et al. A phase 2 study of intravesical mitomycin-C in the treatment of superficial bladder cancer. Br J Urol 1983; 55:676–79.

94. Bracken RB, Swanson DA, Johnson DE, et al. Role of intravesical mitomycin-C in management of superficial bladder tumors. Urology 1980; 16:11–15.

95. Soloway MS. Intravesical and systemic chemotherapy in the management of superficial bladder cancer. Urol Clin North Am 1984; 11:4:623–35.

96. Issell BF, Prout GR Jr, Soloway MS et al. Mitomycin-C intravesical therapy in noninvasive bladder cancer after failure on thio-tepa. Cancer 1984; 53:1025–28.

97. Soloway MS. Followup data on 70 bladder cancer patients treated with intravesical mitomycin-C. J Urol (abstr 288) 1985; 13 (IV) part II.

98. Nissenkorn I, Herrod H, Soloway MS. Side effects associated with intravesical mitomycin-C. J Urol 1981; 126:596–97.

99. Wajsman Z, McGill W, Englander L, et al. Severely contracted bladder following intravesical mitomycin-C therapy. J Urol 1983; 130:340–41.

100. Devonec M, Bouvier R, Sarkissian J, et al. Intravesical instillation of mitomycin-C in the prophylactic treatment of recurring superficial transitional cell carcinoma of the bladder. Br J Urol 1983; 55:382–85.

101. Niijima T, Koiso K, Akaza H, et al. Randomized clinical trial on chemoprophylaxis of recurrence in cases of superficial bladder cancer. Cancer Chemother Pharmacol 11 (suppl.) 1983; S79–S82.

102. Schutz W, Lei HH, Kuntz RM. Topical instillation of mitomycin-C in the treatment of superficial bladder tumors. Urol Assoc 1984; 131 (part II):140A.

103. Huland H, Otto U, Droese M, Kloppel G. Long-term mitomycin-C instillation after transurethral resection of superficial bladder carcinoma: influence on recurrence, progression and survival. J Urol 1984; 132:27–29.

104. Banks MD, Pontes JE, Izbicki RM, et al. Topical instillation of doxorubicin hydrochloride in the treatment of recurring superficial transitional cell carcinoma of the bladder. J Urol 1977; 118:757–60.

105. Eksborg S. Measurements of plasma levels of Adriamycin and Adriamycinol after intravesical instillation of Adriamycin. In: Edsmyr F, ed. Diagnostics and treatment of superficial urinary bladder tumors. Stockholm: Karoliska Hospital, 1978; 55–58.

106. Jacobi GH, Kurth KH. Studies on the intravesical action of topically administered G3 H-doxorubicin hydrochloride in man: plasma uptake and tumor penetration. J Urol 1980; 124:34–37.

107. Garnick MB, Schade D, Israel M, et al. Intravesical doxorubicin for prophylaxis in the management of recurrent superficial bladder carcinoma. J Urol 1984; 131:43–46.

108. Tritton TR, Yee G. The anticancer agent Adriamycin can be actively cytotoxic without entering cells. Science 1982; 217:248–50.

109. Fossberg E, Sander S. Topical Adriamycin treatment of superficial bladder tumors. In: Edsmyr F, ed. Diagnostics and treatment of superficial urinary bladder tumors. Stockholm: Karolinska Hospital, 1978; 99–101.

110. Niijima T. Intravesical therapy with Adriamycin and new trends in the diagnostics and therapy of superficial urinary bladder tumors. In: Edsmyr F, ed. Diagnostics and treatment of superficial urinary bladder tumors. Stockholm: Karolinska Hospital, 1978; 37–46.

111. Edsmyr F, Berlin T, Boman J, et al. Intravesical therapy with Adriamycin in patients with superficial bladder tumors. Eur Urol 1980; 6:132.

112. Pavone-Macaluso M. Intravesical chemotherapy in the treatment and prophylaxis of bladder tumors, with special reference to doxorubicin. In: Muggia FM, Young CW, Carter SK. Anthracycline antibiotics in cancer therapy. The Hague and Boston: M. Nijhoff Publ, 1982.

113. Lamm DL. Intravesical therapy of superficial bladder cancer. AUA update series. Vol. 2, Lesson 20, 1983.

114. Schulman CC, Denis LJ, Costerlinck W, et al. Early adjuvant Adriamycin in superficial bladder carcinoma. In: Progress in clinical and biological research. Alan R. Liss, Inc., 1984; Vol. 162B: 151–62.

115. Abrams PH, Choa RG, Gaches CGC, et al. A controlled trial of single-dose intravesical Adriamycin in superficial bladder tumors. Br J Urol 1981; 53:585–87.

116. Edsmyr F, Andersson L. Chemotherapy in bladder cancer. Urol Res 1978; 6:263–264.

117. Jakse G, Hofstadter F. Intravesical doxorubicin hydrochloride in the management of carcinoma in situ of the bladder. Eur Urol 1980; 6:103–06.

118. Glashan RW, Riley H. Intravesical therapy with Adriamycin in urothelial dysplasia and early carcinoma in situ. Can J Surg 1981; 25:30–32.

119. Zbar B, Rapp HJ. Immunotherapy of guinea pig cancer with BCG. Cancer 1974; 34:1532.

120. Bartlett GL, Zbar B, Rapp HJ. Suppression of murine tumor growth by immune reaction to Bacillus-Calmette-Guerin strain of mycobacterium bovis. JNCI 1972; 48:245–57.

121. Hann MG Jr, Zbar B, Rapp HJ. Histopathology of tumor regression after intralesional injection of mycobacterium bovis: II. Comparative effects of vaccinia virus, oxazolone, and turpentine. JNCI 1972; 48:1697–1703.

122. Zbar B, Bernstein ID, Rapp HJ. Suppression of tumor growth at the site of infection with living Bacillus-Calmette-Guerin. JNCI 1971; 46:831–39.

123. Shapiro A, Ratliff TL, Oakley DM, Catalone WJ. Reduction of bladder tumor growth in mice treated with intravesical Bacillus-Calmette-Guerin and its correlation with Bacillus-Calmette-Guerin viability and natural killer cell activity. Cancer Res 1983; 43:1611.

124. Lamm DL, Thor DE, Stogdill VD, et al. Bladder cancer immunotherapy. J Urol 1982; 128:931–35.

125. Kelley DR, Ratliff TL, Catalona WJ, et al. Intravesical Bacillus-Calmette-Guerin therapy for superficial bladder cancer: effect of Bacillus-Calmette-Guerin viability on treatment results. J Urol 1985; 134:48–53.

126. Herr HW. Editorial comment. J Urol 1985; 134:47.

127. Morales A, Eidinger D, Bruce AW. Intracavitary Bacillus-Calmette-Guerin in the treatment of superficial bladder tumors. J Urol 1976; 116:180–83.

128. Morales A, Ottenhof P, Emerson L. Treatment of residual, noninfiltrating bladder cancer with Bacillus-Calmette-Guerin. J Urol 1981; 125:649–51.

129. Schellhammer PF, Warden SS, Ladaga LE. Bacillus-Calmette-Guerin (BCG) in the treatment of transitional cell carcinoma (TCC) of the bladder. Proc Am Urol Assoc 1984; 139A.

130. DeKernion JB, Huang MY, Lindner A, et al. The management of superficial bladder tumors and carcinoma in situ with intravesical Bacillus-Calmette-Guerin. J Urol 1985; 133:598–601.

131. Morales A. Long-term results of intracavitary Bacillus-Calmette-Guerin therapy for bladder cancer. J Urol 1985; 132:457–59.

132. Herr HW, Pinsky CM, Whitmore WF Jr, et al. Effect of intravesical Bacillus-Calmette-Guerin (BCG) on carcinoma in situ of the bladder. Cancer 1983; 51:1323–26.

133. Herr HW, Pinsky CM, Melamed MO, Whitemore WF Jr. Long-term effect of intravesical BCG on flat carcinoma in situ (CIS) of the bladder. Proc Am Urol Assoc 1984; 139A.

134. Brosman SA. The use of Bacillus-Calmette-Guerin in the therapy of bladder carcinoma in situ. J Urol 1985; 134:36–39.

135. Camacho F, Pinsky C, Kerr D, et al. Treatment of superficial bladder cancer with intravesical BCG. ASCO Abstracts 1980; C – 160.

136. Lamm DL, Thor DE, Winter WD, et al. BCG immunotherapy of bladder cancer: inhibition of tumor recurrence and associated immune response. Cancer 1981; 48:82.

137. Brosman SA. Experience with Bacillus-Calmette-Guerin in patients with superficial bladder carcinoma. J Urol 1982; 128:27–30.

138. Brosman SA. BCG in the management of superficial bladder cancer. Urology 1984; 13(IV-suppl):82.

139. Huffman JL, Pinsky CM, Herr HW, et al. Maintenance intravesical Bacillus-Calmette-Guerin (BCG) in patients with recurrent superficial carcinoma of the urinary bladder. Proc Am Urol Assoc 1985; 304A.

140. Lamm DL, Reichert DF. Long-term protection against bladder cancer produced by immunotherapy. Proc Am Urol Assoc 1982; 92.

141. Lamm DL, Stogdill VD, Stogdill BJ. Complications of BCG immunotherapy in patients with bladder cancer. Proc Am Urol Assoc 1984; 140A.

142. Heney NM, Koontz WK, Bartin B, et al. A comparative study of intravesical thio-tepa and mitomycin-C in patients with superficial bladder carcinoma. Proc Am Urol Assoc 1985; 185A.

143. Zincke H, Benson RC Jr., Fleming TR, et al. Tumor recurrence after intravesical instillation of thio-tepa and mitomycin-C at time of transurethral resection of bladder cancer (Ta TCis) and postoperatively. Proc Am Urol Assoc 1984; 138A.

144. Flanigan RC, Ellison MF, Butler KM, McRoberts JW. Adjuvant intravesical thio-tepa versus mitomycin-C in recurrent or multiple stage 0 and A transitional cell cancers. Am Urol Assoc abstr 285, J Urol 1985; 133 (IV), part II.

145. Zincke H, Utz DC, Taylor WF, et al. Influence of thio-tepa and doxorubicin instillation at time of transurethral surgical treatment of bladder cancer on tumor recurrence: a prospective, randomized, double blind, controlled trial. J Urol 1983; 129:505–09.

146. Denis LJ, Viggiano G, Oosterlinck W, et al. Phase 3 chemotherapy with thio-tepa, Adriamycin and cis-platinum for recurrent superficial bladder tumors. Am Urol Assoc abstr 287. J Urol 1985; 133 (IV), part II.

147. Netto NR Jr., Lemos GC. A comparison of treatment methods for the prophylaxis of recurrent superficial bladder tumors. J Urol 1983; 129:33–34.

148. Lamm DL, Crawford ED. BCG versus Adriamycin in bladder cancer: a Southwest Oncology Group study. Proc ASCO 1985.

149. Hu KN, Kim A, Khan AS, et al. Combined thio-tepa and mitomycin-C instillation therapy for low-grade superficial bladder tumor. Cancer 1985; 55:1654–58.

150. Shortliffe LD, Freiha FS, Hannigan JF, et al. Intravesical interferon therapy for carcinoma in situ and transitional cell carcinoma of the bladder. Am Urol Assoc abstr 271. J Urol 1984; 131 (IV) part II.

151. Koontz WW Jr., Heney N, Soloway M, et al. The ablative effect of mitomycin-C in patients with superficial bladder carcinoma who have previously failed therapy with intravesical thio-tepa. J Urol 1984; 131:238A.

152. McFarlane JR, Tolley DA, Scottish Urological Group. Intravesical mitomycin-C therapy for superficial bladder cancer: report of a multi-centre phase 2 study. Br J Urol 1985; 57:37–39.

References—Chapter 41

1. Goldie JH, Coldman AJ, Gudauskas GA. Rationale for the use of alternating noncross-resistant chemotherapy. Cancer Treat Res 1982; 66:434–49.

2. Kish J, Ensley J, Weaver A, Jacobs J, Cummings G, Al-Sarraf M. Superior response rate with 96-hour 5-fluorouracil (5-FU) infusion vs 5-FU bolus combined with cis-platinum (CACP) in a randomized trial for recurrent and advanced squamous head and neck cancer. (HNG) ASCO Abstr, 1984.

3. Carey RW, Choi NC, Hilgenberg AD, Wilkins WE. Preoperative chemotherapy (5-FU/DDP) as initial component in multimodality treatment programs for esophageal cancer. Proc ASCO 1985; 4:C–301.

4. Heim WJ, et al. Infusional high-dose cis-platinum and 5-fluorouracil in advanced nonsmall-cell lung cancer. Proc ASCO 1986; 5:174.

5. Leichman L, Steiger Z, Seydel HG, et al. Preoperative chemotherapy and radiation therapy for patients with cancer of the esophagus: a potentially curative approach. J Clin Oncol 1984; 2(2):75.

6. Leichman C, Leichman L, Nigro N. Cancer of the anal canal: curative therapy without surgery. Proc ASCO 1984; 3:136.

7. Buroker T, Kim PN, Heilbrun L, Vaitkevicius VK. 5-FU infusion with mitomycin-C vs. 5-FU infusion with methyl CCNU in the treatment of advanced colon cancer. A phase 3 study. ASCO Abstr 1977; C–18.

8. Byfield JE, Barone RM, Sharp TR, Frankel SS. Conservative management without alkylating agents for squamous cell anal cancer using cyclical 5-FU alone and x-ray therapy. Cancer Trat Rep 1983; 67:709–12.

9. Huberman MS, Lokich JJ, Greene R, et al. Vinblastine plus cis-platin in advanced nonsmall-cell lung cancer: lack of advantage for infusion schedule. Cancer Treat Rep 1985 (in press).

10. Bell DR, Woods RL, Levi JA, Fox RM, Tattersall MHN. Advanced ovarian cancer: a prospective randomized trial of chlorambucil versus combined cyclophosphamide and cis-diamminedichloroplatinum. Aust NZ J Med 1982; 12:245–49.

11. Decker DG, Fleming TR, Malkasian GD, Webb MJ, Jefferies JA, Edmonson JH. Cyclophosphamide plus cisplatinum in combination: treatment program for stage 3 or 4 ovarian carcinoma. Obstet Gynecol 1982; 60:481–87.

12. Lokich JJ, Zipoli T, Green R. Infusional cisplatin plus cyclophosphamide in advanced ovarian cancer. J Clin Oncol 1985 (submitted for publication).

13. Hortobagyi G, Frye D, Blumenschein G, et al. FAC with Adriamycin by continuous infusion for treatment of advanced breast cancer. Proc ASCO 1983; 2:105.

14. Legha SS, Benjamin RS, Mackay B, Ewer M, Blumenschein G. Prospects for doxorubicin in adjuvant breast cancer trials. In: Muggia FM, Young CW, Carter SK, eds. Anthracycline antibiotics in cancer therapy. Martinus Nijhoff Publisher, 1982; 432–44.

15. Schell FC, Yap HY, Hortobagyi GN, Issell B, Esparza L. Phase 2 study of VP16-213 (etoposide) in refractory metastatic breast carcinoma. Cancer Chemother Pharmacol 1982; 7:223–25.

16. Matelski HW, Lokich JJ, Huberman MS, et al. Adriamycin, cyclophosphamide, and etoposide (VP-16-213) in extensive-stage small cell lung cancer. Am J Clin Oncol 1984; 7:729–32.

17. O'Connell MJ. Current status of chemotherapy for advanced pancreatic and gastric cancer. J Clin Oncol 1985; 3(7):1032–39.

18. Benz C, DeGregorio M, Saks S, et al. Sequential infusions of methotrexate and 5-fluorouracil in advanced cancer: pharmacology, toxicity, and response. Cancer Res 1985; 45:3354–58.

19. Sweatman T, Israel M (personal communication) 1983.

20. Barlogie B, Smith L, Alexanian R. Effective treatment of advanced multiple myeloma refractory to alkylating agents. N Engl J Med 1984; 310:1353–56.

21. Lokich JJ, Zipoli TE, Moore C, Zonneborn H, Paul S, Greene R. Doxorubicin/vinblastine and doxorubicin/cyclophosphamide combination chemotherapy by continuous infusion. Cancer 1985 (in press).

22. Legha SS, Benjamin RS, Mackay B, Ewer M, Blumenschein G. Role of Adriamycin in breast cancer and sarcomas. In: Muggia FM, Young CW, Carter SK, eds. Anthracycline antibiotics in cancer therapy. Martinus Nijhoff Publishers, 1982.

23. Gaj E, Sesin GP. Compatibility of doxorubicin HCI and vinblastine SO₄. Am J IV Ther Clin Nutr 1984; 11:8–20.

24. Gasparini M, Rouesse J, Van Oosterom A, et al. Phase 2 study of cisplatin in advanced osteogenic sarcoma. Cancer Treat Rep 1985; 69(2):211–13.

25. Eurt G (personal communication) 1983.

26. Lokich JJ, Phillips D, Green R, et al. 5-fluorouracil and methotrexate administered simultaneously as a continuous infusion: a phase 1 study. Cancer Oct. 1985.

References—Chapter 42

1. Bergan T. Pharmacokinetics of tissue penetration of antibiotics. Rev Infect Dis 1981; 3:45–66.

2. Bodey GP, Hersh EM. The problem of infection in children with malignant disease. In: Neoplasia in childhood. Proc 12th Annu Clin Conf at U of Texas M.D. Anderson Hosp and Tumor Inst at Houston. Chicago: Year Book Medical Publishers, Inc., 1969; 135–54.

3. Jaffe RH. Morphology of the inflammatory defense reactions in leukemia. Arch Pathol 1932; 14:177–89.

4. Eagle H, Fleischman R, Musselman AD. The effective concentrations of penicillin in vitro and in vivo for streptococci, pneumococci and *Treponema pallidum*. J Bacteriol 1950; 59:625–43.

5. Eagle H, Fleischman R, Musselman AD. The bactericidal action of penicillin in vivo: the participation of the host, and the slow recovery of the surviving organisms. Ann Intern Med 1950· 33:544–71.

6. Parker RF, Luse S. The action of penicillin on staphylococcus: further observations on the effect of a short exposure. J Bacteriol 1948; 56:75–81.

7. Rolinson GN. Plasma concentrations of penicillin in relation to the antibacteria effect. In: Davies DS, Richard BNC, eds. Biological effects of drugs in relation to their plasma concentration. New York: MacMillan, 1973; 183–89.

8. Wilson DA, Rolinson GN. The recovery period following exposure of bacteria to penicillin. Chemotherapy 1979; 25:14–22.

9. Bodey GP, Pan T. Effect of cephalothin on growth patterns of microorganisms. J Antibiot 1976; 29:1092–95.

10. Bundtzen RW, Gerber AU, Cohn DL, Craig WA. Postantibiotic suppression of bacterial growth. Rev Infect Dis 1981; 3:28–37.

11. Jawetz E. Dynamics of the action of penicillin in experimental animals: observations on mice. Arch Intern Med 1946; 77:1–15.

12. Gibson CD Jr. Comparative effectiveness of two penicillin treatment schedules in pneumococcal infections of mice. Proc Soc Exper Biol Med 1948; 67:278–80.

13. Eagle H, Fleischman R, Levy M. On the duration of penicillin action in relation to its concentration in the serum. J Lab Clin Med 1953; 41:122–32.

14. Eagle H, Fleischman R, Musselman AD. Effect of schedule of administration on the therapeutic efficacy of penicillin. Importance of the aggregate time penicillin remains at effectively bactericidal levels. Am J Med 1950; 9:280–99.

15. Eagle H, Fleischman R, Levy M. 'Continuous' vs. 'discontinuous' therapy with penicillin. The effect of the interval between injections on therapeutic efficacy. N Engl J Med 1953; 248:481–88.

16. Bakker-Woudenberg IAJM, deJohn-Hoenderop JYT, Michel MF. Efficacy of antimicrobial therapy in experimental rat pneumonia: effects of impaired phagocytosis. Infect Immunity 1979; 25:366–75.

17. Bakker-Woudenberg IAJM, deJohn-Hoenderop JYT, Michel MF. Efficacy of antimicrobial therapy in experimental rat pneumonia: antibiotic treatment schedules in rats with impaired phagocytosis. Infect Immunity 1979; 25:376–87.

18. Gerber AU, Craig WA, Brugger H-P, Feller C, Vastola AP, Brandel J. Impact of dosing intervals on activity of gentamicin and ticarcillin against *Pseudomonas aeruginosa* in granulocytopenic mice. J Infect Dis 1983; 147:910–17.

19. Mordenti J. Combination antibiotic therapy: comparison of constant infusion and intermittent bolus dosing in an in vitro kinetic model and an experimental animal model. Thesis, Ph.D. Degree Program, School of Pharm, U of Conn, 1983.

20. Powell SH, Thompson WL, Luthe MA, et al. Once-daily vs. continuous aminoglycoside dosing: efficacy and toxicity in animal and clinical studies of gentamicin, netilmicin, and tobramycin. J Infect Dis 1983; 147:918–32.

21. Bennett WM, Plamp CE, Gilbert DN, Parker RA, Porter GA. The influence of dosage regimen on experimental gentamicin nephrotoxicity: dissociation of peak serum levels from renal failure. J Infect Dis 1979; 140:576–80.

22. Frame PT, Phair JP, Watanakunakorn C, Bannister TWP. Pharmacologic factors associated with gentamicin nephrotoxicity in rabbits. J Infect Dis 1977; 135:952–56.

23. Body GP, Valdivieso M, Yap BS. The role of schedule in antibiotic therapy of the neutropenic patient. Infection 1980; 8(suppl 1):s75–s81.

24. Bodey GP, Rodriguez V, Stewart D. Clinical pharmacological studies of carbenicillin. Am J Med Sci 1969; 257:185–90.

25. Bodey GP, Whitecar JP Jr., Middleman E, Rodriguez V. Carbenicillin therapy of Pseudomonas infections. JAMA 1971; 218:62–66.

26. Rodriguez V, Inagaki J, Bodey GP. Clinical pharmacology of ticarcillin (α-carboxyl-3-thienylmethyl penicillin, BRL-2288). Antimicrob Agents Chemother 1973; 4:31–36.

27. Bodey GP, Rodriguez V. The role of antipseudomonal penicillins in the management of infections in cancer patients. In: Ticarcillin (BRL 2288), Switzerland: Excerpta Medica, 1977; 151–57.

28. Issell BF, Bodey GP, Weaver S. Clinical pharmacology of mezlocillin. Antimicrob Agents Chemother 1978; 13:180–83.

29. Grose WE, Bodey GP, Stewart D. Observations in man on some pharmacologic features of cefamandole. Clin Pharmacol Ther 1976; 20:579–84.

30. Estey EH, Weaver SS, Ho DHW, Bodey GP. Clinical pharmacology of moxalactam in patients with malignant disease. Antimicrob Agents Chemother 1981; 19:639–44.

31. Maksymiuk AW, LeBlanc BM, Brown NS, Ho DH, Bodey GP. Pharmacokinetics of cefoperazone in patients with neoplastic disease. Antimicrob Agents Chemother 1981; 19:1037–41.

32. Salvador P, Smith RG, Weinfeld RE, Ellis DH, Bodey GP. Clinical pharmacology of ceftriaxone in patients with neoplastic disease. Antimicrob Agents Chemother 1983; 23:583–88.

33. Garcia I, Fainstein V, Smith RG, Bodey GP. Multiple-dose pharmacokinetics of ceftazidime in cancer patients. Antimicrob Agents Chemother 1983; 24:141–44.

34. Jones PG, Bodey GP, Swabb EA, Ho DHW, Fainstein V, Pasternak J. Clinical pharmacokinetics of aztreonam in cancer patients. Antimicrob Agents Chemother 1984; 26:455–61.

35. Bodey GP, Yeo E, Ho DH, Rolston K, LeBlanc B. Clinical pharmacology of timentin (ticarcillin and clavulanic acid) (to be published).

36. Rodriguez V, Stewart D, Bodey GP. Gentamicin sulfate distribution in body fluids. J. Clin Pharm Ther 1970; 11:275–81.

37. Horikoshi N, Valdivieso M, Bodey GP. Clinical pharmacology of tobramycin. Amer J Med Sci 1973; 266:453–58.

38. Bodey GP, Valdivieso M, Feld R, Rodriguez V. Pharmacology of amikacin in humans. Antimicrob Agents Chemother 1974; 5:508–12.

39. Yap BS, Stewart D, Bodey GP. Clinical pharmacology of netilmicin. Antimicrob Agents Chemother 1977; 12:717–20.

40. Bodey GP, Chang HY, Rodriguez V, Stewart D. Feasibility of administering aminoglycoside antibiotics by continuous intravenous infusion. Antimicrob Agents Chemother 1975; 8:328–33.

41. Lawson RD, Bodey GP, Pan T, Smith TL. New schedule for tobramycin administration. Antimicrob Agents Chemother 1980; 17:834–37.

42. Bodey GP, Middleman E, Umsawasdi T, Rodriguez V. Infections in cancer patients—results with gentamicin sulfate therapy. Cancer 1972; 29:1697–1701.

43. Valdivieso M, Horikoshi N, Rodriguez V, Bodey GP. Therapeutic trials with tobramycin. Am J Med Sci 1974; 268:149–56.

44. Jackson GG, Riff LJ. Pseudomonas bacteremia: pharmacologic and other bases for failure of treatment with gentamicin. J Infect Dis 1971; 124(suppl):s185–s191.

45. Bodey GP, Rodriguez V, Valdivieso M, Feld R. Amikacin for treatment of infections in patients with malignant diseases: administration by continuous intravenous infusion in the presence of neutropenia. J Infect Dis 1976; S134:421–72.

46. Valdivieso M, Feld R, Rodriguez V, Bodey GP. Amikacin therapy of infections in neutropenic patients. Am J Med Sci 1975; 270:453–63.

47. Yap BS, Bodey GP. Netilmicin in the treatment of infections in patients with cancer. Arch Intern Med 1979; 139:1259–62.

48. Feld R, Valdivieso M, Bodey GP, Rodriguez V. A comparative trial of sisomicin therapy by intermittent versus continuous infusion. Am J Med Sci 1977; 274:179–88.

49. Bodey GP, Cabanillas F, Feld R, et al. Sisomicin therapy of infections in cancer patients. Curr Therap Res 1979; 25:814–26.

50. Feld R, Rachlis A, Tuffnell PG, et al. Empiric therapy for infections in patients with granulocytopenia. Continuous v interrupted infusion of tobramycin plus cefamandole. Arch Intern Med 1984; 144:1005–10.

51. Issell BF, Keating MJ, Valdivieso M, Bodey GP. Continuous infusion tobramycin combined with carbenicillin for infections in cancer patients. Am J Med Sci 1979; 277:311–18.

52. Feld R, Tuffnell PG, Curtis JE, Messner HA, Hasselback R. Empiric therapy for infections in

granulocytopenic cancer patients. Continuous infusion of amikacin plus cephalothin. Arch Intern Med 1979; 139:310–14.

53. Keating MJ, Bodey GP, Valdivieso M, Rodriguez V. A randomized comparative trial of three aminoglycosides – comparison of continuous infusions of gentamicin, amikacin and sisomicin combined with carbenicillin in the treatment of infections in neutropenic patients with malignancies. Medicine 1979; 58:159–70.

54. Middleman EA, Watanabe A, Kaizer H, Bodey GP. Antibiotic combinations for infections in neutropenic patients. Evaluation of carbenicillin plus either cephalothin or kanamycin. Cancer 1972; 30:573–79.

55. Bodey GP, Valdivieso M, Feld R, Rodriguez V, McCredie K. Carbenicillin plus cephalothin or cefazolin as therapy for infections. Amer J Med Sci 1977; 273:309–18.

56. Bodey GP, Ketchel SJ, Rodriguez V. A randomized study of carbenicillin plus cefamandole or tobramycin in the treatment of febrile episodes in cancer patients. Am J Med 1979; 67:608–16.

References—Chapter 43

1. Breedis C, Young G. The blood supply of neoplasms in the liver. Am J Path 1954; 30:969.

2. Healey JE. Vascular patterns in human metastatic liver tumors. Surg Gyn Obst 1965; 120:1187.

3. Ackerman NB, Lien WM, Kondi ES, Silverman NA. The blood supply of experimental liver metastases. I. The distribution of hepatic artery and portal vein blood to "small" and "large" tumors. Surgery 1969; 66:1067.

4. Taylor I, Bennett R, Sherriff S. The blood supply of colorectal liver metastases. Br J Cancer 1979; 39:749.

5. Grage TB, Vassilopoulos PP, Shingleton WW, et al. Results of a prospective randomized study of hepatic artery infusion with 5-fluorouracil versus intravenous 5-fluorouracil in patients with hepatic metastases from colorectal cancer: a Central Oncology Group study. Surgery 1979; 86:550.

6. Bedikian AY. Regional and systemic chemotherapy for advanced colorectal cancer. Dis Col Rect 1983; 26:327.

7. Huberman MS. Comparison of systemic chemotherapy with hepatic arterial infusion in metastatic colorectal carcinoma. Semin Oncol 1983; 10:238.

8. Bedikian AY, Chen TT, Malahy M-A, Patt YZ, Bodey GP. Prognostic factors influencing survival of patients with advanced colorectal cancer: hepatic-artery infusion versus systemic intravenous chemotherapy for liver metastases. J Clin Oncol 1984; 2:17.

9. Bengmark S, Rosengren K. Angiographic study of the collateral circulation to the liver after ligation of the hepatic artery in man. Am J Surg 1970; 119:620.

10. Plengvanit U, Chearanai O, Sindhvananda K, Dambrongsak D, Tuchinda S, Viranuvatti V. Collateral arterial blood supply of the liver after hepatic artery ligation, angiographic study of 20 patients. Ann Surg 1972; 175:105.

11. Tuma RF. The use of degradable starch microspheres for transient occlusion of blood flow and for drug targeting to selected tissues. In: Davis SS, Illum L, McVie JG, Tomlinson E, eds. Microspheres and drug therapy. Pharmaceutical immunology and medical aspects. Elsevier Science Publishers, 1984.

12. Lindberg B, Lote K, Teder H. Biodegradable starch microspheres – a new medical tool. In: Davis SS, Illum L, McVie JG, Tomlinson E, eds. Microspheres and drug therapy. Immunological and medical aspects. Elsevier Science Publishers, 1984.

13. Arfors KE, Forsberg JO, Larsson B, Lewis DH, Rosengren B, Odman S. Temporary intestinal hypoxia induced by degradable microspheres. Nature 1976; 262–500.

14. Forsberg JO. Transient blood flow reduction induced by intra-arterial injection of degradable starch microspheres. Acta Chir Scand 1978; 144:275.

15. Lindell B, Aronsen KF, Rothman U. Repeated arterial embolization of rat livers by degradable microspheres. Eur Surg Res 1977; 9:347.

16. Tuma RF, Forsberg JO, Agerup B. Enhanced uptake of actinomycin D in the dog kidney by simultaneous injection of degradable starch microspheres into the renal artery. Cancer 1982; 50:1.

17. Lote K. Temporary ischaemia induced by degradable starch microspheres. Acta Radiol Oncol 1981; 20:91.

18. Lote K, Myking AO. Starch microspheres induced small intestinal ischaemia. Acta Radiol Oncol 1982; 21:353.

19. Lindell B, Aronsen KF, Nosslin B, Rothman U. Studies in pharmacokinetics and tolerance of substances temporarily retained in the liver by microsphere embolization. Ann Surg 1978; 187:95.

20. Teder H, Aronsen KF, Lindell B, Rothman U. Studies in pharmacokinetics of 5-fluorouracil temporarily retained in the rat liver by degradable microsphere embolization. Acta Chir Scand 1978; 144:71.

21. Lorelius LE, Benedetto AR, Blumhardt R, Gaskill HV, Lancaster JL, Stridbeck H. Enhanced drug retention in VX2 tumors by use of degradable starch microspheres. Invest Radiol 1984; 19:212.

22. Dakhill S, Ensminger W, Cho K, Niederhuber J, Doan K, Wheeler R. Improved regional selectivity of hepatic arterial BCNU with degradable microspheres. Cancer 1982; 50:631.

23. Teder H, Nilsson B, Jonsson K, Hellekant C, Aspegren K, Aronsen KF. Hepatic arterial administration of doxorubicin (Adriamycin) with or without degradable starch microspheres: a pharmacokinetic study in man. In: Hansen H, ed. Anthracyclines and cancer therapy. Amsterdam: Excerpta Medica, 1983.

24. Gyves JW, Ensminger WD, VanHarken D, Niederhuber J, Stetson P, Walker S. Improved regional selectivity of hepatic arterial mitomycin by starch microspheres. Clin Pharmacol Ther 1983; 34:259.

25. Svedberg J, Ekberg S, Håkansson L, Leander E, Starkhammar H. Effect of degradable starch microspheres on the passage of intra-arterially injected labeled tracer to the systemic circulation. A methodological study (in press).

26. Starkhammar H, Hakansson L, Morales O, Persliden J, Svedberg J, Sjödahl R. Effect of microspheres (Spherex[R]) on the arterial liver blood flow studied in tumour patients and in an experimental model. Acta Chir Scand 1983; suppl 516.

27. Starkhammar H, Håkansson L, Morales O, Svedberg J. Intra-arterial mitomycin-C treatment of unresectable liver tumours. Preliminary results on the effect of degradable starch microspheres. Acta Radiol Oncol (in press).

28. Starkhammar H, Håkansson L, Sjödahl R, Svedberg J, Ekberg S. Effect of portal blood flow and intra-arterially injected degradable starch microspheres on the passage of a radiolabeled tracer through the liver. An experimental study in the pig. Acta Radiol Oncol (in press).

29. Starkhammar H, Håkansson L, Morales O, Svedberg L. Factors affecting the effect of degradable starch microspheres in intra-arterial chemotherapy of liver tumours. A radionuclide study (in press).

30. Starkhammar H, Hakansson L, Morales O, Sjödahl R, Ekberg S, Svedberg J. Degradable starch microspheres in cancer treatment. Effect on regional blood flow and uptake of cytostatic drugs. 14th Int Cong Chemother, Kyoto, Japan 1985.

31. Starkhammar H, Hakansson L, Morales O, Sjödahl R, Svedberg J. Degradable starch microspheres in intra-arterial chemotherapy of inoperable primary or secondary liver cancer. Proc ASCO 1985; (abstr 98).

32. Starkhammar H, Hakansson L, Ekberg S, Svedberg J, Morales O. Degradable starch microspheres in intra-arterial chemotherapy. Influence of A-V shunting and size of the vascular bed. Proc 3rd Eur Conf Clin Oncol and Cancer Nursing (abstract 77).

References—Chapter 44

1. Cullinan S, Moertel C, Fleming T, Everson L, Krook J, Schutt A. A randomized comparison of 5-FU alone, 5-FU + Adriamycin, and 5-FU + Adriamycin + mitomycin-C in gastric and pancreas cancer. Proc ASCO 1984; 3:137.

740

2. Hodgson TA Jr. The economic costs of cancer. In: Shottenfield D, ed. Cancer epidemiology and prevention. Springfield, IL: Charles C. Thomas, 1975; 29–59.

3. Houts P, Lipton A, Harvey H, Martin B. A method for collecting detailed data on direct and indirect medical expenses of cancer patients. Presented at Progress in Cancer Control III Conf Washington DC, March 1982.

4. Houts PS, Lipton A, Harvey HA, et al. Nonmedical costs to patients and their families associated with outpatient chemotherapy. Cancer 1984; 53:2388–92.

5. Stagg R, Vielw C, Lewis B, Ignoffo R, Hohn D. A comparison of external pumps (EP) vs implantable pumps (IP) for continuous infusion chemotherapy: compliance, complications, and costs. Proc ASCO (abstr C-1031) March 1985; 4:265.

References—Chapter 45

1. Bonadonna G, Valagussa P. Adjuvant systemic therapy for resectable breast cancer. J Clin Oncol 1985; 3(2):259.

2. Gastrointestingal Tumor Study Group. Douglas HO Jr., Stablein DM. Controlled trial of adjuvant chemotherapy following curative resection of gastric cancer. In: Jones SE, Salmon SE, eds. Adjuvant therapy of cancer IV. New York: Grune & Stratton, Inc., 1984; 457–64.

3. Kalser MH, Ellenberg SS. Pancreatic cancer. Adjuvant combined radiation and chemotherapy following curative resection. Arch Surg 1985; 120:899–903.

4. Gastrointestinal Tumor Study Group. Prolongation of the disease-free interval in surgically treated rectal carcinoma. N Engl J Med 1985; 312(23):1465–72.

5. Gastrointestinal Tumor Study Group. Lessner HE, Mayer R, Ellenberg SS. Adjuvant therapy of colon cancer: results of a prospectively randomized trial. N Engl J Med 1984; 310:737–43.

6. Tiver KW, Langlands AO. Synchronous chemotherapy and radiotherapy for carcinoma of the anal canal—an alternative to abdominoperineal resection. Aust NZ J Surg 1984; 54:101–08.

7. Weichselbaum RR, Clark JR, Miller D, et al. Combined modality treatment of head and neck cancer with cisplatin, bleomycin, methotrexate with leucovorin rescue chemotherapy. Cancer 1985; 55:2149–55.

8. Fram R, Skarin A, Balikian J, et al. Upfront CAP chemotherapy followed by radiotherapy (XRT) in stage 3 M_o nonsmall-cell lung cancer (NSCLC). Proc ASCO 1984; C–855.

9. Ragaz J, Baird R, Rebbeck P, Goldie J, Coldman A, Spinelli J. Neoadjuvant (preoperative) chemotherapy for breast cancer. Cancer 1985; 56:719–24.

10. Boice JD Jr., Greene MH, Killen JY Jr., Ellenberg SS, et al. Leukemia and preleukemia after adjuvant treatment of gastrointestinal cancer with methyl-CCNU. N Engl J Med 1983; 309:1079.

11. Grossi CE, Wolffe WI, Nealon TF Jr., Pasternack B, Ginzburg L, Rousselot LM. Intraluminal fluorouracil chemotherapy adjunct to surgical procedure for resectable carcinoma of the colon and rectum. Surg Gynecol Obstet 1977; 145:549–54.

12. Lawrence W Jr., Terz JJ, Horsley JS III, Brown PW, Romero C. Chemotherapy as an adjuvant to surgery for colorectal cancer. Arch Surg 1978; 113:164–68.

13. Taylor I, Brooman P, Rowling JT. Adjuvant liver perfusion in colorectal cancer: initial results of a clinical trial. Br Med J 1977; 2:1320–22.

14. Taylor I, Cooke T, Machin D, Harman M. Adjuvant therapy of colorectal cancer with portal vein cytotoxic perfusion. In: Jones SE, Salmon SE, eds. Adjuvant therapy of cancer IV. New York: Grune & Stratton, Inc., 1984.

15. Metzger UF, Mermillod B, Aeberhard P, et al. Adjuvant liver perfusion with 5-fluorouracil and mitomycin-C following curative large bowel cancer surgery. In: Kimura K, Fujii S, Ogawa M, Bodey GP, Alberto P, eds. Fluoropyrimidines in cancer therapy. Elsevier Science Publishers B.V., 1984.

16. Patt YV, Boddie I, Charnasangavez C, et al. Arterial therapy in the management of resectable and

unresectable metastatic colon and rectal cancer in the liver. In: Eigner K, Patt YV, eds. Proc Second Conf on Advances in Regional Cancer Therapy. New York: Springer Verlag, 1986.

17. McCracken JD, Weatherall TJ, Oishi Noboru, Janaki L, Boyer C. Adjuvant intrahepatic chemotherapy with mitomycin and 5-FU combined with hepatic irradiation in high risk patients with carcinoma of the colon: a Southwest Oncology Group phase 2 pilot study. Cancer Treat Rep 1985; 69(1):129-31.

18. O'Connell MJ, Adson MA, Schutt AJ, Rubin J, Moertel CG, Ilstrup DM. Clinical trial of adjuvant chemotherapy after surgical resection of colorectal cancer metastatic to the liver. Mayo Clin Proc 1985; 60:517-20.

19. Fortner JG, Silva JS, Golbey RB, Cox EB, MacLean BJ. Multivariate analysis of a personal series of 247 consecutive patients with liver metastases from colorectal cancer. Ann Surg 1984; 199:306.

20. Kemeny MM, Goldberg DA, Browning S, Metter GE, Miner PA, Terz JJ. Experience with continuous regional chemotherapy and hepatic resection as treatment of hepatic metastases from colorectal primaries. A prospective randomized study. Cancer 1985; 55:1265-70.

21. Patt Y, Mavligit GM, Chuang VP, et al. Percutaneous hepatic arterial infusion of mitomycin-C and floxuridine: an effective treatment for metastatic colorectal carcinoma in the liver. Cancer Treat Rep 1984; 68.

22. Speyer JL, Sugarbaker PH, Collins JM, Dedrick RL, Klecker RW, Meyers CE. Portal levels and hepatic chance of 5-fluorouracil after intraperitoneal administration in humans. Cancer Res 1981; 41:1916-22.

23. Sugarbaker PH, Gianola FJ, Speyer JC, Wesley R, Barofsky I, Myers CE. Prospective randomized trial of intravenous vs. intraperitoneal 5-FU in patients with advanced primary colon or rectal cancer. Surgery (in press).

24. Mayer J. Adjuvant therapy in rectal cancer: a protocol proposal. Semin Oncol 1985; 12(3) suppl 4:116-20.

25. Rich TA, Lokich JJ, Chaffey JT. A pilot study of protracted venous infusion of 5-fluorouracil and concomitant radiation therapy. J Clin Oncol 1985; 3(5):710-17.

26. Lokich JJ, Phillips D, Greene R, Paul S, Sonneborn H, Zipoli TE, Curt G. 5-fluorouracil and methotrexate administered simultaneously as a continuous infusion: a phase 1 study. Cancer 1985; 56:2395-98.

27. Lokich JJ, Zipoli T, Moore C, Sonneborn H, Paul S, Greene R. Doxorubicin/vinblastine and doxorubicin/cyclophosphamide combination chemotherapy by continuous infusion. Cancer 1986; 58:1020-23.

28. Douglass HO Jr. Gastric cancer: overview of current therapies. Semin Oncol 1985; 12(3) suppl 4:57-62.

29. Mallinson CN, Rake MO, Cocking JB, et al. Chemotherapy in pancreatic cancer: results of a controlled, prospective, randomized, multicentre trial. Br Med J 1980; 281:1589-91.

30. Lokich JJ, Zipoli T, Greene R. Infusional cisplatin plus cyclophosphamide in advanced ovarian cancer (in press).

31. Heim W, et al. Infusional 5-fluorouracil and cisplatinum in advanced nonsmall-cell lung cancer. Protocol in progress. Mid Atlant Oncol Program. Nov. 1985.

32. Liechman L, Steiger Z, Seydel HG, et al. Preoperative chemotherapy and radiation therapy for patients with cancer of the esophagus: a potentially curative approach. J Clin Oncol 1984; 2(2):75-79.

33. Leichman C, Leichman L, Nigro N. Cancer of the anal canal: curative therapy without surgery. Proc ASCO 1984; 3:136.

34. Legha SS, Benjamin RS, Mackay B, Ewer M, Blumenschein G. Role of Adriamycin in breast cancer and sarcomas. In: Muggia FM, Young CW, Carter SK, eds. Anthracycline antibiotics in cancer therapy. Martinus Nijhoff Publishers, 1982.

35. Gasparini M, Rouesse J, Van Oosterom A, et al. Phase 2 study of cisplatin in advanced osteogenic sarcoma. Cancer Treat Rep 1985; 69(2):211-13.

36. Gonzales MF, Valdivieso JG, Sartiano GP. Continuous intravenous infusion combination chemotherapy for head and neck squamous cell carcinoma. Oncology 1984; 41:377-82.

INDEX

743